Clinical Gastroenterology

Series Editor

George Y. Wu, Divison of Gastroenterology-Hepatology
University of Connecticut School of Medicine
Farmington, CT, USA

Clinical Gastroenterology is a series of concise monographs on diseases commonly encountered in the clinical practice of Internal Medicine and Gastroenterology. Particular emphasis is placed on areas in which knowledge is advancing rapidly. Each volume is concise, concentrating on "clinical pearls," and new advances in diagnostic and therapeutic technology.

Volumes in the series include practical information of companies or laboratories that perform specialized testing, relative costs of diagnostic and therapeutic options. An emphasis is placed on illustrations, especially diagrams and diagnostic/ therapeutic algorithms to permit rapid acquisition of practical information that is not readily available in the major texts.Additional unique features include summaries of key points, recommendations, and indications for requesting GI subspecialty consultation.

The series is of great value to Gastroenterologists and Hepatologists interested in the latest practical developments in the field as well as Internists who have particular interests or large numbers of patients with particular diseases in the field of Gastroenterology-Hepatology.

Micheal Tadros • Lee Shapiro
Tracy Frech • George Y. Wu
Editors

GI Diseases Associated with Rheumatological and Vasculitic Conditions

Springer

Editors
Micheal Tadros
Division of Gastroenterology-Hepatology
Albany Medical Center Hospital
Niskayuna, NY, USA

Lee Shapiro
Division of Rheumatology
Albany Medical College
Albany, NY, USA

Tracy Frech
Rheumatology
Vanderbilt University Medical Center
Nashville, TN, USA

George Y. Wu
Division of Gastroenterology-Hepatology
Univ Connecticut Health Ctr
Farmington, CT, USA

ISSN 2197-7399 ISSN 2197-7704 (electronic)
Clinical Gastroenterology
ISBN 978-3-032-07867-4 ISBN 978-3-032-07868-1 (eBook)
https://doi.org/10.1007/978-3-032-07868-1

This Springer imprint is published by the registered company Springer Nature Switzerland AG
The registered company address is: Gewerbestrasse 11, 6330 Cham, Switzerland

Contents

Chapter 1
Introduction

Tracy Frech

The gastrointestinal tract can be affected by rheumatologic and vasculitic conditions and is an important cause of morbidity and mortality in this patient population [1]. General symptoms of weight loss, fever, and change in bowel symptoms are critical aspect of a rheumatologic history [2]. Prompt diagnosis is important for targeted treatment [3]. The evaluation should determine whether disease activity or damage is responsible for symptoms, which often diagnostically approached by anatomical location. The approach for targeted assessment of gastrointestinal tract symptoms may include a combination of physical exam, questionnaires, laboratory, and imaging studies. While physical exam can be quite limited with regards to diagnosis, the oropharyngeal exam can be supportive of a diagnosis of Sjogren's disease or systemic sclerosis, the rectal exam can identify the etiology of incontinence, and an abdominal exam can help guide urgent imaging needs for complications of rheumatologic and vasculitic conditions (Fig. 1.1). A methodical approach to gastrointestinal tract symptoms is necessary in patients with rheumatologic disease to guide treatment.

Gastrointestinal tract symptoms may be due to rheumatic or vasculitic disease, or from the treatment of these diseases. Parotid involvement from Sjogren's syndrome; esophageal symptoms from systemic sclerosis or mixed connective disease; bowel ischemia from vasculitides including polyarteritis nodosa and systemic lupus erythematosus; liver disease from sarcoidosis; and gastrointestinal tract bleeding from vascular ectasias in systemic sclerosis require a rheumatologist to understand diagnostic testing and targeted management strategies. Ancillary services, such a dietician referral and speech therapy evaluation may be required. Thus, the proper

T. Frech (✉)
Department of Medicine, Division of Rheumatology and Immunology, Vanderbilt University Medical Center, Nashville, TN, USA
e-mail: tracy.frech@vumc.org

M. Tadros et al. (eds.), *GI Diseases Associated with Rheumatological and Vasculitic Conditions*, Clinical Gastroenterology,
https://doi.org/10.1007/978-3-032-07868-1_1

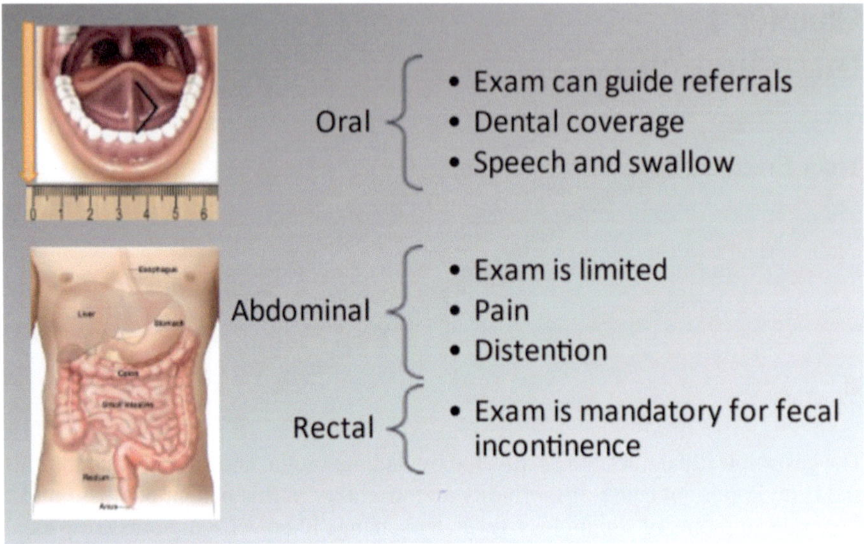

Fig. 1.1 Aspects of physical exam in rheumatic patients

approach to gastrointestinal tract management in rheumatic disease requires an understanding of symptom assessment as well as diagnostic tests and procedures.

Patient reported outcomes (PRO) regarding bowel symptoms can often be completed prior to a scheduled appointment to identify moderate to severe gastrointestinal tract symptoms, however barriers for PRO implementation may include time constraints and lack of electronic medical record integration that limit effective incorporation into clinical practice [4]. PRO which captures components of the gastrointestinal complications that can negatively impact quality of life are particularly important. Importantly, questionnaires allow symptom quantification and at no cost can guide care decisions particularly in diseases that may longitudinally and progressively affect the gastrointestinal tract. The simple use of categorical severity scores for certain symptoms may help the direct the treating physician to the urgency of evaluation [5]. Testing guided by PRO may help clarify the role of serial noninvasive testing may help clarify the effect of long-term immunosuppression on the gastrointestinal tract.

Diagnostics for rheumatic disease gastrointestinal tract symptoms can be performed in either the outpatient or inpatient setting. In most cases, outpatient assessment is appropriate for diagnostics, however concern for an acute abdomen or computed tomography imaging suggesting necrotic lesions; pneumatosis cystoides intestinalis; or free air in the peritoneal cavity mandate hospital admission for fluids and electrolyte management, intestinal 'rest', and consideration of parenteral nutrition, antibiotics, and supplemental oxygen [6, 7]. Inpatient assessment should include coordinated services of rheumatology, gastroenterology, and surgical services consultation, though unnecessary surgery should be avoided [8]. In necrotizing vasculitides, peritonitis, bowel perforation, gastrointestinal ischemia or infarctions and intestinal occlusion are associated with higher mortality in rheumatic disease, thus are critical to diagnosis and manage in the inpatient setting.

Esophageal assessment is particularly important in rheumatic patients with interstitial lung disease [9]. Patients identified as having heartburn, regurgitation, or dysphagia should receive education on management (Fig. 1.2). Long-term use of acid suppression and refractory esophageal symptoms requires co-management of a rheumatic disease patient with a gastroenterologist to help direct additional diagnostic needs that may require direct tissue visualization or biopsy. Evaluation of nutritional needs and diet are important. Specifically, concurrent gastroparesis has additional behavioral management considerations for rheumatic disease patient education (Fig. 1.3). Laboratories, such as serum carotene, vitamin D, B12, and iron, may be helpful in identifying malnutrition in rheumatic disease [10].

Lower gastrointestinal tract evaluation may include imaging, motility testing, and endoscopy (Fig. 1.4). Organ based evaluation, such as liver or pancreas, is guided by indication of function abnormality or injury tests. However, most diagnostic testing is guided by suspicion of whether luminal injury, peritoneal involvement, perfusion abnormalities, or nervous system dysfunction is the etiology. Urgent imaging is indicated for suspected bowel ischemia with computed tomographic angiography (CTA) and contrast-enhanced magnetic resonance angiography (MRA) are noninvasive screening techniques for patients suspected of having mesenteric ischemia [11]. Understanding the indications and urgency of gastrointestinal tract testing are an important aspect of caring for rheumatic disease patients.

In this book the treating rheumatologist and gastroenterologist are provided a framework for assessment of oropharynx, esophagus, small bowel, liver, biliary tract, pancreas, and anorectum when caring for a patient with rheumatic disease. The importance of diet and medication review is discussed. A goal of rheumatic disease management is to optimize gastrointestinal tract health and promptly identify complications.

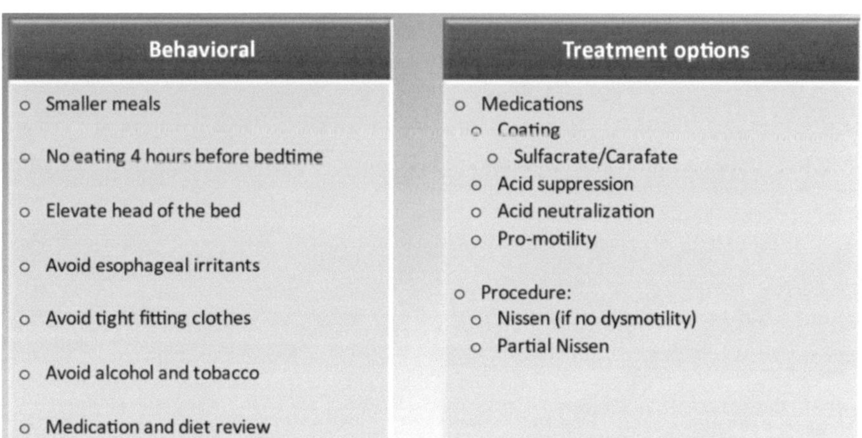

Fig. 1.2 Reflux management considerations

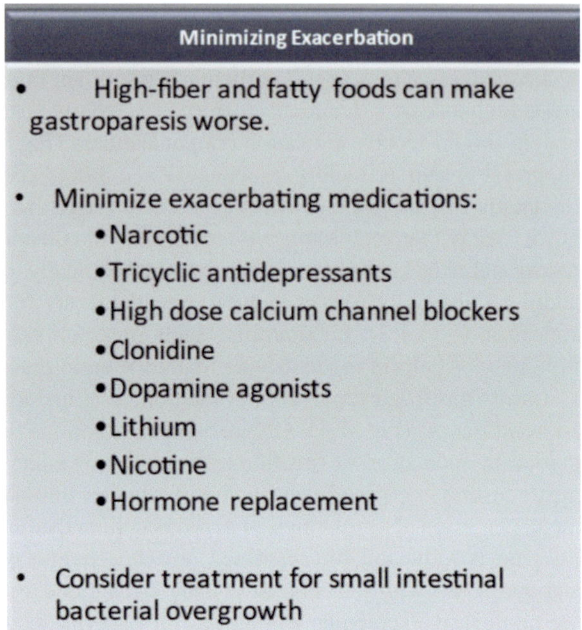

Fig. 1.3 Considerations if gastroparesis

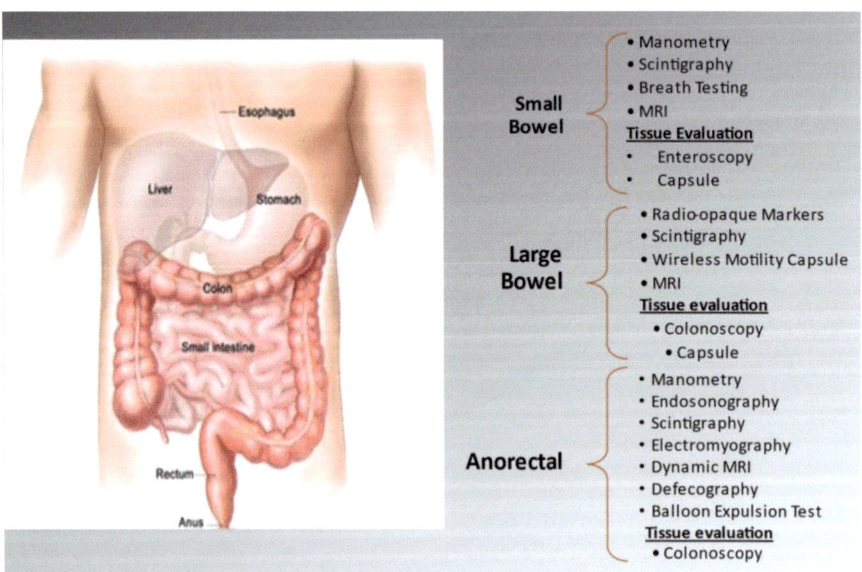

Fig. 1.4 Lower tract gastrointestinal tract evaluation

References

1. Hatemi I, Hatemi G, Celik AF. Systemic vasculitis and the gut. Curr Opin Rheumatol. 2017;29(1):33–8.
2. Perera LAM, Chopra A, Shaw AL. Approach to patients with unintentional weight loss. Med Clin North Am. 2021;105(1):175–86.
3. Nassar M, Ghernautan V, Nso N, Nyabera A, Castillo FC, Tu W, Medina L, Ciobanu C, Alfishawy M, Rizzo V, et al. Gastrointestinal involvement in systemic sclerosis: an updated review. Medicine (Baltimore). 2022;101(45):e31780.
4. Horrigan JM, Louis E, Spinelli A, Travis S, Moum B, Salwen-Deremer J, Halfvarson J, Panaccione R, Dubinsky MC, Munkholm P, et al. The real-world global use of patient-reported outcomes for the care of patients with inflammatory bowel disease. Crohns Colitis 360. 2023;5(2):otad006.
5. Kumar A, Marwaha V, Grover R. Emergencies in rheumatology. J Indian Med Assoc. 2003;101(9):520, 522, 524 passim.
6. Oiwa H, Taniguchi K, Miyoshi N, Sasaki K, Ichimura K, Kubota T, Sato D. Polyarteritis nodosa with marked eosinophilia, associated with severe gastrointestinal tract involvement and recurrent venous thrombosis. Intern Med. 2019;58(20):3051–5.
7. Balbir-Gurman A, Brook OR, Chermesh I, Braun-Moscovici Y. Pneumatosis cystoides intestinalis in scleroderma-related conditions. Intern Med J. 2012;42(3):323–9.
8. Bernardi MP, Warrier S, Lynch AC, Heriot AG. Acute and chronic pseudo-obstruction: a current update. ANZ J Surg. 2015;85(10):709–14.
9. Vaezi MF, Sifrim D. Assessing old and new diagnostic tests for gastroesophageal reflux disease. Gastroenterology. 2018;154(2):289–301.
10. Nagaraja V, McMahan ZH, Getzug T, Khanna D. Management of gastrointestinal involvement in scleroderma. Curr Treatm Opt Rheumatol. 2015;1(1):82–105.
11. Shih MC, Hagspiel KD. CTA and MRA in mesenteric ischemia: part 1, role in diagnosis and differential diagnosis. AJR Am J Roentgenol. 2007;188(2):452–61.

Part I
Organ Involvement

Chapter 2
Oral Cavity

David M. Leader, Martin Hogan, Nawar Issac, Allison R. Leader, Luis Del Castillo, Jonathan Garlick, and Carole A. Palmer

D. M. Leader (✉)
Dental Division, North Shore Community Health, Salem, MA, USA

Department of Comprehensive Care, Tufts University School of Dental Medicine, Boston, MA, USA
e-mail: David.Leader@tufts.edu

M. Hogan
Department of Surgery, General Practice Residency, Division of Dental Medicine, Loyola University Medical Center, Maywood, IL, USA

N. Issac
Oral Health Policy and Epidemiology, Harvard School of Dental Medicine, Boston, MA, USA

Dental International Student Program, Tufts University School of Dental Medicine, Boston, MA, USA

A. R. Leader
Dental Hygienist, D2 Dental Associates, Malden, MA, USA

L. Del Castillo
Postgraduate Prosthodontics Department of Restorative Sciences & Biomaterials Henry M Goldman School of Dental Medicine Boston University, Boston, MA, USA

J. Garlick
Division of Cancer Biology and Tissue Engineering, Science Communications, Tufts CTSI, Tufts Initiative In Civic Science (TICS), Tufts University School of Dental Medicine, Tufts University School of Medicine/Tufts University School of Engineering, Boston, MA, USA

C. A. Palmer
Department of Comprehensive Care, Tufts University School of Dental Medicine, Boston, MA, USA

Tufts University Friedman School of Nutrition Science and Policy, Boston, MA, USA

M. Tadros et al. (eds.), *GI Diseases Associated with Rheumatological and Vasculitic Conditions*, Clinical Gastroenterology,
https://doi.org/10.1007/978-3-032-07868-1_2

2.1 Introduction

The oral cavity is the entrance to the GI system. The oral cavity includes a complex system of hard and soft tissues extending to the oropharynx that help to initiate and mediate intake and output of a wide range of gasses, fluids, and solids that maintain the health of the mammalian corpus. Rheumatologic and vasculitic diseases affect the control and balance of this system. The changes and effects on health and quality of life are not always obvious. In this chapter, we will review the normal physiology of the oral cavity, discuss effects of autoimmune and rheumatic diseases, and describe considerations by types of autoimmune disease and condition.[1, 2, 3, 4]

2.2 Normal Anatomy

2.2.1 Oral Mucosa

There are three types of oral mucosa: lining mucosa, masticatory mucosa, and specialized mucosa. All oral mucosa is covered by stratified squamous epithelium. Typical, healthy lining mucosa is soft, elastic, non-keratinized tissue.[5] It is found on the inside of the lips and cheeks, soft palate, lining of the esophagus,[6] and alveolar mucosa. Masticatory mucosa or gingiva, when healthy, is firm and rubbery in texture, and tightly attached to the bone below it; this tissue includes the hard palate and the attached gingiva. Around the teeth, the sulcus or the pocket, provides a home for bacteria that causes inflammation. Inflammation from infection and tension on the gingiva denudes tooth roots resulting in irritation, pain and tooth loss.

---

[1] Ahola K, Saarinen A, Kuuliala A, Leirisalo-Repo M, Murtomaa H, Meurman JH. Impact of rheumatic diseases on oral health and quality of life. Oral Dis. 2015 Apr;21(3):342–8. doi: 10.1111/odi.12285. Epub 2014 Sep 22. PMID: 25158802.

[2] Schmalz G, Noack S, Patschan S, Patschan D, Müller GA, Rupprecht A, Schmickler J, Haak R, Ziebolz D. Disease activity, morning stiffness and missing teeth are associated with oral health-related quality of life in individuals with rheumatoid arthritis. Clin Oral Investig. 2020 Oct;24(10):3559–3566. doi: 10.1007/s00784-020-03226-3. Epub 2020 Feb 6. PMID: 32025884.

[3] Schmalz G, Patschan D, Schmickler J, Bethke N, Scherzinger E, Müller GA, Ziebolz D, Patschan S. Oral health-related quality of life in different rheumatic diseases. Oral Dis. 2020 Nov;26(8):1783–1792. doi: 10.1111/odi.13464. Epub 2020 Jun 29. PMID: 32510714.

[4] Skeie MS, Gil EG, Cetrelli L, Rosén A, Fischer J, Åstrøm AN, Luukko K, Shi X, Feuerherm AJ, Sen A, Frid P, Rygg M, Bletsa A. Oral health in children and adolescents with juvenile idiopathic arthritis - a systematic review and meta-analysis. BMC Oral Health. 2019 Dec 19;19(1):285. doi: 10.1186/s12903-019-0965-4. PMID: 31856793; PMCID: PMC6921440.

[5] Brizuela M, Winters R. Histology, Oral Mucosa. [Updated 2021 Jun 9]. In: StatPearls [Internet]. Treasure Island (FL): StatPearls Publishing; 2022 Jan-. Available from: https://www.ncbi.nlm.nih.gov/books/NBK572115/

[6] "Esophagus." *Histology at SIU*, Souther Illinois University, 26 Aug. 2021, https://histology.siu.edu/erg/esoph.htm#:~:text=The%20esophageal%20lining%20is%20protected,provides%20peristaltic%20propulsion%20of%20food

Aphthae, aphthous ulcers, or recurrent aphthous stomatitis (RAS) are painful benign lesions. Aphthae may be round, oval or irregular. The lesion is gray in the center with an erythematous border. Common triggers include stress, infection including COVID-19, medications, autoimmunity, and nutritional deficits. Aphthae may affect otherwise healthy people, and there is a strong association with irritable bowel disease (IBD) including Crohn's Disease.[7, 8, 9, 10, 11, 12]

Three categories of aphthae include minor, major, and herpetiform. Up to five minor RAS lesions appear on the mucosa of the lips, cheek, tongue, and the floor of the mouth. These lesions are under 10 mm in diameter, resolve without treatment in less than 2 weeks, and heal without scarring. Major RAS denotes the occurrence of up to ten lesions at once and lesions that are greater than 10 mm in diameter. Major RAS is less likely to affect the floor of the mouth and may affect the soft palate. Major lesions heal within 3 months and may scar. Minor and major RAS affects all genders equally. Herpetiform RAS affects the soft tissue of the oral cavity including the gingiva (an important difference). Eruptions include many deep ulcers up to 3 mm in diameter. Herpetiform lesions start as small bullae that break open and may coalesce into larger lesions. Herpetiform lesions are do not scar when healing.[13, 14, 15, 16]

---

[7] Papageorgiou, Spyridon N et al. "Inflammatory bowel disease and oral health: systematic review and a meta-analysis." *Journal of clinical periodontology* vol. 44,4 (2017): 382–393. doi:10.1111/jcpe.12698

[8] Gajendran, Mahesh et al. "A comprehensive review and update on ulcerative colitis." *Disease-a-month : DM* vol. 65,12 (2019): 100851. doi:10.1016/j.disamonth.2019.02.004

[9] Tan, Christopher X W et al. "A self-reported survey on oral health problems in patients with inflammatory bowel disease with a stoma." *Oral surgery, oral medicine, oral pathology and oral radiology* vol. 130,3 (2020): e80–e86. doi:10.1016/j.oooo.2020.04.816

[10] Vasovic, Miroslav et al. "The relationship between the immune system and oral manifestations of inflammatory bowel disease: a review." *Central-European journal of immunology* vol. 41,3 (2016): 302–310. doi:10.5114/ceji.2016.63131

[11] Barta, Zsolt. "Apical Periodontitis in Patients With Inflammatory Bowel Disease: A Puppet Master?." *Inflammatory bowel diseases* vol. 26,2 (2020): 280–282. doi:10.1093/ibd/izz129

[12] Flynn, Sean, and Samuel Eisenstein. "Inflammatory Bowel Disease Presentation and Diagnosis." *The Surgical clinics of North America* vol. 99,6 (2019): 1051–1062. doi:10.1016/j.suc.2019.08.001

[13] Edgar, Natalie Rose et al. "Recurrent Aphthous Stomatitis: A Review." *The Journal of clinical and aesthetic dermatology* vol. 10,3 (2017): 26–36.

[14] Saikaly, Sami Kameel et al. "Recurrent aphthous ulceration: a review of potential causes and novel treatments." *The Journal of dermatological treatment* vol. 29,6 (2018): 542–552. doi:10.1080/09546634.2017.1422079

[15] Chiang, Chun-Pin et al. "Recurrent aphthous stomatitis - Etiology, serum autoantibodies, anemia, hematinic deficiencies, and management." *Journal of the Formosan Medical Association = Taiwan yi zhi* vol. 118,9 (2019): 1279–1289. doi:10.1016/j.jfma.2018.10.023

[16] Sánchez-Bernal, J et al. "Recurrent Aphthous Stomatitis." "Aftosis oral recidivante." *Actas dermo-sifiliograficas* vol. 111,6 (2020): 471–480. doi:10.1016/j.ad.2019.09.004

2.2.2 Teeth

The normal complement of teeth includes 32 succedaneous or adult teeth and 20 deciduous, milk or baby teeth. Enamel, the hard material found on the surface of the crown of the tooth, is a nonrenewable, crystalline structure primarily composed of 90% calcium hydroxyapatite (Ca10(PO4)6(OH)2).[17] Enamel is acellular, avascular, and highly mineralized.[18] Dentin, the layer deep to enamel, is about 70% inorganic.[19] Deeper, odontoblasts line up in a "picket fence" pattern, extending from the pulp of the tooth to the surface of the dentin in contact with the enamel. The pulp, an active mass of connective tissue supplied by nerves and small capillaries, is at the core of the tooth.[20] The layers of the pulp, dentin, and enamel are identifiable in both 2D and 3D dental x-ray imaging.

A feature of tooth enamel is the cycle of demineralization and remineralization. Teeth lose calcium when exposed to dietary or stomach acid (as in gastro-esophageal reflux disease). Calcium ions in saliva remineralize enamel restoring integrity. In healthy individuals with a low acid diet, this cycle maintains a steady state. Diet, health, and medication may tip the balance in favor of loss of calcium and dental caries by increasing acidity or decreasing saliva (xerostomia).[21, 22]

Xerostomia or dry mouth is a common and serious finding for patients with autoimmune diseases and conditions. Xerostomia creates challenges with eating and digesting food and places the dentition at an increased risk of caries.[23]

2.2.3 Alveolar Bone

An area of spongy bone surrounded by thin, cancellous bone forms the alveoli of the mandible and the maxilla. Alveolar bone supports the teeth. Teeth attach to the bone of the alveolus by the periodontal ligament. Infection or constant pressure on teeth

[17] Abou Neel, Ensanya Ali et al. "Demineralization-remineralization dynamics in teeth and bone." *International journal of nanomedicine* vol. 11 4743–4763. 19 Sep. 2016, doi:10.2147/IJN.S107624

[18] Farci F, Soni A. Histology, Tooth. [Updated 2021 Jul 5]. In: StatPearls [Internet]. Treasure Island (FL): StatPearls Publishing; 2022 Jan-. Available from: https://www.ncbi.nlm.nih.gov/books/NBK572055/

[19] Farci F, Soni A. Histology, Tooth. [Updated 2021 Jul 5]. In: StatPearls [Internet]. Treasure Island (FL): StatPearls Publishing; 2022 Jan-. Available from: https://www.ncbi.nlm.nih.gov/books/NBK572055/

[20] Farci F, Soni A. Histology, Tooth. [Updated 2021 Jul 5]. In: StatPearls [Internet]. Treasure Island (FL): StatPearls Publishing; 2022 Jan-. Available from: https://www.ncbi.nlm.nih.gov/books/NBK572055/

[21] Abou Neel, Ensanya Ali et al. "Demineralization-remineralization dynamics in teeth and bone." *International journal of nanomedicine* vol. 11 4743–4763. 19 Sep. 2016, doi:10.2147/IJN.S107624

[22] Papas, Athena et al. "Caries clinical trial of a remineralising toothpaste in radiation patients." *Gerodontology* vol. 25,2 (2008): 76–88. doi:10.1111/j.1741-2358.2007.00199.x

[23] Beaty KL, Gurenlian JR, Rogo EJ. Oral Health Experiences of the Limited Scleroderma Patient. J Dent Hyg. 2021 Aug;95(4):59–69. PMID: 34376545.

(as in malocclusion or orthodontic treatment), results in remodeling of the bone by the mechanisms of bone resorption and formation.[24] Untreated loss of alveolar bone by periodontal or autoimmune disease results in tooth loss.

2.2.4 The Tongue

The tongue is a small but prominent organ in that it is easy for subjects to see and feel. The tongue is muscular. Three types of papillae cover the dorsal mucosa of the tongue giving it a rough appearance. The tongue's gustatory cells (taste receptor cells or taste buds) provide taste sensation. The tongue provides touch and temperature sensation. The tongue mechanically cleans the mouth of food and plaque. It is important for speech, swallowing, and physical expression of affection. Lesions and conditions that affect the tongue may dramatically affect quality of life.

Glossodynia (burning tongue or burning mouth syndrome) is a pernicious condition that is difficult to treat. It is more common in patients with IBD,[25, 26, 27] and up to seven times more prevalent in patients who are biologically female. Most patients are perimenopausal. The mean age of diagnosis is 59–61 years. Current theory is that glossodynia is primarily a neuropathy. There is no known cure. Management (symptomatic treatment) includes a variety of topical and systemic medications and dietary supplements. Cognitive behavioral therapy may improve the course of this condition.[28, 29]

Effects of medications and disease may result in alteration, reduction, and loss of taste sensation (dysgeusia, hypogeusia, and ageusia). Primary causes include damage to sensory organs (taste buds), neurological, and xerostomia. Secondary causes include aging, disease (including autoimmunity and viruses), side effects of medications, malnutrition, smoking (tobacco and marijuana), and exposure to chemicals. Taste alteration lowers patients' sense of wellbeing and is associated with loss of appetite and poor nutrition.[30]

---

[24] Hadjidakis, Dimitrios J, and Ioannis I Androulakis. "Bone remodeling." *Annals of the New York Academy of Sciences* vol. 1092 (2006): 385–96. doi:10.1196/annals.1365.035

[25] de Vries, Silvia A G et al. "Salivary Function and Oral Health Problems in Crohn's Disease Patients." *Inflammatory bowel diseases* vol. 24,6 (2018): 1361–1367. doi:10.1093/ibd/izy017

[26] Tan, Christopher X W et al. "A self-reported survey on oral health problems in patients with inflammatory bowel disease with a stoma." *Oral surgery, oral medicine, oral pathology and oral radiology* vol. 130,3 (2020): e80–e86. doi:10.1016/j.oooo.2020.04.816

[27] Vasovic, Miroslav et al. "The relationship between the immune system and oral manifestations of inflammatory bowel disease: a review." *Central-European journal of immunology* vol. 41,3 (2016): 302–310. doi:10.5114/ceji.2016.63131

[28] Klein, Brittany et al. "Burning Mouth Syndrome." *Dermatologic clinics* vol. 38,4 (2020): 477–483. doi:10.1016/j.det.2020.05.008

[29] Teruel, Antonia, and Seena Patel. "Burning mouth syndrome: a review of etiology, diagnosis, and management." *General dentistry* vol. 67,2 (2019): 24–29.

[30] Risso, Davide et al. "Alteration, Reduction and Taste Loss: Main Causes and Potential Implications on Dietary Habits." *Nutrients* vol. 12,11 3284. 27 Oct. 2020, doi:10.3390/nu12113284

2.2.5 *The Oral Microbiome*

The oral microbiome (OMB) is the second most complex in humans after the intestine.[31] The healthy OMB may include bacteria, viruses, fungi, archaea, and protozoa.[32] The bacteria of the healthy OMB comprise core and variable subsets. 96% of the core OMB includes the following microbial phyla: Firmicutes, Actinobacteria, Proteobacteria, Fusobacteria, Bacteroidetes, and Spirochaetes. The balance of the core OMB (4%) includes Actinomyces, Atopobium, Corynebacterium, Prevotella of Bacteroidetes, Granulicatella, Streptococcus and Veillonella of Firmicutes, Campylobacter, Cardiobacterium, Haemophilus, Neisseria of Proteobacteria, TM7, and Fusobacteria (add Derxia and Leptotrichia with high throughput sequencing). The variable OMB may include Chryseobacterium, Anaeroglobus, Filifactor, Lactobacillus, Johnsonella, Shuttleworthia, OD2 (not classified), Brachymonas, Propiniovibrio, Scardovia, Olsenella, and Cryptobacterium. Environment (geography and climate), medication, illness, and diet affect the OMB. Smokers may have a higher count of anaerobes compared to non-smokers.[33]

The OMB is a component of the bidirectional relationship between oral and systemic health. Changes in the OMB may contribute to pathogenesis of autoimmune disease including Sjögren's syndrome (SS), rheumatoid arthritis (RA), systemic lupus erythematosus (SLE), inflammatory bowel disease[34] including Crohn's disease (CD).[35]

2.3 Rheumatic Diseases and Conditions and Oral Health Effects

2.3.1 *Collagen Vascular Diseases*

Collagen vascular diseases (CVD) affect connective tissue. CVDs include systemic lupus erythematosus (SLE), Sjögren's syndrome (SS), systemic sclerosis or scleroderma and related conditions (SSC), Sarcoidosis, rheumatoid arthritis (RA) and mixed connective tissue disorders. The effects of CVDs may be localized as in morphea, or systemic as in SLE.

[31] Zorba, Matina et al. "The role of oral microbiome in pemphigus vulgaris." *Archives of microbiology* vol. 203,5 (2021): 2237–2247. doi:10.1007/s00203-021-02199-5

[32] Khor, Brandon et al. "Interconnections Between the Oral and Gut Microbiomes: Reversal of Microbial Dysbiosis and the Balance Between Systemic Health and Disease." *Microorganisms* vol. 9,3 496. 26 Feb. 2021, doi:10.3390/microorganisms9030496

[33] Verma, Digvijay et al. "Insights into the human oral microbiome." *Archives of microbiology* vol. 200,4 (2018): 525–540. doi:10.1007/s00203-018-1505-3

[34] Khor, Brandon et al. "Interconnections Between the Oral and Gut Microbiomes: Reversal of Microbial Dysbiosis and the Balance Between Systemic Health and Disease." *Microorganisms* vol. 9,3 496. 26 Feb. 2021, doi:10.3390/microorganisms9030496

[35] Nikitakis, N G et al. "The autoimmunity-oral microbiome connection." *Oral diseases* vol. 23,7 (2017): 828–839. doi:10.1111/odi.12589

Signs and symptoms of CVDs inform diagnoses. Some of these findings are specific to oral health. Dentists may aid in the diagnosis of SSC by reading dental radiographs. Radiographic findings in SSC include widening of the periodontal ligament (PDL) and resorption of the angles of the mandible, the alveolus, teeth, and rarely, the condyles and fossae of the temporo-mandibular joint (TMJ). The extent of widening of the PDL may be related to the seriousness of the disease.[36, 37] Note that widening of the periodontal ligament space is the most common radiographic finding in scleroderma found in about two-thirds of patients;[38] it is not evidence of periodontal disease and does not indicate a need for periodontal treatment.

There may be an association between periodontal disease and CVDs. Experimental studies and systematic reviews that compare the risk of periodontal disease for patients with SLE and SS with variable results. The relationship may be due to genetics, immunity, medications, environmental factors, or xerostomia. Systematic reviews recommend answering this research question with large prospective studies.[39, 40, 41, 42, 43]

Dentists often note external resorption of the roots of teeth in scleroderma.[44, 45, 46] This finding is uncommon in non-scleroderma patients. Epidemiological research on this association with SSC does not exist. Research by Memida et. al.[47]

---

[36] Baron, Murray et al. "Relationship Between Disease Characteristics and Oral Radiologic Findings in Systemic Sclerosis: Results From a Canadian Oral Health Study." *Arthritis care & research* vol. 68,5 (2016): 673–80. doi:10.1002/acr.22739

[37] Bhaskar 1981.

[38] Yalcin, Eda Didem et al. "Evaluation of radiomorphometric indices and bone findings on panoramic images in patients with scleroderma." *Oral surgery, oral medicine, oral pathology and oral radiology* vol. 127,1 (2019): e23–e30. doi:10.1016/j.oooo.2018.08.007

[39] Rutter-Locher, Zoe et al. "Association between Systemic Lupus Erythematosus and Periodontitis: A Systematic Review and Meta-analysis." *Frontiers in immunology* vol. 8 1295. 17 Oct. 2017, doi:10.3389/fimmu.2017.01295

[40] Sojod, Bouchra et al. "Systemic Lupus Erythematosus and Periodontal Disease: A Complex Clinical and Biological Interplay." *Journal of clinical medicine* vol. 10,9 1957. 2 May. 2021, doi:10.3390/jcm10091957

[41] Calderaro, Débora Cerqueira et al. "Is chronic periodontitis premature in systemic lupus erythematosus patients?." *Clinical rheumatology* vol. 36,3 (2017): 713–718. doi:10.1007/s10067-016-3385-8

[42] Sete, Manuela Rubim Camara et al. "Periodontitis and systemic lupus erythematosus." *Revista brasileira de reumatologia* vol. 56,2 (2016): 165–70. doi:10.1016/j.rbre.2015.09.001

[43] Wu, Shih-Yun et al. "Periodontal conditions in patients with Sjögren's syndrome: A meta-analysis." *Journal of dental sciences* vol. 16,4 (2021): 1222–1232. doi:10.1016/j.jds.2020.11.015

[44] de Figueiredo, Maria Antonia Zancanaro et al. "Root resorption associated with mandibular bone erosion in a patient with scleroderma." *Journal of endodontics* vol. 34,1 (2008): 102–3. doi:10.1016/j.joen.2007.10.021

[45] Memida, Takumi et al. "Multiple External Root Resorption of Teeth as a New Manifestation of Systemic Sclerosis-A Cross-Sectional Study in Japan." *Journal of clinical medicine* vol. 8,10 1628. 4 Oct. 2019, doi:10.3390/jcm8101628

[46] Arroyo-Bote, Sebastiana et al. "External Cervical Resorption: A New Oral Manifestation of Systemic Sclerosis." *Journal of endodontics* vol. 43,10 (2017): 1740–1743. doi:10.1016/j.joen.2017.03.040

[47] Memida T, Matsuda S, Kajiya M, Mizuno N, Ouhara K, Fujita T, Hirata S, Yoshida Y, Sugimoto T, Nishi H, Kawaguchi H, Sugiyama E, Kurihara H. Multiple external root resorption of teeth as a

demonstrates a frequency of external resorption of dental roots of 9.8% in a small study of scleroderma patients in Japan. An unpublished report of a case of external resorption in a scleroderma patient involves a single tooth. As demonstrated in this pair of radiographs, the lesion is below the level of the attached gingiva on the labial facing surface of the root of the upper left canine (Fig. 2.1). The dentist excised the soft tissue lesion from within the root defect. The biopsy specimen was preserved in 10% formalin. In the lab, Hematoxylin and Eosin staining was performed following paraffin-embedding of soft tissues from the lesion. Upper left—Low power magnification (4×), tissues displayed focally dense inflammatory infiltrate scattered in a loose connective tissue stroma. Figure 2.2, Upper Right—Higher power magnification (10×) revealed the presence of fused phagocytic macrophages forming multinucleated giant cells. Figure 2.2, Lower Center—These giant cells demonstrated typical features of cells known to resorb tooth surfaces and bone under highest magnification (40×) (Fig. 2.2).[48] There is no known preventive or curative treatment for external tooth resorption.

2.3.2 *Raynaud's Phenomenon*

Raynaud's Phenomenon, the dramatic reduction of blood flow through capillaries when exposed to low temperatures is a common finding with collagen vascular disease. The effect of Raynaud's Phenomenon on digits is mirrored in oral structures. Papers document effects of Raynaud's on the tongue.[49, 50, 51, 52] There is a case report of the effect of Raynaud's on capillary rich dental pulps resulting in the need for endodontic treatment (root canal treatment) of 8 teeth in a single patient.[53]

A 2021 study demonstrates an association between periapical pathology (indicating a need for endodontic treatment) with SLE. Authors propose the following

---

new manifestation of systemic sclerosis-a cross-sectional study in Japan. J Clin Med. 2019;8(10):1628. https://doi.org/10.3390/jcm8101628. PMID: 31590327; PMCID: PMC6832113.

[48] Jonathan Garlick, DDS, PhD; Jason DiFuria, PhD, and David Leader, DMD, MPH. Case report: scleroderma and external resorption of a tooth root, treatment and pathology. Autoimmuniity in 2017—Where are We Now?. April 2017. Poster presentation.

[49] Grémain, Vincent et al. "Raynaud's phenomenon of the tongue." *Joint bone spine* vol. 84,2 (2017): 231. doi:10.1016/j.jbspin.2016.02.031

[50] Cohen, Justin C et al. "Raynaud's phenomenon of the tongue." *The Journal of rheumatology* vol. 40,3 (2013): 336. doi:10.3899/jrheum.121093

[51] Rosato, Edoardo, and Felice Salsano. "Raynaud phenomenon of the tongue in a patient with scleroderma." *Journal of clinical rheumatology : practical reports on rheumatic & musculoskeletal diseases* vol. 16,4 (2010): 201. doi:10.1097/RHU.0b013e3181e08d65

[52] Bridges, M J, and C A Kelly. "Raynaud's phenomenon affecting the tongue of a patient with scleroderma." *Annals of the rheumatic diseases* vol. 61,5 (2002): 472. doi:10.1136/ard.61.5.472

[53] Rankin, Charles H. "A case report of a patient with Raynaud's phenomenon undergoing multiple endodontic procedures." *Journal of endodontics* vol. 33,2 (2007): 187–90. doi:10.1016/j.joen.2006.08.010

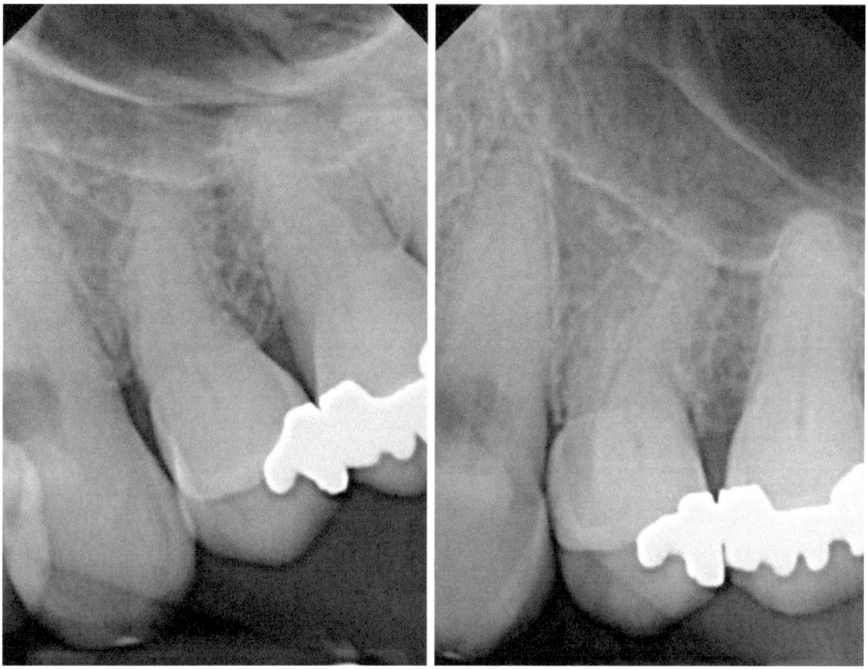

Fig. 2.1 Radiography by David M Leader, DMD, MPH, Tufts University School of Dental Medicine, 2014

mechanisms for this relationship. Patients with SLE generally have a higher risk of infection over controls. Patients with SLE are more likely to have a variety of blood dyscrasias, C reactive protein (CRP), diabetes, and renal involvement. These conditions are associated with periapical disease. Additionally, chronic use of glucocorticoids contributes to risk for periapical lesions.[54]

Telangiectasia is a common finding in scleroderma and one of the diagnostic criteria in the classification of scleroderma and CREST syndrome.[55] Oral telangiectasias on the tongue, palate, lips, and mucosa do not seem to cause spontaneous hemorrhage. However, there may be surgical implications.[56]

[54] Rotstein, Ilan, and Joseph Katz. "Prevalence of periapical abscesses in patients with systemic lupus erythematosus." Special care in dentistry : official publication of the American Association of Hospital Dentists, the Academy of Dentistry for the Handicapped, and the American Society for Geriatric Dentistry, 10.1111/scd.12630. 8 Jul. 2021, doi:10.1111/scd.12630

[55] Johnson, Sindhu R. "New ACR EULAR guidelines for systemic sclerosis classification." *Current rheumatology reports* vol. 17,5 (2015): 32. doi:10.1007/s11926-015-0506-3

[56] Stanford, T W Jr et al. "CREST syndrome and periodontal surgery: a case report." *Journal of periodontology* vol. 70,5 (1999): 536–41. doi:10.1902/jop.1999.70.5.536

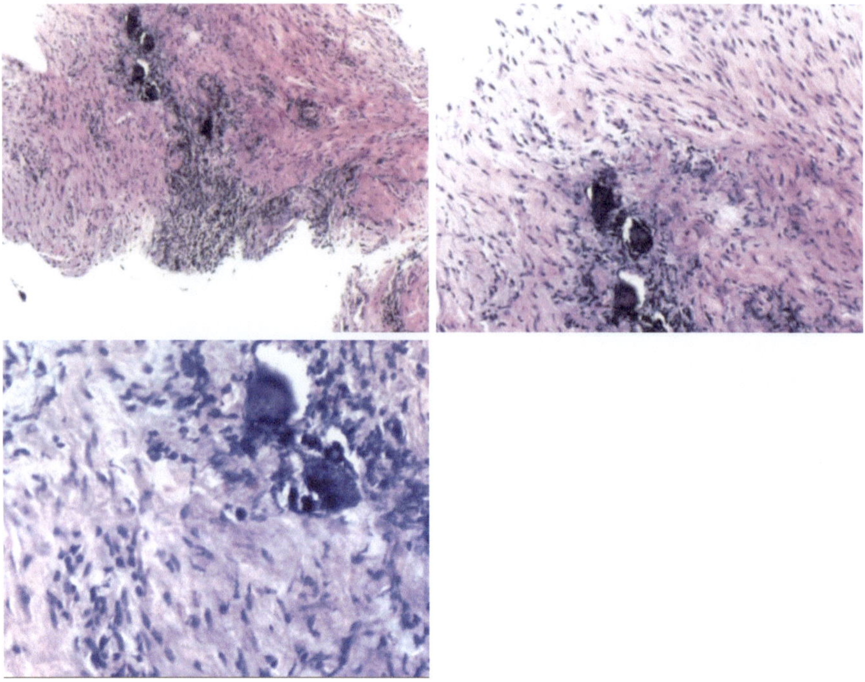

Fig. 2.2 Microscopy by Jonathan Garlick, DDS, PhD and Jason DiFuria, PhD, Tufts University School of Dental Medicine 2014

CVDs may affect the tongue. There may be loss of the papillae resulting in loss of taste sensation and associated with burning tongue syndrome.[57] There may be loss of motility due to fibrosis of the tongue and surrounding tissues particularly in scleroderma. And there may be atrophy of the tongue itself.[58, 59]

[57] Abrão ALP, Santana CM, Bezerra ACBet al. What rheumatologists should know about orofacial manifestations of autoimmune rheumatic diseases. Rev Bras Reumatol 2016 56: 441–450.

[58] Burch, J et al. "Myasthenia gravis--a rare presentation with tongue atrophy and fasciculation." *Age and ageing* vol. 35,1 (2006): 87–8. doi:10.1093/ageing/afj001

[59] Zampeli, Evangelia et al. "Tongue Atrophy in Sjögren Syndrome Patients with Mucosa-associated Lymphoid Tissue Lymphoma: Autoimmune Epithelitis beyond the Epithelial Cells of Salivary Glands?." *The Journal of rheumatology* vol. 45,11 (2018): 1565–1571. doi:10.3899/jrheum.180101

2.3.3 Sarcoidosis

Sarcoidosis is a granulomatous disease which commonly affects the lungs, liver, spleen, skin, eyes, and parotid glands. Intra-oral effects are uncommon.[60, 61] In one study, only three of 104 patients with recurrent facial swelling had a diagnosis of sarcoidosis.[62] Oral sarcoidosis appears as granulomatous lesions of the buccal mucosa, gingiva, lips, floor of the mouth, tongue, palate, and major salivary glands. There are few reports of intraosseous sarcoid lesions.[63] Diagnosis involves histopathology and ruling out other causes of granulomatous inflammation.[64] Intraosseous lesions respond well to excision and curettage.[65] Other causes may include infection, autoimmune, toxic, allergic, medication, and neoplastic conditions.[66] Treat individual lesions by surgical excision.[67] Many cases will resolve without intervention or medical treatment.

Sarcoidosis of oral soft tissue may be an incidental finding with little or no symptomatology. However, sarcoidosis of the salivary glands may result in swelling and xerostomia resulting in extensive caries. Sarcoid lesions in the alveolar bone may affect alveolar bone and the roots of teeth resulting in tooth loss.[68]

---

[60] Wilder, Elizabeth G et al. "Spectrum of orocutaneous disease associations: Genodermatoses and inflammatory conditions." *Journal of the American Academy of Dermatology* vol. 77,5 (2017): 809–830. doi:10.1016/j.jaad.2017.02.017

[61] Motswaledi, M H et al. "Oral sarcoidosis: a case report and review of the literature." *Australian dental journal* vol. 59,3 (2014): 389–94. doi:10.1111/adj.12196

[62] Miest, Rachel Y et al. "A Diagnostic Approach to Recurrent Orofacial Swelling: A Retrospective Study of 104 Patients." *Mayo Clinic proceedings* vol. 92,7 (2017): 1053–1060. doi:10.1016/j.mayocp.2017.03.015

[63] James, Martin et al. "Prosthetic Rehabilitation of a Patient Diagnosed With Sarcoidosis Using Dental Implants: A Clinical Case Report." *The Journal of oral implantology* vol. 46,3 (2020): 235–243. doi:10.1563/aaid-joi-D-18-00309

[64] Wilder, Elizabeth G et al. "Spectrum of orocutaneous disease associations: Genodermatoses and inflammatory conditions." *Journal of the American Academy of Dermatology* vol. 77,5 (2017): 809–830. doi:10.1016/j.jaad.2017.02.017

[65] James, Martin et al. "Prosthetic Rehabilitation of a Patient Diagnosed With Sarcoidosis Using Dental Implants: A Clinical Case Report." *The Journal of oral implantology* vol. 46,3 (2020): 235–243. doi:10.1563/aaid-joi-D-18-00309

[66] Kabeer K. Shah, Bobbi S. Pritt, Mariam P. Alexander, Histopathologic review of granulomatous nflammation, Journal of Clinical Tuberculosis and Other Mycobacterial Diseases, Volume 7, 2017, Pages 1–12, ISSN 2405-5794, https://doi.org/10.1016/j.jctube.2017.02.001

[67] James, Martin et al. "Prosthetic Rehabilitation of a Patient Diagnosed With Sarcoidosis Using Dental Implants: A Clinical Case Report." *The Journal of oral implantology* vol. 46,3 (2020): 235–243. doi:10.1563/aaid-joi-D-18-00309

[68] Motswaledi, M H et al. "Oral sarcoidosis: a case report and review of the literature." *Australian dental journal* vol. 59,3 (2014): 389–94. doi:10.1111/adj.12196

2.3.4 The Periodontium and Rheumatoid Arthritis

There is a documented relationship between periodontal disease and autoimmune diseases including IBD[69, 70, 71, 72, 73, 74, 75] and rheumatoid arthritis (RA). Periodontal disease and RA are characterized by increased secretion of pro-inflammatory mediators. Both diseases share common risk factors such as genetic predisposition, abnormal host inflammatory response, infection and inflammation, and smoking.[76] There is a higher prevalence of periodontitis in RA patients than in controls. Both conditions share the over-expression of pro-inflammatory cytokines. The severity of RA is reduced with the non-surgical treatment of periodontal disease (dental prophylaxis and scaling). TNF blockers are not as effective against RA when periodontitis is present.[77, 78]

Pathobiologic processes are common between RA and periodontitis including osteoclast-mediated bone destruction. RA develops through a loss of tolerance for proteins that have undergone citrullination. Citrullination is the posttranslational modification of a positively charged arginine into a neutral citrulline group. *P*

---

[69] Papageorgiou, Spyridon N et al. "Inflammatory bowel disease and oral health: systematic review and a meta-analysis." *Journal of clinical periodontology* vol. 44,4 (2017): 382–393. doi:10.1111/jcpe.12698

[70] de Vries, Silvia A G et al. "Salivary Function and Oral Health Problems in Crohn's Disease Patients." *Inflammatory bowel diseases* vol. 24,6 (2018): 1361–1367. doi:10.1093/ibd/izy017

[71] Tan, Christopher X W et al. "A self-reported survey on oral health problems in patients with inflammatory bowel disease with a stoma." *Oral surgery, oral medicine, oral pathology and oral radiology* vol. 130,3 (2020): e80–e86. doi:10.1016/j.oooo.2020.04.816

[72] Keskin, Mutlu et al. "Two Cheers for Crohn's Disease and Periodontitis: Beta-Defensin-2 as an Actionable Target to Intervene on Two Clinically Distinct Diseases." *Omics : a journal of integrative biology* vol. 19,8 (2015): 443–50. doi:10.1089/omi.2015.0077

[73] Vasovic, Miroslav et al. "The relationship between the immune system and oral manifestations of inflammatory bowel disease: a review." *Central-European journal of immunology* vol. 41,3 (2016): 302–310. doi:10.5114/ceji.2016.63131

[74] She, Yang-Yang et al. "Periodontitis and inflammatory bowel disease: a meta-analysis." *BMC oral health* vol. 20,1 67. 12 Mar. 2020, doi:10.1186/s12903-020-1053-5

[75] Barta, Zsolt. "Apical Periodontitis in Patients With Inflammatory Bowel Disease: A Puppet Master?." *Inflammatory bowel diseases* vol. 26,2 (2020): 280–282. doi:10.1093/ibd/izz129

[76] Radwan-Oczko M, Duś-Ilnicka I, Richards P, Thomsen AM, Rasmussen C. Rheumatoid arthritis patients' oral health and disease activity. Int J Rheum Dis. 2019 Aug;22(8):1538–1543. doi: 10.1111/1756-185X.13590. Epub 2019 May 7. PMID: 31062938.

[77] Gualtierotti R, Marzano AV, Spadari F, Cugno M. Main Oral Manifestations in Immune-Mediated and Inflammatory Rheumatic Diseases. J Clin Med. 2018 Dec 25;8(1):21. doi: 10.3390/jcm8010021. PMID: 30585183; PMCID: PMC6351952.

[78] Radwan-Oczko M, Duś-Ilnicka I, Richards P, Thomsen AM, Rasmussen C. Rheumatoid arthritis patients' oral health and disease activity. Int J Rheum Dis. 2019 Aug;22(8):1538–1543. doi: 10.1111/1756-185X.13590. Epub 2019 May 7. PMID: 31062938.

gingivalis is the only oral bacteria that possesses peptidylarginine deiminase (PAD) activity which causes citrullination of arginine.[79, 80, 81, 82, 83, 84, 85, 86]

2.3.5 *Vasculitides*

2.3.5.1 Giant Cell Granuloma (and Horton Giant Cell Arteritis), Wegener's Granulomatosis (WG), and Polyarteritis Nodosa (PAN)

Although rare, giant cell arteritis and related conditions are the most common cause of lingual necrosis. Giant cell arteritis itself has a prevalence in people over 50-year-old of 51.74 [42.04, 61.43] cases per 100,000.[87] Typically, patients present with pain and visible necrosis of the tongue. Glossodynia may precede visible signs of disease. When present, lingual necrosis may inform an early diagnosis of giant cell arteritis. Often, early treatment with high doses of corticosteroids is curative, but the

[79] Sedghi L, DiMassa V, Harrington A, Lynch SV, Kapila YL. The oral microbiome: Role of key organisms and complex networks in oral health and disease. Periodontol 2000. 2021 Oct;87(1):107–131. doi: 10.1111/prd.12393. PMID: 34463991; PMCID: PMC8457218.

[80] Gualtierotti R, Marzano AV, Spadari F, Cugno M. Main Oral Manifestations in Immune-Mediated and Inflammatory Rheumatic Diseases. J Clin Med. 2018 Dec 25;8(1):21. doi: 10.3390/jcm8010021. PMID: 30585183; PMCID: PMC6351952.

[81] Bingham CO 3rd, Moni M. Periodontal disease and rheumatoid arthritis: the evidence accumulates for complex pathobiologic interactions. *Curr Opin Rheumatol.* 2013;25(3):345–353. doi:10.1097/BOR.0b013e32835fb8ec

[82] Sedghi L, DiMassa V, Harrington A, Lynch SV, Kapila YL. The oral microbiome: Role of key organisms and complex networks in oral health and disease. Periodontol 2000. 2021 Oct;87(1):107–131. doi: 10.1111/prd.12393. PMID: 34463991; PMCID: PMC8457218.

[83] Sedghi L, DiMassa V, Harrington A, Lynch SV, Kapila YL. The oral microbiome: Role of key organisms and complex networks in oral health and disease. Periodontol 2000. 2021 Oct;87(1):107–131. doi: 10.1111/prd.12393. PMID: 34463991; PMCID: PMC8457218.

[84] Sedghi L, DiMassa V, Harrington A, Lynch SV, Kapila YL. The oral microbiome: Role of key organisms and complex networks in oral health and disease. Periodontol 2000. 2021 Oct;87(1):107–131. doi: 10.1111/prd.12393. PMID: 34463991; PMCID: PMC8457218.

[85] Sedghi L, DiMassa V, Harrington A, Lynch SV, Kapila YL. The oral microbiome: Role of key organisms and complex networks in oral health and disease. Periodontol 2000. 2021 Oct;87(1):107–131. doi: 10.1111/prd.12393. PMID: 34463991; PMCID: PMC8457218.

[86] Nair S, Faizuddin M, Dharmapalan J. Role of autoimmune responses in periodontal disease. Autoimmune Dis. 2014;2014:596824. doi: 10.1155/2014/596824. Epub 2014 May 25. PMID: 24963400; PMCID: PMC4055614.

[87] Li, K., Semenov, D., Turk, M. et al. A meta-analysis of the epidemiology of giant cell arteritis across time and space. *Arthritis Res Ther* **23,** 82 (2021). https://doi.org/10.1186/s13075-021-02450-w

patient may retain mild scarring and deformity of the tongue.[88, 89, 90, 91, 92, 93, 94, 95, 96, 97, 98, 99, 100, 101, 102]

There are oral findings in up to 10% of patients with Wegener's granulomatosis (WG).[103] Oral findings may include "strawberry gingivitis" characterized by marked

---

[88] Kumarasinghe, Anuttara Panchali et al. "Temporal arteritis presenting with tongue necrosis." *BMJ case reports* vol. 2012 bcr2012007241. 19 Nov. 2012, doi:10.1136/bcr-2012-007241

[89] Lobato-Berezo, Alejandro et al. "Tongue necrosis: an unusual clinical presentation of giant cell arteritis." *Arthritis & rheumatology (Hoboken, N.J.)* vol. 66,10 (2014): 2803. doi:10.1002/art.38767

[90] Truffaut, Laurent, and Philippe Lefebvre. "Tongue Necrosis in Giant-Cell Arteritis." *The New England journal of medicine* vol. 378,26 (2018): 2517. doi:10.1056/NEJMicm1709412

[91] Lima, Filipa Bacalhau et al. "Tongue ischemia - an unusual presentation of Giant Cell Arteritis." "Tongue ischemia—an unusual presentation of Giant Cell Arteritis." *Acta reumatologica portuguesa* vol. 44,3 (2019): 273–275.

[92] Truffaut, Laurent, and Philippe Lefebvre. "Tongue Necrosis in Giant-Cell Arteritis." *The New England journal of medicine* vol. 378,26 (2018): 2517. doi:10.1056/NEJMicm1709412

[93] Dilly, Baptiste, and Charlene Bomahou. "Tongue Necrosis in Giant-Cell Arteritis." *The New England journal of medicine* vol. 385,25 (2021): 2377. doi:10.1056/NEJMicm2105150

[94] Zaragoza, Jose R et al. "Tongue necrosis as an initial manifestation of giant cell arteritis: case report and review of the literature." *Case reports in rheumatology* vol. 2015 (2015): 901795. doi:10.1155/2015/901795

[95] Sobrinho, Rafael Alex Barbosa de Siqueira et al. "Tongue Necrosis Secondary to Giant Cell Arteritis: A Case Report and Literature Review." *Case reports in medicine* vol. 2017 (2017): 6327437. doi:10.1155/2017/6327437

[96] Saadi, Altaf et al. "Tongue infarction due to giant cell arteritis." *Practical neurology* vol. 16,3 (2016): 231. doi:10.1136/practneurol-2015-001304

[97] Cockey, George et al. "Giant Cell Arteritis Presenting with a Tongue Lesion." *The American journal of medicine* vol. 132,5 (2019): 576–578. doi:10.1016/j.amjmed.2018.12.026

[98] Tago, Masaki et al. "Tongue Necrosis: An Atypical Sign of Giant-cell Arteritis." *Internal medicine (Tokyo, Japan)* vol. 60,20 (2021): 3347–3348. doi:10.2169/internalmedicine.7096-21

[99] Wang, Sijie Jason et al. "A Picture's Worth: Giant Cell Arteritis." *The American journal of medicine* vol. 129,9 (2016): 942–4. doi:10.1016/j.amjmed.2016.04.029

[100] Dos Reis, Leonardo Amaral et al. "Lingual necrosis leading to the diagnosis of giant cell arteritis." Special care in dentistry : official publication of the American Association of Hospital Dentists, the Academy of Dentistry for the Handicapped, and the American Society for Geriatric Dentistry vol. 41,3 (2021): 408–410. doi:10.1111/scd.12571

[101] Fongaufier, Christelle et al. "Tongue and Scalp Necrosis: Simultaneous Initial Complications Revealing Giant Cell Arteritis." *The Journal of rheumatology* vol. 45,6 (2018): 873–874. doi:10.3899/jrheum.171321

[102] Husein-Elahmed, Husein et al. "Tongue infarction as first symptom of temporal arteritis." *Rheumatology international* vol. 32,3 (2012): 799–800. doi:10.1007/s00296-009-1355-z

[103] Xing, Xianghui et al. "Pediatric Wegener's granulomatosis with oral ulcers and progressive periodontitis: a case report." *Oral surgery, oral medicine, oral pathology, oral radiology, and endodon-*

dark reddish purple swelling of the gingiva with petechiae,[104, 105, 106] and lingual necrosis.[107]

Polyarteritis nodosa (PN) is a rare autoimmune disease that results in necrotizing inflammatory lesions as a result of vasculitis. PN rarely affects the tongue as demonstrated in two case reports, one in an adult and one in a child. Course, treatment, and outcomes are akin to other types of arteritis that affect the tongue.[108, 109]

There are similarities among arteritis diseases and conditions. For example, Winiwarter-Buerger Disease (Thromboangiitis Obliterans) is indicated in some cases of lingual necrosis. Thromboangiitis obliterans is not classified as an autoimmune condition; it may be due to another cause such as infection,[110, 111] and may be related to periodontitis.[112, 113]

---

tics vol. 112,4 (2011): e1–5. doi:10.1016/j.tripleo.2011.05.030

[104] Ruokonen, Hellevi et al. "Strawberry like" gingivitis being the first sign of Wegener's granulomatosis." *European journal of internal medicine* vol. 20,6 (2009): 651–3. doi:10.1016/j.ejim.2009.04.007

[105] Hanisch, Marcel et al. "Gingival hyperplasia as first sign of recurrence of granulomatosis with polyangiitis (Wegener's granulomatosis): case report and review of the literature." *BMC oral health* vol. 17,1 33. 2 Aug. 2016, doi:10.1186/s12903-016-0262-4

[106] Muller, Romain, and Gaetan Lebrun. "Strawberry gingivitis." *Kidney international* vol. 100,6 (2021): 1353. doi:10.1016/j.kint.2021.04.013

[107] Carter, Lachlan M, and Eitan Brizman. "Lingual infarction in Wegener's Granulomatosis: a case report and review of the literature." *Head & face medicine* vol. 4 19. 21 Aug. 2008, doi:10.1186/1746-160X-4-19

[108] Mondal, Rakesh et al. "Necrotic tongue ulcer: an unusual presentation of childhood polyarteritis nodosa." *Indian journal of pediatrics* vol. 80,11 (2013): 974–5. doi:10.1007/s12098-012-0936-0

[109] Ciurtin, Coziana et al. "Polyarteritis nodosa associated with necrosis of the tongue: a rare presentation in an adult patient." *The British journal of oral & maxillofacial surgery* vol. 53,9 (2015): 883–5. doi:10.1016/j.bjoms.2015.06.009

[110] Li, Meng-di et al. "Risk Factors, Mechanisms and Treatments of Thromboangiitis Obliterans: An Overview of Recent Research." *Current medicinal chemistry* vol. 27,35 (2020): 6057–6072. doi:10.2174/0929867326666190816233042

[111] Fazeli, Bahare et al. "Recent Updates and Advances in Winiwarter-Buerger Disease (Thromboangiitis Obliterans): Biomolecular Mechanisms, Diagnostics and Clinical Consequences." *Diagnostics (Basel, Switzerland)* vol. 11,10 1736. 22 Sep. 2021, doi:10.3390/diagnostics11101736

[112] Igari, Kimihiro et al. "The Epidemiologic and Clinical Findings of Patients with Buerger Disease." *Annals of vascular surgery* vol. 30 (2016): 263–9. doi:10.1016/j.avsg.2015.07.014

[113] Li, Meng-di et al. "Risk Factors, Mechanisms and Treatments of Thromboangiitis Obliterans: An Overview of Recent Research." *Current medicinal chemistry* vol. 27,35 (2020): 6057–6072. doi:10.2174/0929867326666190816233042

2.3.5.2 Behçet's Disease

Patients who have Behçet's disease (BD) have oral findings in 97–100% of cases.[114] BD occurs in any decade of life but is more common in the third and fourth decades. Oral lesions in BD are similar to recurrent aphthous stomatitis (RAS). Ulcerations begin as small papules that coalesce into round or oval lesions one to several millimeters in diameter. They usually occur on the non-keratinized mucous membrane such as the inside of the cheeks and lips and the floor of the mouth. Lesions may occur on the soft palate and in the pharynx. The painful ulcerations have an erythematous halo and may be covered with a yellowish membrane.[115]

Clinical criteria inform the diagnosis of BD; there are no pathognomonic diagnostic criteria, no lab tests, or pathology. Diagnostic criteria of the International Criteria for Behçet's Disease (ICBD) have high selectivity and specificity. The ICBD scores findings thusly: 2 points each for ocular lesions, genital aphthosis, and oral aphthosis; one point each for skin lesions, neurological manifestations, vascular manifestations, and an optional extra point for a positive pathergy test.[116] Pathergy refers to the insertion of a fine needle into the skin. A positive result is when a small red bump or pustule forms within two days. This test is not 100% specific and is positive for less than half of patients. [117] Additionally, per ICBD guidelines oral aphthae must appear at least three times within 12 months.[118]

2.4 Vitamins and Oral Health

"Vitamins are a group of organic compounds that are essential for growth and nutrition and are required in small quantities in the diet because they are not synthesized in the body [except for vitamin D which is inadequately synthesized with exposure to sunlight]."[119] Chronic illness and autoimmunity challenge nutrition in two ways.

[114] Bulur, Isil, and Meltem Onder. "Behçet disease: New aspects." *Clinics in dermatology* vol. 35,5 (2017): 421–434. doi:10.1016/j.clindermatol.2017.06.004

[115] Bulur, Isil, and Meltem Onder. "Behçet disease: New aspects." *Clinics in dermatology* vol. 35,5 (2017): 421–434. doi:10.1016/j.clindermatol.2017.06.004

[116] Kiafar, Mina et al. "Diagnosis of Behçet's disease: clinical characteristics, diagnostic criteria, and differential diagnoses." *BMC rheumatology* vol. 5,1 2. 15 Jan. 2021, doi:10.1186/s41927-020-00172-1

[117] "Diagnosis of Behcet's Disease: American Behcets Disease Association." *American Behcets Disease Association—Support, Education, Advocacy, Research*, American Behcet's Disease Association—ABDA, 31 Mar. 2019, https://www.behcets.com/basics-of-behcets/diagnosis/#:~:text=The%20pathergy%20test%20is%20a,test%20constitutes%20a%20positive%20result

[118] Bulur, Isil, and Meltem Onder. "Behçet disease: New aspects." *Clinics in dermatology* vol. 35,5 (2017): 421–434. doi:10.1016/j.clindermatol.2017.06.004

[119] *OED Online*, Oxford University Press, December 2021, www.oed.com/viewdictionaryentry/Entry/11125. Accessed 29 January 2022

People who are chronically ill face difficulties consuming food. Consumption may be physically challenging and less enjoyable. This may be due to tooth loss, xerostomia, microstomia, TMJ function and pain, trouble swallowing, convenience, and difficulty manipulating food. Additionally, many illnesses, aging, and conditions limit absorption of nutrients. Vitamin deficiency often causes oral findings in advance of other findings thanks to rapid turnover of oral tissues, visibility, and concentration of sensory receptor cells.

Although patients may experience vitamin deficiencies due to diet and health, it is important not to overcompensate. Over consumption of most vitamins can be deleterious. For most patients including those who are chronically ill, the dosage of vitamins in a daily multivitamin is usually enough.[120] Patients with autoimmunity may work closely with a nutritionist or dietician and with an occupational therapist to ensure a healthy diet.

2.4.1 Oral Findings That Indicate Vitamin Deficiency

Vitamin B refers to a group of water-soluble vitamins including B1 (thiamine), B2 (riboflavin), B3 (niacin), B6, and B12. Based on data from large surveys, the prevalence of Vitamin B12 deficiency in subjects 60 years old and older, is approximately 6%; the prevalence increases with age.[121] Deficiency of B vitamins is associated with recurrent aphthous stomatitis, enamel hypomineralization, cheilosis, cheilitis [cracking in the corners of the mouth], halitosis, gingivitis (including hemorrhagic gingivitis), periodontal disease, glossitis, glossodynia (burning mouth syndrome), atrophy of the lingual papillae, stomatitis, rashes around the nose, dysphagia, salivary gland dysfunction (xerostomia), and pallor.[122, 123]

Deficiency in vitamin C, another water-soluble vitamin, may cause changes in the bone, gingiva, and salivary glands resulting in xerostomia.[124, 125] Vitamin C is an

---

[120] Palmer, Carole A., and Linda D. Boyd. Diet and Nutrition in Oral Health. Third edition., Pearson Prentice Hall, 2016.

[121] Allen, Lindsay H. "How common is vitamin B-12 deficiency?" *The American journal of clinical nutrition* vol. 89,2 (2009): 693S–6S. doi:10.3945/ajcn.2008.26947A

[122] Gutierrez Gossweiler, Ana, and E Angeles Martinez-Mier. "Chapter 6: Vitamins and Oral Health." *Monographs in oral science* vol. 28 (2020): 59–67. doi:10.1159/000455372

[123] Sheetal, Aparna et al. "Malnutrition and its oral outcome—a review." *Journal of clinical and diagnostic research : JCDR* vol. 7,1 (2013): 178–80. doi:10.7860/JCDR/2012/5104.2702

[124] Gutierrez Gossweiler, Ana, and E Angeles Martinez-Mier. "Chapter 6: Vitamins and Oral Health." *Monographs in oral science* vol. 28 (2020): 59–67. doi:10.1159/000455372

[125] Palmer, Carole A., and Linda D. Boyd. Diet and Nutrition in Oral Health. Third edition., Pearson Prentice Hall, 2016.

important component of bone metabolism.[126] Extreme deficiency of vitamin C results in scurvy.

For young patients, vitamin D deficiency disrupts tooth development. These patients may exhibit non-syndromic amelogenesis and dentinogenesis imperfecta, hypoplasia, and dysplasia.[127] Conversely, consumption of excess vitamin D may result in calcification of the dental pulp and counterintuitively, enamel hypoplasia.[128]

Low vitamin K increases hemorrhage which may be observed as gingival bleeding with little or no provocation.[129]

Excess vitamin A may be diagnosed by an orange dermal hue. It is reversible by adjusting diet. Without treatment, excess vitamin A may result in bone loss.[130]

2.5 Summary

Recognize normal oral findings in the oral cavity, request guidance or referral when in doubt. Patients with autoimmune conditions benefit from regular examination of the oral cavity by oral and systemic healthcare providers. Look for changes in the mucosa including the floor of the mouth and soft palate, the tongue, teeth, and the periodontium (gingiva and masticatory mucosa). Abnormal findings may be subtle. Oral healthcare providers are instrumental in identifying and treating effects of xerostomia, GERD, aphthae, and osteogenic changes. Systemic healthcare providers identify changes in vascularity, and provide treatment or alter treatment of xerostomia, GERD, dysgeusia (when possible), aphthae, osteogenic changes, and changes in vascularity. Patients benefit when their providers collaborate.

The final section of this chapter identifies the way specific autoimmune diseases and conditions affect the oral cavity. Autoimmunity effects diet and absorption of nutrients; therefore, this chapter includes a section on oral findings that indicate vitamin deficiency.

The authors of this chapter include a nutritionist, a dental hygienist, two general dentists, an oral surgeon, an oral pathologist, and a prosthodontist. We thank Dr Mark Lerman, Professor and Interim Chair, Department of Diagnostic Sciences, Tufts University School of Dental Medicine, and Amy Lapidow, Research and Instruction Librarian, for their guidance in research and writing this chapter.

---

[126] Bellissimo, Moriah P et al. "Metabolomic Associations with Serum Bone Turnover Markers." *Nutrients* vol. 12,10 3161. 16 Oct. 2020, doi:10.3390/nu12103161

[127] Gutierrez Gossweiler, Ana, and E Angeles Martinez-Mier. "Chapter 6: Vitamins and Oral Health." *Monographs in oral science* vol. 28 (2020): 59–67. doi:10.1159/000455372

[128] Palmer, Carole A., and Linda D. Boyd. Diet and Nutrition in Oral Health. Third edition., Pearson Prentice Hall, 2016.

[129] Gutierrez Gossweiler, Ana, and E Angeles Martinez-Mier. "Chapter 6: Vitamins and Oral Health." *Monographs in oral science* vol. 28 (2020): 59–67. doi:10.1159/000455372

[130] Palmer, Carole A., and Linda D. Boyd. Diet and Nutrition in Oral Health. Third edition., Pearson Prentice Hall, 2016.

Chapter 3
Salivary Manifestations of Rheumatologic and Vasculitic Conditions

Lisa Rosenberg, Vivek Mehta, and Ruben Peredo-Wende

3.1 Introduction

Salivary glands are differentiated structures that ensure the secretion of fluid into the oral cavity. With the primary function of keeping oral structures lubricated and moist, they enable the preservation of the integrity of the oral mucosa, gums, teeth, gustatory papillae, and other structures [1]. They facilitate feeding by their fluidification and digestive properties. Additional functions include an adjuvant feature for mastication, taste, digestion, and speech [2]. The protective immunity provided relies on the release of immunoglobulins, lactoferrin, lysozyme, peroxidase, and mucins [3, 4].

Salivary glands group into major and minor glands, which ultimately drain into the same compartment, the oral cavity. The first category of major glands comprises the parotid, submandibular, and lingual glands, which are distributed symmetrically on each side, being six in total [2]. Minor salivary glands are dispersed within the oral mucosa, mainly in the labial mucosa, at the base of the mouth, palate, and tongue. The minor salivary glands, numbered at an estimated 750 glands within the oral cavity, supply an estimated 10% of saliva, whereas the major, and mainly the parotid glands, provide the principal amount of saliva [5, 6]. As described, parotid glands secrete serous saliva, rich in α-amylase, while sublingual glands secrete mucous, mucin-rich saliva. Submandibular glands secrete a mixed serous-mucus saliva [7].

L. Rosenberg
Division of Rheumatology, University of Vermont Medical Center, Burlington, VT, USA

V. Mehta
Rheumatology, Alaska Native Medical Center, Anchorage, AK, USA

R. Peredo-Wende (✉)
Division of Rheumatology, Department of Medicine, Stratton VA Medical Center, Albany, NY, USA
e-mail: ruben.peredo-wende@va.gov

M. Tadros et al. (eds.), *GI Diseases Associated with Rheumatological and Vasculitic Conditions*, Clinical Gastroenterology,
https://doi.org/10.1007/978-3-032-07868-1_3

Each one of the major salivary glands has a similar structure, connected to a secretory duct. The parotid glands, each located under and in front of each ear, connect via the Stensen's duct into the oral cavity. The latter localizes in the upper posterior aspect of the cheek mucosa [6]. The submandibular glands, each one located between the mandible and the root of the trachea, communicate through the Wharton's duct into the opening located under the tongue, at the sublingual caruncula. Finally, the sublingual glands, located at the base of the mouth, end up in an opening mediated by Bartholin's ducts. These latter connect with the Warthon's duct before its ending at the oral cavity [6]. Additionally, a series of undersized ducts, known as Rivinus ducts, connect to the sublingual glands and have their openings located under the tongue [5].

The morphology of salivary glands follows a pattern replicated among all glands (Fig. 3.1). It consists of acini grouped within lobules. Acini confluence into ducts that, in turn, will merge into larger ducts. Depending on the epithelial cell layering, ducts will subdivide into intercalated ducts, within which cells have a cuboidal appearance, followed by the striated ducts, which have a peculiar feature: invaginations within the basal membrane of the cells [5, 8].

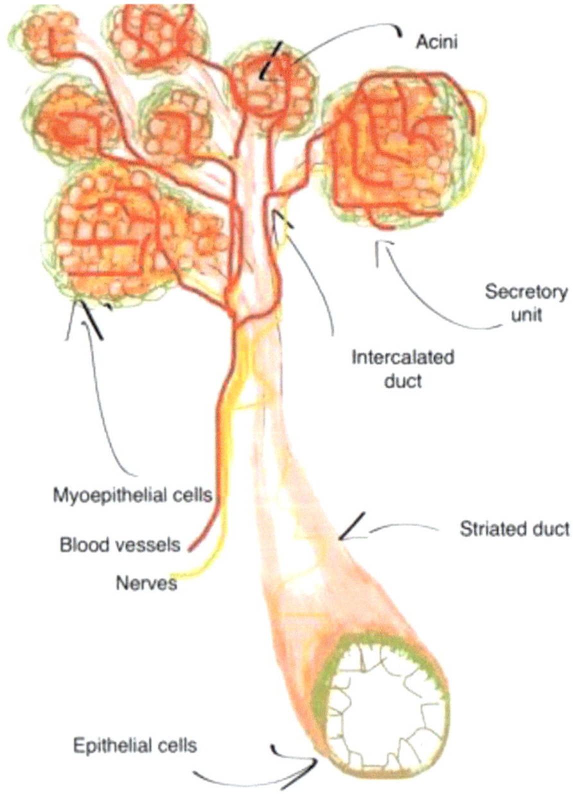

Fig. 3.1 Schematic structure of salivary glands. Acini gather together to form lobules. They generate and concentrate saliva, which, after neurologic impulses, will secrete the fluid into the intermediate ducts. The ducts will merge into the larger ducts or striated ducts. The final destination will end at the papilla next to the opening to the oral cavity. Myoepithelial cells surrounding the acini units have contractile properties and will help the saliva flow by constricting the acini. Rich innervation parallels the vascularization and will provide the cholinergic and adrenergic neurotransmission necessary for the sequential saliva production and secretion

3.2 Embryogenesis and Morphology

The origin of salivary glands derives from the epithelial placode. Between weeks 4 and 12 of embryogenesis, the placode embeds within the mesenchymal tissue. Along the differentiation, the placode grows to form a bud, which in turn will be the source for further branching to form independent buds. Each of the buds will carry a vessel that supplies sufficient nutrients for further growth [6]. Similarly, cholinergic neurons follow the arborizing subdivisions, which appear to participate in salivary gland development actively, and this is mediated by an influx of acetylcholine [8]. Each bud is composed of epithelial layers to form the acini. The inner layer will differentiate into either the stalk at the proximal aspect or the tips at the distal aspect. In the mature stages, the stalk will develop into a duct, and the tips will form acini. The outer layer differentiates into myoepithelial cells. They will grow into smooth muscle cell-like features surrounding the acini, which will participate in the secretory activity. The interphase between the epithelial and mesenchymal cells will constitute the basement membrane, distinguishing it from the surrounding matrix. Acinar branching will depend on the composition of the matrix. Grouped acini form a lobule, which then merges into the ducts [6, 8].

Innervation, by the autonomic nervous system, follows an anatomically organized subdivision. The parasympathetic nerves will innervate the submandibular and sublingual glands through the facial nerve (CN VII) [5, 9]. In contrast, the glossopharyngeal nerve (CN IX) will extend the branching terminals to the parotid gland [9]. The parasympathetic nerve fibers release acetylcholine, which subsequently binds to muscarinic receptors, enabling the salivary gland to produce fluid-rich saliva. The sympathetic nerves, arising from the upper thoracic spinal centers, will supply the innervation via the superior cervical ganglion. This latter system will release noradrenaline and activate the alpha-and beta-adrenergic receptors, inducing the gland to produce a protein-rich secretion [5, 10, 11]. The terminal nerves are myelinated by Schwann cells, which encroach on the salivary glands [12].

3.3 Physiology of Salivation and Enzymatic Activity

Salivation consists of a coordination of simultaneous processes, including: myoepithelial cell contraction of salivary glands, initial cholinergic influx shifting fluid to run from vessels to the glands via aquaporin channels (AQP5) [13] and secretory material from within the cytoplasm [5]. Saliva collection starts at the acinar lumen. Fluid will be pumped out of the acinar cells once the Na^+/K-ATPase develops a gradient by pumping sodium out into the extracellular space. At the same time, Na will simultaneously outflow to the paracellular space. Cholinergic impulses activate the G-protein-mediated cascade, leading to the subsequent activation of phospholipase C, and through hydrolytic mechanisms, an increase in inositol triphosphate (IP3) concentrations [5, 9]. By binding to receptors on the endoplasmic reticulum, IP3 increases intracytosolic Ca^{2+}. They, in turn, will activate the Cl^- channel, allowing fluid to flow down the gradient into the extracellular space. Further Ca^{2+} supply will depend on store-operated calcium entry (SOCE) [9, 14–16].

Fluid will undergo a transformation along the ducts. In striated-cell ducts, the Na^+/ K ATPase and carbonic/Cl^- pumps reabsorb NaCl from the forming saliva [17]. The impermeability of the fluid to cross the duct cell lining prevents further saliva from shifting to re-enter the gland [5]. The final saliva quality remains depleted in NA^+ and favors alkalinity to preserve tissues within the oral cavity. Salivary acinar cells contain cytoplasmic granules, which are protein-rich and primarily serve enzymatic purposes, and are released upon stimulation. Once the degranulated acinar cells change, gland volumes may change. Subsequently, the parotid and submandibular glands will undergo functional shrinkage [18]. In the serous and seromucous glands (mainly parotid and submandibular), the sympathetic system, mediated by the β-adrenoreceptors and via the cAMP mechanism, will activate the degranulation [5].

In contrast, the sublingual glands contain granules rich in mucins that ultimately receive impulses from the muscarinic system [5]. Each one of the glands has a prevailing type of cytoplasmic granules. The sublingual glands contain mucins, mainly sialic acid-rich, while the parotid glands are rich in α-amylase [19]. The submandibular glands contain two types of cytoplasmic granules: mucin- and serous-rich, as well as other types of enzymatically rich granules, primarily lysozymes. The latter enzyme plays a significant role in the immune system by targeting different types of microorganisms [20, 21]. Sialic acid, released from mucin-rich glands (sublingual), is a unique characteristic of salivary glands compared to other secretory glands within the organism [22]. During the degranulation phase, and following a nerve stimulatory impulse, myoepithelial cells contract the acinar glands, facilitating a synergistic impulse for saliva secretion and progressive flow [5, 23]. The sizes of salivary glands will therefore functionally change, differing from situations when the glands remain enlarged [18]. In such circumstances, the evaluation of the underlying etiology should follow a systematic approach as described below.

3.4 Salivary Gland Exam

Evaluation of major salivary glands ensues recognition of any anomaly in a particular gland or multiple glands. During the inspection, while placing the patient in front of the examiner, they may identify possible asymmetries in parotid gland sizes [24–26]. Color changes and sweating over the parotid glands occur while the individual eats, related to the re-anastomosis of the auriculotemporal nerve after surgery (i.e., parotid resection) or salivary gland injury, known as Frey syndrome [27]. Palpation will identify texture, size, pain sensation, fluctuation, and possible attachment to underlying tissues (i.e., malignancy) [24, 26]. By squeezing the gland, the examiner should enquire intact duct patency by determining any fluid protruding out of the papilla as the oral duct terminal of the Stensen's duct. The papilla is localized adjacent to the upper second molar tooth on each side. Similarly, the examiner should palpate each one of the glands and papillae of the submandibular (localized below the jaw) and the sublingual glands (at the floor of the mouth). For the latter purpose, the examiner should sweep the roof of the mouth with one digit while the patient keeps the tongue upward [24–26]. The examiner should document the fluid type or any other material protruding out of the papillae. Examples of saliva include mucoid, purulent discharge, plugs, sialoliths, and other debris [4, 5]. In addition, the examiner should evaluate the ear canal for sensation response, as it is part of the sensory terminal of cranial nerve VII.

Additionally, cranial nerve V, which is mainly sensorial, might be compromised in the presence of parotid gland anomalies. Finally, the marginal mandibular branch of CN VII, in the presence of submandibular gland enlargement, might show a motor dysfunction seen at the mouth commissure [28]. Examining the salivary glands should enable the discrimination of adjacent anatomic structures, particularly nearby lymph nodes. If enlarged, they are preauricular, within the parotid gland, and just below it, next to the jawbone angle [25]. Additional lymph nodes to explore are the anterior, lateral, and posterior chains of cervical lymph nodes [25, 26].

3.5 Salivary Gland Enlargement

Depending on the type of presentation, it is classified as acute, if it is abrupt, and usually painful, either as a unique or polyglandular presentation, or as a chronic presentation. This latter case is generally painless, compromising either one or several glands. Associated symptomatology, including habits (alcohol use), review of systems, history of sicca symptoms in other mucosae (i.e., eyes), pharmacologic drug use, history of iodine exposure, radiation surgery, comorbidities (i.e., psychiatric disorders such as bulimia nervosa), and other relevant history should be reviewed as part of the comprehensive history [24–26, 29].

Common problems associated with unilateral single salivary gland enlargement might relate to infections or primary salivary gland neoplasms, including lymphomas. Chronic sialadenitis or obstruction is also considered if they present acutely [24, 25]. Whenever they are bilateral and present as a recent onset, a systemic illness is considered that includes viral infections (cytomegalovirus, influenza, parainfluenza, coxsackie B8, mumps, and other viruses) [24]. In a chronic progression, systemic illnesses to consider include IgG4-related disease, granulomatous diseases (such as infectious diseases like tuberculosis, leprosy, and atypical tuberculosis), and sarcoidosis. HIV related diffuse idiopathic lymphocytosis syndrome (DILS) presents chronically as well, as does Sjogren's disease, and is usually symmetric. The evaluation of bilateral, symmetric salivary enlargement, idiopathic causes, chronic liver disease, and endocrine problems, including acromegaly, type 2 diabetes mellitus, gonadal hypofunction, hyperlipoproteinemia, alcoholism, and chronic pancreatitis, among others, should be considered [24].

3.6 Ancillary Imaging Tests to Evaluate the Salivary Gland

Different radiographic imaging modalities will have advantages in exploring the salivary glands. Overall, each one of them will help define the underlying pathology, and the combination of them will narrow down diagnoses and determine the extent of lesions (e.g., tumors, calculi, etc.) [25].

3.7 Ultrasonography

The advantages of performing bedside and onsite ultrasound of major salivary glands include defining the gland's texture, ductal system, and masses. Inhomogeneity, which details parenchymal focal hypo- or anechoic round areas, defines the degree of inflammation, blood flow, and the description of margins, has been systematically and standardized to assess Sjögren's disease [30]. This modality is used for diagnostic purposes and monitoring of responses to therapies. Moreover, the utility of the US for determining Sjögren's disease from other etiologies has been proposed [31]. As a result, applications of the US as a diagnostic criterion for SJD are considered [32]. Its validation may help define early SJD and potentially substitute for the minor salivary gland biopsy [33]. Sialoliths are identifiable and can be accurately identified, which is an advantage compared to other study modalities and may help guide future invasive procedures. The sensitivity and specificity of a US are comparable to those of sialography in terms of duct imaging (ectasia, dilatation, obstruction), favoring its use due to its less invasive techniques [34].

Additionally, it may be helpful for guidance on draining abscesses and following up on them [25]. The Doppler modality might help determine the magnitude of inflammation based on the vascularity magnitude [30, 35]. Limitations to clearly differentiate low-grade malignant neoplasms from benign lesions might be overcome with the use of combined fine needle aspiration for cytology analysis [25].

3.8 Computed Tomography

It is the preferred modality without contrast for determining calculi, masses, fatty deposits, or even tumors. The best utility is applied in sialolithiasis and calcifications [36]. In the parenchymal granulomatous pattern, for example, the CT scan shows sufficient sensitivity for its recognition [37]. Additionally, it may define the size and other adjacent tissues [38]. Combined with ultrasound, the CT scan with contrast will define the extent of strictures and accurately localize calculi. Other modalities are also available for the latter, such as sialography and sialendoscopy [37]. The latter two procedures are reserved for cases with undefined outcomes using ultrasound and for the treatment of calculi [24, 25]. Computed Tomography with contrast is the preferred imaging modality for identifying malignancies, sometimes even over PET/

CT, as some tumors may not exhibit avid uptake, and in cases where MRI is contraindicated [37].

3.9 Magnetic Resonance

This technique is the preferred imaging modality for defining neoplasms. The MRI has the best contrast resolution, enabling differentiation of various tissues, such as fat, lymph nodes, and parenchymal pathology [36]. Additional benefits are the lack of radiation exposure [37]. It helps determine the extension and adjacent tissue invasion, including intraglandular and paraglandular lymph nodes [39]. Promising features of this modality include the capability to define anatomic features and the potential recognition of possible associated pathologies based on readings in minor salivary glands [40].

3.10 Positron Emission Tomography

This modality may determine features of salivary gland lymphoma, with distant extension of metastasis. Increased standardized uptake value (SUVmax), however, is indistinguishable in patients with Sjögren's disease, regardless of whether they have lymphoma or not. Clues to define lymphoma in SJD associate with a high SUVmax in the parotid glands of ≥4.7 and coexisting focal lung lesions [41]. High uptake in the submandibular glands, albeit at a lower degree compared to malignancy, is seen in IgG4-RD, in addition to revealing other distant affected areas [42].

Specific entities that we will describe below should be considered whenever there is a first approach to determine etiologies for the underlying enlarged salivary glands.

3.11 Sialadenosis

Swelling of mainly the parotid, but rarely the submandibular glands, in the absence of a specific pathogenic disorder, is known as sialadenosis. Multiple ethologists account for this phenomenon, including alcoholism, type 2 diabetes mellitus, nutritional deficiencies, and idiopathic. A neurogenic component plays a leading role, with a demyelinating nerve process responsible for regulating the pooling and flow of saliva [43]. The outcome will determine an imbalance between the excretion and accumulation of fluid in the salivary glands. In histopathology, clusters of zymogen granules within enlarged cells (hypertrophic) with an excess of fluid retention within acini characterize sialadenosis [44]. Dysfunction in aquaporin channels appears to contribute to the imbalance of fluid accumulation [45]. A history, examination, and comorbidities, along with a salivary gland CT scan, will reveal an enlarged parotid gland with increased density [24]. The approach should address the underlying cause.

3.12 Bulimia Nervosa

Mostly present in young women, it refers to an eating disorder. Alternating bursts of eating binges with anorexic episodes, and intercurrent self-provoked emetic events, is a behavior overlying a psychiatric composite of depression, obsessive-compulsive disorder, altered body image perception, and past stressors. Self-inflicted episodic emesis appears to be a self-motivating action that provides patients with relief. Complications include enamel destruction and mainly salivary gland enlargement [24]. Electrolyte depletion, weight fluctuations, and obsessive-compulsive disorder (OCD) patterns may highlight the underlying eating irregularity. Salivary gland enlargement bears similarities to sialadenosis.

3.13 Celiac Disease

Celiac disease is an autoimmune disorder caused by the ingestion of gluten in a genetically susceptible individual [46]. The small intestine is largely affected, but the salivary glands can also be involved. Typically, inflammation primarily affects the minor rather than the major salivary glands in celiac disease [47]. Patients can present with impaired mucosal lubrication, with xerostomia and labial dryness [48]. Labial salivary gland tissue biopsies can show more extensive, diffuse chronic inflammation, focal lymphocytic infiltration, acinar atrophy, and glandular fibrosis [47]. Tissue transglutaminase 2 (TG2) contributes to the disease process by deamidating glutamine residues in gluten peptides, thereby increasing the ability of these peptides to bind to the HLA-DQ2 or HLA-DQ8 groove of antigen-presenting cells [46]. It also facilitates crosslinking to form TG2-gluten complexes, which can activate B cells to produce autoantibodies [46]. These autoantibodies are sensitive and specific and are used as the preferred serologic test for diagnosis [49]. Management of celiac disease usually requires a gluten-free diet [50]. Clinicians should be aware of an overlap between celiac disease and other coexisting autoimmune diseases, such as autoimmune thyroiditis, Sjögren's disease, type I diabetes mellitus, and, in the context of autoimmune hepatitis and inflammatory diseases, among others [51, 52]. It is worth noting that the shared genetic background among these entities, primarily due to the two genes mentioned above, accounts for their simultaneous and coexisting presence [53].

3.14 IgG4–Related Disease

IgG4-related disease is a rare, immune-mediated systemic disease characterized by soft tissue lymphocyte infiltration and resultant fibrosis [54]. Patients can exhibit a variety of manifestations, ranging from multi-organ involvement, including acute pancreatitis and biliary stenosis; however, the salivary glands are the most commonly affected organs, leading to subacute submandibular and/or parotid swelling and sialadenitis [54]. A patient is said to have Mikulicz's disease (MD) if they exhibit symmetrical enlargement of the lacrimal, parotid, and submandibular glands, as well as the sublingual glands, accompanied by symptoms of dry mouth and ocular dryness [55]. Swelling mainly involving the submandibular glands with predominance of fibrosis, sclerosing sialadenitis, and salivary duct destruction is described as Küttner's tumor [55]. In the inflammatory phase, polyclonal B and T cell subpopulations infiltrate affected tissues and undergo mutual activating, antigen-mediated interactions leading to the secretion of profibrotic cytokines such as IL-1β, IL-6, interferon-γ, transforming growth factor-β, and platelet-derived growth factor B. Lymphocyte subpopulations including plasmablasts/plasma cells, cytotoxic T lymphocytes, and CD4 $^{+}$ T follicular helper cells are involved in causing the disease [54]. T-helper type 2 responses have also been implicated in the pathogenesis of IgG4-related disease. Thus, IgG4-related disease should be suspected in patients with a history of atopy who present with salivary gland swelling, a long-standing history of allergies, peripheral blood eosinophilia, and elevated serum IgE levels [56].

Diagnosis incorporates clinical, serologic, radiologic, and pathologic findings; however, histological examination is crucial for a definitive diagnosis, as it is more specific [54, 57]. Histopathological features include a dense, polyclonal, lymphoplasmacytic infiltrate rich in IgG4+ plasma cells, storiform fibrosis, and obliterative phlebitis [58]. However, obtaining optimal biopsy samples can be challenging, as it may require invasive procedures [57]. A complete picture of the disease involvement can be obtained with a whole-body computed tomography scan or an ^{18}F-fluorodeoxyglucose positron emission tomography (^{18}F-FDG-PET) scan, both for staging purposes and for identifying sites that can be sampled more easily [57].

Treatment usually depends on the pattern and extent of organ involvement. Glucocorticoids are generally the first line for inducing disease remission [57, 58]. Variables to consider as predictors of compromised response include multi-organ involvement, high serum IgG4 and IgE levels, and peripheral blood eosinophilia, for which disease-modifying anti-rheumatic drugs (DMARDs) such as rituximab are recommended in addition to glucocorticoid therapy to increase the likelihood of achieving disease remission [57, 58].

3.15 Sarcoidosis

Sarcoidosis is a chronic granulomatous disease that can affect any organ or tissue [59]. Salivary gland involvement is usually rare and presents as painless, persistent, bilateral parotid gland enlargement, accompanied by xerostomia and reduced salivary flow [60]. The submandibular glands can also be affected [60]. Glandular swelling can occur in conjunction with systemic signs of sarcoidosis [24]. For instance, Heerfordt's syndrome, a subtype of sarcoidosis, includes disease features of parotid gland enlargement, uveitis, facial palsy, and low-grade fever [59]. Diagnosis of sarcoidosis is usually made by integrating clinical, radiographic, and histologic findings [24]. The histopathological feature of sarcoidosis is the presence of non-caseating granulomas that need to be differentiated from granulomas of other causes; however, sarcoid granulomas lack unique histologic features to distinguish them from granulomas of different causes [60, 61]. Even so, some features in the histopathology are worth mentioning, giving some hints towards sarcoidosis as etiology. Among multiple inflammatory cells, T helper CD4+ cells prevail in the early granuloma, followed by CD8+ lymphocytes in later stages. Epithelioid cells of monocytic origin may sometimes merge to form giant multinucleated cells, which are localized within the center of the granuloma or in its periphery. Large giant cells containing over 20 small nuclei in the cytoplasmic periphery, or named as Langerhans-type, may differentiate from foreign body-like giant cells in which nuclei are dispersed in the cytoplasm [62]. In the central area, fibrinoid necrosis may be present in 6–35% of cases, indistinguishable from other necrotizing granulomas [63]. Schauman bodies, also known as conchoidal bodies, localized within the cytoplasm of giant cells, are composed of laminated dense proteins or calcium and with birefringence properties under polarizing light microscopy, unlike the asteroid bodies, or stellate inclusions that are birefringent negative; finally Hamazaki-Wesenberg bodies, of probably lysosomal origin have an oval or fusiform shape and brownish coloration [64]; the lung biopsy with bronchoscopy or biopsy of intrathoracic lymph nodes may also be necessary to confirm the diagnosis [61]. A detailed history, clinical presentation, serologic studies, special stains and cultures for acid-fast bacilli and fungi, current tumor or histologic evidence supporting malignant cause of granulomas like Reed-Sternberg cells, radiologic findings, and PET scanning can help delineate between the various etiologies of granulomas including infectious, occupational and environmental, malignant, drug-induced, vasculitides/connective tissue diseases, and granulomatous reactions to foreign substances [61, 65]. An elevated angiotensin-converting enzyme can help differentiate sarcoid granulomas from other granulomas, but it is a nonspecific serologic marker [24]. Usually, no treatment is required, as glandular swellings can often spontaneously regress [24, 66]. A variety of conventional immunosuppressants (azathioprine, methotrexate, mycophenolate mofetil, etc.) may provide anti-inflammatory effects while sparing the undesired side effects of glucocorticoids. Biologic drugs, and mainly TNF-alpha blocking therapy (such as infliximab), can be used to manage refractory cases [24, 66]. Patients should also be closely monitored for the development of lymphomas [24].

3.16 Sjögren's Disease

Described in the early 1900s, it was initially identified in patients with keratoconjunctivitis sicca and active inflammatory arthritis [67]. Initially, there was no apparent difference between Mikulicz's disease, which was later identified as IgG4-related disease [68].

Sjögren's disease (SJD) is defined as a chronic inflammatory systemic illness, affecting mainly the exocrine glands, particularly the salivary and lacrimal glands, and resulting in dryness (sicca) in the mouth and eyes [69]. Lymphocytes invade the glands (and mainly the ducts) in clusters known as focal lymphocytic sialadenitis (FSL), which eventually leads to their destruction [70]. The number of FSLs over the measured salivary gland surface of minor salivary gland samples, times 4mm^2, will define a Focus Score. A Focus Score is the main feature in the histopathology of SJD [71]. The associated serology, primarily anti-SSA/Ro and anti-SSB/La antibodies, supports the autoimmune nature of the pathogenesis [72]. Homing lymphocytes, mainly T cells but also B cells and other inflammatory cells, surround the epithelial cells of the salivary ducts and exhibit a similar morphology in other distant organs, such as primary biliary cholangitis (PBC). Based on the similarities and the coexistence of both SJD and PBC, a concept of autoimmune epithelitis was formulated [73, 74]. The etiology of SJD is still not fully understood. Possibly initiated by an invading virus and via the interferon signature released by plasmacytoid dendritic cells, the immune system activates an intricate chain of processes aimed at clearing the virus. In genetically susceptible individuals (carriers of mainly but not only HLA-DR3-DQ1, and polymorphisms in STAT4 and IRF5 genes) [75], the immune activity will acquire an autonomous pattern, procuring the continuation of a local (and probably distant) inflammation, independent of the initial ignition (viruses) [76–78]. Difficulties in understanding the pathogenesis made it cumbersome to define the disease. The difficulties reflect the numerous changes to the SJD classification criteria that have occurred over the last few decades [79]. Overall, gathering information regarding mucosal dryness in the eyes and mouth, along with objective sicca findings, has been the pivotal concept in defining SJD. The current European League against Arthritis (EULAR) and the American College of Rheumatology (ACR) define the disease based on the weight of the objective but not the subjective components. They include objective evidence of dry eyes and dry mouth, as well as positive anti-SSA/Ro antibodies but not anti-SSB/LA antibodies, and finally, the previously described abnormal histopathology [80]. Histopathology with focus scoring has been the gold standard for defining the underlying disease, although an estimated 15% of healthy individuals may have positive focus scoring without meeting the criteria for Sjögren's disease [81]. Conversely, patients meeting with criteria for SJD but with negative histopathology are 20% [82]. Sjögren's disease affects mainly middle-aged women 9:1, with an estimated prevalence of 1.02 per 10,000 adults [83]. Approximately one-third of patients with SJD may experience extra-glandular manifestations, including involvement in the peripheral and central nervous systems, as well as the respiratory, endocrine, renal, musculoskeletal, cutaneous, hematologic (with cytopenia), immunological, and lymphatic systems, along with constitutional features [84]. If presenting alone, SJD is defined as primary and in the context of another autoimmune, mainly connective tissue disease, as secondary [69]. Patients might experience xerostomia, even years before the diagnosis, requiring the provider's curiosity to complete the criteria for diagnosis. With the ultrasound pairing, the equivalency of a minor salivary gland biopsy will yield a more accurate diagnosis sooner, increasing the SJD frequency. Sjögren's disease typically presents with symmetrical, non-tender, soft, swollen glands (parotids are more visible than submandibular glands) and some features of dry mouth and ocular dryness. In addition to the sicca symptoms, fatigue, polyarthralgia, and fibromyalgia-like symptoms are the most common presentations. Even though it is considered a benign and rare disorder, it may carry a burden of morbidity, not only due to corneal complications (keratitis sicca), but also since SJD associates with extra-glandular manifestations (i.e., polyneuropathy, interstitial lung disease, polyarthritis, uveitis, etc.) and malignancy. Among the connective tissue diseases, SJD is considered to be the most frequently linked disorder with lymphomas. Analogous to *H. pillory* Mucosal-Associated Lymphatic [85, 86] Tissue (MALT) lymphomas, SJD has a preponderance to develop lymphomas in salivary glands. MALT lymphomas originate from marginal zone B-cells that surround the mantle zone and germinal centers, and are classified as non-Hodgkin lymphomas. Predictors for this complication are found under the presence of enlarged salivary (parotid) glands, vasculitis and skin ulcers, palpable purpura, lymphadenopathy (mainly but not only cervical), peripheral neuropathy, higher markers of ESSDAI-score (European League Against Rheumatism, Disease Activity Index) representing a higher interferon signature, disease duration, and Raynaud's phenomenon. The laboratory profile suggesting lymphoma prediction includes low C4, cryoglobulinemia, leukopenia with low CD4 counts, highly positive rheumatoid factor, monoclonal gammopathy (IgM kappa), and positive serology for anti-SSA/Ro, anti-SSB/La, and centromere antibodies, as well as additional anemia and elevated β-2 microglobulin levels [85–87]. The evaluation of dry mouth (xerostomia) should consider chronic complications, including gum retraction, mucosal frailty, dental caries at the neck of teeth, and various forms of *Candida albicans* growth, which can overlap with the severity of dryness and contribute to burning mouth syndrome [29, 88]. In the assessment, unexplained weight loss, early dysphagia, voice changes, odynophagia, and trouble with teeth and dentures should also be considered [89].

3.17 ANCA-Associated Vasculitis (AAV)

Anti-Neutrophilic Cytoplasmic Antibody (ANCA)-associated vasculitis with three main clinicopathologic variants- microscopic polyangiitis (MPA), granulomatosis with polyangiitis (GPA), and eosinophilic granulomatosis with polyangiitis (EGPA) [90]. All three are necrotizing small vessel vasculitides with some distinct clinical and serological differences, but often with overlapping clinical features. Salivary gland involvement in AAV is uncommon but well-documented [91] . It can often lead to diagnostic delays due to similarities in presentation with infections, malignancies, and other rheumatologic diseases, such as Sjögren's Disease, sarcoidosis, and IgG4-related disease.

Most reported cases of salivary gland involvement have been documented primarily in GPA and EGPA. The parotid glands are the most common target tissue, followed by the submandibular glands. Targeted sublingual glands are less commonly affected. Half of the patients with this presentation in AAV may complain of pain, and rarely, parotid gland ulceration has been observed [91].

The swollen glands can be identified through a physical exam or with imaging techniques, such as ultrasound, CT scan, MRI, or PET-CT scans. Usually, a histopathology is needed to determine the underlying pathology. AAV usually shows necrotizing granulomatous inflammation of small vessels; however, nonspecific chronic inflammation is also a possible finding [91]. Histopathological findings, combined with other organ involvement, examination findings, and ANCA serology, usually aid in diagnosis. One should be cautious in overreliance on serology, as it can often be positive in infections and malignancies, and approximately 20% of patients with AAV may be negative for ANCA. ANCA-negative is more common in patients with EGPA [92]. Data on treatment for salivary gland involvement in AAV are limited and may vary based on the severity of the involvement in other glands. Glucocorticoids, Cyclophosphamide, Rituximab, Methotrexate, and other immune modulators or suppressors are effective in treating AAV [93].

3.18 Inflammatory Bowel Disease (IBD)

Inflammatory Bowel Disease (IBD) comprises two major disorders, Ulcerative Colitis(UC) and Crohn's disease (CD). There is limited data regarding salivary gland involvement in IBD. However, salivary gland dysfunction has been reported, suggesting a probable alteration in the function of salivary glands in IBD [94, 95]. Compared with patients with Crohn's disease who do not have orofacial granulomatosis, or those carriers of CD with orofacial manifestations or only orofacial granulomatosis, the latter two groups secreted higher concentrations of IgA from parotid glands and whole saliva compared to the former group. Furthermore, in this study, the high whole-salivary IgA against *Saccharomyces cerevisiae* or IgA2 in saliva may reflect oral, but not intestinal, inflammation [96]. In case reports of CD affecting the parotid glands, salivary duct fistula may present as another oral manifestation among the many others reported in CD [90]. There is also a report of a cystic mass in the sublingual gland in a CD patient, which revealed non-caseating granulomas on histopathology and was responsive to azathioprine therapy [97]. In a similar case, infliximab was also of great benefit [98]. Since this appears to be a rare occurrence, it is crucial that alternative infectious, occlusive, and malignant pathologies be ruled out in an IBD patient presenting with salivary gland involvement, and a tissue sample be examined before initiating immunosuppressive therapy. It is also relevant to mention the presence of sialadenosis in patients with IBD (i.e., CD) who may have nutritional deficiencies or comorbid entities (i.e., alcoholism, type 2 diabetes mellitus) accountable for this presentation.

3.19 Eosinophilic Sialodochitis

Eosinophilic Sialodochitis is a rare disorder characterized by recurrent swelling of the salivary glands. It has been previously described with several different names, including "sialodochitis fibrinosa", "allergic parotitis", "Kussmaul disease", "chronic sialodochitis with eosinophilia", and "idiopathic eosinophilic parotitis" [99, 100].

Eosinophilic Sialodochitis is a chronic inflammatory allergic disease of salivary glands with a background of atopy, intermittent, recurrent swelling, and mucus plugging. The preferred age range is middle-aged patients, with a predominance of East Asian women [100]. Patients typically present with recurrent salivary gland inflammation, often accompanied by pruritus of the overlying skin. They frequently have a history of atopic and allergic diseases like asthma, rhinitis, and eczema. String-like mucous discharge and increased meal-time symptoms are often reported. Eosinophil-rich mucus plugs vary in consistency, and rarely, Charcot-Leyden crystals have been reported. The parotid glands appear to be the most commonly affected target organs, followed by the submandibular glands. Presentation of multiple and bilateral major salivary glands is often seen, but in a small fraction, unilateral presentation has been reported. Elevated IgE and peripheral eosinophilia are often observed in blood work [99, 100].

On Ultrasound imaging of the affected salivary gland, heterogeneous and hypoechoic gland changes can be seen. Generalized dilatation of the salivary duct system has been reported [99] . Contrast sialography and magnetic resonance imaging often reveal intra- and/or extraglandular dilatation of the main duct; usually, segmental involvement is seen, which is occasionally severe [100]. Histopathology often shows dense eosinophil-rich periductal inflammatory infiltrate with periductal fibrosis; the background of lymphoplasmacytic infiltrate shows a prevailing population of CD4-positive T cells and occasional lymphoid follicle formation [100]. The fibrosis is usually focally dense and does not exhibit the storiform pattern seen in IGG4-related disease [101].

Variable treatment responses are seen with both surgical and medical treatments. High-dose antihistamines, leukotriene receptor antagonists, mucolytic agents, and short courses of prednisone have been used for treatment. No treatment is consistently successful, often leading to glandular resection in severe cases [100].

3.20 Conclusions

Salivary glands are specialized structures that secrete saliva within the oral cavity, primarily for moisturizing the oral components,, including mucosae, teeth, tongue, and other soft tissues. The anatomy closely linked to functionality explains most of the salivary glands' roles in digestion and the immune system. Given the high blood flow and direct communication with the oral cavity, the glands become susceptible to insults from environmental, food-related, and infectious sources. The immune system will actively participate in evolving into inflammatory and autoimmune processes that target the salivary glands. Understanding the primary pathogenic and clinical features of these inflammatory and immune diseases will enable the accurate diagnosis of the underlying systemic illness, upon which appropriate pharmacological and non-pharmacological interventions can follow. Awareness of each of the described diseases will help prevent potential long-term complications resulting from salivary gland damage.

References

1. Dawes C, Pedersen AM, Villa A, Ekstrom J, Proctor GB, Vissink A, et al. The functions of human saliva: a review sponsored by the world workshop on Oral medicine VI. Arch Oral Biol. 2015;60(6):863–74.
2. Farnaud SJ, Kosti O, Getting SJ, Renshaw D. Saliva: physiology and diagnostic potential in health and disease. ScientificWorldJournal. 2010;10:434–56.

3. Smith DJ, Taubman MA, King WF. Immunological features of minor salivary gland saliva. J Clin Immunol. 1987;7(6):449–55.
4. de Almeida PV, Gregio AM, Machado MA, de Lima AA, Azevedo LR. Saliva composition and functions: a comprehensive review. J Contemp Dent Pract. 2008;9(3):72–80.
5. Porcheri C, Mitsiadis TA. Physiology, pathology and regeneration of salivary glands. Cells. 2019;8(9)
6. Carlson GW. The salivary glands. Embryology, anatomy, and surgical applications. Surg Clin North Am. 2000;80(1):261–73. xii
7. Humphrey SP, Williamson RT. A review of saliva: normal composition, flow, and function. J Prosthet Dent. 2001;85(2):162–9.
8. Patel VN, Rebustini IT, Hoffman MP. Salivary gland branching morphogenesis. Differentiation. 2006;74(7):349–64.
9. Proctor GB, Carpenter GH. Salivary secretion: mechanism and neural regulation. Monogr Oral Sci. 2014;24:14–29.
10. Lee MG, Ohana E, Park HW, Yang D, Muallem S. Molecular mechanism of pancreatic and salivary gland fluid and HCO3 secretion. Physiol Rev. 2012;92(1):39–74.
11. Carpenter GH. The secretion, components, and properties of saliva. Annu Rev Food Sci Technol. 2013;4:267–76.
12. Garrett JR, Kidd A. The innervation of salivary glands as revealed by morphological methods. Microsc Res Tech. 1993;26(1):75–91.
13. Delporte C, Bryla A, Perret J. Aquaporins in salivary glands: from basic research to clinical applications. Int J Mol Sci. 2016;17(2)
14. Melvin JE, Yule D, Shuttleworth T, Begenisich T. Regulation of fluid and electrolyte secretion in salivary gland acinar cells. Annu Rev Physiol. 2005;67:445–69.
15. Mikoshiba K, Hisatsune C, Futatsugi A, Mizutani A, Nakamura T, Miyachi K. The role of Ca2+ signaling in cell function with special reference to exocrine secretion. Cornea. 2008;27(Suppl 1):S3–8.
16. Putney JW, Bird GS. Calcium signaling in lacrimal glands. Cell Calcium. 2014;55(6):290–6.
17. Nizamuddin I, Koulen P, McArthur CP. Contribution of HIV infection, AIDS, and antiretroviral therapy to exocrine pathogenesis in salivary and lacrimal glands. Int J Mol Sci. 2018;19(9)
18. Segawa A, Terakawa S, Yamashina S, Hopkins CR. Exocytosis in living salivary glands: direct visualization by video-enhanced microscopy and confocal laser microscopy. Eur J Cell Biol. 1991;54(2):322–30.
19. Vreugdenhil AP, Nieuw Amerongen AV, de Lange GL, Roukema PA. Localization of amylase and mucins in the major salivary glands of the mouse. Histochem J. 1982;14(5):767–80.
20. Ibrahim HR, Thomas U, Pellegrini A. A helix-loop-helix peptide at the upper lip of the active site cleft of lysozyme confers potent antimicrobial activity with membrane permeabilization action. J Biol Chem. 2001;276(47):43767–74.
21. Laible NJ, Germaine GR. Bactericidal activity of human lysozyme, muramidase-inactive lysozyme, and cationic polypeptides against streptococcus sanguis and Streptococcus faecalis: inhibition by chitin oligosaccharides. Infect Immun. 1985;48(3):720–8.
22. Garrett JR, Thulin A. Changes in parotid acinar cells accompanying salivary secretion in rats on sympathetic or parasympathetic nerve stimulation. Cell Tissue Res. 1975;159(2):179–93.
23. Garrett JR, Emmelin N. Activities of salivary myoepithelial cells: a review. Med Biol. 1979;57(1):1–28.
24. Mandel L. Salivary gland disorders. Med Clin North Am. 2014;98(6):1407–49.
25. Mehanna H, McQueen A, Robinson M, Paleri V. Salivary gland swellings. Clin Otolaryngol. 2013;38(1):58–65.
26. Brown JE. Salivary gland diseases: presentation and investigation. Prim Dent J. 2018;7(1):48–57.
27. Dulguerov P, Marchal F, Gysin C. Frey syndrome before Frey: the correct history. Laryngoscope. 1999;109(9):1471–3.
28. Jorquera Moya M, Merino Menendez S, Porta Etessam J, Escribano Vera J, Yus FM. Cranial nerve disorders: clinical manifestations and topography. Radiologia (Engl Ed). 2019;61(2):99–123.
29. Mariette X, Criswell LA. Primary Sjogren's syndrome. N Engl J Med. 2018;378(10):931–9.

30. Martire MV, Santiago ML, Cazenave T, Gutierrez M. Latest advances in ultrasound assessment of salivary glands in Sjogren syndrome. J Clin Rheumatol. 2018;24(4):218–23.
31. Lee KA, Lee SH, Kim HR. Diagnostic and predictive evaluation using salivary gland ultrasonography in primary Sjogren's syndrome. Clin Exp Rheumatol. 2018;36 Suppl 112(3):165–72.
32. Jonsson MV, Baldini C. Major salivary gland ultrasonography in the diagnosis of Sjogren's syndrome: a place in the diagnostic criteria? Rheum Dis Clin N Am. 2016;42(3):501–17.
33. Mossel E, Delli K, van Nimwegen JF, Stel AJ, Kroese FGM, Spijkervet FKL, et al. Ultrasonography of major salivary glands compared with parotid and labial gland biopsy and classification criteria in patients with clinically suspected primary Sjogren's syndrome. Ann Rheum Dis. 2017;76(11):1883–9.
34. Jager L, Menauer F, Holzknecht N, Scholz V, Grevers G, Reiser M. Sialolithiasis: MR sialography of the submandibular duct--an alternative to conventional sialography and US? Radiology 2000;216(3):665–671.
35. Nieto-Gonzalez JC, Serrano Benavente B, Molina CJ. Salivary gland ultrasound: update. Med Clin (Barc). 2021;156(2):81–7.
36. Wang KY, Wintermark M, Penta M. Imaging characteristics of Sjogren's syndrome. Clin Imaging. 2022;92:7–18.
37. Mar D, Fairchild RM. Imaging of the major salivary glands in rheumatic disease. Rheum Dis Clin N Am. 2024;50(4):701–20.
38. D'Arco F, Ugga L. Computed tomography and magnetic resonance imaging in pediatric salivary gland diseases: a guide to the differential diagnosis. Pediatr Radiol. 2020;50(9):1293–307.
39. Agarwal AK, Kanekar SG. Imaging of submandibular and sublingual salivary glands. Neuroimaging Clin N Am. 2018;28(2):227–43.
40. Abdel Razek AAK, Mukherji SK. Imaging of minor salivary glands. Neuroimaging Clin N Am. 2018;28(2):295–302.
41. Keraen J, Blanc E, Besson FL, Leguern V, Meyer C, Henry J, et al. Usefulness of (18) F-labeled Fluorodeoxyglucose-positron emission tomography for the diagnosis of lymphoma in primary Sjogren's syndrome. Arthritis Rheumatol. 2019;71(7):1147–57.
42. Takano K, Yajima R, Kamekura R, Yamamoto M, Takahashi H, Yama N, et al. Clinical utility of (18) F-fluorodeoxyglucose/positron emission tomography in diagnosis of immunoglobulin G4-related sclerosing sialadenitis. Laryngoscope. 2018;128(5):1120–5.
43. Chilla R. Sialadenosis of the salivary glands of the head. Studies on the physiology and pathophysiology of parotid secretion. Adv Otorhinolaryngol. 1981;26:1–38.
44. Donath K, Seifert G. Ultrastructural studies of the parotid glands in sialadenosis. Virchows Arch A Pathol Anat Histol. 1975;365(2):119–35.
45. Teymoortash A, Wiegand S, Borkeloh M, Bette M, Ramaswamy A, Steinbach-Hundt S, et al. Variations in the expression and distribution pattern of AQP5 in acinar cells of patients with sialadenosis. In Vivo. 2012;26(6):951–5.
46. Catassi C, Verdu EF, Bai JC, Lionetti E. Coeliac disease. Lancet. 2022;399(10344):2413–26.
47. Liu J, Lundemann AJ, Reibel J, Pedersen AML. Salivary gland involvement and oral health in patients with coeliac disease. Eur J Oral Sci. 2022;130(3):e12861.
48. Borghini R, Donato G, Alvaro D, Picarelli A. New insights in IBS-like disorders: Pandora's box has been opened; a review. Gastroenterol Hepatol Bed Bench. 2017;10(2):79–89.
49. Lewis NR, Scott BB. Meta-analysis: deamidated gliadin peptide antibody and tissue transglutaminase antibody compared as screening tests for coeliac disease. Aliment Pharmacol Ther. 2010;31(1):73–81.
50. Lebwohl B, Ludvigsson JF, Green PH. Celiac disease and non-celiac gluten sensitivity. BMJ. 2015;351:h4347.
51. Vigren L, Tysk C, Strom M, Kilander AF, Hjortswang H, Bohr J, et al. Celiac disease and other autoimmune diseases in patients with collagenous colitis. Scand J Gastroenterol. 2013;48(8):944–50.
52. Lauret E, Rodrigo L. Celiac disease and autoimmune-associated conditions. Biomed Res Int. 2013;2013:127589.
53. Lundin KE, Wijmenga C. Coeliac disease and autoimmune disease-genetic overlap and screening. Nat Rev Gastroenterol Hepatol. 2015;12(9):507–15.

54. Skillington SA, Ogden MA. IgG4-related disease and the salivary glands: a review of pathophysiology, diagnosis, and management. Otolaryngol Clin N Am. 2021;54(3):497–508.
55. Kamiński B, Błochowiak K. Mikulicz's disease and Küttner's tumor as manifestations of IgG4-related diseases: a review of the literature. Reumatologia. 2020;58(4):243–50.
56. Della Torre E, Mattoo H, Mahajan VS, Carruthers M, Pillai S, Stone JH. Prevalence of atopy, eosinophilia, and IgE elevation in IgG4-related disease. Allergy. 2014;69(2):269–72.
57. Lanzillotta M, Mancuso G, Della-Torre E. Advances in the diagnosis and management of IgG4 related disease. BMJ. 2020;369:m1067.
58. Maritati F, Peyronel F, Vaglio A. IgG4-related disease: a clinical perspective. Rheumatology (Oxford). 2020;59(Suppl 3):iii123–i31.
59. Sève P, Pacheco Y, Durupt F, Jamilloux Y, Gerfaud-Valentin M, Isaac S, et al. Sarcoidosis: a clinical overview from symptoms to diagnosis. Cells. 2021;10(4)
60. Carubbi F, Alunno A, Gerli R, Giacomelli R. Histopathology of salivary glands. Reumatismo. 2018;70(3):146–54.
61. Iannuzzi MC, Rybicki BA, Teirstein AS. Sarcoidosis. N Engl J Med. 2007;357(21):2153–65.
62. Lehmuskallio E, Hannuksela M, Halme H. The liver in sarcoidosis. Acta Med Scand. 1977;202(4):289–93.
63. Rosen Y. Pathology of sarcoidosis. Semin Respir Crit Care Med. 2007;28(1):36–52.
64. Tana C, Donatiello I, Caputo A, Tana M, Naccarelli T, Mantini C, et al. Clinical features, histopathology and differential diagnosis of sarcoidosis. Cells. 2021;11(1)
65. Judson MA. Granulomatous Sarcoidosis Mimics. Front Med (Lausanne). 2021;8:680989.
66. Mandel L, Wolinsky B, Chalom EC. Treatment of refractory sarcoidal parotid gland swelling in a previously reported unresponsive case. J Am Dent Assoc. 2005;136(9):1282–5.
67. Holm S, Sjogren H, et al. Studies on keratoconjunctivitis sicca, based on examination of 500 subjects affected with rheumatism and an equally large control material. Acta Ophthalmol. 1948;26(2):269–73.
68. Morgan WS, Castleman B. A clinicopathologic study of Mikulicz's disease. Am J Pathol. 1953;29(3):471–503.
69. Fox RI. Sjogren's syndrome. Lancet. 2005;366(9482):321–31.
70. Parke AL, Buchanan WW. Sjogren's syndrome: history, clinical and pathological features. Inflammopharmacology. 1998;6(4):271–87.
71. Fisher BA, Jonsson R, Daniels T, Bombardieri M, Brown RM, Morgan P, et al. Standardisation of labial salivary gland histopathology in clinical trials in primary Sjogren's syndrome. Ann Rheum Dis. 2017;76(7):1161–8.
72. Rischmueller M, Tieu J, Lester S. Primary Sjogren's syndrome. Best Pract Res Clin Rheumatol. 2016;30(1):189–220.
73. Skopouli FN, Moutsopoulos HM. Autoimmune epitheliitis: Sjogren's syndrome. Clin Exp Rheumatol. 1994;12(Suppl 11):S9–11.
74. Selmi C, Meroni PL, Gershwin ME. Primary biliary cirrhosis and Sjogren's syndrome: autoimmune epithelitis. J Autoimmun. 2012;39(1–2):34–42.
75. Imgenberg-Kreuz J, Rasmussen A, Sivils K, Nordmark G. Genetics and epigenetics in primary Sjogren's syndrome. Rheumatology (Oxford). 2021;60(5):2085–98.
76. Garcia-Carrasco M, Fuentes-Alexandro S, Escarcega RO, Salgado G, Riebeling C, Cervera R. Pathophysiology of Sjogren's syndrome. Arch Med Res. 2006;37(8):921–32.
77. Mariette X, Gottenberg JE. Pathogenesis of Sjogren's syndrome and therapeutic consequences. Curr Opin Rheumatol. 2010;22(5):471–7.
78. Igoe A, Scofield RH. Autoimmunity and infection in Sjogren's syndrome. Curr Opin Rheumatol. 2013;25(4):480–7.
79. Bautista-Vargas M, Vivas AJ, Tobon GJ. Minor salivary gland biopsy: its role in the classification and prognosis of Sjogren's syndrome. Autoimmun Rev. 2020;19(12):102690.
80. Shiboski CH, Shiboski SC, Seror R, Criswell LA, Labetoulle M, Lietman TM, et al. 2016 American College of Rheumatology/European league against rheumatism classification criteria for primary Sjogren's syndrome: a consensus and data-driven methodology involving three international patient cohorts. Ann Rheum Dis. 2017;76(1):9–16.
81. Radfar L, Kleiner DE, Fox PC, Pillemer SR. Prevalence and clinical significance of lymphocytic foci in minor salivary glands of healthy volunteers. Arthritis Rheum. 2002;47(5):520–4.

82. Sharma R, Chaudhari KS, Kurien BT, Grundahl K, Radfar L, Lewis DM, et al. Sjogren syndrome without focal lymphocytic infiltration of the salivary glands. J Rheumatol. 2020;47(3):394–9.
83. Maciel G, Crowson CS, Matteson EL, Cornec D. Prevalence of primary Sjogren's syndrome in a US population-based cohort. Arthritis Care Res (Hoboken). 2017;69(10):1612–6.
84. Seror R, Bootsma H, Saraux A, Bowman SJ, Theander E, Brun JG, et al. Defining disease activity states and clinically meaningful improvement in primary Sjogren's syndrome with EULAR primary Sjogren's syndrome disease activity (ESSDAI) and patient-reported indexes (ESSPRI). Ann Rheum Dis. 2016;75(2):382–9.
85. De Vita S, Gandolfo S, Zandonella Callegher S, Zabotti A, Quartuccio L. The evaluation of disease activity in Sjogren's syndrome based on the degree of MALT involvement: glandular swelling and cryoglobulinaemia compared to ESSDAI in a cohort study. Clin Exp Rheumatol. 2018;36 Suppl 112(3):150–6.
86. De Vita S, Gandolfo S. Predicting lymphoma development in patients with Sjogren's syndrome. Expert Rev Clin Immunol. 2019;15(9):929–38.
87. Brito-Zeron P, Kostov B, Fraile G, Caravia-Duran D, Maure B, Rascon FJ, et al. Characterization and risk estimate of cancer in patients with primary Sjogren syndrome. J Hematol Oncol. 2017;10(1):90.
88. Tanasiewicz M, Hildebrandt T, Obersztyn I. Xerostomia of various etiologies: a review of the literature. Adv Clin Exp Med. 2016;25(1):199–206.
89. Epstein JB, Villines DC, Sroussi HY. Oral symptoms and oral function in people with Sjogren's syndrome. Clin Exp Rheumatol. 2015;33(1):132–3.
90. Almaani S, Fussner LA, Brodsky S, Meara AS, Jayne D. ANCA-associated Vasculitis: an update. J Clin Med. 2021;10(7)
91. Akiyama M, Takanashi S, Takeuchi T, Kaneko Y. Salivary gland involvement in ANCA-associated vasculitis. Autoimmun Rev. 2021;20(11):102940.
92. Trivioli G, Terrier B, Vaglio A. Eosinophilic granulomatosis with polyangiitis: understanding the disease and its management. Rheumatology (Oxford). 2020;59(Suppl 3):iii84–94.
93. Samman KN, Ross C, Pagnoux C, Makhzoum JP. Update in the management of ANCA-associated Vasculitis: recent developments and future perspectives. Int J Rheumatol. 2021;2021:5534851.
94. Goldinova A, Tan CX, Bouma G, Duijvestein M, Brand HS, de Boer NK. Oral health and salivary function in ulcerative colitis patients. United European Gastroenterol J. 2020;8(9):1067–75.
95. de Vries SAG, Tan CXW, Bouma G, Forouzanfar T, Brand HS, de Boer NK. Salivary function and Oral health problems in Crohn's disease patients. Inflamm Bowel Dis. 2018;24(6):1361–7.
96. Savage NW, Barnard K, Shirlaw PJ, Rahman D, Mistry M, Escudier MP, et al. Serum and salivary IgA antibody responses to Saccharomyces cerevisiae, Candida albicans and Streptococcus mutans in orofacial granulomatosis and Crohn's disease. Clin Exp Immunol. 2004;135(3):483–9.
97. Schnitt SJ, Antonioli DA, Jaffe B, Peppercorn MA. Granulomatous inflammation of minor salivary gland ducts: a new oral manifestation of Crohn's disease. Hum Pathol. 1987;18(4):405–7.
98. Blasco Patino F, Nicolae MV, Navarro E. Acute submandibular sialadenitis in a patient with Crohn's disease being treated with infliximab. Gastroenterol Hepatol. 2021;44(1):49–50.
99. Carey B, O'Neill N, Brown J, Escudier M, Hullah E, Beneng K, et al. Eosinophilic sialodochitis: an emerging atopic condition. Oral Dis. 2022;28(3):648–56.
100. Baer AN, Okuhama A, Eisele DW, Tversky JR, Gniadek TJ. Eosinophilic sialodochitis: redefinition of 'allergic parotitis' and 'sialodochitis fibrinosa'. Oral Dis. 2017;23(7):840–8.
101. Deshpande V, Zen Y, Chan JK, Yi EE, Sato Y, Yoshino T, et al. Consensus statement on the pathology of IgG4-related disease. Mod Pathol. 2012;25(9):1181–92.

Chapter 4
Pharyngeal Dysphagia Associated with Rheumatological and Vasculitic Conditions

Promila Banerjee, Fahad Abu Abbasi, Anne M. Lunkes, and Dia Shah

4.1 Introduction

Oropharyngeal dysphagia is considered a symptom of many complex medical conditions and may significantly impact healthcare expenditure. The presence of dysphagia is associated with reduced quality of life, malnutrition, dehydration, and poor healthcare outcomes, including aspiration pneumonia, which is the second leading cause of death in the elderly [1]. Many medical centers have introduced a nursing screener to detect dysphagia at admission. Primary care physicians know to inquire about dysphagia if the individual has a history of stroke, head and neck cancer, or pulmonary disease on an outpatient basis. Physicians need to know about the less common diseases that may result in oropharyngeal dysphagia. This chapter will focus on vasculitic and rheumatological diseases.

P. Banerjee (✉)
Loyola Stritch School of Medicine, Maywood, IL, USA

Edward Hines Jr VA Hospital, Hines, IL, USA
e-mail: Promila.Banerjee@va.gov

F. A. Abbasi
Mercy Health Hospital, University of Illinois, Rockford, IL, USA

A. M. Lunkes
Edward Hines Jr VA Hospital, Hines, IL, USA

D. Shah
Albany Medical College, Albany, NY, USA

M. Tadros et al. (eds.), *GI Diseases Associated with Rheumatological and Vasculitic Conditions*, Clinical Gastroenterology,
https://doi.org/10.1007/978-3-032-07868-1_4

4.2 The Pharynx

The Pharynx is an important structure of both the respiratory and digestive tracts as well as secretion production and vocal resonance. The pharynx can be divided into the nasopharynx, oropharynx, and laryngopharynx and is composed of longitudinal and circular muscles [2]. The nasopharynx runs from the nares and the soft palate to the oral cavity and includes the adenoids and tonsils. The oropharynx begins at the uvula and runs to the hyoid bone. The hypopharynx, or laryngopharynx, lies from inferior hyoid to the lower margin of the larynx and then separates into the respiratory and digestive pathways. Other important structures are the pyriform sinuses and the lateral and posterior pharyngeal walls and the posterior surface rim of the larynx.

4.3 Anatomy and Physiology of Deglutition

Deglutition, also known as the process of swallowing, is a highly coordinated system for the consumption of food and liquids. The phases of the swallow are the pre-oral phase, which includes oral awareness and acceptance, and the oral phase, which includes bolus manipulation, lingual control, and oral clearance. Pharyngeal swallow initiates as the head of the bolus passes the ramus of the mandible. Multiple components have to occur to ensure the bolus travels safely and efficiently through the pharynx. A combination of the action of the pharyngeal constrictor muscles, laryngeal elevation, and tongue base retraction results in epiglottic retroversion, which helps clear the vallecular space and aids in laryngeal protection. Hyolaryngeal elevation and anterior excursion relax the cricopharyngeal muscle and open the upper esophageal sphincter. The bolus then enters the esophagus, which begins the esophageal phase of the swallow.

Cranial Nerves 5, 7, 9, 10, 12 are involved in swallowing. Cranial Nerve V, the Trigeminal Nerve is integral for the muscles of mastication, such as the masseter muscle, and the sensation of the face, mouth and teeth [3]. The Facial Nerve, CNVII, provides sensation to the anterior 2/3 of the tongue, the soft palate and upper pharyngeal wall [4]. This nerve is responsible for facial movement and salivary and lacrimal glands for the production of secretions and tears [5]. The Glossopharyngeal Nerve, Cranial Nerve IX supplies taste and sensation to posterior 1/3 of tongue, inner ear, outside walls of pharynx, pharyngeal swallow initiation and innervates the stylopharyngeus muscle, which elevates and dilates the larynx and pharynx [6]. The Vagus Nerve, CN X is another mixed motor and sensory cranial nerve with 3 branches, the Pharyngeal branch, the Recurrent and Superior branches [4]. The pharyngeal branch innervates all muscles of the soft palate except Tensor V Palatini (CNV) and then recurrent branch innervates all intrinsic laryngeal muscles, except cricothyroid. Lastly, the superior branch provides sensory input to the inside of the larynx, base of tongue, epiglottis and aryepiglottic folds and the external branch innervates the cricothyroid muscle, which controls vocal pitch [3]. The Hypoglossal Nerve, CNXII provides motor innervation to all the intrinsic and all but 1 extrinsic lingual muscle, specifically the genioglossus, styloglossus, hypoglossus, strap muscles, and geniohyoid [6].

4.4 The Evaluation of Oropharyngeal Swallow

Ongoing discussion of the physiology of the swallow will be covered under this section as most assessments include ratings of this. The oropharyngeal swallow can be evaluated with a modified barium swallow exam, which uses videofluoroscopy (AKA a videofluoroscopic swallow study, VFSS), a Fiberoptic Endoscopic Swallow Study (FEES), or high resolution pharyngeal manometry (HRPM).

Pharyngeal manometry evaluates for oropharyngeal dysphagia by measuring pharyngeal muscle contraction and bolus propulsion. Upper esophageal sphincter relaxation and pharyngeal pressures are some of the components of this exam [8]. This was traditionally completed by Gastroenterologists, but now gaining momentum with Speech-Language Pathologists and may be used for therapeutic purposes, specifically biofeedback as well.

FEES uses flexible endoscopy to visualize the pharynx and larynx. This is an excellent exam for assessing the surface anatomy of the three regions of the pharynx, as well as secretion management. FEES may be used in the acute care setting to obtain quick information regarding swallow safety and readiness to initiate a PO diet. A frequent clinical scenario demonstrating the utility of FEES is a patient with respiratory failure who was recently extubated, and the medical team desires to know if the patient is safe to introduce a diet. Occasional incidental findings of structural abnormalities are common in this population, for example, laryngeal findings of reflux or a granuloma associated with intubation. PO may be dyed with food coloring to improve visualization. Oral containment, the timing of pharyngeal swallow initiation, airway closure and protection, and bolus clearance are all seen with a FEES. Although future research is needed to test the validity, the Visual Analysis of Swallowing Efficiency and Safety (VASES) is a new standardized FEES rating method to enhance the subjective analysis of pharyngeal residue, penetration, and aspiration [9]. FEES is diagnostic tool but is considered a valuable therapy tool as well.

The view of the fiberoptic endoscopic evaluation of the swallow. Thin liquids visualized around the laryngeal rim. Image from [10], "Fiberoptic Endoscopic Evaluation of Swallowing Across the Age Spectrum" by Miller et al. 2020. American Journal of Speech Lang Pathology. 29(2S):967–978.

The VFSS is a radiographic procedure that provides a direct and dynamic view of the oral, pharyngeal and esophageal function [11]. The VFSS is typically completed by speech-language pathologists in Xray and uses 30 frames per second of videofluoroscopy while feeding the patient various consistencies and textures with barium as the contrast agent.

Although not the only tool, the Modified Barium Swallow Impairment Profile (MBSImP) is a widely used standardized protocol to interpret and communicate swallowing impairment in VFSS in a manner that is specific, consistent, accurate and objective [12]. There are 17 physiologic components to the swallow and each component score on the MBSIMP is 0 to 3 or 5. The physiologic components lend to a severity score. The table below shows all the physiologic components of the swallow from the MBImp. The MBSImp is widely used by Speech-Language Pathologists as it has been found to have "clinical practicality, favorable inter- and intrarater reliability following standardized training, content, and external validity." [12] This tool allowed for standardization of quantifying oropharyngeal swallowing impairment. This is considered the gold standard in the interpretation of the video-fluoroscopic swallow study.

4.5 Disordered Deglutition

A breakdown in the highly coordinated process of swallowing can occur at any time. Speech-language pathologists are trained in the interpretation of the endoscopic or videofluoroscopic findings. For example, a dementia diagnosis may result in poor oral bolus awareness [14]. Reduced lingual control and spillage into the pharynx or larynx prior to initiation of the swallow may be due to an injury to the hypoglossal nerve [4]. If the base of tongue does not fully contact the posterior pharyngeal wall and epiglottis fails to retrovert, residue in the valleculae can remain after the swallow [11]. Reduced elevation and anterior excursion of the hyolaryngeal complex can result in reduced laryngeal closure/ aspiration and reduced cricopharyngeal relaxation/ upper esophageal sphincter opening [11]. Safety and efficiency of the swallow are the 2 main areas of focus.

Image demonstrating a pharyngeal swallow delay from, [12], "MBS measurement tool for swallow impairment--MBSImp: establishing a standard." By Martin-Harris, B. et al, 2008, Dysphagia. [4]:392–405.

4.6 Dysphagia Management

Multiple interventions have been used to manage dysphagia, which extend from texture-modified foods and thickened fluids, swallowing therapy, drug therapy, neuromuscular stimulation, and botulinum toxin therapy [15]. The International Dysphagia Diet Standardization Initiative (IDDSI) began in 2013 intending to promote patient safety and facilitate evolution of the field to deliver better treatment outcomes [16]. Thickening liquids alter the bolus viscosity and increase sensory input and oral transit time, improving control through the oropharyngeal space [17].

The below chart [18] describes some of the postural adjustments, maneuvers, and facilitatory techniques and strengthening exercises and their rationale. The supraglottic swallow maneuver was initially designed for a patient status post supraglottic laryngectomy, which involves a breath hold and then a throat clear as these patients have reduced structural airway protection.

Not all patients are appropriate for maneuvers given cognitive or physical limitations, and they may be ineffective, so maneuvers should be trialed under fluoroscopy or endoscopy to ensure effectiveness. A combination of indirect and direct approaches to dysphagia therapy should be considered. Direct treatment may follow the principles of exercise physiology with the goal of increasing muscle strength and endurance. The targeted groups include the oral, hyolaryngeal, and respiratory musculature. There is a gap in the literature regarding the treatment dosage [19]. There are some device-facilitated therapies on the market to improve dysphagia, such as the Iowa Oral Pressure Instrument (IOPI) may improve lingual pressures, and the Expiratory Strength Trainer (EMST) to improve cough strength and hyolaryngeal movement [20].

With all dysphagia management, quality of life is the most important aspect. Modifying the diet may have a great impact on a patient's daily life, or a patient may not be able to complete an exercise regimen. Multidisciplinary management and consideration of the patient and family goals of care is essential for the best outcomes. A team may include primary and specialty physicians, a speech-language pathologist, and registered dietitian (Table 4.1).

Table 4.1 Maneuvers to ease swallowing in the geriatric population

Technique	Execution (rationale)	Indication	Limitations in geriatric patients
Maneuvers			
Supraglottic swallow	Breath hold, double swallow, forceful expiration (closes vocal folds before and during swallow)	Reduced/late vocal fold closure	Problematic in patients with cardiovascular disease
Supersupraglottic swallow	Effortful breath hold, swallow, cough, swallow (closes vocal folds before and during swallow)	Reduced/late vocal fold closure	Problematic in patients with cardiovascular disease
Effortful swallow	Effortful tongue action (increases posterior motion of tongue base)	Poor posterior tongue base motion	May cause fatigue of swallowing
Mendelsohn maneuver	Prolong hyoid excursion guided by manual palpation (prolongs upper esophageal sphincter opening)	Poor pharyngeal clearance and laryngeal movement	May cause fatigue of swallowing

(continued)

Table 4.1 (continued)

Technique	Execution (rationale)	Indication	Limitations in geriatric patients
Postural adjustments			
Head tilt	Head tilt posteriorly at swallow initiation (gravity clears oral cavity)	Poor tongue control	Increases aspiration risk in most older subjects
	Head tilt laterally to unaffected side (directs bolus down stronger side)	Unilateral pharyngeal weakness	May have limitations in patients with cervical spine disease
Chin tuck	Chin down (displaces tongue base and epiglottis posteriorly)	Delayed pharyngeal swallow response	May have limitations in patients with cervical spine disease
Head rotation	Rotate head to affected side (isolates damaged side from bolus path)	Unilateral pharyngeal weakness	May have limitations in patients with cervical spine disease
Facilitatory techniques			
Thermal stimulation	Cold tactile stimulation to anterior faucial pillar	Delayed/absent swallow response	Poor evidence, especially in stroke patients
Gustatory stimulation	Sour or spicy bolus, capsaicin (facilitates swallow response)	Reduced oral sensitivity, delayed/absent swallow response	Promising approach
Strengthening exercises			
Shaker exercise	Repeated head lifting while lying (strengthening of neck and laryngeal muscles)	Enhanced opening of the upper esophageal sphincter	May have limitations in patients with cervical spine disease; the suggested intensity may not be feasible for geriatric patients

Chart from reference: [18], Oropharyngeal dysphagia in older persons—from pathophysiology to adequate intervention: A review and summary of an international expert meeting. Clinical Interventions in Aging. 11. 189. 10.2147/CIA.S97481

Notes: Adapted from Gastroenterology, Volume 116/Edition 2, Cook IJ, Kahrilas PJ, AGA technical review on management of oropharyngeal dysphagia, Pages 455–478, Copyright 1999, with permission from Elsevier

4.7 Rheumatological Conditions Resulting in an Oropharyngeal Dysphagia

Most common conditions resulting in dysphagia are stroke, degenerative diseases and the head and neck cancers. There are many vasculitic and rheumatologic diseases that result in symptoms of dysphagia. In this section we will go over these diseases briefly while highlighting their oropharyngeal manifestations.

Rheumatoid arthritis is an autoimmune disorder characterized by synovial hyperplasia that induces cartilage and bone erosions and joint destruction. Rheumatoid arthritic patients may have prolonged oral passage time with higher oral residual levels often originating from several factors including crico-arytenoid joint dysfunction, cervical vertebra, and mandibular inflammation [1]. Dysphagia is noted to be associated with increased morbidity in RA patients [1]. Pharyngeal dysfunction can be caused by non-ideal muscular attachments and inflamed turning joints. In particular, vertical dislocation of the C1–C2 has led to increased pharyngeal transit times [2]. In clinical practice, ankylosis of cervical spine in severe RA has been noted to cause difficulty during general anesthesia intubation procedures due to narrowing of the pharynx [3]. Addition to dysphagia, rheumatic arthritis patients may experience transient episodes of upper airway obstruction due to pharyngeal obstruction; usually caused by severe arthritic destruction inflammation of the temporomandibular joints [4]. In addition, decreased peristaltic pressure has been demonstrated in RA, indicating possible involvement of striated muscles [5].

Myasthenia Gravis is an autoimmune disorder where the formation of autoantibodies against the specific postsynaptic acetylcholine receptor consequently causes muscle weakness. Manometry studies revealed suboptimal swallowing pressures throughout the pharynx; edrophonium administration had partial reversal and increased swallowing speeds [6]. Flaccidity of the pharyngeal muscles produces dysphagia; a major source of morbidity in MG [7]. Most myasthenia crisis episodes are caused by aspiration pneumonia in patients with severe dysphagia, who were at risk of aspiration [8].

Systemic sclerosis causes fibrosis and atrophy does not usually involve the striated muscle in the pharynx. Etiology of dysphagia is unknown and theorized to be from impaired vagus function [9]. Prolonged pharyngeal transit times have been demonstrated using videofluoroscopy in patients with Sjögren's syndrome [10]. When oropharyngeal dysphagia occurs, very rare, it is life-threatening; treatable if nutrition is maintained by PEG-tube and steroid therapy to assist muscle function [11]. Additionally, hyposalivation in systemic sclerosis leads to increased oropharyngeal infections as saliva assists in epithelial repair of the oropharynx [12].

Hypoperistalsis and aperistalsis have been noted in over 70% of patients with SLE. Prolonged pharyngeal transit times have been recorded in patients with SLE [13]. Swallowing disorder is mainly related to recurrent mouth ulcers. While the majority of oral mucosal lesions are typically located on the hard palate, less than 10% of lesions are found on the pharynx [13]. In addition, lupus encephalitis has resulted in transient neurological dysphagia due to interference with the vagus resolving with intravenous dexamethasone [14]. A potential cause of dysphagia in SLE patients is *Candida albicans*, especially in patients treated with chronic steroid therapy.

Idiopathic inflammatory myopathies (IIM) are a group of chronic, autoimmune processes affecting proximal muscles. The most common types are dermatomyositis (DM), polymyositis (PM) and inclusion body myositis (IBM). Dysphagia is commonly seen in IIM and symptoms include choking and pharyngeal bolus sticking [15]. Over 70% of IIM patients exhibit pharyngeal dysmotility; most commonly

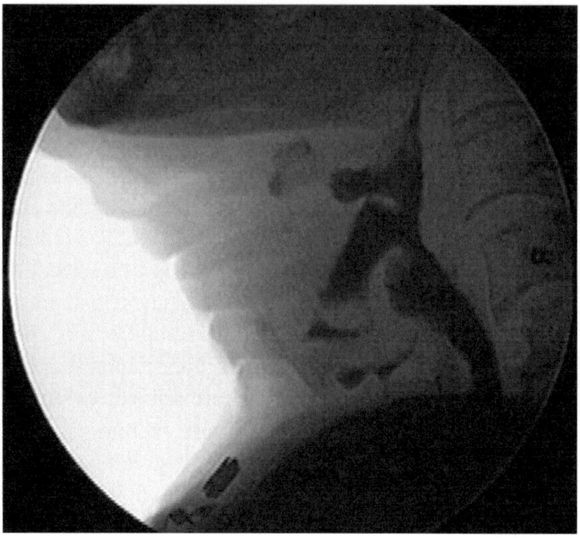

Fig. 4.1 Eighty year old veteran with Dermatomyocitis and diffuse pharyngeal edema

delayed swallow initiation. Currently, in refractory IIM, myotomy has been given in definitive treatment; however, further investigation of pre- and post-myotomy are needed [15]. The involvement of striated muscle of the pharynx or esophagus also contributes to the occurrence of dysphagia. Severity of dysphagia correlates with mortality (Fig. 4.1) [16].

Granulomatosis with polyangiitis (GPA), formerly Wegener's Granulomatosis, is a vasculitis affecting small vessels. Features include necrotizing granulomas and pauci-immune vasculitis affecting the upper respiratory tract, lungs, and kidneys [17]. The pharynx is affected in 6–10% of individuals with GPA [18, 19]. Of the pharynx, the nasopharynx is commonly affected in 60–80% of cases, with the next common subtype being oropharynx and may present with dysphasia [20, 21]. Soft nasal tissue mass may present on CT in GPA [22]. In addition, there may be ulcerations of the pharynx which respond well to cyclophosphamide and steroids [23]. Rarely, severe nasopharyngeal necrosis impacts surrounding structures as nasopharyngeal lesion can cause atlantoaxial instability requiring posterior spinal fusion C1–C2 [24].

Churg-Strauss syndrome is a vasculitis affecting small- to medium-sized blood vessels. Churg-Strauss is characterized by asthma, eosinophilia, and involvement of various organ systems including the respiratory tract, peripheral nervous system, kidney, and gastrointestinal tract [25]. Dysphagia is a very unusual symptom in Churg-Strauss due to delayed oral transit time with delayed pharyngeal trigger [26].

Behcet disease is a chronic and relapsing inflammatory disorder typically characterized by oral aphthous ulcers, genital ulcerations, ocular manifestations, and systemic involvement [27]. Dysphagia is an unusual symptom in Behcet's syndrome due to either pharyngeal stenosis or pharyngeal webs [28–30]. Pharyngeal stenosis presented with obstructive airway symptoms in addition to dysphagia [28, 29]. Oropharyngeal intubation has been reported to be extremely difficult due to the extensive scarring and adhesion formation in the pharynx [31]. In addition to aphthous ulcers, Behcet's syndrome may present with pharyngeal ulcers [32].

Psoriasis is a chronic inflammatory dermatology condition. It is characterized by erythematous raised plaques surrounded by silvery scales typically on extensor surfaces, scalp, and lumbosacral region [33]. Involvement of the mucous membrane in psoriasis is extremely unusual; however there are instances of psoriasis on the hypopharynx [34]. Psoriasis exacerbation has been associated with pharyngitis. Over 40% of patients with plaque psoriasis, 67% of patients with guttate psoriasis, and 70% of patients with a history of both guttate and plaque psoriasis have had a predisposing pharyngitis episode [35]. Additionally, there are reported significant differences in the bacterial microbiome of the pharynx and skin in patients with psoriasis compared with healthy controls.Further research is needed as the pharynx and skin microbiome may be of relevant to the pathogenesis of psoriasis [36].

Crohn disease (CD) and ulcerative colitis (UC) are two conditions commonly referred to as inflammatory bowel disease (IBD) that may present with rare pharyngeal symptoms [37]. Oropharyngeal lesions in Crohn's disease are well concealed during initial endoscopy, resulting in delay of diagnosis, and the associated odynophagia [37, 38]. These lesions are a good prognosis as 25% of lesions in Crohn's resolve without steroid usage [38]. Crohn's is well-known for fistula formation in the GI tract due to continuous inflammation in the epithelial and the activation of matrix metalloproteinase, TNF, and IL-13 [39]. There has been a report of pharyngeal perforation in Crohn's disease during intubation; potentially a weakened pharynx from premature fistula formation which perforated [40]. The role for oropharyngeal bacteria is emphasized as oral Klebsiella may exacerbate IBD as they colonize and create gut dysbiosis [41]. In addition, a microbial analysis of an intra-abdominal abscess revealed a specific species of streptococcus and peptostreptococcus predominantly found in the oropharyngeal [42, 43].

Sarcoidosis is a multisystem characterized by non-caseating granulomas in young females. Pharyngeal involvement affects less than 5% of those with sarcoidosis [44, 45]. Barium swallow in patients with sarcoidosis may reveal delayed transit times and incomplete pharyngeal clearance. Skeletal muscle is involved in 50–80% of patients with sarcoidosis and may contribute to dysphagia [46]. The skeletal muscle of the pharynx is replaced by non-caseating granulomatous inflammation and fibrosis [46]. A muscle biopsy in patients suffering unexplained pharyngeal dysphagia would be a definitive test [44, 46].

Bullous pemphigoid is an autoimmune subepidermal blistering disorder classically presenting with tense bullae, with mucosal lesions happening in 17% of patients [47]. Bullous pemphigoid may uniquely present with mild pharyngeal ulcers [48]; however, further testing is needed. In refractory pharyngolaryngeal lesions, bullous pemphigoid should be considered in differential diagnosis [49].

References

1. Attrill S, White S, Murray J, et al. Impact of oropharyngeal dysphagia on healthcare cost and length of stay in hospital: a systematic review. BMC Health Serv Res. 2018;18:594. https://doi.org/10.1186/s12913-018-3376-3. Accessed 15 May 2022.
2. Massey BT. Physiology of oral cavity, pharynx and upper esophageal sphincter. GI Motility Online. 2006. https://doi.org/10.1038/gimo2. https://www.nature.com/gimo/contents/pt1/full/gimo2.html. Accessed 15 May 2022.
3. Florie MGMH, Pilz W, Dijkman RH, et al. The effect of cranial nerve stimulation on swallowing: a systematic review. Dysphagia. 2021;36:216–30. https://doi.org/10.1007/s00455-020-10126-x. Accessed 15 May 2022.
4. Jones B. Normal and abnormal swallowing. 2. New York: Springer; 2002.
5. Dulak D, Naqvi IA. Neuroanatomy, cranial nerve 7 (Facial) [Updated 2021 Jul 31]. In: StatPearls [Internet]. Treasure Island: StatPearls Publishing; 2022. Available from: https://www.ncbi.nlm.nih.gov/books/NBK526119/.
6. Walker HK. Cranial Nerves IX and X: the glossopharyngeal and vagus nerves. In: Walker HK, Hall WD, Hurst JW, editors. Clinical methods: the history, physical, and laboratory examinations, 3rd edn. Boston: Butterworths; 1990. Chapter 63. Available from: https://www.ncbi.nlm.nih.gov/books/NBK386/.
7. Smith JC, Goldberg SJ, Shall MS. Phenotype and contractile properties of mammalian tongue muscles innervated by the hypoglossal nerve. Resp Physiol Neurobiol. 2005;147(2–3, 253):–62.
8. Cock C, Omari T. Diagnosis of swallowing disorders: how we interpret pharyngeal manometry. Curr Gastroenterol Rep. 2017;19:11.
9. Curtis JA, Borders JC, Perry SE, et al. Visual Analysis of Swallowing Efficiency and Safety (VASES): a standardized approach to rating pharyngeal residue, penetration, and aspiration during FEES. Dysphagia. 2022;37:417–35. https://doi.org/10.1007/s00455-021-10293-5.
10. Miller CK, Schroeder JW Jr, Langmore S. Fiberoptic endoscopic evaluation of swallowing across the age spectrum. Am J Speech Lang Pathol. 2020;29(2S):967–78. https://doi.org/10.1044/2019_AJSLP-19-00072. Epub 2020 Jul 10. PMID: 32650653
11. Logemann JA. Manual for the videofluorographic study of swallowing. Little, Brown; 1986.
12. Martin-Harris B, Brodsky MB, Michel Y, Castell DO, Schleicher M, Sandidge J, Maxwell R, Blair J. MBS measurement tool for swallow impairment—MBSImp: establishing a standard. Dysphagia. 2008;23(4):392–405. https://doi.org/10.1007/s00455-008-9185-9. Epub 2008 Oct 15. PMID: 18855050; PMCID: PMC4217120.
13. Hazelwood RJ, Armeson KE, Hill EG, Bonilha HS, Martin-Harris B. Identification of swallowing tasks from a modified barium swallow study that optimize the detection of physiological impairment. J Speech Lang Hear Res. 2017;60(7):1855–63. https://doi.org/10.1044/2017_JSLHR-S-16-0117. PMID: 28614846; PMCID: PMC5831085
14. Payne M, Morley JE. Dysphagia, dementia and frailty. J Nutr Health Aging. 2018;22(5):562–5.
15. Steele SJ, Ennis SL, Dobler CC. Treatment burden associated with the intake of thickened fluids. Breathe (Sheff). 2021;17(1):210003. https://doi.org/10.1183/20734735.0003-2021. PMID: 34295407; PMCID: PMC8291955

16. Cichero JAY, Lam P, Steele CM, et al. Development of international terminology and definitions for texture-modified foods and thickened fluids used in dysphagia management: the IDDSI framework. Dysphagia. 2017;32:293–314. https://doi.org/10.1007/s00455-016-9758-y.
17. Newman R, Vilardell N, Clavé P, et al. Effect of bolus viscosity on the safety and efficacy of swallowing and the kinematics of the swallow response in patients with oropharyngeal dysphagia: white paper by the European Society for Swallowing Disorders (ESSD). Dysphagia. 2016;31:232–49. https://doi.org/10.1007/s00455-016-9696-8.
18. Wirth R, Dziewas R, Beck AM, Clavé P, Heppner H, Langmore S, Leischker A, Martino R, Pluschinski P, Rösler A, Shaker R, Warnecke T, Sieber C, Volkert D, Hamdy S. Oropharyngeal dysphagia in older persons—from pathophysiology to adequate intervention: a review and summary of an international expert meeting. Clin Intervent Aging. 2016;11:189. https://doi.org/10.2147/CIA.S97481.
19. Krekeler BN, Rowe LM, Connor NP. Dose in exercise-based dysphagia therapies: a scoping review. Dysphagia. 2021;36(1):1–32. https://doi.org/10.1007/s00455-020-10104-3. Epub 2020 Mar 5. PMID: 32140905; PMCID: PMC7483259
20. Troche MS, Okun MS, Rosenbek JC, Musson N, Fernandez HH, Rodriguez R, Romrell J, Pitts T, Wheeler-Hegland KM, Sapienza CM. Aspiration and swallowing in Parkinson disease and rehabilitation with EMST: a randomized trial. Neurology. 2010;75(21):1912–9. https://doi.org/10.1212/WNL.0b013e3181fef115. PMID: 21098406; PMCID: PMC2995389
21. Doğan M, Gündoğan F, Hira İ, Bayram A, Kaya A, Erdoğan Z, Mutlu C, Öz. Scintigraphic evaluation of swallowing function in patients with rheumatoid arthritis Romatoid artritli hastalarda yutma fonksiyonunun sintigrafik olarak değerlendirilmesi. 2019;7:97–101. https://doi.org/10.5606/kbbu.2019.40085.
22. Ekberg O, Redlund-Johnell I, Sjöblom KG. Pharyngeal function in patients with rheumatoid arthritis of the cervical spine and temporomandibular joint. Acta Radiol. 1987;28(1):35–9. PMID: 2952139
23. Gu J, Xu K, Ning J, Yi B, Lu K. GlideScope-assisted fiberoptic bronchoscope intubation in a patient with severe rheumatoid arthritis. Acta Anaesthesiol Taiwan. 2014;52(2):85–7. https://doi.org/10.1016/j.aat.2014.04.002. Epub 2014 Jun 18. PMID: 25016513
24. Redlund-Johnell I. Upper airway obstruction in patients with rheumatoid arthritis and temporomandibular joint destruction. Scand J Rheumatol. 1988;17(4):273–9. https://doi.org/10.3109/03009748809098796. PMID: 3187458
25. Geterud A, Bake B, Bjelle A, Jonsson R, Sandberg N, Ejnell H. Swallowing problems in rheumatoid arthritis. Acta Oto-Laryngol. 1991;111(6):1153–61. https://doi.org/10.3109/00016489109100771. PMID: 1763639
26. Joshita Y, Yoshida M, Yoshida Y, Kimura K. [Manometric study of the pharynx and pharyngoesophageal sphincter in myasthenia gravis]. Rinsho Shinkeigaku. 1990;30(9):944–51. Japanese. PMID: 2265503.
27. Colton-Hudson A, Koopman WJ, Moosa T, Smith D, Bach D, Nicolle M. A prospective assessment of the characteristics of dysphagia in myasthenia gravis. Dysphagia. 2002;17(2):147–51. https://doi.org/10.1007/s00455-001-0114-4. PMID: 11956840
28. Cohen MS, Younger D. Aspects of the natural history of myasthenia gravis: crisis and death. Ann N Y Acad Sci. 1981;377:670–7. https://doi.org/10.1111/j.1749-6632.1981.tb33765.x. PMID: 6951491
29. Mandl T, Ekberg O, Wollmer P, Manthorpe R, Jacobsson LT. Dysphagia and dysmotility of the pharynx and oesophagus in patients with primary Sjögren's syndrome. Scand J Rheumatol. 2007;36(5):394–401. https://doi.org/10.1080/03009740701607638. PMID: 17963171
30. Fraticelli P, Pisani AM, Benfaremo D, De Marino L, Campioni D, Carboni N, Fischetti C, Manfredi L, Gabrielli A, Giovagnoni A. Videofluorography swallow study in patients with systemic sclerosis: correlation with clinical and radiological features. Clin Exp Rheumatol. 201; 119(4):108–14. Epub 2019 Oct 3. PMID: 31587696.

31. Das L, Bowden A, Cooper RG, Mitchell W, O'Sullivan M, Herrick AL. Percutaneous endoscopic gastrostomy feeding—a life-saving intervention in SSc-myositis overlap with pharyngeal dysfunction. Rheumatology (Oxford). 2012;51(8):1518–20. https://doi.org/10.1093/rheumatology/kes020. Epub 2012 Mar 29. PMID: 22461389
32. Abrão AL, Santana CM, Bezerra AC, Amorim RF, Silva MB, Mota LM, Falcão DP. What rheumatologists should know about orofacial manifestations of autoimmune rheumatic diseases. Rev Bras Reumatol. 2016:S0482-5004(16)00021-8. https://doi.org/10.1016/j.rbr.2015.08.011. English, Portuguese. Epub ahead of print. PMID: 26947177.
33. Sultan SM, Ioannou Y, Isenberg DA. A review of gastrointestinal manifestations of systemic lupus erythematosus. Rheumatology. 1999;38(10):917–32. https://doi.org/10.1093/rheumatology/38.10.917.
34. Yu KH, Yang CH, Chu CC. Swallowing disturbance due to isolated vagus nerve involvement in systemic lupus erythematosus. Lupus. 2007;16(9):746–9. https://doi.org/10.1177/0961203307080632. PMID: 17728370
35. Claire Langdon P, Mulcahy K, Shepherd KL, et al. Pharyngeal dysphagia in inflammatory muscle diseases resulting from impaired suprahyoid musculature. Dysphagia. 2012;27:408–17. https://doi.org/10.1007/s00455-011-9384-7.
36. Abrão ALP, Santana CM, Bezerra ACB, Batista RF, de Amorim M, da Silva B, Henrique LM, da Mota D, Falcão P. What rheumatologists should know about orofacial manifestations of autoimmune rheumatic diseases. Rev Bras Reumatol (English Ed). 2016;56(5):441–50. https://doi.org/10.1016/j.rbre.2016.02.006. ISSN 2255-5021
37. Garlapati P, Qurie A. Granulomatosis with polyangiitis. [Updated 2021 Dec 7]. In: StatPearls [Internet]. Treasure Island: StatPearls Publishing; 2022. Available from: https://www.ncbi.nlm.nih.gov/books/NBK557827.
38. Galli J, Corina L, Larocca LM. Su di un raro caso di granulomatosi di Wegener a localizzazione faringo-laringea [Unusual case of pharyngeal-laryngeal Wegener's granulomatosis]. Acta Otorhinolaryngol Ital. 2001;21(3):187–91. Italian. PMID: 11677846.
39. Manna R, Cadoni G, Ferri E, Verrecchia E, Giovinale M, Fonnesu C, Calò L, Armato E, Paludetti G. Wegener's granulomatosis: an update on diagnosis and therapy. Exp Rev Clin Immunol. 2008;4(4):481–95.
40. Morales-Angulo C, García-Zornoza R, Obeso-Agüera S, Calvo-Alén J, González-Gay MA. [Ear, nose and throat manifestations of Wegener's granulomatosis (granulomatosis with polyangiitis)]. Acta Otorrinolaringol Esp. 2012;63:206–11.
41. Polychronopoulos VS, Prakash UB, Golbin JM, Edell ES, Specks U. Airway involvement in Wegener's granulomatosis. Rheum Dis Clin North Am. 2007;33:755–75.
42. Panwar J, et al. A case of Wegener granulomatosis with unprecedented hypopharyngeal and splenic involvement. Austin J Otolaryngol. 2015. https://austinpublishinggroup.com/otolaryngology/fulltext/ajo-v2-id1062.
43. Ayache S, Smail A, Stramandinoli E, Pichon JC, Strunski V. A propos d'un cas de forme pharyngée de maladie de Wegener [Pharyngeal Wegener's disease: a case report]. Ann Otolaryngol Chir Cervicofac. 2001;118(3):187–92. French. PMID: 11431593
44. Mohapatra A, Holekamp T, Diaz JA, Zebala L, Brasington R. FACP|| Atlantoaxial subluxation and nasopharyngeal necrosis complicating suspected granulomatosis with polyangiitis. JCR J Clin Rheumatol. 2015;21(3):156–9. https://doi.org/10.1097/RHU.0000000000000236.
45. Chakraborty RK, Aeddula NR. Churg Strauss Syndrome. [Updated 2022 Jan 4]. In: StatPearls [Internet]. Treasure Island: StatPearls Publishing; 2022. Available from: https://www.ncbi.nlm.nih.gov/books/NBK537099/.
46. Park J, Im S, Moon SJ, Park GY, Jang Y, Kim Y. Churg-Strauss Syndrome as an unusual cause of dysphagia: case report. Ann Rehabil Med. 2015;39(3):477–81. https://doi.org/10.5535/arm.2015.39.3.477.
47. Adil A, Goyal A, Quint JM. Behcet disease. [Updated 2022 Feb 10]. In: StatPearls [Internet]. Treasure Islan: StatPearls Publishing; 2022. Available from: https://www.ncbi.nlm.nih.gov/books/NBK470257/.

48. Hamza M, Ferjaoui M, Elleuch M, Bergaoui N, Souilem J, Atallah M, Benayed H. Sténose pharyngée dans un cas de maladie de Behçet [Pharyngeal stenosis in a case of Behçet's disease]. Ann Otolaryngol Chir Cervicofac. 1985;102(6):465–7. French. PMID: 4091396
49. Brookes GB. Pharyngeal stenosis in Behçet's syndrome. The first reported case. Arch Otolaryngol. 1983;109(5):338–40. https://doi.org/10.1001/archotol.1983.00800190060015. PMID: 6847487

Chapter 5
Esophageal Manifestations of Rheumatologic Disease

Sonia B. Samuel, Lisa Rosenberg, Anusha Agarwal, Alla Turshudzhyan, and Micheal Tadros

5.1 Anatomy and Physiology of the Esophagus

5.1.1 Introduction

Involvement of the esophagus, a multilayered organ, has been reported in many rheumatologic conditions. The major role of the esophagus is to transport food into the stomach and prevent gastroesophageal reflux. As such, rheumatologic conditions can lead to the impairment of the esophagus to transport food and impact antireflux mechanisms. Mechanisms related to inflammation, infiltration, fibrosis, immune dysfunction, and neuronal abnormality have been implicated in the onset of esophageal dysfunction. Systemic lupus erythematosus (SLE), rheumatoid arthritis (RA), sarcoidosis, systemic sclerosis, among others are conditions that are commonly associated with esophageal dysfunction. Complications of these

S. B. Samuel
Department of Internal Medicine, Albany Medical Center, Albany, NY, USA

L. Rosenberg
Division of Rheumatology, Department of Internal Medicine, The University of Vermont Medical Center, Burlington, VT, USA

A. Agarwal
Albany Medical College, Albany, NY, USA

A. Turshudzhyan
Division of Gastroenterology, Department of Internal Medicine, NIH/University of Maryland, Bethesda, MD, USA

M. Tadros (✉)
Division of Gastroenterology, Department of Internal Medicine, Albany Medical Center, Albany, NY, USA
e-mail: Tadrosm1@amc.edu

M. Tadros et al. (eds.), *GI Diseases Associated with Rheumatological and Vasculitic Conditions*, Clinical Gastroenterology,
https://doi.org/10.1007/978-3-032-07868-1_5

rheumatologic conditions can greatly impact patients' quality of life, thus careful focus on normal esophagus physiology, early detection of symptoms, appropriate diagnosis, and timely intervention is paramount for optimal management and in prevention of disease progression.

5.1.2 Esophagus Anatomy and Physiology

The esophagus is a tubular organ with a multilayered wall that functions to transport food into the stomach while also preventing gastroesophageal reflux [1]. The esophageal wall is made up of the mucosa, submucosa and muscularis propria layers; the outer wall is bounded by a thin layer of connective tissue, the adventitia [1, 2]. The mucosal layer of the esophageal body is composed of a stratified squamous epithelium and can be further broken down into three sublayers: mucus membrane, lamina propria, and muscularis mucosa [1, 2]. The submucosal layer consists of glands that secrete water, bicarbonate, mucins, epidermal growth factor, and prostaglandins. These secretions aid in mucosal clearance, peristalsis, and protection against gastroesophageal reflux [1]. Other structures within the submucosa include nerves, blood vessels, and lymph vessels [2]. The muscularis propria is composed of both an inner circular muscle layer and an outer longitudinal muscle layer [1, 2]. The proximal one-third of the esophagus is made up of striated muscle while the distal two-third is made up of smooth muscle [1, 2].

Primary peristalsis is the coordinated muscle contraction by the esophagus during the act of swallowing [1]. The food bolus travels through the relaxed upper esophageal sphincter into the esophageal body after the pharyngeal phase of swallowing [1, 3]. Once in the esophagus, the bolus is propelled by progressive contractions beginning in the upper esophagus and proceeding distally [1, 3]. The muscle contractions are triggered by esophageal distension, and allow the bolus to travel towards the stomach [4]. While primary peristalsis generally results in clearance of food from esophagus into stomach, there may be residual food. For this reason, there is a secondary wave, or secondary peristalsis, which occurs due to residual food or reflux events [1, 4]. Secondary peristalsis involves contractions of the lower esophagus to clear remnants of the bolus and remove refluxed gastric contents [4].

5.1.3 Anti-reflux Mechanism

Gastroesophageal (GE) reflux occurs when gastric contents flow into the esophagus. While reflux can often be normal and physiologic, gastroesophageal reflux disease (GERD) develops when there are symptoms or complications related to this retrograde flow of contents [5]. In a normal esophagus, there are multiple defenses in place to protect against GE reflux. The anatomic barriers include the lower esophageal sphincter (LES) and the supporting extrinsic crural diaphragm [4, 5].

Mechanisms that result in reflux include transient LES relaxations (TLESR), low LES pressure, LES relaxation due to swallowing, straining, and molecular changes [5]. TLESR is a physiologic process that occurs after meals due to gastric distension and allows for release of gas from the stomach through belching [6]. However, gastric contents may also simultaneously reflux during these episodes resulting in GERD [6]. This mechanism is thought to be the most common, accounting for up to 90% of reflux events in GERD patients without a hiatal hernia [7]. For patients with a hiatal hernia, low LES pressure, LES relaxation during swallowing, or straining-induced LES relaxation can contribute to GERD [8].

Other barriers that protect against reflux include secondary peristalsis, which rapidly clears refluxed materials, bicarbonate in swallowed saliva, local bicarbonate and mucus secretion, and epithelium resistance [1, 4]. Impaired anti-reflux barriers precipitate increased reflux events, with the severity of reflux correlating with the extent of dysfunction of the barriers [5]. The injury caused by this reflux is then determined by the duration of exposure and causticity of contents. Ineffective esophageal clearance increases the duration of exposure which then puts patients at a higher risk of GERD and esophagitis [5].

5.2 Discussion of Rheumatologic Conditions

5.2.1 Systemic Sclerosis

Systemic sclerosis (SSc) is a chronic autoimmune disorder characterized by vascular and fibrotic changes affecting both the skin and internal organs. SSc has a wide spectrum of presentation, severity, and outcomes. Regardless of subtype, approximately 90% of patients with SSc present with gastrointestinal manifestations, with esophageal dysmotility being the most frequently reported [9]. Esophageal dysmotility affects about 70–75% of SSc patients [10]. Most cases of esophageal dysmotility result in loss of peristalsis and a hypotensive LES [11]. The inflammatory changes cause smooth muscle atrophy in the lower two-thirds of the distal esophagus and lower esophageal sphincter, leading to replacement of normal muscle tissue with fibrosed tissue. Histopathology demonstrates increased collagen deposition within the lamina propria and submucosa and evidence of esophagitis. In some cases, neuronal abnormality may also lead to an incompetent LES. This pathology coupled with abnormal peristaltic contractions causes delayed esophageal transit, increased gastric acid exposure and stricture formation [11, 12]. Such pathologic changes precipitate early signs of esophageal manifestations of SSc, including dysphagia and choking, substernal pain, heartburn, cough, and hoarseness. Patients may also experience reflux, pseudo-obstruction, nausea, vomiting and aspiration [10, 13]. Symptoms may become very severe, leading to poor appetite, weight loss and impaired quality of life [13, 14].

Patients with longer disease duration can develop interstitial lung disease (ILD) secondary to micro-aspiration, which is a major cause of morbidity and mortality [13, 15]. Presenting signs include chronic cough and asthma-like symptoms [13]. Due to the similar presentations of ILD and pulmonary disease secondary to reflux, it is important to rule out this important differential diagnosis after optimized treatment of reflux disease [16]. Patients whose symptoms do not improve with immunosuppressant therapy intended for ILD should be further evaluated for GERD as the underlying cause of their pulmonary symptoms [16].

Esophageal pH monitoring, with or without impedance, is considered the gold standard for gastroesophageal reflux detection and should be used early in SSc patients with early-stage lung disease. The test identifies those who should undergo intense anti-reflux therapy to prevent detrimental reflux effects while awaiting lung transplantation [17]. Twenty-four-hour ambulatory pH monitor with impedance monitoring and manometry can demonstrate ineffective esophageal motility with subsequent stasis of acidic contents in the esophagus. It documents prolonged esophageal acidity compared to acid exposure in the stomach. Esophageal pH monitoring was performed in a study of 10 SSc patients referred for lung transplantation and severe reflux. It concluded abnormal pH was a better predictor of survival than abnormal pulmonary function tests.

In addition to pulmonary disease, other complications from incompetent LES and abnormal peristalsis with secondary GERD include Barrett's esophagus, strictures, erosive esophagitis, and adenocarcinoma [11, 12]. Barrett's esophagus has been documented in up to 37% of patients with SSc (Fig. 5.1) [18]. Increased impaired LES tone and longer periods of dysphagia are often seen in patients with Barrett's esophagus [19]. Though less common, the resultant metaplasia and dysplasia contributes to the development of adenocarcinoma in SSc patients with

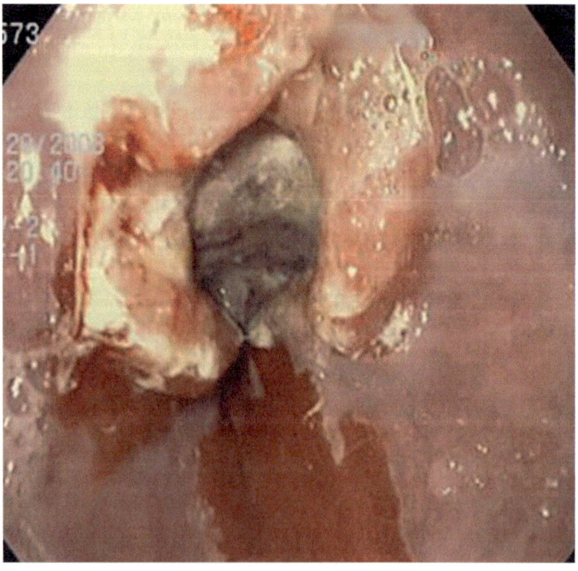

Fig. 5.1 Barrett's Esophagus with low grade dysplasia

Barrett's esophagus. The incidence of esophageal adenocarcinoma is 0.7% per year in patients with SSc and Barrett's esophagus whereas in patients with Barrett's esophagus without SSc, the incidence is 0.45% [20]. While these complications are rare, symptoms of mechanical obstruction, such as dysphagia, warrant further investigation to rule out Barret's esophagus and esophageal adenocarcinoma.

Additionally, it is more common for SSc patients to develop erosive esophagitis and stricture formation. About 30–60% of patients develop erosive esophagitis [21–23]. Erosive esophagitis results from increased acid exposure due to impaired acid clearance in the esophagus, impaired LES tone and pathologic nighttime GER [21, 22]. The presence of a hiatal hernia likely exacerbates the severity of GERD symptoms and may be found more commonly in SSc patients than the general population, which can lead to erosive esophagitis [24, 25]. Chronic GER leads to repeated injury to the esophageal mucosa and subsequent erosive esophagitis. During the healing phase, excess collagen deposition may result in stricture formation [26]. Strictures are a major culprit of dysphagia found in 17–29% of SSc patients [27]. Strictures may cause obstructive dysphagia by the narrowing of the esophageal lumen and reduced esophageal distensibility [28]. This sequence of events further predisposes SSc patients to more esophageal insult, which can precipitate the complications of Barrett's esophagus and adenocarcinoma, if left untreated.

5.2.2 *Systemic Lupus Erythematosus*

Systemic lupus erythematous (SLE) is a chronic systemic autoimmune disorder with a complex pathophysiology [29, 30]. It involves immune system dysregulation along with associated genetic, epigenetic, hormonal, and environmental factors [29, 30]. It is a multifactorial process involving an inflammatory reaction in esophageal muscles, muscle atrophy, and ischemic vasculitis [31]. GI involvement is seen in about half of the patients [32]. Esophageal dysmotility can affect 21–72% of SLE patients [31]. Symptoms most commonly include dysphagia, heartburn, and regurgitation [31]. Less commonly, SLE patients with dysphagia and chest pain may have manometry findings of peaked, broad primary contractions consistent with diffuse esophageal spasm. Symptoms resembling esophageal spasm may also indicate a neurogenic component in the pathophysiology, potentially related to degeneration of the vagus nerve [33]. Other findings including decreased saliva production, inflammation of upper esophageal muscles, or aperistalsis in the lower esophagus with hypotony of LES may also contribute to dysphagia and suggest a concomitant inflammatory disease or mixed connective tissue disease [31]. Further complications that can arise are peptic esophagitis with ulceration or rarely, esophageal perforation [34].

5.2.3 Rheumatoid Arthritis

Rheumatoid arthritis (RA), the most common inflammatory arthritis, is a chronic, systemic autoimmune disorder that is characterized by inflammatory arthritis of synovial joints and extraarticular manifestation [35]. GI derangements are rare extraarticular manifestations of RA. Several studies have documented manometric esophageal changes in RA, including lower peristaltic motion in the lower two thirds of the esophagus, reduced LES pressure, and abnormal peristalsis [36]. However, there were several limitations associated with these studies, including a small sample size and confounding variables [37]. They lacked appropriate controls for medications and associated comorbidities that can independently affect esophageal function. Furthermore, a study with over 2000 subjects showed no subjective association between RA and dysphagia or GERD, when controlling for prednisone or NSAIDs [37].

5.2.4 Sarcoidosis

Sarcoidosis is a multisystem inflammatory disease characterized by noncaseating granulomas. This condition typically has an indolent course that affects young African American females who classically present with bilateral hilar adenopathy on chest imaging. Gastrointestinal disease may occur in 0.1–0.9% of patients, though it is possible that these patients may have subclinical GI disease that is more indolent and undetectable at greater rates [38]. Approximately 80% of GI sarcoidosis affects the esophagus, stomach, and the duodenum [38].

Esophageal sarcoidosis is not often diagnosed in asymptomatic patients, making it important to be cognizant of its presenting symptoms. Patients commonly present with dysphagia. Less common symptoms include weight loss, odynophagia, anemia, and hoarseness. Several mechanisms have been described in the pathogenesis of esophageal sarcoidosis. Superficial mucosal infiltration typically affects the upper esophagus and can form esophageal nodules and strictures, leading to dysphagia [38]. Infiltration of the skeletal muscle in the upper esophagus may also impact function of the cricopharyngeal muscle, leading to oropharyngeal dysphagia. The lower esophagus may also be involved, where damage to the myenteric plexus leads to achalasia-like symptoms. Although uncommon, esophageal perforation secondary to enlarged periesophageal lymph nodes can occur. One case report demonstrated a patient with dysphagia was found to have extrinsic compression of the esophagus by enlarged mediastinal lymph nodes which showed noncaseating granulomas on biopsy [39]. Additionally, a patient had a perforated esophagus with necrosis of the esophageal wall from mediastinal nodal hypertrophy secondary to sarcoidosis [40].

5.2.5 *Myositis*

Inflammatory myopathies, or myositis, describe multiple inflammatory disorders of skeletal muscles including polymyositis, dermatomyositis, necrotizing myositis and inclusion body myositis [41]. Over 50% of myositis patients present with GI involvement. Dysphagia is a common presenting symptom of esophageal involvement in myositis [41]. Prevalence of dysphagia is variable in myositis but may be as high as 73% [42]. Dysphagia may range from mild, with coughing during eating, to severe impairment of food passage with choking [41]. Hoarseness, reflux symptoms, and laryngitis are also common symptoms [42]. Complications of severe dysphagia include malnutrition and aspiration pneumonia [42]. The mortality risk is increased greatly in patients with dysphagia, with the most common cause of death being respiratory failure from aspiration pneumonia [42]. Myositis may also be related to development of hiatal hernia, which could worsen reflux symptoms [43]. Fibromuscular degeneration leads to decreased elasticity in the structures surrounding the diaphragmatic hiatus, lending to the formation of hiatal hernia [43].

5.2.6 *Ehler's Danlos Syndrome*

Ehler's Danlos Syndrome (EDS) represents a group of heritable disorders that affect the connective tissue due to defects in collagen synthesis. EDS typically presents with skin hyperextensibility, joint hypermobility and skin fragility, but also leads to changes in GI anatomy and physiology [44, 45]. In one retrospective review of 687 EDS patients, 56% had associated GI manifestations [46]. Connective tissue and autonomic dysfunctions predispose patients with EDS to GERD due to the development of a hiatal hernia, reduced LES tone and decreased GI motility. More serious complications can occur in the EDS vascular subtype [46, 47]. Diagnostic studies can be performed to assess for GI impairment. Esophagogastroduodenoscopy (EGD) can detect the presence of a hiatal hernia [48]. Endoscopic biopsies may reveal reflux-related changes such as reflux esophagitis or Barrett's esophagus [46]. Furthermore, manometry and an esophageal pH study can assess for esophageal dysmotility and reflux [46]. These diagnostic tests should also be performed for concern of epiphrenic esophageal diverticula, a rare esophageal finding [49]. These result from esophageal motor dysfunction or weakness in esophageal muscles and may present either asymptomatically or with symptoms of dysphagia and regurgitation [49].

5.2.7 Sjogren's Syndrome

Sjogren's syndrome (SS) is a chronic autoimmune disease in which inflammatory changes of the salivary and lacrimal glands lead to diminished glandular function and subsequent dryness of the mouth and eyes. SS commonly occurs in women between the ages of 45–50 years and can overlap with other autoimmune diseases such as rheumatoid arthritis or lupus [50]. Disease severity varies and manifestations are typically characterized into two classes: extra-glandular or exocrine glandular features. GI involvement is typically considered extra-glandular involvement of systemic disease. Esophageal involvement may be due to poor salivary flow rates; however further mechanisms of symptom onset remain to be investigated [50, 51]. Some studies revealed decreased contractility in the upper one third of the esophagus is likely precipitated by decreased lubrication of the esophagus. This leads to prolonged esophageal transit times, reduced clearance of acid and caustic substances and impairment of anti-reflux barriers [52]. SS patients may experience dysphagia, acid reflux and pharyngitis. Severe forms of SS can lead to GERD, esophagitis and esophageal dysmotility [52].

5.2.8 Plummer-Vinson Syndrome

Plummer Vinson syndrome presents with a triad of symptoms: dysphagia, iron-deficiency anemia and esophageal webs [53]. The classic presentation includes post-cricoid dysphagia of solid foods with progression to liquids over time [54]. Severe dysphagia can be complicated by aspiration pneumonia [55]. Plummer-Vinson syndrome is also a risk factor for squamous cell carcinoma of the upper GI tract. It is estimated that 3–15% of patients develop esophageal or pharyngeal cancer [56, 57].

5.2.9 Overlap Syndrome and Mixed Connective Tissue Disorder

Overlap syndrome has an ambiguous clinical presentation in which individuals must meet the selection criteria for more than one of the defined autoimmune connective tissue diseases [58]. These include SLE, scleroderma, myositis, RA, and Sjogren's syndrome [59]. Yet the most well-defined overlap syndrome is mixed connective tissue disease [58]. Mixed connective tissue disease (MCTD) is a rare autoimmune disease diagnosed when a specific antibody, anti-U1-ribonucleoprotein, is present and there are features of at least two connective tissue diseases [60].

With respect to GI manifestations of the disease, the esophagus was implicated in almost 85% of cases [61]. In MCTD, there is esophageal involvement of the upper one third of striated muscle and/or lower two thirds of smooth muscle. Although the proximal segment can be involved, esophageal manometry typically demonstrates aperistalsis in the lower two thirds of the esophagus [61]. Complications include esophagitis, strictures and Barrett's esophagus [60]. It is proposed that autoantibodies attack the smooth and striated muscle tissue, the ganglion cells of the Auerbach plexus, vascular walls, and squamous epithelium contributing to dysphasia [61].

5.2.10 Diffuse Idiopathic Skeletal Hyperostosis (DISH)

Diffuse idiopathic skeletal hyperostosis (DISH) is the ossification and calcification of tendons and ligaments in the skeletal system, commonly involving the spine and manifests with pain and stiffness. It is characterized by the flowing ossification of at least three successive vertebral levels at the anterolateral spine or four continuous vertebrae [62].

In DISH, the involvement of the esophagus is a result of mechanical obstruction. Given the presence of new bone growth anterior to the cervical vertebral bodies, the esophagus can be compressed, leading to dysphagia [63].

5.2.11 Amyloidosis

Amyloidosis is a heterogenous group of diseases characterized by extracellular deposition of abnormal protein, which aggregate and disrupt normal tissue architecture and function, resulting in a wide variety of symptoms [64, 65]. This disease can be further broken down into systemic or localized amyloidosis, with potential GI manifestations in both subtypes [26]. Commonly, amyloidosis presents with gastrointestinal dysmotility in a stasis syndrome [21]. Pathogenesis likely includes gastrointestinal myopathic and neuropathic dysfunction from amyloid infiltration of both muscles and autonomic nerves [21, 22] Predominating esophageal symptoms include nausea, vomiting, dysphagia and GERD [21]. Though uncommon, esophageal variceal bleeding may occur resulting from portal hypertension due to sinusoidal amyloid deposits [23, 27, 66]. With extensive esophageal involvement and invasion through the entire wall of the esophagus, perforation may also result [28].

5.2.12 Pemphigus Vulgaris, Steven-Johnson Syndrome and Toxic Epidermal Necrolysis

Several ulcerating and blistering diseases with esophageal manifestations include pemphigus vulgaris, toxic epidermal necrolysis, and Steven-Johnson syndrome. Pemphigus vulgaris is a rare autoimmune blistering disease of the skin and mucous membranes that involves IgG1 and IgG4 autoantibodies against glycoproteins desmoglein 1 and desmoglein 3 [19, 67]. This can lead to rupture of intercellular bridges and subsequent acantholysis, a phenomenon that results in easily ruptured blisters and a clinical sign known as Nikolsky sign [19, 68]. Esophageal disease is rare but usually occurs in the context of previously diagnosed cutaneous pemphigus [67]. Symptoms can include odynophagia and dysphagia [20].

Toxic epidermal necrolysis (TEN) and Steven-Johnson syndrome (SJS) are acute mucocutaneous vesiculobullous disorders characterized by life-threatening, widespread full-thickness cutaneous and mucosal necrosis [69]. TEN is defined as the involvement of at least 30% total body surface area (TBSA) of the skin, with SJS involving <10%. SJS/TEN overlap when there is between 10% and 30% TBSA involvement. These immune-complex-mediated diseases usually occur as an adverse reaction to a medication or an infection [70, 71]. Patients with esophageal involvement usually complain of odynophagia, dysphagia and poor oral intake [71, 72]. Endoscopy with biopsy will demonstrate necrotic epithelial detachment [73].

5.2.13 Vasculitis

Vasculitis are characterized by inflammation of blood vessels and affect vessels of varying sizes and locations. Overall, the esophagus is rarely implicated in vasculitis, but certain vasculitides have been associated with esophageal dysfunction. Primary esophageal involvement is observed in granulomatosis with polyangiitis (GPA), eosinophilic granulomatosis with polyangiitis and IgA vasculitis [74–76]. GPA is an ANCA-mediated necrotizing granulomatous vasculitis affecting the small vessels [77]. The GI tract is not commonly affected in GPA and the esophagus is rarely implicated with less than 8 documented cases [76, 78]. Upper endoscopy typically reveals discrete, punched out lesions, however, circumferential ulcerations of the esophagus may also occur [76]. In approximately half of the cases, dysphagia was the presenting symptom. Interestingly, one case initially presented with odynophagia which improved after GPA was diagnosed and treated [78]. Thus, it is important to consider GPA as a cause of esophageal ulcerations in challenging cases.

Eosinophilic granulomatosis with polyangiitis is a necrotizing vasculitis that involves small- and medium-sized vessels. The esophagus is rarely involved, but there have been several case reports demonstrating esophagitis with markedly thickened esophageal wall and esophageal ulcers which resolved after treatment of the vasculitis [75].

Additionally, IgA vasculitis is a small vessel vasculitis that involves the joints, skin, kidneys and GI tract [79]. The GI tract is affected up to 40% of patients. The typical presentation includes abdominal pain, arthralgias, renal involvement and palpable purpura. Complications of intussusception, perforation and hemorrhage can arise [79]. The esophagus is not commonly involved, but there have been a few cases of esophageal cancer in individuals with IgA vasculitis [74, 80]. Neoplasia is an established but rare cause of vasculitides especially with IgA vasculitis [74]. Although the esophagus is not commonly affected by vasculitis, systemic vasculitis should be consider in those presenting with dysphagia of unclear etiology.

5.2.14 Behcet's Disease

Behcet's disease is a systemic inflammatory vasculitis typically characterized by recurrent oral aphthous and genital ulcerations. Manifestations of Behcet's disease may involve additional organ systems resulting in uveitis, gastrointestinal ulcers and/or skin lesions [81]. Mucosal ulcerations can generally occur in the esophagus, terminal ileum, colon and cecum [82]. Esophageal complications of Behcet's are quite rare, affecting approximately 2–11% of patients [36]. Esophageal symptoms include retrosternal chest pain, dysphagia, odynophagia and upper and lower GI bleeding due to ulcerative lesions [82]. Further complications includes stenosis, perforation and dysmotility [36]. Endoscopy may reveal single or multiple ulcers [83].

5.3 Secondary Complications of Rheumatologic Conditions with Esophageal Involvement

Patients with chronic rheumatologic conditions with esophageal involvement are at an increased risk of complications. Secondary complications may be related to the therapeutic interventions or from the chronic disease itself. Understanding of possible sequelae of long-term esophageal damage can help facilitate early intervention and timely therapy.

5.3.1 Opportunistic Infections: Candida, CMV, HSV-1

Candida, an opportunistic fungus, remains the most common cause of infectious esophagitis, with an incidence of up to 88% [84, 85]. In immunocompromised patients who have an impaired host-defense system, uncontrolled growth of *Candida* in the esophageal mucosa may occur. Candida esophagitis (CE) may be attributed to immunosuppressive therapy, delayed esophageal transit, and poor esophageal emptying, all of which are commonly seen in rheumatologic conditions [86]. Fungal colonization of the esophagus appears as characteristic adhesive plaques on endoscopy. Initiating appropriate anti-fungal treatment is crucial for limiting CE progression to major esophageal complications such as necrotizing Candida esophagitis and stricture formation [87, 88].

Cytomegalovirus or CMV infection is most commonly seen in immunocompromised patients [89]. Following the colon, the esophagus is the most common affected site in the GI tract [90]. Patients often present with odynophagia or substernal chest pain. Other accompanying symptoms include dysphagia, nausea, vomiting, abdominal pain, weight loss and diarrhea [90, 91]. In endoscopy, CMV esophagitis appears as well-demarcated, linear, vertical or horizontal shallow ulcers at the mid-to-distal esophagus [90]. Ulcerations may be singular or multiple and are associated with mucosal edema and nodularity. The most reliable diagnostic tool is endoscopic biopsy demonstrating CMV inclusion bodies [90]. Treatment options for active disease include ganciclovir and valganciclovir, with foscarnet as an alternative if resistance develops [91].

Herpes simplex virus (HSV) can affect the esophagus and tends to present in the immunocompromised host. HSV type 1 is implicated in most cases. This occurs due to the reactivation of the virus and spread to the esophagus via the vagus nerve or direct extension of oropharyngeal infection [92]. Patients typically experience dysphagia, odynophagia, fever and retrosternal chest pain [93]. Diagnosis is generally achieved via endoscopic visualization of the esophagus, followed by histopathological confirmation, which shows multinucleated giant cells, ground glass nuclei and eosinophilic inclusion bodies [92]. Lesions may appear as a vesicle early in the disease course that coalesces to form well circumcised, "volcano-like" ulcers that may present with exudates, plaques or diffuse erosive esophagitis [93]. Patients with HSV esophagitis can have concomitant herpes labialis and oropharyngeal ulcers. The treatment of choice is oral acyclovir. Famciclovir and valacyclovir are considered for those who cannot tolerate oral therapy; however, there is limited evidence for these alternatives in esophagitis [93].

5.3.2 Pill-Induced Esophagitis

Pill-induced esophagitis occurs from direct injury to the esophageal mucosa due to ingestion of certain medications. Presenting symptoms include dysphagia, heartburn, retrosternal pain, and odynophagia. Notable culprit medications include non-steroidal anti-inflammatory drugs (NSAIDs), aspirin, bisphosphonates, potassium chloride and antibiotics, specifically clindamycin and tetracycline. Medications commonly used in the management of rheumatologic conditions, such as methotrexate and quinidine are also implicated in pill-induced esophagitis [94]. Mechanisms that lead to this pathology include caustic injury, disruption of the cytoprotective prostaglandin layer of the mucosa and vascular injury secondary to hyperosmotic properties of the pill [94–97]. Additionally, anatomic changes to the esophagus seen in rheumatologic conditions often lead to stasis and delayed esophageal transit time, which increases exposure of offending medications to the esophageal mucosa [97]. For instance, in scleroderma patients, pill-induced esophagitis may occur more frequently at the site of esophageal narrowing due to decreased LES tone, decreased esophageal peristalsis, or stricture formation. If untreated, complications such as ulceration and perforation can occur [98]. Importantly, additional patient-related risk factors that delay transit time of medications include saliva production, amount of water ingested while taking the pill, pill size and position of patient with ingestion [97]. As such, treatment of pill-induced esophagitis requires a comprehensive approach for patients with rheumatologic disorders. Appropriate pharmacologic regimen and patient education for proper pill-ingesting strategies should be simultaneously conducted to reduce the risk of pill-induced esophagitis.

5.3.3 Effect of Opioids on the Esophagus

Patients with esophageal dysmotility secondary to chronic opioid use can present with symptoms of nausea, vomiting, reflux and dyspepsia [99]. Opioids impair esophagogastric junction relaxation and cause spastic and vigorous esophageal body contractions [100]. In a retrospective study at the Yale Gastrointestinal Motility Lab, manometric abnormalities were found in 56.4% of 218 chronic opioid users compared to 47.5% of 1053 non-chronic opioid users. Esophagogastric junction outflow obstruction (EGJOO) was identified in 17.9% of chronic opioid users compared to 11.2% nonusers [101]. Further, a retrospective study conducted by Ratuapli and colleagues demonstrated that EGJOO was significantly more prevalent in patients using opioids within 24 h of esophageal pressure topography compared with those who did not (27% of 66 patients on opioids vs. 7% of 55 patients off opioids) [99]. Thus, it was concluded that chronic opioid use in rheumatologic diseases increases the risk of EGJOO.

5.4 Diagnosis and Intervention

5.4.1 Diagnostic Modalities

Multiple diagnostic testing can be performed to evaluate for esophageal symptoms, deeming it important to understand the diagnostic utility of each test. Esophagography is the primary radiologic modality for esophageal imaging [102]. It involves swallowing a barium suspension with imaging to evaluate esophageal anatomy and motility [102]. This is often done for individuals with dysphagia or reflux, and can reveal structural lesions of the esophagus, motility disorders such as achalasia or diffuse esophageal spasms, or reflux disease [102]. EGD is one of the most common procedures used to visualize the oropharynx up to the proximal duodenum [103]. It may be used as a diagnostic procedure to further evaluate symptoms such as dysphagia, GERD, persistent abdominal pain or emesis [103, 104]. It can also be used therapeutically for foreign body removal, dilation or stenting of strictures, variceal ligation, upper GI bleeds or achalasia management [103, 104]. The gold standard in the evaluation of esophageal motility disorders is high-resolution manometry [105]. This test is often recommended after structural or obstructive causes of dysphagia have been excluded [105]. It can classify diseases such as achalasia, diffuse esophageal spasm, and hypomotility by identifying motility patterns [105]. Another well-tolerated and quantifiable test to evaluate motility is esophageal transit scintigraphy by monitoring a swallowed radioactive bolus [106]. To investigate GERD symptoms, the 24-h esophageal pH monitoring is a conventional diagnostic test [107]. While this was previously considered the gold standard for reflux, it is now known that some types of reflux may go undetected [108]. Esophageal impedance-pH monitoring is a more novel technique used for the evaluation of GERD. It monitors both bolus transport and types of reflux based on acidity and therefore identifies reflux that may have been undetected by other testing modalities [108].

5.4.2 Lifestyle Management

While optimal management of dysphagia include targeted therapies of the underlying cause, lifestyle management such as dietary modifications and rehabilitative exercise maneuvers may be beneficial. It can further ensure adequate nutrition, reduce aspiration risk and improve quality of life. For example, individuals with dysphagia can benefit from a soft and easily chewable diet, thus reducing the aspiration risk [109]. Close follow-up with a nutritionist can enable greater adherence to the dysphagia diet, while also ensuring nutritional goals. Additional compensatory methods can also be useful such as postural techniques. Altering the chin and head position will prevent swallowing discomfort and aspiration [109]. Furthermore, rehabilitative maneuvers such as the super supraglottic swallow can improve the underlying physiological function [110]. Individual preferences, social determinants of health, and cultural and religious values are important factors to consider as these can significantly impact the patient's overall prognosis and health.

5.4.3 Medications

While rheumatologic and vasculitic conditions demonstrate great variability, pharmacologic management often involves the use of similar drug classes. Medications such as NSAIDs, methotrexate, quinidine, etanercept, and infliximab are frequently used. When considering medical management of esophageal manifestations, the approach often involves treating the underlying pathology, symptomatic management, or both. With symptomatic management, first line treatment includes a trial of proton pump inhibitors (PPIs) or histamine H2 receptor antagonists. Lifestyle intervention in addition to medical management can optimize symptomatic relief. In cases of refractory symptoms after a trial of PPIs and H2 receptor blockers, minimally invasive imaging studies may be warranted. Endoscopic or surgical intervention should also be carefully considered especially if esophageal symptoms acutely worsen. Additionally, buspirone, a serotonin 5-HT1A receptor agonist and anxiolytic, can be used for GERD in SSc patients. The drug binds the endogenous neurotransmitter serotonin (5-hydroxytryptamine) and increases LES pressure, reducing reflux symptoms [13].

5.4.4 Endoscopic and Surgical Intervention

The endoscopic and surgical treatment options for dysphagia and other esophageal symptoms are tailored to the underlying etiology. Mechanical obstructions including intraluminal rings, webs, and strictures can be endoscopically managed via mechanical or balloon dilation [111]. Benign strictures are commonly treated with endoscopic dilators. As an adjunctive therapy, intra-lesion steroid injections or oral steroid gel can help decrease the inflammatory-related injury from dilation and reduce the risk of re-stenosis [112]. In benign strictures resistant to dilation or malignant strictures, esophageal stents may be considered [111]. In general, intraluminal masses, diverticula, or extrinsic compression of the esophagus require surgical intervention to remove the obstruction when conservative measures fail [113].

Fundoplication is considered for SSc patients with severe GERD, repeated aspiration pneumonia or asthma, Barrett's esophagus, failed pharmacological therapy, medication noncompliance, or intolerable side effects [114]. These surgeries may be performed via an open or laparoscopic approach. Laparoscopic approach is as safe and effective in treating GERD as open surgery with the added benefit of shorter hospital stays and fewer complications [114]. Absolute contraindications for laparoscopic anti-reflux surgeries are the inability to tolerate anesthesia and uncorrectable coagulopathy [114]. Additional relative contraindications include prior abdominal surgery, severe morbid obesity and esophageal dysmotility [114]. Some studies suggest that esophageal dysmotility, as seen in SSc patients, is associated with an increased incidence of post-operative dysphagia, especially in Nissen fundoplication due to the tight wrapping of the gastroesophageal junction [115]. Early literature demonstrated mixed results in SSc patients with complete aperistalsis undergoing fundoplication. Orringer and colleagues reported improvement of GERD symptoms in SSc patients after Collis-Belsey fundoplication [116]. Unfortunately, 41% of these patients had symptom recurrence during a 42-month period, which prompted experts to favor a Collis-Nissen repair, which demonstrated a 25% recurrence at 22 months postoperatively [116]. Mansour and Malone tried an array of fundoplication techniques to treat reflux in 11 SSc patients, and esophagitis reoccurred in all patients at a mean follow-up of 7.4 years [116].

Partial fundoplication procedures are becoming increasingly popular to treat GERD in SSc. During these procedures, the fundus of the stomach is wrapped to different degrees around the intraabdominal esophagus to strengthen the LES [115]. In a small study, four of five patients experienced a 90% improvement in GERD symptoms after undergoing the Dor fundoplication [115]. In a comparative cohort study, 17 patients with SSc were matched to 526 non-SSc patients, and they all underwent partial fundoplication [117]. Surgery was equally effective at controlling heartburn in both groups of patients, and satisfaction scores were comparable [117]. These results suggest that partial fundoplication procedures are safe and effective in SSc patients with medically refractory GERD.

5.5 Conclusion

While esophageal involvement can vary greatly in rheumatologic and vasculitis conditions, the resultant symptoms have a profound impact on quality of life. Pathophysiologic changes that precipitate the onset of symptoms differ from disease to disease, evident by differences in histopathology. It is also important to consider the secondary complications of rheumatologic diseases when managing patients with esophageal involvement. Multiple diagnostic imaging modalities are used for evaluation for esophageal symptoms; however, it is important to be cognizant of the clinical utility, sensitivity, and specificity of each test based on the patient's history and symptomatology. It is imperative to recognize esophageal symptoms such as acid reflux may be secondary to underlying rheumatologic disorders. Early recognition can help prevent disease progression and provide symptomatic and long-term relief through lifestyle, pharmacologic, and procedural interventions. Further studies of the underlying etiology and pathogenesis of GI manifestations in these conditions can lead to development of targeted therapy or repurposing of pipeline drugs used to treat rheumatologic conditions.

References

1. Yazaki E, Sifrim D. Anatomy and physiology of the esophageal body. Dis Esophagus. 2012;25(4):292–8.
2. Oezcelik A, DeMeester SR. General anatomy of the esophagus. Thorac Surg Clin. 2011;21(2):289–97.
3. Sasegbon A, Hamdy S. The anatomy and physiology of normal and abnormal swallowing in oropharyngeal dysphagia. Neurogastroenterol Motil. 2017;29(11).
4. Barrett KE, Barrett KE. Gastrointestinal physiology. 2nd ed. New York: McGraw Hill Medical Publishing Division; 2014.

5. Tack J, Pandolfino JE. Pathophysiology of gastroesophageal reflux disease. Gastroenterology. 2018;154(2):277–88.
6. Herregods TV, Bredenoord AJ, Smout AJ. Pathophysiology of gastroesophageal reflux disease: new understanding in a new era. Neurogastroenterol Motil. 2015;27(9):1202–13.
7. van Herwaarden MA, Samsom M, Smout AJ. Excess gastroesophageal reflux in patients with hiatus hernia is caused by mechanisms other than transient LES relaxations. Gastroenterology. 2000;119(6):1439–46.
8. Lin S, Ke M, Xu J, Kahrilas PJ. Impaired esophageal emptying in reflux disease. Am J Gastroenterol. 1994;89(7):1003–6.
9. McMahan ZH. Gastrointestinal involvement in systemic sclerosis: an update. Curr Opin Rheumatol. 2019;31(6):561–8.
10. Shreiner AB, Murray C, Denton C, Khanna D. Gastrointestinal manifestations of systemic sclerosis. J Scleroderma Relat Disord. 2016;1(3):247–56.
11. D'Angelo WA, Fries JF, Masi AT, Shulman LE. Pathologic observations in systemic sclerosis (scleroderma). A study of fifty-eight autopsy cases and fifty-eight matched controls. Am J Med. 1969;46(3):428–40.
12. Cohen S, Fisher R, Lipshutz W, Turner R, Myers A, Schumacher R. The pathogenesis of esophageal dysfunction in scleroderma and Raynaud's disease. J Clin Invest. 1972;51(10):2663–8.
13. Frech TM, Mar D. Gastrointestinal and hepatic disease in systemic sclerosis. Rheum Dis Clin N Am. 2018;44(1):15–28.
14. Sierakowska M, Doroszkiewicz H, Sierakowska J, Olesinska M, Grabowska-Jodkowska A, Brzosko M, et al. Factors associated with quality of life in systemic sclerosis: a cross-sectional study. Qual Life Res. 2019;28(12):3347–54.
15. McFarlane IM, Bhamra MS, Kreps A, Iqbal S, Al-Ani F, Saladini-Aponte C, et al. Gastrointestinal manifestations of systemic sclerosis. Rheumatology (Sunnyvale). 2018;8(1).
16. Montes RA, Mazolli Veiga N, Lanzieri PG, Mocarzel LO. Pulmonary disease secondary to reflux mimicking interstitial pneumonia in systemic sclerosis: case report and literature review. Case Rep Rheumatol. 2016;2016:5926327.
17. Denaxas K, Ladas SD, Karamanolis GP. Evaluation and management of esophageal manifestations in systemic sclerosis. Ann Gastroenterol. 2018;31(2):165–70.
18. Katzka DA, Reynolds JC, Saul SH, Plotkin A, Lang CA, Ouyang A, et al. Barrett's metaplasia and adenocarcinoma of the esophagus in scleroderma. Am J Med. 1987;82(1):46–52.
19. de Macedo AG, Bertges ER, Bertges LC, Mendes RA, Bertges T, Bertges KR, et al. Pemphigus vulgaris in the mouth and esophageal mucosa. Case Rep Gastroenterol. 2018;12(2):260–5.
20. Gannavarapu B, Hanson JA, Elwood H, Gavin M. Hard to swallow: a rare cause. Dig Dis Sci. 2015;60(9):2608–11.
21. Petre S, Shah IA, Gilani N. Review article: gastrointestinal amyloidosis—clinical features, diagnosis and therapy. Aliment Pharmacol Ther. 2008;27(11):1006–16.
22. Battle WM, Rubin MR, Cohen S, Snape WJ Jr. Gastrointestinal-motility dysfunction in amyloidosis. N Engl J Med. 1979;301(1):24–5.
23. Kapp JP. Hepatic amyloidosis with portal hypertension. JAMA. 1965;191:497–9.
24. Zuber-Jerger I, Muller A, Kullmann F, Gelbmann CM, Endlicher E, Muller-Ladner U, et al. Gastrointestinal manifestation of systemic sclerosis--thickening of the upper gastrointestinal wall detected by endoscopic ultrasound is a valid sign. Rheumatology (Oxford). 2010;49(2):368–72.
25. Petcu A, Ghib LJ, Grad SM, Popovici C, Rogojan L, Rednic NV, et al. Upper gastrointestinal involvement in systemic sclerosis: findings in a real-life setting. Exp Ther Med. 2019;18(6):5095–100.
26. Cowan AJ, Skinner M, Seldin DC, Berk JL, Lichtenstein DR, O'Hara CJ, et al. Amyloidosis of the gastrointestinal tract: a 13-year, single-center, referral experience. Haematologica. 2013;98(1):141–6.
27. Zeijen RN, Sels JP, Flendrig JA, Arends JW. Portal hypertension and intrahepatic cholestasis in hepatic amyloidosis. Neth J Med. 1991;38(5-6):257–61.

28. Heitzman EJ, Heitzman GC, Elliott CF. Primary esophageal amyloidosis. Report of a case with bleeding, perforation, and survival following resection. Arch Intern Med. 1962;109:595–600.
29. Tsokos GC. Systemic lupus erythematosus. N Engl J Med. 2011;365(22):2110–21.
30. Fortuna G, Brennan MT. Systemic lupus erythematosus: epidemiology, pathophysiology, manifestations, and management. Dent Clin N Am. 2013;57(4):631–55.
31. Ebert EC, Hagspiel KD. Gastrointestinal and hepatic manifestations of systemic lupus erythematosus. J Clin Gastroenterol. 2011;45(5):436–41.
32. Bailey M, Chapin W, Licht H, Reynolds JC. The effects of vasculitis on the gastrointestinal tract and liver. Gastroenterol Clin N Am. 1998;27(4):747–82, v–vi.
33. Peppercorn MA, Docken WP, Rosenberg S. Esophageal motor dysfunction in systemic lupus erythematosus. Two cases with unusual features. JAMA. 1979;242(17):1895–6.
34. Sultan SM, Ioannou Y, Isenberg DA. A review of gastrointestinal manifestations of systemic lupus erythematosus. Rheumatology (Oxford). 1999;38(10):917–32.
35. Chauhan K, Jandu JS, Goyal A, Bansal P, Al-Dhahir MA. Rheumatoid arthritis. StatPearls. Treasure Island: StatPearls Publishing. Copyright © 2021, StatPearls Publishing LLC; 2021.
36. Halabi H, AlDabbagh A, Alamoudi A. Gastrointestinal manifestations of rheumatic diseases. In: Almoallim H, Cheikh M, editors. Skills in rheumatology. Singapore: Springer; 2021. p. 475–99.
37. Craig E, Cappelli LC. Gastrointestinal and hepatic disease in rheumatoid arthritis. Rheum Dis Clin N Am. 2018;44(1):89–111.
38. Brito-Zeron P, Bari K, Baughman RP, Ramos-Casals M. Sarcoidosis involving the gastrointestinal tract: diagnostic and therapeutic management. Am J Gastroenterol. 2019;114(8):1238–47.
39. Abraham A, Hajar R, Virdi R, Singh J, Mustacchia P. Esophageal sarcoidosis: a review of cases and an update. ISRN Gastroenterol. 2013;2013:836203.
40. Rustagi T, Majumder S. Dysphagia and spontaneous esophageal perforation in sarcoidosis. Dig Dis Sci. 2013;58(1):282–5.
41. Schmidt J. Current classification and management of inflammatory myopathies. J Neuromuscul Dis. 2018;5(2):109–29.
42. Gadiparthi C, Hans A, Potts K, Ismail MK. Gastrointestinal and hepatic disease in the inflammatory myopathies. Rheum Dis Clin N Am. 2018;44(1):113–29.
43. Menon S, Trudgill N. Risk factors in the aetiology of hiatus hernia: a meta-analysis. Eur J Gastroenterol Hepatol. 2011;23(2):133–8.
44. Yen JL, Lin SP, Chen MR, Niu DM. Clinical features of Ehlers-Danlos syndrome. J Formos Med Assoc. 2006;105(6):475–80.
45. Callewaert B, Malfait F, Loeys B, De Paepe A. Ehlers-Danlos syndromes and Marfan syndrome. Best Pract Res Clin Rheumatol. 2008;22(1):165–89.
46. Nelson AD, Mouchli MA, Valentin N, Deyle D, Pichurin P, Acosta A, et al. Ehlers Danlos syndrome and gastrointestinal manifestations: a 20-year experience at Mayo Clinic. Neurogastroenterol Motil. 2015;27(11):1657–66.
47. Curci JA, Melman LM, Thompson RW, Soper NJ, Matthews BD. Elastic fiber depletion in the supporting ligaments of the gastroesophageal junction: a structural basis for the development of hiatal hernia. J Am Coll Surg. 2008;207(2):191–6.
48. Beckers AB, Keszthelyi D, Fikree A, Vork L, Masclee A, Farmer AD, et al. Gastrointestinal disorders in joint hypermobility syndrome/Ehlers-Danlos syndrome hypermobility type: a review for the gastroenterologist. Neurogastroenterol Motil. 2017;29(8).
49. van der Peet DL, Klinkenberg-Knol EC, Berends FJ, Cuesta MA. Epiphrenic diverticula: minimal invasive approach and repair in five patients. Dis Esophagus. 2001;14(1):60–2.
50. Carsons SE, Patel BC. Sjogren syndrome. StatPearls. Treasure Island; 2021.
51. Sheikh SH, Shaw-Stiffel TA. The gastrointestinal manifestations of Sjogren's syndrome. Am J Gastroenterol. 1995;90(1):9–14.

52. Chun-Yu Lin K-LW, Yao C-C, Tsai C-E, Tai W-C, Liang C-M, Chou Y-P, Chuah S-K. Clinical characteristics and esophageal motility in Sjögren's syndrome: a single-center study in Taiwan. Adv Digest Med. 2021;8:218–23.
53. Wynder EL, Hultberg S, Jacobsson F, Bross IJ. Environmental factors in cancer of the upper alimentary tract; a Swedish study with special reference to Plummer-Vinson (Paterson-Kelly) syndrome. Cancer. 1957;10(3):470–87.
54. Hoffman RM, Jaffe PE, Plummer-Vinson syndrome. A case report and literature review. Arch Intern Med. 1995;155(18):2008–11.
55. Verma S, Mukherjee S. Plummer Vinson Syndrome. StatPearls. Treasure Island; 2021.
56. Chisholm M. The association between webs, iron and post-cricoid carcinoma. Postgrad Med J. 1974;50(582):215–9.
57. Messmann H. Squamous cell cancer of the oesophagus. Best Pract Res Clin Gastroenterol. 2001;15(2):249–65.
58. Greidinger EL. Chapter 48—Overlap syndromes. In: Tsokos GC, editor. Systemic lupus erythematosus. Boston: Academic; 2016. p. 425–30.
59. Pepmueller PH. Undifferentiated connective tissue disease, mixed connective tissue disease, and overlap syndromes in rheumatology. Mo Med. 2016;113(2):136–40.
60. Sapkota B, Al Khalili Y. Mixed connective tissue disease. StatPearls. Treasure Island; 2021.
61. Gyorffy JB, Marowske J, Gancayco J. A rare cause of dysphagia and weight loss. Case Rep Gastroenterol. 2018;12(3):640–5.
62. Luo TD, Varacallo M. Diffuse idiopathic skeletal hyperostosis. StatPearls. Treasure Island; 2021.
63. Karaarslan N, Gurbuz MS, Caliskan T, Simsek AT. Forestier syndrome presenting with dysphagia: case report of a rare presentation. J Spine Surg. 2017;3(4):723–6.
64. Westermark P. Aspects on human amyloid forms and their fibril polypeptides. FEBS J. 2005;272(23):5942–9.
65. Levine RA. Amyloid disease of the liver. Correlation of clinical, functional and morphologic features in forty-seven patients. Am J Med. 1962;33:349–57.
66. Serra L, Poppi MC, Criscuolo M, Zandomeneghi R. Primary systemic amyloidosis with giant hepatomegaly and portal hypertension: a case report and a review of the literature. Ital J Gastroenterol. 1993;25(8):435–8.
67. Al-Janabi A, Greenfield S. Pemphigus vulgaris: a rare cause of dysphagia. BMJ Case Rep. 2015;2015.
68. Leal C, Silva M, Barbeiro S, Vasconcelos H. Pemphigus vulgaris presenting as esophageal ulceration. Report of an underdiagnosed manifestation. Acta Gastroenterol Belg. 2021;84(2):365–6.
69. Charlton OA, Harris V, Phan K, Mewton E, Jackson C, Cooper A. Toxic epidermal necrolysis and Steven-Johnson syndrome: a comprehensive review. Adv Wound Care (New Rochelle). 2020;9(7):426–39.
70. Brown CS, Defazio JR, An G, O'Connor A, Whitcomb E, Hart J, et al. Toxic epidermal necrolysis with gastrointestinal involvement: a case report and review of the literature. J Burn Care Res. 2017;38(1):e450–e5.
71. Bakshi SS. Stevens-Johnson syndrome. Intern Emerg Med. 2019;14(2):323–4.
72. Clayton NA, Kennedy PJ. Management of dysphagia in toxic epidermal necrolysis (TEN) and Stevens-Johnson syndrome (SJS). Dysphagia. 2007;22(3):187–92.
73. Gendreau S, Amiot A, Le Baleur Y, Charpy C, Wolkenstein P, Chosidow O, et al. Gastrointestinal involvement in Stevens-Johnson syndrome and toxic epidermal necrolysis: a retrospective case series. Br J Dermatol. 2019;180(5):1234–5.
74. Chen H, Li C, Ye W, Ye W, Xu H, Jiang Q, et al. Henoch-Schonlein purpura in a patient with oesophageal cancer: a case report. Medicine (Baltimore). 2020;99(49):e23492.
75. Mir O, Nazal EM, Cohen P, Vignaux O, Krivitzky A, Christoforov B, et al. Esophageal involvement as an initial manifestation of Churg-Strauss syndrome. Presse Med. 2007;36(1 Pt 1):57–60.

76. Alexander S, Simon EG, Burad D, Varughese S, David VG, Jacob S, et al. Esophageal vasculitis in granulomatosis with polyangiitis. Trop Gastroenterol. 2015;36(2):132–4.
77. Garlapati P, Qurie A. Granulomatosis with polyangiitis. StatPearls. Treasure Island; 2021.
78. Fallows GA, Hamilton SF, Taylor DS, Reddy SB. Esophageal involvement in Wegener's granulomatosis: a case report and review of the literature. Can J Gastroenterol. 2000;14(5):449–51.
79. Roache-Robinson P, Hotwagner DT. Henoch Schonlein Purpura. StatPearls. Treasure Island; 2021.
80. Weiler-Bisig D, Ettlin G, Brink T, Arnold W, Glatz-Krieger K, Fischer A. Henoch-schonlein purpura associated with esophagus carcinoma and adenocarcinoma of the lung. Clin Nephrol. 2005;63(4):302–4.
81. Adil A, Goyal A, Bansal P, Quint JM. Behcet disease. StatPearls. Treasure Island; 2021.
82. Yi SW, Cheon JH, Kim JH, Lee SK, Kim TI, Lee YC, et al. The prevalence and clinical characteristics of esophageal involvement in patients with Behcet's disease: a single center experience in Korea. J Korean Med Sci. 2009;24(1):52–6.
83. Kokturk A. Clinical and pathological manifestations with differential diagnosis in Behcet's disease. Pathol Res Int. 2012;2012:690390.
84. Kliemann DA, Pasqualotto AC, Falavigna M, Giaretta T, Severo LC. Candida esophagitis: species distribution and risk factors for infection. Rev Inst Med Trop Sao Paulo. 2008;50(5):261–3.
85. Walsh TJ, Hamilton SR, Belitsos N, Esophageal candidiasis. Managing an increasingly prevalent infection. Postgrad Med. 1988;84(2):193–6, 201–5.
86. Ebert EC. Esophageal disease in scleroderma. J Clin Gastroenterol. 2006;40(9):769–75.
87. Adarsh MB, Sharma SK, Sinha SK, Bhattacharya A, Rana S, Dhir V, et al. Gastrointestinal dysmotility and infections in systemic sclerosis- an Indian scenario. Curr Rheumatol Rev. 2018;14(2):172–6.
88. Natsui K, Tsuchiya A, Terai S. Refractory hemorrhagic esophageal ulcers by Candida esophagitis with advanced systemic sclerosis. JGH Open. 2020;4(5):1007–8.
89. Schottstedt V, Blümel J, Burger R, Drosten C, Gröner A, Gürtler L, et al. Human Cytomegalovirus (HCMV)—revised. Transfus Med Hemother. 2010;37(6):365–75.
90. Li L, Chakinala RC. Cytomegalovirus esophagitis. StatPearls. Treasure Island; 2022.
91. Gupta M, Shorman M. Cytomegalovirus. StatPearls. Treasure Island; 2022.
92. Eymard D, Martin L, Doummar G, Piché J. Herpes simplex esophagitis in immunocompetent hosts. Can J Infect Dis. 1997;8(6):351–3.
93. Canalejo E, García Durán F, Cabello N, García Martínez J. Herpes esophagitis in healthy adults and adolescents: report of 3 cases and review of the literature. Medicine (Baltimore). 2010;89(4):204–10.
94. Zografos GN, Georgiadou D, Thomas D, Kaltsas G, Digalakis M. Drug-induced esophagitis. Dis Esophagus. 2009;22(8):633–7.
95. Carlborg B, Densert O, Lindqvist C. Tetracycline induced esophageal ulcers. a clinical and experimental study. Laryngoscope. 1983;93(2):184–7.
96. de Groen PC, Lubbe DF, Hirsch LJ, Daifotis A, Stephenson W, Freedholm D, et al. Esophagitis associated with the use of alendronate. N Engl J Med. 1996;335(14):1016–21.
97. Saleem F, Sharma A. Drug induced esophagitis. StatPearls. Treasure Island; 2020.
98. Jaspersen D. Drug-induced oesophageal disorders: pathogenesis, incidence, prevention and management. Drug Saf. 2000;22(3):237–49.
99. Ratuapli SK, Crowell MD, DiBaise JK, Vela MF, Ramirez FC, Burdick GE, et al. Opioid-induced esophageal dysfunction (OIED) in patients on chronic opioids. Am J Gastroenterol. 2015;110(7):979–84.
100. Snyder DL, Crowell MD, Horsley-Silva J, Ravi K, Lacy BE, Vela MF. Opioid-induced esophageal dysfunction: differential effects of type and dose. Am J Gastroenterol. 2019;114(9):1464–9.

101. Sanchez MJ, Olivier S, Gediklioglu F, Almeida M, Gaeta M, Nigro M, et al. Chronic opioid use is associated with obstructive and spastic disorders in the esophagus. Neurogastroenterol Motil. 2022;34(3):e14233.
102. Levine MS, Rubesin SE. Diseases of the esophagus: diagnosis with esophagography. Radiology. 2005;237(2):414–27.
103. Ahlawat R, Hoilat GJ, Ross AB. Esophagogastroduodenoscopy. StatPearls. Treasure Island; 2021.
104. Committee ASoP, Early DS, Ben-Menachem T, Decker GA, Evans JA, Fanelli RD, et al. Appropriate use of GI endoscopy. Gastrointest Endosc. 2012;75(6):1127–31.
105. Yazaki E, Woodland P, Sifrim D. Uses of esophageal function testing: dysphagia. Gastrointest Endosc Clin N Am. 2014;24(4):643–54.
106. Klein HA. Esophageal transit scintigraphy. Semin Nucl Med. 1995;25(4):306–17.
107. Jamieson JR, Stein HJ, DeMeester TR, Bonavina L, Schwizer W, Hinder RA, et al. Ambulatory 24-h esophageal pH monitoring: normal values, optimal thresholds, specificity, sensitivity, and reproducibility. Am J Gastroenterol. 1992;87(9):1102–11.
108. Sifrim D, Fornari F. Esophageal impedance-pH monitoring. Dig Liver Dis. 2008;40(3):161–6.
109. Eyigor S. Dysphagia in rheumatological disorders. World J Rheumathol. 2013;3(3):45–50.
110. Wheeler-Hegland K, Ashford J, Frymark T, McCabe D, Mullen R, Musson N, et al. Evidence-based systematic review: Oropharyngeal dysphagia behavioral treatments. Part II—impact of dysphagia treatment on normal swallow function. J Rehabil Res Dev. 2009;46(2).
111. Chilukuri P, Odufalu F, Hachem C. Dysphagia. Mo Med. 2018;115(3):206–10.
112. Desai JP, Moustarah F. Esophageal stricture. StatPearls. Treasure Island: StatPearls Publishing. Copyright © 2022, StatPearls Publishing LLC; 2022.
113. Shama L, Connor NP, Ciucci MR, McCulloch TM. Surgical treatment of dysphagia. Phys Med Rehabil Clin N Am. 2008;19(4):817–35. ix
114. Seeras K, Bittar K, Siccardi MA. Nissen fundoplication. StatPearls. Treasure Island; 2022.
115. Loganathan P, Gajendran M, Davis B, McCallum R. Efficacy and safety of robotic dor fundoplication on severe gastroesophageal reflux disease in patients with scleroderma. J Investig Med High Impact Case Rep. 2021;9:23247096211051211.
116. Bakhos CT, Petrov RV, Parkman HP, Malik Z, Abbas AE. Role and safety of fundoplication in esophageal disease and dysmotility syndromes. J Thorac Dis. 2019;11(Suppl 12):S1610–S7.
117. Hii A, Liu DS, Kholmurodova F, Irvine T, Bright T, Watson DI, et al. Partial fundoplication is effective treatment for female patients with gastroesophageal reflux and scleroderma: a multicenter comparative cohort study. World J Surg. 2022;46(1):147–53.

Chapter 6
Gastric Diseases in Rheumatology

Amjad Waseem, Ethan Pearlstein, Dharma Ayer, and Asra Batool

Rheumatic diseases (RD) can involve any organ in the body, including the stomach. It can be challenging to diagnose RD based upon gastric manifestations because the presentation can be nonspecific, slowly progressive and intermittent [1]. The chronicity and severity of the disease can be debilitating. The gastrointestinal manifestations during the course of RD are insidious, which can delay the diagnosis [2]. The common mechanisms leading to gastric symptoms involve systemic inflammation, disrupted motility, autonomic nervous system impairment, vascular damage, smooth muscle atrophy and fibrosis [3, 4].

It is important to identify the RD which can alter gastric physiology. The known gastric pathologies seen in these patients are gastroparesis, Gastric Antral Vascular Ectasia (GAVE), arteriovenous malformation (AVM) and gastric diseases due to chronic non-steroidal anti-inflammatory drugs (NSAIDS) [5]. The literature lacks prospective studies and systematic reviews on gastric pathology in RD. The impact of bariatric surgery on RD will also be discussed later in this chapter.

A. Waseem
Albany Medical Center, Albany, NY, USA

E. Pearlstein
Gastro Health, Miami, FL, USA

D. Ayer
Albany Medical College, Albany, NY, USA

A. Batool (✉)
Wellstar Gastroenterology, Marietta, GA, USA

M. Tadros et al. (eds.), *GI Diseases Associated with Rheumatological and Vasculitic Conditions*, Clinical Gastroenterology,
https://doi.org/10.1007/978-3-032-07868-1_6

6.1 Gastric Antral Vascular Ectasia (GAVE)

Gastric antral vascular ectasia (GAVE) is uncommon but can present with major upper gastrointestinal (GI) bleeding. A retrospective study showed that 4% of cases of nonvariceal upper GI bleeding are due to GAVE with or without portal hypertension [6]. The majority of these cases are idiopathic and the known etiologies include cirrhosis and systemic sclerosis (SSc) [7]. A case series showed that 5.7% of SSc patients had watermelon stomach [8]. Other comorbid conditions with possible association to GAVE include chronic kidney disease, ischemic heart disease, bone marrow transplantation and valvular heart disease [9]. GAVE is diagnosed based upon the characteristic appearance of longitudinal rugal folds or stripes radiating toward the pylorus with each fold containing convoluted vessels, with an appearance similar to a watermelon. These stripes constitute areas of vascular malformation [10]. It can also present as a coalescence of gastric angiodysplasias in the antrum, called 'honeycomb stomach' [8]. The presence of portal hypertension (PH) is associated with more diffuse vascular malformation. The characteristic biopsy findings are gastric ectasia, vasodilation, thrombi, fibrohylanosis and increased spindle cells [9]. GAVE is more prevalent in early diffuse cutaneous SSc and late onset anti-centromere positive limited cutaneous SSc. The presence of rapidly progressing cutaneous SSc or positive RNA polymerase III antibodies may suggest early development of GAVE [11]. In a small study, the median time interval from SSc diagnosis to GAVE was 3 years [8]. This suggests that SSc patients with iron deficiency anemia or gastric symptoms should undergo endoscopic evaluation to identify GAVE.

6.1.1 Pathophysiology

The exact mechanism underlying the development of vascular ectasias is poorly understood. Cutaneous telangiectasia is seen commonly with GAVE and SSc, and a few of these cases have coexisting GI telangiectasia. The histological appearance of gastric and cutaneous telangiectasias is similar, and the presence of GAVE may rarely be the presenting sign of SSc [8]. SSc and CREST syndrome are connective tissue diseases, and can involve microvascular dysfunction. Endothelial cell dysfunction is also demonstrated in those with no cutaneous disease manifestations, which suggests microvascular disease progression before the onset of clinical symptoms [12]. Studies examining GI disease in SSc show lower mucosal blood flow, which can lead to tissue hypoxia in the stomach [13]. SSc causes vascular damage and submucosal ischemia in the setting of poor gastric motility, which can be explained by the histological presence of fibromuscular hyperplasia, capillary dilation in the lamina propria and thrombi [3, 8, 14].

The presence of GAVE in SSc could be immune mediated, as literature shows clinical improvement in sporadic cases with the use of cyclophosphamide [15, 16].

The anti scl-70 Ab and anti-U1 ribonucleoprotein (RNP) are negative in the presence of GAVE whereas anti-RNA pol III may remain positive in a few cases [17, 18]. It is proposed that cross reaction of these antibodies against gastric mucosal proteins can lead to vascular dysfunction and the clinical findings of GAVE [19].

6.2 Arteriovenous Malformation

Gastric arteriovenous malformation (AVM) is a rarer cause of upper GI bleeding. GAVE is associated with abnormal vasodilation, ectasia, thrombosis and fibrinolysis in the blood vessel walls, whereas AVM causes an abnormal shunt between the arteries and veins which bypass the capillary bed; therefore, this direct communication can complicate the oxygen supply to the tissue and occasionally present as major hemorrhage [9, 20]. Other vascular malformations seen in the stomach are angiodysplasia, and hemangioma. AVMs are usually diagnosed on endoscopy or angiography [21]. The endoscopic management of AVMs can be challenging. AVM's can present endoscopically as flat red, telangiectatic or submucosal nodular lesions [21]. AVMs are classified into one of three patterns: I (flat and red lesions), II (telangiectatic form) and III (submucosal nodular form); the latter is associated with a higher risk of acute gastrointestinal bleeding. A retrospective study shows that mucosal telangiectasias were one of the common causes of upper gastrointestinal bleeding in SSc and calcinosis, Raynaud's phenomenon, esophageal disease, sclerodactyly, and limited scleroderma (CREST) syndrome [13]. There can be misuse of the term AVM for other GI mucosal lesions, including angioma, angioectasia and telangiectasia [22].

6.2.1 *Pathophysiology*

The AVM is a congenital lesion caused by the incomplete maturation of the vascular plexus of the gastrointestinal tract and can present later in life, with bleeding. The arteries are directly connected to the veins which causes relatively high pressures, and can lead to major bleeding. Early literature on AVMs suggests an acquired nature of these lesions which are more common in the elderly population. Degeneration of the GI wall and increased tension can lead to these vascular abnormalities [23]. Another report states that AVMs are a congenital lesion which can grow with aging [22]. The smaller lesions can be treated with endoscopic ablation, and the larger lesions can be treated surgically [22]. Hypoxia due to intermittent vascular obstruction can lead to congestion of the capillaries. This congestion causes induction of neovascular growth factors including vascular endothelial growth factor (VEGF) and basic fibroblast growth factor (bFGF), and formation of collaterals [24]. High expression of VEGF is reported in angiodysplasia which can serve as a therapeutic target for the AVM [25]. Thalidomide, which has antiangiogenic properties, and suppresses neovascular growth factors, shows efficacy in the treatment of refractory bleeding from gastrointestinal vascular malformation [26].

6.3 Gastroparesis

Gastroparesis (GP) is a complex, debilitating disorder, usually presenting with postprandial fullness or abdominal pain, nausea, and vomiting. Gastroparesis is characterized by delayed gastric emptying in the absence of mechanical obstruction [27]. Most cases of gastroparesis are not diagnosed. The Olmstead community study showed an estimated prevalence of gastroparesis of nearly 2%, which was higher than the national prevalence; therefore, the identified cases can be considered the tip of the iceberg [28]. The etiologies of gastroparesis include diabetes mellitus, postsurgical, neuromuscular disease, post infectious, drug induced, and idiopathic [27]. Gastroparesis is common among RD, including SSc, polymyositis, dermatomyositis, and systemic lupus erythematosus (SLE) [1, 29]. Gastroparesis is seen in most SSc patients (50–75%) and can be a major cause of discomfort in these patients [30, 31]. These disorders not only effect the motility of the GI tract, but also absorption of vital nutrients [13].

Poor oral intake in gastroparesis patients can lead to malnutrition, which causes frequent hospitalizations and increases the disease burden on the health system [32–34]. The Rochester Epidemiology project shows that gastroparesis was associated with a higher rate of mortality than the general population (33% in 5 years) [35]. The solid gastric emptying scintigraphy test is the most utilized diagnostic test. Based on the Togas protocol [36], a gastric retention rate of >10% at 4 h is used to identify gastroparesis patients. Wireless capsule gastric motility testing is used in patients who are unable to tolerate the gastric emptying test meal [37]. The Carbon radiolabeled breath test is another alternative diagnostic modality [38].

Management of gastroparesis in RD is not different from the general population, and includes dietary modification with small meal portions, and a diet low in fat and fiber. In a few cases, liquid emptying is preserved, and the intake of nutrients and appropriate calories in liquid form is recommended. For those who cannot tolerate a solid or liquid diet, alternatives may include tube feeding or total parenteral nutrition. The use of alcohol, cigarette smoking and carbonated drinks should be discouraged as these can worsen gastric emptying [32, 39, 40]. Better glycemic control in those with diabetes mellitus is recommended and amylin analogs and glucagon like peptide-1 agonists can worsen gastric emptying; therefore, alternative hypoglycemic agents should be considered [41, 42]. Prokinetic agents including metoclopramide, domperidone and erythromycin alongside anti-nausea and non-opiate pain medications can be used for treatment. If the above measures fail, additional interventions, including botulinum injection, gastroesophageal stimulator implantation, pyloroplasty, venting gastrostomy and partial gastrectomy should be considered [27].

6.3.1 Pathophysiology

The strict regulation of emptying of semi-digested food (chyme) from the stomach to the small intestine is crucial for the digestion of food and absorption of nutrients, as this process is a complex interplay of signals from the nervous system and the intrinsic gut hormones. Inhibitory and excitatory neurons in the nucleus tractus solitarius are responsible for sending signals through vagus motor circuits and thereby control gastric emptying [43]. The small intestine releases hormones as feedback responses which can also affect gastric emptying. Ghrelin and motilin are accelerating peptides and stimulate gastrointestinal motility, whereas leptin, cholecystokinin, glucagon like peptide-1, peptide PYY, oxyntomodulin, gastrin releasing peptide, pancreatic amylin and pancreatic polypeptide are inhibitory and slow gastric motility [44]. The gastric emptying rate depends on food volume, chemical composition and energy density [45]. The gastric fundus and proximal body serve as a pressure pump, the distal body and antrum function as a peristaltic pump, and the pylorus grinds the tenderized food and converts it into chyme. Liquids can bypass solid food along the lesser curvature via a functional canal, "*magenstrasse*", and therefore have relatively faster gastric emptying [44, 46]. The impaired relaxation of the pressure pump and pylorus, and the decreased strength of the peristaltic pump is associated with delayed gastric emptying [47]. Increased relaxation of the pylorus leads to the duodeno-gastric reflux and reduced relaxation, which causes gastric outlet obstruction [48]. During the inter-digestive phase, the low amplitude waves in the antrum and phasic large contractions move the residual food towards the pylorus [49]. The interstitial cells of Cajal (ICC), or pacemaker cells, play a major role in gastric emptying by affecting the activity of smooth muscle [43]. The ICC are electrically active cells which generate slow waves, and these slow waves lead to a contractility response via activated smooth muscle channels including L-type calcium. The ICC determine the contractility strength and frequency, and interact with the enteric nerves to generate inhibitory and excitatory responses which result in smooth muscle contractility and relaxation [50]. Neuronal Nitric oxide synthetase (nNOS) in enteric nerves produce nitric oxide (NO), which causes relaxation of the longitudinal and circular smooth muscles of the pylorus [51]. The sympathetic nervous system does not play an important role in controlling gastric motility. The vagus nerve controls stomach emptying via non-cholinergic inhibitory and cholinergic excitatory circuits.

The proposed pathophysiology of gastroparesis includes the extrinsic denervation and altered function of immune cells, leading to damage of ICC and smooth muscles. Decreased function of ICC leads to decreased smooth muscle contractility [27]. The Grover M. et al. study showed a decreased number of ICC in gastroparesis. The number of ICC were inversely related to the level of gastric retention in diabetics, and the presence of myenteric immune infiltrates in idiopathic gastroparesis was associated with severity of symptoms [52]. A study based on the The NIDDK Gastroparesis Clinical Research Consortium showed that ICC damage was greater in idiopathic gastroparesis, and that the loss of kit gene expression and increased CD45 and CD68 immunoreactivity was seen in gastroparesis [53]. The inhibition of nNOS can also lead to increased tension in the pylorus which delays gastric motility [54, 55].

The exact mechanism of gastroparesis in RD is not certain. An immune infiltrate leading to inflammatory cell activation seems to be the most agreed upon mechanism. Systemic inflammation can cause ICC damage, smooth muscle atrophy and inhibition of pylorus relaxation. Vascular involvement can cause intermittent ischemia, which leads to hypoxic neuropathy that can affect gastric motility [56]. Immune system activation can lead to the production of antibodies against muscarinic receptor mediated cholinergic neurotransmission [57, 58]. Autonomic dysfunction, smooth muscle damage, and fibrotic tissue are formed in the stomach wall, and lead to progressive and refractory disease [59]. Electrophysiologic, proteomic and histological studies are recommended in animal models and patients with rheumatological diseases to better understand the pathogenesis.

6.4 Henoch-Schönlein Purpura and *Helicobacter pylori* Infection

Henoch- Schönlein purpura (HSP) is commonly seen in children under 10 years of age and uncommonly in adults. It is an immune complex mediated vasculitis which typically presents with palpable purpura, abdominal pain and arthritis. Most cases of HSP resolve spontaneously and are treated supportively, while a minority of cases can lead to renal disease [60]. Historically, there is an observed association between HSP and *Helicobacter pylori* (*H. pylori)* infection, which is reported predominantly in Chinese studies, and eradication of the infection leads to decreased recurrence [61–63]. Those patients with HSP who present with epigastric pain and bloating should be screened for *H. pylori* infection.

6.4.1 Pathophysiology

The exact mechanism of HSP in *H. pylori* is unclear. The clinical manifestations of HSP are due to leukocytoclastic vasculitis with deposition of IgA, activated complements and fibrin/fibrinogen. IgA1 plays an important role in the pathogenesis of HSP, and the pathogens which induce type III allergic reactions are associated with high IgA1 levels and hence lead to systematic vasculitis [64, 65].

H. pylori mainly infects the gastric mucosa. It invades the gastric mucosa and activates the humoral and cellular immunity to attack the bacterial antigen and neutralize the toxin. It is possible that this immune response produces extra-gastrointestinal immune complexes which can lead to autoimmunity [66]. A small retrospective study shows the presence of high *H. pylori* IgG in the acute phase of HSP and high IgA levels in the chronic phase of the disease [67].

6.5 Hiatal Hernia

Hiatal hernia is a condition when the abdominal contents, mainly gastroesophageal junction (GEJ) and part of the proximal stomach slides through the esophageal hiatus into the thoracic cavity [68]. Normally the phreno-esophageal membrane anchors the distal portion of the esophagus and prevents the displacement of GEJ or stomach into the mediastinum [69]. The hiatal hernia can be sliding/axial and para-esophageal, and can be divided into four types. Type I is the sliding hernia which is the most common type. In the type I sliding hernia, GEJ and part of the stomach (cardia) slides above the diaphragm. The type II hernia is para-esophageal, where the gastric fundus slides into the thoracic cavity and the GEJ is not herniated. The type III hernia includes a paraoesophageal hernia with GEJ displacement above the diaphragm and the type IV hernia includes other intraabdominal organs, including the spleen and pancreas which slide into the posterior mediastinum [70]. Hiatal hernia is more commonly seen in patients with systemic sclerosis and Ehlers-Danlos syndrome (EDS) [71–75].

6.5.1 Pathophysiology

The endothoracic and endo-abdominal fascia form a phreno-esophageal ligament which inserts into the esophagus circumferentially. The phreno-esophageal ligament secures the esophagus and prevents the GEJ and abdominal contents from entering into the posterior mediastinum [76]. During swallowing, the longitudinal muscles of the esophagus contract, the esophagus shortens, and the phreno-esophageal membrane stretches. When food is swallowed, the membrane recoils and the abdominal organs are prevented from entering the thoracic cavity [77]. The phreno-esophageal ligament can lose elasticity due to age, pregnancy, genetic predisposition and intensive exercise, which can lead to sliding of the GEJ and stomach into the mediastinum [70].

EDS is associated with deformity of collagen fibers in the extracellular matrix, which leads to weakness and laxity of the diaphragm and phreno-esophageal ligament, and is a possible cause of hiatal hernia [78, 79]. The literature also shows sporadic cases of spontaneous rupture of the diaphragm, causing herniation of abdominal contents into the thoracic cavity [80, 81]. Systemic sclerosis leads to a structural alteration of the esophagus, and the muscle atrophy leads to decreased tone, dilation of the esophagus, an incompetent lower esophageal sphincter and hiatal hernia.

6.6 Gastric Ulcer

Peptic ulcer disease (PUD) is acid related mucosal damage which is commonly located in the stomach and proximal duodenum and is predominantly caused by non-steroidal anti-inflammatory drugs (NSAIDs) and *Helicobacter pylori* infection. The lifetime prevalence of PUD in the general population is estimated to be 5–10%, whereas incidence is 0.1–0.3% per year [82]. GI bleeding can be the presenting complaint in 15–20% of PUD cases and can lead to surgery or death in this population. NSAIDs are commonly used in RD, which will be discussed later in detail. PUD is also associated with rheumatoid arthritis (RA), SLE and polyarteritis nodosa [83–86].

6.6.1 Pathophysiology

The gastric mucosa is able to sustain a high proton concentration with a pH of 1–2 due to a protective gastric mucosal surface composed of two mucus layers [87]. The inner attached mucus (MUC5AC) is produced by the endothelial cells, which acts as barrier to hydrochloric acid and luminal pepsin. The sodium bicarbonate produced by the epithelial cells also serve as a protective mechanism against hydrochloric acid by neutralizing the mucosal surface [88]. Hydrochloric acid is produced with pepsin and MUC6, and it is able to cross the mucus membrane through temporary canals which are immediately closed [89]. MUC6 also forms the inner mucus membrane and adds to the protection against the gastric acid [90].

The microvascular lesions in SSc can cause damage of the gastric endothelium leading to ulcer formation [13]. Polyarteritis nodosa is a focal segmental necrotizing vasculitis which involves medium sized arteries. Immune complex deposition in the arteries leads to inflammation, edema and eventually necrosis of the tunica intima, media, ulcers and perforation [86].

6.7 Atrophic Gastritis

Atrophic gastritis is a chronic inflammatory condition which is characterized by the loss of glandular structure and secretory function. The mucosal surface is either replaced by scarring or glandular tissue in an unsuitable location which is called metaplasia and is associated with *H. pylori* infection and autoimmune conditions. Atrophic gastritis can present with iron deficiency anemia, megaloblastic anemia, hyperhomocysteinemia and peripheral neuropathy [91]. Atrophic gastritis can also lead to delayed gastric emptying [92]. Additionally, atrophic gastritis is a risk factor for gastric cancer [93–95]. Atrophic gastritis is commonly associated with Sjogren syndrome, and should be considered in those patients presenting with epigastric pain, nausea and other dyspeptic symptoms [96–101].

A Japanese study shows that atrophic gastritis in SSc could be induced by H. pylori infection, and that H. pylori infection was associated with mucosal damage due to the parietal cell antibody [102]. *H. pylori* gastritis can be divided into type A (localized to the gastric body), type B (gastric antrum) and type AB (both gastric body and antrum). A small study shows decreased acid secretion in type A and AB infection, compared to increased gastrin levels in type A [103].

6.7.1 Pathophysiology

The parietal cell in the gastric mucosa produces hydrochloric acid and intrinsic factor. The parietal cell antibodies attack these cells in autoimmune gastritis, leading to hypochlorhydria (increased pH) and decreased intrinsic factor production, leading to poor absorption of iron and vitamin B12.

The exact mechanism of autoimmune gastritis in Sjogren syndrome patients is unclear. The complement dependent cytotoxic activity of anti-parietal antibodies and the subsequent loss of parietal cells from the gastric mucosa may be one possible mechanism of atrophic gastirits [104]. The loss of parietal cells via this mechanism does not explain the pathology in antibody negative autoimmune gastritis nor does it explain the presence of disease in immunodeficient individuals. In these situations, the autoimmune diseases are likely mediated by the CD4 T cells [105]. Most of these auto-reactive cells are located in the gastric mucosa, exhibit phenotype T_H17 (T helper cells) and T_H1, and secrete IL-21 and tumor necrosis factor (TNF) [106]. Patients with pernicious anemia have also shown the presence of IgG4 producing plasma cells in the gastric mucosa [107].

The enterochromaffin cells (ECL) induce the production of acid and intrinsic factor via histamine. Due to atrophy of the gastric mucosa, parietal cell damage causes hyperplasia of ECL cells, which is initially linear but can advance to nodular hyperplasia and type 1 neuroendocrine tumor (NET) [106].

6.8 Amyloidosis

Localized gastric amyloidosis is very uncommon. A retrospective study shows that among gastrointestinal local amyloidosis, type ALλ is the most common, followed by transthyretin (ATTR) and type serum amyloid A (AA) [108]. Amyloidosis is rarely associated with chronic inflammatory conditions like RA, where serum amyloid protein A (AA) can be deposited in the intestinal wall [109]. Approximately 0.6–1.1% of rheumatoid arthritis patients can develop this form of reactive AA amyloidosis [110, 111]. Amyloidosis of the stomach presents with upper gastrointestinal bleeding and delayed gastric motility [109], and can be a diagnostic challenge because of the variable presentation. Amyloidosis in such cases is managed by treatment of the underlying inflammatory condition [112, 113].

6.8.1 Pathophysiology

Extracellular proteins misfold and get deposited as toxic protein aggregate in the gastrointestinal wall [114]. In chronic inflammatory conditions, cytokines leads to the production of acute phase reactant serum protein A (AA) by the liver. The serum protein A leads to aggregation of amyloid into β-sheet fibrillar sheets [115], and deposition of these AA proteins in the gastric wall leads to organ damage.

6.9 Steroid Use and Gastropathy

The glucocorticoids are commonly used in inflammatory and autoimmune diseases. The use of steroids has increased in the field of rheumatology in the last few decades. A large European study shows shown that long term steroid use has increased in rheumatoid arthritis from use in 10.3% of patients in 1989 to 13.6% in 2008 and from 57.6% to 66.5% of patients in polymyalgia rheumatica/giant cell arteritis [116]. Long term steroid use is associated with several adverse outcomes. The association of steroid use and peptic ulcer disease is controversial and there is still a thought that steroid use is ulcerogenic [117]. Steroid use can lead to an increased risk of GI bleeding and perforation in the inpatient setting, and this could be due to use of higher doses and addition of other factors contributing to peptic ulcer formation [118, 119].

6.9.1 Pathophysiology

The mucosal surface in the stomach protects the epithelium from pepsin induced proteolytic damage. Additionally, bicarbonate is secreted in the adherent mucosal surface, protecting the epithelium from the damage of luminal acid [88]. Steroids reduce bicarbonate and mucus production and as a result, the natural defense mechanism is impaired. Steroids also decrease the gastric protective prostaglandins and increase leukotriene production, which damages gastric mucosa [120]. Angiogenesis is impaired in these patients, leading to impaired regeneration and ulcer healing [121, 122].

6.10 Nonsteroidal Anti-inflammatory Drugs Gastropathy

Nonsteroidal anti-inflammatory drugs (NSAIDs) are exceedingly used for symptom relief in rheumatoid arthritis patients. It is estimated that this class of medication is used daily by almost 30 million people, and this number continues to rise as the medicine is readily available over the counter [123]. These agents are associated with gastric ulcers and erosions [124]. Gastric ulcers are seen in 15–40% of patients with long term use of NSAIDs [125]. The damage to the gastric mucosa can be prostaglandin (PG) dependent or PG independent. The judicial use of NSAIDs, topical NSAIDs, use of cyclo-oxygenase 2 specific inhibitors and/ or concomitant use of proton pump inhibitors or H2 receptor antagonists can lower the rate of these complications but will not eliminate the risk [126]. Patients with advanced age, prolonged use or higher doses of NSAIDs , or use in combination with corticosteroids have shown a higher risk of developing peptic ulcer disease [127].

6.10.1 Pathophysiology

Gastric mucosal defense mechanisms include mucus, bicarbonate, surface phospholipids, surface epithelial cells and microcirculation. Prostaglandins play an important role in the secretion of bicarbonate and mucus and also inhibit gastric acid secretion and increase mucosal blood flow [128]. Prostaglandin and nitric oxide also inhibit leukocyte adhesion in the endothelial surface of blood vessels [129].

Aspirin inhibits cyclooxygenase (COX) irreversibly whereas NSAIDs are a reversible inhibitor. COX inhibition leads to decreased prostaglandin production. The use of NSAIDs induces the expression of adhesion molecules on the endothelial surface, and can compromise the microcirculation, which leads to tissue damage with hypoxia [129]. Two COX isoforms are seen in humans: COX-1 and COX-2. The COX-1 protein is abundant in the gastrointestinal tract and is involved in production of prostaglandins, which is an integral part of the gastric defense mechanism. The release of COX-2 is mediated by inflammation and is found in various tissues throughout the body. This led to the introduction of COX-2 specific inhibitors for pain control [128, 130]. COX-2 plays a supportive role in situations where COX-1 is blocked. Combined COX-1 and COX-2 inhibition will cause more damage. The COX-2 inhibitors reduce the risk of NSAID associated gastric ulcers [131].

Gastric mucosal damage with NSAIDs can be prostaglandin independent. The NSAIDs diffuse across the gastric mucosa and enter the epithelial cell cytoplasm. These molecules are acidic and they can accumulate within the cell, leading to cellular damage [132]. The NSAIDs also uncouple the oxidative phosphorylation of the mitochondria which can cause ulcerative damage, increased permeability and low-grade inflammation [129].

6.11 Bariatric Surgery and Connective Tissue Disorders

Bariatric surgery is the most effective therapeutic intervention to treat obesity and related comorbid conditions. It reduces mortality, cardiovascular diseases, diabetes mellitus and cancer [133]. Obesity is an inflammatory state, which not only increases the prevalence of osteoarthritis due to mechanical stress on musculoskeletal tissue but is also associated with RA, psoriatic arthritis and SLE [134–138]. Obesity has a negative impact on quality of life, disease activity and progression in RD. [139] Weight loss with bariatric surgery can lead to decreased disease activity, reduction in inflammatory markers and less utilization of disease specific medications [140]. Despite the benefits of bariatric surgery, only a small portion (<1%) of qualifying patients undergo the surgery. This could be due to the patient's fear, patient physician interactions, physician perceptions and cost burden. The long-term maintenance of weight loss after initial success is also a challenge [141].

6.11.1 Pathophysiology

The adipose tissue is not an innocent bystander. It contains not only adipocytes and pre-adipocytes but also T cells, eosinophils and B- regulatory cells [142]. These cells and inflammatory macrophages result in production of pro-inflammatory cytokines including tumor necrosis factor alpha and interleukin 6 [143]. The pro-inflammatory adipokines also produced by adipose tissue are leptin, adiponectin, resistin and visfatin which lead to a pro-inflammatory state. Adipokines are also increased in RD including RA, SLE, psoriatic arthritis and ankylosing spondylitis [139, 143].

Reduction in fat mass with bariatric surgery reduces inflammation. Post-operatively, leptin and visfatin levels are decreased whereas adiponectin levels are increased [144, 145]. The increased adiponectin/leptin ratio is associated with reduced inflammation and more cardiometabolic benefits [146]. The alteration of gut hormones, including glucagon like peptide (increased), ghrelin (decreased), gastric inhibitory peptide (increased), and pancreatic peptide YY (increased) also play a role in reduction of the inflammatory state [147]. Another hypothesis underlying the reduction in the inflammatory response post-operatively is the change in gut that occurs after surgery [148]. In addition to this multitude of beneficial effects, the durable weight loss with bariatric surgery leads to a reduction of medications for treatment of metabolic disorders and RD, and can further improve the health outcomes of this patient population [140].

The healing difficulties in connective tissue diseases like Ehlers-Danlos Syndrome, rheumatoid arthritis, and vasculitis are major concerns when it comes to bariatric surgery [149–151]. This could be due to structural changes or prolonged use of steroids [152]. The surgical risk can be higher than that of the average population for these individuals, and could limit utilization of this promising intervention. Data about the use of immunosuppressive drugs before and after the surgery is sparse. Although the data is limited, the outcomes are reassuring in terms of safety of the procedure in the setting of RD. [140, 153–155]

Connective tissue disorders and RD are risk factors for developing malnutrition [156, 157]. Bariatric surgery changes the gastrointestinal anatomy and physiology, which makes patients susceptible to the development of nutritional deficiencies. In sleeve gastrectomy, the risk of nutritional deficiency is lower, though still present [158]. Interventions to address the nutritional deficiencies in patients with RD are important considerations in those patients undergoing gastric bypass surgery.

6.12 Percutaneous Gastrostomy in Rheumatic Diseases

Enteral feeding can be challenging in those patients that may have impaired GI motility as a consequence of their RD. [159] SSc patients with dysphagia may benefit from a percutaneous gastrostomy (PEG) tube, but these benefits are questionable if the patient is also suffering from malabsorption and delayed gastric emptying. PEG tubes can be utilized for enteral feeding in SSc patients whose primary problem is esophageal dysfunction [160].

PEG tube venting can be used for decompression of the stomach. There is limited data on the utilization of a gastric stimulator in gastroparesis patients with refractory gastroparesis due to SSc. PEG decompression can be considered in patients when all other treatment modalities have failed [161]. SSc can be present with chronic intestinal pseudo-obstruction and in some severe cases, decompression can be achieved with placement of a PEG tube [162].

6.13 Conclusion

In summary, gastric manifestations are commonly seen in RD. The presence of anemia and upper GI bleeding should raise the suspicion of GAVE, peptic ulcers due to chronic NSAID use, and AVM. The damage of smooth muscles, pacemaker cells (ICC) and the autonomic nervous system due to gastric inflammation can lead to gastroparesis, which is associated with malnutrition and increased comorbidities. Sjogren syndrome is associated with atrophic gastritis which commonly presents with abdominal pain and anemia. The global prevalence of obesity is increasing, and it can add to the progression of RD due to the mechanical effect on the musculoskeletal system and associated inflammation. Bariatric surgery is underutilized nationally in the morbidly obese population and in obese patients with RD.

References

1. Kröner PT, Tolaymat OA, Bowman AW, Abril A, Lacy BE. Gastrointestinal manifestations of rheumatological diseases. Am J Gastroenterol. 2019;114(9):1441–54. https://doi.org/10.14309/ajg.0000000000000260.
2. Ebert EC, Hagspiel KD. Gastrointestinal and hepatic manifestations of systemic lupus erythematosus. J Clin Gastroenterol. 2011;45(5):436–41. https://doi.org/10.1097/MCG.0b013e31820f81b8.
3. Sjogren RW. Gastrointestinal motility disorders in scleroderma. Arthritis Rheum. 1994;37(9):1265–82. https://doi.org/10.1002/art.1780370902.
4. Wegener M, Adamek RJ, Wedmann B, Jergas M, Altmeyer P. Gastrointestinal transit through esophagus, stomach, small and large intestine in patients with progressive systemic sclerosis. Dig Dis Sci. 1994;39(10):2209–15. https://doi.org/10.1007/BF02090373.
5. Sultan SM, Ioannou Y, Isenberg DA. A review of gastrointestinal manifestations of systemic lupus erythematosus. Rheumatology. 1999;38(10):917–32. https://doi.org/10.1093/rheumatology/38.10.917.
6. Dulai GS, Jensen DM, Kovacs TOG, Gralnek IM, Jutabha R. Endoscopic treatment outcomes in watermelon stomach patients with and without portal hypertension. Endoscopy. 2004;36(1):68–72. https://doi.org/10.1055/s-2004-814112.
7. Gostout CJ, Viggiano TR, Ahlquist DA, Wang KK, Larson MV, Balm R. The clinical and endoscopic spectrum of the watermelon stomach. J Clin Gastroenterol. 1992;15(3):256–63. https://doi.org/10.1097/00004836-199210000-00019.
8. Marie I, Ducrotte P, Antonietti M, Herve S, Levesque H. Watermelon stomach in systemic sclerosis: its incidence and management. Aliment Pharmacol Ther. 2008;28(4):412–21. https://doi.org/10.1111/j.1365-2036.2008.03739.x.
9. Burak KW, Lee SS, Beck PL. Portal hypertensive gastropathy and gastric antral vascular ectasia (GAVE) syndrome. Gut. 2001;49(6):866–72. https://doi.org/10.1136/gut.49.6.866.
10. Jabbari M, Cherry R, Lough JO, Daly DS, Kinnear DG, Goresky CA. Gastric antral vascular ectasia: the watermelon stomach. Gastroenterology. 1984;87(5):1165–70.
11. Ingraham KM, O'Brien MS, Shenin M, Derk CT, Steen VD. Gastric antral vascular ectasia in systemic sclerosis: demographics and disease predictors. J Rheumatol. 2010;37(3):603–7. https://doi.org/10.3899/jrheum.090600.
12. Freemont AJ, Hoyland J, Fielding P, Hodson N, Jayson MI. Studies of the microvascular endothelium in uninvolved skin of patients with systemic sclerosis: direct evidence for a generalized microangiopathy. Br J Dermatol. 1992;126(6):561–8. https://doi.org/10.1111/j.1365-2133.1992.tb00100.x.
13. Duchini A, Sessoms SL. Gastrointestinal hemorrhage in patients with systemic sclerosis and CREST syndrome. Am J Gastroenterol. 1998;93(9):1453–6. https://doi.org/10.1111/j.1572-0241.1998.00462.x.
14. Gilliam JH 3rd, Geisinger KR, Wu WC, Weidner N, Richter JE. Endoscopic biopsy is diagnostic in gastric antral vascular ectasia. The "watermelon stomach". Dig Dis Sci. 1989;34(6):885–8. https://doi.org/10.1007/BF01540274.
15. Lorenzi AR, Johnson AH, Davies G, Gough A. Gastric antral vascular ectasia in systemic sclerosis: complete resolution with methylprednisolone and cyclophosphamide. Ann Rheum Dis. 2001;60(8):796–8. https://doi.org/10.1136/ard.60.8.796.
16. Schulz SW, O'Brien M, Maqsood M, Sandorfi N, Del Galdo F, Jimenez SA. Improvement of severe systemic sclerosis-associated gastric antral vascular ectasia following immunosuppressive treatment with intravenous cyclophosphamide. J Rheumatol. 2009;36(8):1653–6. https://doi.org/10.3899/jrheum.081247.
17. Hung EW, Mayes MD, Sharif R, et al. Gastric antral vascular ectasia and its clinical correlates in patients with early diffuse systemic sclerosis in the SCOT trial. J Rheumatol. 2013;40(4):455–60. https://doi.org/10.3899/jrheum.121087.

18. Ceribelli A, Cavazzana I, Airò P, Franceschini F. Anti-RNA polymerase III antibodies as a risk marker for early gastric antral vascular ectasia (GAVE) in systemic sclerosis. J Rheumatol. 2010;37(7):1544. https://doi.org/10.3899/jrheum.100124.
19. Parrado RH, Lemus HN, Coral-Alvarado PX, Quintana López G. Gastric antral vascular ectasia in systemic sclerosis: current concepts. Int J Rheumatol. 2015;2015:762546. https://doi.org/10.1155/2015/762546.
20. Fleetwood IG, Steinberg GK. Arteriovenous malformations. Lancet (London, England). 2002;359(9309):863–73. https://doi.org/10.1016/S0140-6736(02)07946-1.
21. Moretó M, Figa M, Ojembarrena E, Zaballa M. Vascular malformations of the stomach and duodenum: an endoscopic classification. Endoscopy. 1986;18(6):227–9. https://doi.org/10.1055/s-2007-1018385.
22. Ng SC, Thomas-Gibson S, Harbin LJ, Gupta A, Gould SWT, Jacyna M. Gastric arteriovenous malformation: a rare cause of upper GI bleed. Gastrointest Endosc. 2009;69(1):155–6; discussion 156. https://doi.org/10.1016/j.gie.2008.07.013.
23. Boley SJ, Sammartano R, Adams A, DiBiase A, Kleinhaus S, Sprayregen S. On the nature and etiology of vascular ectasias of the colon. Degenerative lesions of aging. Gastroenterology. 1977;72(4 Pt 1):650–60.
24. Szilagyi A, Ghali MP. Pharmacological therapy of vascular malformations of the gastrointestinal tract. Can J Gastroenterol. 2006;20(3):171–8. https://doi.org/10.1155/2006/859435.
25. Junquera F, Saperas E, de Torres I, Vidal MT, Malagelada JR. Increased expression of angiogenic factors in human colonic angiodysplasia. Am J Gastroenterol. 1999;94(4):1070–6. https://doi.org/10.1111/j.1572-0241.1999.01017.x.
26. Ge Z-Z, Chen H-M, Gao Y-J, et al. Efficacy of thalidomide for refractory gastrointestinal bleeding from vascular malformation. Gastroenterology. 2011;141(5):1624–9. https://doi.org/10.1053/j.gastro.2011.07.018.
27. Camilleri M, Parkman HP, Shafi MA, Abell TL, Gerson L. Clinical guideline: management of gastroparesis. Am J Gastroenterol. 2013;108(1):18–37; quiz 38. https://doi.org/10.1038/ajg.2012.373.
28. Rey E, Choung RS, Schleck CD, Zinsmeister AR, Talley NJ, Locke GR 3rd. Prevalence of hidden gastroparesis in the community: the gastroparesis "iceberg". J Neurogastroenterol Motil. 2012;18(1):34–42. https://doi.org/10.5056/jnm.2012.18.1.34.
29. Cozzi F, Parisi G, Ciprian L, et al. Gastric dysmotility after liquid bolus ingestion in systemic sclerosis: an ultrasonographic study. Rheumatol Int. 2012;32(5):1219–23. https://doi.org/10.1007/s00296-010-1779-5.
30. Omair MA, Lee P. Effect of gastrointestinal manifestations on quality of life in 87 consecutive patients with systemic sclerosis. J Rheumatol. 2012;39(5):992–6. https://doi.org/10.3899/jrheum.110826.
31. Maddern GJ, Horowitz M, Jamieson GG, Chatterton BE, Collins PJ, Roberts-Thomson P. Abnormalities of esophageal and gastric emptying in progressive systemic sclerosis. Gastroenterology. 1984;87(4):922–6.
32. Abell TL, Bernstein RK, Cutts T, et al. Treatment of gastroparesis: a multidisciplinary clinical review. Neurogastroenterol Motil. 2006;18(4):263–83. https://doi.org/10.1111/j.1365-2982.2006.00760.x.
33. Wadhwa V, Mehta D, Jobanputra Y, Lopez R, Thota PN, Sanaka MR. Healthcare utilization and costs associated with gastroparesis. World J Gastroenterol. 2017;23(24):4428–36. https://doi.org/10.3748/wjg.v23.i24.4428.
34. Wang YR, Fisher RS, Parkman HP. Gastroparesis-related hospitalizations in the United States: trends, characteristics, and outcomes, 1995–2004. Am J Gastroenterol. 2008;103(2):313–22. https://doi.org/10.1111/j.1572-0241.2007.01658.x.
35. Jung H-K, Choung RS, Locke GR 3rd, et al. The incidence, prevalence, and outcomes of patients with gastroparesis in Olmsted County, Minnesota, from 1996 to 2006. Gastroenterology. 2009;136(4):1225–33. https://doi.org/10.1053/j.gastro.2008.12.047.

36. Tougas G, Eaker EY, Abell TL, et al. Assessment of gastric emptying using a low fat meal: establishment of international control values. Am J Gastroenterol. 2000;95(6):1456–62. https://doi.org/10.1111/j.1572-0241.2000.02076.x.
37. Kuo B, McCallum RW, Koch KL, et al. Comparison of gastric emptying of a nondigestible capsule to a radio-labelled meal in healthy and gastroparetic subjects. Aliment Pharmacol Ther. 2008;27(2):186–96. https://doi.org/10.1111/j.1365-2036.2007.03564.x.
38. Szarka LA, Camilleri M, Vella A, et al. A stable isotope breath test with a standard meal for abnormal gastric emptying of solids in the clinic and in research. Clin Gastroenterol Hepatol. 2008;6(6):635–43.e1. https://doi.org/10.1016/j.cgh.2008.01.009.
39. Camilleri M. Appraisal of medium- and long-term treatment of gastroparesis and chronic intestinal dysmotility. Am J Gastroenterol. 1994;89(10):1769–74.
40. Pfeiffer A, Högl B, Kaess H. Effect of ethanol and commonly ingested alcoholic beverages on gastric emptying and gastrointestinal transit. Clin Investig. 1992;70(6):487–91. https://doi.org/10.1007/BF00210229.
41. Kolterman OG, Kim DD, Shen L, et al. Pharmacokinetics, pharmacodynamics, and safety of exenatide in patients with type 2 diabetes mellitus. Am J Heal Pharm AJHP. 2005;62(2):173–81. https://doi.org/10.1093/ajhp/62.2.173.
42. Vella A, Lee JS, Camilleri M, et al. Effects of pramlintide, an amylin analogue, on gastric emptying in type 1 and 2 diabetes mellitus. Neurogastroenterol Motil. 2002;14(2):123–31. https://doi.org/10.1046/j.1365-2982.2002.00311.x.
43. Travagli RA, Anselmi L. Vagal neurocircuitry and its influence on gastric motility. Nat Rev Gastroenterol Hepatol. 2016;13(7):389–401. https://doi.org/10.1038/nrgastro.2016.76.
44. Goyal RK, Guo Y, Mashimo H. Advances in the physiology of gastric emptying. Neurogastroenterol Motil. 2019;31(4):e13546. https://doi.org/10.1111/nmo.13546.
45. Hunt JN, Smith JL, Jiang CL. Effect of meal volume and energy density on the gastric emptying of carbohydrates. Gastroenterology. 1985;89(6):1326–30. https://doi.org/10.1016/0016-5085(85)90650-x.
46. Ramkumar D, Schulze KS. The pylorus. Neurogastroenterol Motil. 2005;17(Suppl 1):22–30. https://doi.org/10.1111/j.1365-2982.2005.00664.x.
47. Bharucha AE, Manduca A, Lake DS, et al. Gastric motor disturbances in patients with idiopathic rapid gastric emptying. Neurogastroenterol Motil. 2011;23(7):617-e252. https://doi.org/10.1111/j.1365-2982.2011.01710.x.
48. Sivarao DV, Mashimo H, Goyal RK. Pyloric sphincter dysfunction in nNOS-/- and W/Wv mutant mice: animal models of gastroparesis and duodenogastric reflux. Gastroenterology. 2008;135(4):1258–66. https://doi.org/10.1053/j.gastro.2008.06.039.
49. Takahashi T. Mechanism of interdigestive migrating motor complex. J Neurogastroenterol Motil. 2012;18(3):246–57. https://doi.org/10.5056/jnm.2012.18.3.246.
50. Farrugia G. Interstitial cells of Cajal in health and disease. Neurogastroenterol Motil. 2008;20(Suppl 1):54–63. https://doi.org/10.1111/j.1365-2982.2008.01109.x.
51. Liu N, Abell T. Gastroparesis updates on pathogenesis and management. Gut Liver. 2017;11(5):579–89. https://doi.org/10.5009/gnl16336.
52. Grover M, Bernard CE, Pasricha PJ, et al. Clinical-histological associations in gastroparesis: results from the Gastroparesis Clinical Research Consortium. Neurogastroenterol Motil. 2012;24(6):531–9, e249. https://doi.org/10.1111/j.1365-2982.2012.01894.x.
53. Grover M, Farrugia G, Lurken MS, et al. Cellular changes in diabetic and idiopathic gastroparesis. Gastroenterology. 2011;140(5):1575–85.e8. https://doi.org/10.1053/j.gastro.2011.01.046.
54. Vittal H, Farrugia G, Gomez G, Pasricha PJ. Mechanisms of disease: the pathological basis of gastroparesis—a review of experimental and clinical studies. Nat Clin Pract Gastroenterol Hepatol. 2007;4(6):336–46. https://doi.org/10.1038/ncpgasthep0838.
55. Plourde V, Quintero E, Suto G, Coimbra C, Taché Y. Delayed gastric emptying induced by inhibitors of nitric oxide synthase in rats. Eur J Pharmacol. 1994;256(2):125–9. https://doi.org/10.1016/0014-2999(94)90236-4.

56. Zhu J, Frech T. Gut disease in systemic sclerosis—new approaches to common problems. Curr Treat Options Rheumatol. 2019;5(1):11–9. https://doi.org/10.1007/s40674-019-00117-x.
57. Goldblatt F, Gordon TP, Waterman SA. Antibody-mediated gastrointestinal dysmotility in scleroderma. Gastroenterology. 2002;123(4):1144–50. https://doi.org/10.1053/gast.2002.36057.
58. Iovino P, Valentini G, Ciacci C, et al. Proximal stomach function in systemic sclerosis: relationship with autonomic nerve function. Dig Dis Sci. 2001;46(4):723–30. https://doi.org/10.1023/a:1010779729184.
59. Greydanus MP, Camilleri M. Abnormal postcibal antral and small bowel motility due to neuropathy or myopathy in systemic sclerosis. Gastroenterology. 1989;96(1):110–5. https://doi.org/10.1016/0016-5085(89)90770-1.
60. Reamy BV, Williams PM, Lindsay TJ. Henoch-Schönlein purpura. Am Fam Physician. 2009;80(7):697–704.
61. Reinauer S, Megahed M, Goerz G, et al. Schönlein-Henoch purpura associated with gastric Helicobacter pylori infection. J Am Acad Dermatol. 1995;33(5 Pt 2):876–9. https://doi.org/10.1016/0190-9622(95)90426-3.
62. Cecchi R, Torelli E. Schönlein-Henoch purpura in association with duodenal ulcer and gastric Helicobacter pylori infection. J Dermatol. 1998;25(7):482–4. https://doi.org/10.1111/j.1346-8138.1998.tb02440.x.
63. Xiong L-J, Tong Y, Wang Z-L, Mao M. Is Helicobacter pylori infection associated with Henoch-Schonlein purpura in Chinese children? A meta-analysis. World J Pediatr. 2012;8(4):301–8. https://doi.org/10.1007/s12519-012-0373-1.
64. Touchard G, Maire P, Beauchant M, et al. Vascular IgA and C3 deposition in gastrointestinal tract of patients with Henoch-Schoenlein purpura. Lancet (London, England). 1983;1(8327):771–2. https://doi.org/10.1016/s0140-6736(83)92065-2.
65. Xiong L-J, Mao M. Current views of the relationship between Helicobacter pylori and Henoch-Schonlein purpura in children. World J Clin Pediatr. 2016;5(1):82–8. https://doi.org/10.5409/wjcp.v5.i1.82.
66. Gasbarrini A, Franceschi F. Autoimmune diseases and Helicobacter pylori infection. Biomed Pharmacother. 1999;53(5-6):223–6. https://doi.org/10.1016/S0753-3322(99)80092-4.
67. Novák J, Szekanecz Z, Sebesi J, et al. Elevated levels of anti-Helicobacter pylori antibodies in Henoch-Schönlein purpura. Autoimmunity. 2003;36(5):307–11. https://doi.org/10.1080/08916930232000114535.
68. Marchand P. The anatomy of esophageal hiatus of the diaphragm and the pathogenesis of hiatus herniation. J Thorac Surg. 1959;37(1):81–92.
69. Eliska O. Phreno-oesophageal membrane and its role in the development of hiatal hernia. Acta Anat (Basel). 1973;86(1):137–50.
70. Hyun JJ, Bak Y-T. Clinical significance of hiatal hernia. Gut Liver. 2011;5(3):267–77. https://doi.org/10.5009/gnl.2011.5.3.267.
71. Petronovich JJ, Bock JM. Systemic sclerosis and reflux. Ear Nose Throat J. 2013;92(4–5):192–4. https://doi.org/10.1177/014556131309200410.
72. McFarlane IM, Bhamra MS, Kreps A, et al. Gastrointestinal manifestations of systemic sclerosis. Rheumatology (Sunnyvale). 2018;8(1). https://doi.org/10.4172/2161-1149.1000235.
73. Beighton PH, Murdoch JL, Votteler T. Gastrointestinal complications of the Ehlers-Danlos syndrome. Gut. 1969;10(12):1004–8. https://doi.org/10.1136/gut.10.12.1004.
74. Ignoto A, Ambrogio M, Distefano N, et al. Acute para-esophageal hernia in Ehlers-Danlos Syndrome. Chir Ital. 2006;58(6):797–801.
75. Nelson AD, Mouchli MA, Valentin N, et al. Ehlers Danlos syndrome and gastrointestinal manifestations: a 20-year experience at Mayo Clinic. Neurogastroenterol Motil. 2015;27(11):1657–66. https://doi.org/10.1111/nmo.12665.
76. Bombeck CT, Dillard DH, Nyhus LM. Muscular anatomy of the gastroesophageal junction and role of phrenoesophageal ligament; autopsy study of sphincter mechanism. Ann Surg. 1966;164(4):643–54. https://doi.org/10.1097/00000658-196610000-00011.

77. Edmundowicz SA, Clouse RE. Shortening of the esophagus in response to swallowing. Am J Phys. 1991;260(3 Pt 1):G512–6. https://doi.org/10.1152/ajpgi.1991.260.3.G512.
78. Malfait F, Francomano C, Byers P, et al. The 2017 international classification of the Ehlers-Danlos syndromes. Am J Med Genet C: Semin Med Genet. 2017;175(1):8–26. https://doi.org/10.1002/ajmg.c.31552.
79. Lin IC, Ko SF, Shieh CS, Huang CF, Chien SJ, Liang CD. Recurrent congenital diaphragmatic hernia in Ehlers-Danlos syndrome. Cardiovasc Intervent Radiol. 2006;29(5):920–3. https://doi.org/10.1007/s00270-005-0154-5.
80. Hamaoui K, Riaz A, Hay A, Botha A. Massive spontaneous diaphragmatic rupture in Ehlers-Danlos syndrome. Ann R Coll Surg Engl. 2012;94(1):e5–7. https://doi.org/10.1308/003588412X13171221499306.
81. Amin R, Waibel BH. Spontaneous diaphragmatic rupture in hypermobile type Ehlers-Danlos syndrome. Case Rep Surg. 2017;2017:2081725. https://doi.org/10.1155/2017/2081725.
82. Lanas A, Chan FKL. Peptic ulcer disease. Lancet (London, England). 2017;390(10094):613–24. https://doi.org/10.1016/S0140-6736(16)32404-7.
83. Farah D, Sturrock RD, Russell RI. Peptic ulcer in rheumatoid arthritis. Ann Rheum Dis. 1988;47(6):478–80. https://doi.org/10.1136/ard.47.6.478.
84. Lin Y-T, Chuang Y-S, Wang J-W, Wu P-H. High risk of gastrointestinal hemorrhage in patients with systemic sclerosis. Arthritis Res Ther. 2019;21(1):301. https://doi.org/10.1186/s13075-019-2078-5.
85. Narusako T, Ueyama H, Tsunetomi N, et al. Multiple hemorrhagic gastric ulcers due to polyarteritis nodosa. Intern Med. 1997;36(9):657–60. https://doi.org/10.2169/internalmedicine.36.657.
86. Ebert EC, Hagspiel KD, Nagar M, Schlesinger N. Gastrointestinal involvement in polyarteritis nodosa. Clin Gastroenterol Hepatol. 2008;6(9):960–6. https://doi.org/10.1016/j.cgh.2008.04.004.
87. Atuma C, Strugala V, Allen A, Holm L. The adherent gastrointestinal mucus gel layer: thickness and physical state in vivo. Am J Physiol Gastrointest Liver Physiol. 2001;280(5):G922–9. https://doi.org/10.1152/ajpgi.2001.280.5.G922.
88. Allen A, Flemström G. Gastroduodenal mucus bicarbonate barrier: protection against acid and pepsin. Am J Phys Cell Physiol. 2005;288(1):C1–19. https://doi.org/10.1152/ajpcell.00102.2004.
89. Johansson M, Synnerstad I, Holm L. Acid transport through channels in the mucous layer of rat stomach. Gastroenterology. 2000;119(5):1297–304. https://doi.org/10.1053/gast.2000.19455.
90. Ho SB, Takamura K, Anway R, Shekels LL, Toribara NW, Ota H. The adherent gastric mucous layer is composed of alternating layers of MUC5AC and MUC6 mucin proteins. Dig Dis Sci. 2004;49(10):1598–606. https://doi.org/10.1023/b:ddas.0000043371.12671.98.
91. Rodriguez-Castro KI, Franceschi M, Noto A, et al. Clinical manifestations of chronic atrophic gastritis. Acta Biomed. 2018;89(8-S):88–92. https://doi.org/10.23750/abm.v89i8-S.7921.
92. Kalkan Ç, Soykan I, Soydal Ç, Özkan E, Kalkan E. Assessment of gastric emptying in patients with autoimmune gastritis. Dig Dis Sci. 2016;61(6):1597–602. https://doi.org/10.1007/s10620-015-4021-1.
93. de Vries AC, Haringsma J, Kuipers EJ. The detection, surveillance and treatment of premalignant gastric lesions related to Helicobacter pylori infection. Helicobacter. 2007;12(1):1–15. https://doi.org/10.1111/j.1523-5378.2007.00475.x.
94. Joo Y-E, Park H-K, Myung D-S, et al. Prevalence and risk factors of atrophic gastritis and intestinal metaplasia: a nationwide multicenter prospective study in Korea. Gut Liver. 2013;7(3):303–10. https://doi.org/10.5009/gnl.2013.7.3.303.
95. Uemura N, Okamoto S, Yamamoto S, et al. Helicobacter pylori infection and the development of gastric cancer. N Engl J Med. 2001;345(11):784–9. https://doi.org/10.1056/NEJMoa001999.

96. Sheikh SH, Shaw-Stiffel TA. The gastrointestinal manifestations of Sjögren's syndrome. Am J Gastroenterol. 1995;90(1):9–14.
97. Ostuni PA, Germana B, Di Mario F, et al. Gastric involvement in primary Sjögren's syndrome. Clin Exp Rheumatol. 1993;11(1):21–5.
98. Collin P, Karvonen AL, Korpela M, Laippala P, Helin H. Gastritis classified in accordance with the Sydney system in patients with primary Sjögren's syndrome. Scand J Gastroenterol. 1997;32(2):108–11. https://doi.org/10.3109/00365529709000179.
99. Dai S-M, Han X-H, Li Z-S. Hypertrophic gastritis in early stages of primary Sjögren's syndrome. Arthritis Rheum. 2008;59(8):1191–3. https://doi.org/10.1002/art.23926.
100. Bouomrani S, Ghribi M, Masmoudi I, Benteber S. Diffuse nodular gastritis revealing primary Sjogren's syndrome in young woman. 2019;4(1):27–9.
101. van Leeuwen ML, Tjiong HL, van Blankenstein M, Mulder AH, Bakker CM. Phlegmonous gastritis: an unusual presenting symptom of Sjögren's syndrome. Gut. 1993;34(8):1142–4. https://doi.org/10.1136/gut.34.8.1142.
102. Sugaya T, Sakai H, Sugiyama T, Imai K. [Atrophic gastritis in Sjögren's syndrome]. Nihon Rinsho. 1995;53(10):2540–4.
103. Pokorny G, Karácsony G, Lonovics J, Hudák J, Németh J, Varró V. Types of atrophic gastritis in patients with primary Sjögren's syndrome. Ann Rheum Dis. 1991;50(2):97–100. https://doi.org/10.1136/ard.50.2.97.
104. De Aizpurua HJ, Cosgrove LJ, Ungar B, Toh BH. Autoantibodies cytotoxic to gastric parietal cells in serum of patients with pernicious anemia. N Engl J Med. 1983;309(11):625–9. https://doi.org/10.1056/NEJM198309153091102.
105. Marshall ACJ, Alderuccio F, Murphy K, Toh B-H. Mechanisms of gastric mucosal cell loss in autoimmune gastritis. Int Rev Immunol. 2005;24(1–2):123–34. https://doi.org/10.1080/08830180590884567.
106. Lenti MV, Rugge M, Lahner E, et al. Autoimmune gastritis. Nat Rev Dis Prim. 2020;6(1):56. https://doi.org/10.1038/s41572-020-0187-8.
107. Pikkarainen S, Martelius T, Ristimäki A, Siitonen S, Seppänen MRJ, Färkkilä M. A high prevalence of gastrointestinal manifestations in common variable immunodeficiency. Am J Gastroenterol. 2019;114(4):648–55. https://doi.org/10.14309/ajg.0000000000000140.
108. Freudenthaler S, Hegenbart U, Schönland S, Behrens H-M, Krüger S, Röcken C. Amyloid in biopsies of the gastrointestinal tract-a retrospective observational study on 542 patients. Virchows Arch. 2016;468(5):569–77. https://doi.org/10.1007/s00428-016-1916-y.
109. Craig E, Cappelli LC. Gastrointestinal and hepatic disease in rheumatoid arthritis. Rheum Dis Clin N Am. 2018;44(1):89–111. https://doi.org/10.1016/j.rdc.2017.09.005.
110. Carmona L, González-Alvaro I, Balsa A, Angel Belmonte M, Tena X, Sanmartí R. Rheumatoid arthritis in Spain: occurrence of extra-articular manifestations and estimates of disease severity. Ann Rheum Dis. 2003;62(9):897–900. https://doi.org/10.1136/ard.62.9.897.
111. Calgüneri M, Ureten K, Akif Oztürk M, et al. Extra-articular manifestations of rheumatoid arthritis: results of a university hospital of 526 patients in Turkey. Clin Exp Rheumatol. 2006;24(3):305–8.
112. Inoue D, Arima H, Kawanami C, et al. Excellent therapeutic effect of tocilizumab on intestinal amyloid a deposition secondary to active rheumatoid arthritis. Clin Rheumatol. 2010;29(10):1195–7. https://doi.org/10.1007/s10067-010-1422-6.
113. Gottenberg J-E, Merle-Vincent F, Bentaberry F, et al. Anti-tumor necrosis factor alpha therapy in fifteen patients with AA amyloidosis secondary to inflammatory arthritides: a followup report of tolerability and efficacy. Arthritis Rheum. 2003;48(7):2019–24. https://doi.org/10.1002/art.11163.
114. Merlini G, Bellotti V. Molecular mechanisms of amyloidosis. N Engl J Med. 2003;349(6):583–96. https://doi.org/10.1056/NEJMra023144.
115. Westermark GT, Fändrich M, Westermark P. AA amyloidosis: pathogenesis and targeted therapy. Annu Rev Pathol. 2015;10:321–44. https://doi.org/10.1146/annurev-pathol-020712-163913.

116. Fardet L, Petersen I, Nazareth I. Prevalence of long-term oral glucocorticoid prescriptions in the UK over the past 20 years. Rheumatology (Oxford). 2011;50(11):1982–90. https://doi.org/10.1093/rheumatology/ker017.
117. Martínek J, Hlavova K, Zavada F, et al. "A surviving myth"—corticosteroids are still considered ulcerogenic by a majority of physicians. Scand J Gastroenterol. 2010;45(10):1156–61. https://doi.org/10.3109/00365521.2010.497935.
118. Nielsen GL, Sørensen HT, Mellemkjoer L, et al. Risk of hospitalization resulting from upper gastrointestinal bleeding among patients taking corticosteroids: a register-based cohort study. Am J Med. 2001;111(7):541–5. https://doi.org/10.1016/s0002-9343(01)00941-x.
119. Narum S, Westergren T, Klemp M. Corticosteroids and risk of gastrointestinal bleeding: a systematic review and meta-analysis. BMJ Open. 2014;4(5):e004587. https://doi.org/10.1136/bmjopen-2013-004587.
120. Guslandi M. Steroid ulcers: any news? World J Gastrointest Pharmacol Ther. 2013;4(3):39–40. https://doi.org/10.4292/wjgpt.v4.i3.39.
121. Luo JC, Shin VY, Liu ESL, et al. Dexamethasone delays ulcer healing by inhibition of angiogenesis in rat stomachs. Eur J Pharmacol. 2004;485(1–3):275–81. https://doi.org/10.1016/j.ejphar.2003.11.038.
122. Carpani de Kaski M, Rentsch R, Levi S, Hodgson HJ. Corticosteroids reduce regenerative repair of epithelium in experimental gastric ulcers. Gut. 1995;37(5):613–6. https://doi.org/10.1136/gut.37.5.613.
123. Singh G, Triadafilopoulos G. Epidemiology of NSAID induced gastrointestinal complications. J Rheumatol Suppl. 1999;56:18–24.
124. Burmester G, Lanas A, Biasucci L, et al. The appropriate use of non-steroidal anti-inflammatory drugs in rheumatic disease: opinions of a multidisciplinary European expert panel. Ann Rheum Dis. 2011;70(5):818–22. https://doi.org/10.1136/ard.2010.128660.
125. Geis GS, Stead H, Wallemark CB, Nicholson PA. Prevalence of mucosal lesions in the stomach and duodenum due to chronic use of NSAID in patients with rheumatoid arthritis or osteoarthritis, and interim report on prevention by misoprostol of diclofenac associated lesions. J Rheumatol Suppl. 1991;28:11–4.
126. Goldstein JL, Cryer B. Gastrointestinal injury associated with NSAID use: a case study and review of risk factors and preventative strategies. Drug Healthc Patient Saf. 2015;7:31–41. https://doi.org/10.2147/DHPS.S71976.
127. Drini M. Peptic ulcer disease and non-steroidal anti-inflammatory drugs. Aust Prescr. 2017;40(3):91–3. https://doi.org/10.18773/austprescr.2017.037.
128. Matsui H, Shimokawa O, Kaneko T, Nagano Y, Rai K, Hyodo I. The pathophysiology of non-steroidal anti-inflammatory drug (NSAID)-induced mucosal injuries in stomach and small intestine. J Clin Biochem Nutr. 2011;48(2):107–11. https://doi.org/10.3164/jcbn.10-79.
129. Bjarnason I, Scarpignato C, Holmgren E, Olszewski M, Rainsford KD, Lanas A. Mechanisms of damage to the gastrointestinal tract from nonsteroidal anti-inflammatory drugs. Gastroenterology. 2018;154(3):500–14. https://doi.org/10.1053/j.gastro.2017.10.049.
130. Kargman S, Charleson S, Cartwright M, et al. Characterization of Prostaglandin G/H Synthase 1 and 2 in rat, dog, monkey, and human gastrointestinal tracts. Gastroenterology. 1996;111(2):445–54. https://doi.org/10.1053/gast.1996.v111.pm8690211.
131. Laine L, Takeuchi K, Tarnawski A. Gastric mucosal defense and cytoprotection: bench to bedside. Gastroenterology. 2008;135(1):41–60. https://doi.org/10.1053/j.gastro.2008.05.030.
132. Laine L. Nonsteroidal anti-inflammatory drug gastropathy. Gastrointest Endosc Clin N Am. 1996;6(3):489–504.
133. Sjöström L. Review of the key results from the Swedish Obese Subjects (SOS) trial—a prospective controlled intervention study of bariatric surgery. J Intern Med. 2013;273(3):219–34. https://doi.org/10.1111/joim.12012.
134. Wearing SC, Hennig EM, Byrne NM, Steele JR, Hills AP. Musculoskeletal disorders associated with obesity: a biomechanical perspective. Obes Rev. 2006;7(3):239–50. https://doi.org/10.1111/j.1467-789X.2006.00251.x.

135. Voigt LF, Koepsell TD, Nelson JL, Dugowson CE, Daling JR. Smoking, obesity, alcohol consumption, and the risk of rheumatoid arthritis. Epidemiology. 1994;5(5):525–32.
136. Crowson CS, Matteson EL, Davis JM 3rd, Gabriel SE. Contribution of obesity to the rise in incidence of rheumatoid arthritis. Arthritis Care Res. 2013;65(1):71–7. https://doi.org/10.1002/acr.21660.
137. Bhole VM, Choi HK, Burns LC, et al. Differences in body mass index among individuals with PsA, psoriasis, RA and the general population. Rheumatology (Oxford). 2012;51(3):552–6. https://doi.org/10.1093/rheumatology/ker349.
138. Katz P, Yazdany J, Julian L, et al. Impact of obesity on functioning among women with systemic lupus erythematosus. Arthritis Care Res. 2011;63(10):1357–64. https://doi.org/10.1002/acr.20526.
139. Nikiphorou E, Fragoulis GE. Inflammation, obesity and rheumatic disease: common mechanistic links. A narrative review. Ther Adv Musculoskelet Dis. 2018;10(8):157–67. https://doi.org/10.1177/1759720X18783894.
140. Sparks JA, Halperin F, Karlson JC, Karlson EW, Bermas BL. Impact of bariatric surgery on patients with rheumatoid arthritis. Arthritis Care Res. 2015;67(12):1619–26. https://doi.org/10.1002/acr.22629.
141. Westerveld D, Yang D. Through thick and thin: identifying barriers to bariatric surgery, weight loss maintenance, and tailoring obesity treatment for the future. Surg Res Pract. 2016;2016:8616581. https://doi.org/10.1155/2016/8616581.
142. Nishimura S, Manabe I, Takaki S, et al. Adipose natural regulatory B cells negatively control adipose tissue inflammation. Cell Metab. 2013;18(5):759–66. https://doi.org/10.1016/j.cmet.2013.09.017.
143. Gremese E, Tolusso B, Gigante MR, Ferraccioli G. Obesity as a risk and severity factor in rheumatic diseases (autoimmune chronic inflammatory diseases). Front Immunol. 2014;5:576. https://doi.org/10.3389/fimmu.2014.00576.
144. Beckman LM, Beckman TR, Earthman CP. Changes in gastrointestinal hormones and leptin after Roux-en-Y gastric bypass procedure: a review. J Am Diet Assoc. 2010;110(4):571–84. https://doi.org/10.1016/j.jada.2009.12.023.
145. Unamuno X, Izaguirre M, Gómez-Ambrosi J, et al. Increase of the adiponectin/leptin ratio in patients with obesity and type 2 diabetes after Roux-en-Y gastric bypass. Nutrients. 2019;11(9). https://doi.org/10.3390/nu11092069.
146. Frühbeck G, Catalán V, Rodríguez A, et al. Adiponectin-leptin ratio is a functional biomarker of adipose tissue inflammation. Nutrients. 2019;11(2). https://doi.org/10.3390/nu11020454.
147. Chen C-Y, Tsai C-Y. From endocrine to rheumatism: do gut hormones play roles in rheumatoid arthritis? Rheumatology (Oxford). 2014;53(2):205–12. https://doi.org/10.1093/rheumatology/ket255.
148. Sweeney TE, Morton JM. The human gut microbiome: a review of the effect of obesity and surgically induced weight loss. JAMA Surg. 2013;148(6):563–9. https://doi.org/10.1001/jamasurg.2013.5.
149. Fogel S. Surgical failures: is it the surgeon or the patient? The all too often missed diagnosis of Ehlers-Danlos syndrome. Am Surg. 2013;79(6):608–13.
150. Tada M, Inui K, Sugioka Y, et al. Delayed wound healing and postoperative surgical site infections in patients with rheumatoid arthritis treated with or without biological disease-modifying antirheumatic drugs. Clin Rheumatol. 2016;35(6):1475–81. https://doi.org/10.1007/s10067-016-3274-1.
151. Shanmugam VK. Vasculitic diseases and prothrombotic states contributing to delayed healing in chronic wounds. Curr Dermatol Rep. 2016;5(4):270–7. https://doi.org/10.1007/s13671-016-0157-2.
152. van den Hoogen FH, Boerbooms AM, Swaak AJ, Rasker JJ, van Lier HJ, van de Putte LB. Comparison of methotrexate with placebo in the treatment of systemic sclerosis: a 24 week randomized double-blind trial, followed by a 24 week observational trial. Br J Rheumatol. 1996;35(4):364–72. https://doi.org/10.1093/rheumatology/35.4.364.

153. Verdure L, Genser L, Rebibo L, et al. Bariatric surgery is feasible in patients with Ehlers-Danlos Syndrome. Surg Obes Relat Dis. 2020;16(9):1328–31. https://doi.org/10.1016/j.soard.2020.03.033.
154. Gerogiannis IN, Gkegkes ID, Dempster NJ, Gillies RS, Sgromo B. Obesity surgery and Ehlers-Danlos syndrome: challenges and considerations based on a case report. Ann R Coll Surg Engl. 2020;102(1):e7–e11. https://doi.org/10.1308/rcsann.2019.0122.
155. Corcelles R, Daigle CR, Talamas HR, Batayyah E, Brethauer SA, Schauer PR. Bariatric surgery outcomes in patients with systemic lupus erythematosus. Surg Obes Relat Dis. 2015;11(3):684–8. https://doi.org/10.1016/j.soard.2014.10.006.
156. Helliwell M, Coombes EJ, Moody BJ, Batstone GF, Robertson JC. Nutritional status in patients with rheumatoid arthritis. Ann Rheum Dis. 1984;43(3):386–90. https://doi.org/10.1136/ard.43.3.386.
157. Elshebini E, Elsawah H, Fathy T, et al. Assessment of nutritional deficiency manifestations in patients with rheumatic diseases. Egypt Rheumatol. 2021;43(2):167–71. https://doi.org/10.1016/j.ejr.2020.06.009.
158. Lupoli R, Lembo E, Saldalamacchia G, Avola CK, Angrisani L, Capaldo B. Bariatric surgery and long-term nutritional issues. World J Diabetes. 2017;8(11):464–74. https://doi.org/10.4239/wjd.v8.i11.464.
159. Shreiner AB, Murray C, Denton C, Khanna D. Gastrointestinal manifestations of systemic sclerosis. J Scleroderma Relat Disord. 2016;1(3):247–56. https://doi.org/10.5301/jsrd.5000214.
160. Fynne L, Kruse A, Borre M, Søndergaard K, Krogh K. Percutaneous endoscopic gastrostomy in patients with systemic sclerosis. Scand J Rheumatol. 2010;39(3):266–8. https://doi.org/10.3109/03009740903468990.
161. Nagaraja V, McMahan ZH, Getzug T, Khanna D. Management of gastrointestinal involvement in scleroderma. Curr Treat Options Rheumatol. 2015;1(1):82–105. https://doi.org/10.1007/s40674-014-0005-0.
162. Nunokawa T, Yokogawa N, Ohtsuka H, Shimada K, Sugii S. Transgastric long tube placement following percutaneous endoscopic gastrostomy for severe chronic intestinal pseudo-obstruction related to systemic sclerosis. Mod Rheumatol. 2015;25(6):958–61. https://doi.org/10.3109/14397595.2013.844385.

Chapter 7
Small Bowel Disease Associated with Rheumatologic and Vasculitic Conditions

Tracy Frech, Madeleine E. Frech, Rishi D. Naik, and Laura Pace

7.1 Introduction

Small bowel abnormalities are reported in rheumatologic and vasculitic conditions. The most critical role of the small intestine, which is the longest organ in the gastrointestinal tract, is digestion, absorption, immune system training, and immune system regulation. As such, electrolyte balance, water balance, nutrient uptake, endocrine secretion, and immune barrier function can all be affected by inflammation, immune dysfunction, fibrosis, and vascular disease of the small bowel. In assessment of patients with rheumatic disease and gastrointestinal tract symptomatology, an understanding of normal small intestine physiology as well as the mechanism of immune dysfunction is critical.

Altered physiology of the small intestine is reported in systemic lupus erythematosus (SLE), sarcoidosis, polyarteritis nodosum (PAN) and other forms of mesenteric vasculitis, Degos, and systemic sclerosis (SSc) (Table 7.1). Complications of

T. Frech (✉)
Department of Internal Medicine, Division of Rheumatology and Immunology, Vanderbilt University Medical Center, Nashville, TN, USA
e-mail: Tracy.frech@vumc.org

M. E. Frech
University of Utah School of Medicine, Salt Lake City, UT, USA

R. D. Naik
Department of Gastroenterology, Hepatology, and Nutrition, Vanderbilt University Medical Center, Nashville, TN, USA

L. Pace
Division of Gastroenterology and Hepatology, Department of Medicine, Stanford University, Stanford, CA, USA
e-mail: lapace@stanford.edu

M. Tadros et al. (eds.), *GI Diseases Associated with Rheumatological and Vasculitic Conditions*, Clinical Gastroenterology,
https://doi.org/10.1007/978-3-032-07868-1_7

Table 7.1 Small bowel pathology with rheumatological and vasculitic conditions

Lupus
Enteritis
Pseudo-obstruction
Mesenteric thrombosis
Encapsulating peritoneal sclerosis
Sarcoidosis
Gastrointestinal sarcoid
Protein losing enteropathy
Mesenteric venous insufficiency
Terminal ileum infiltration
Encapsulating peritoneal sclerosis
Polyarteritis nodosa and vasculitis
Pain
Infarction
Bowel perforation
Degos
Ischemic microperforation
Systemic sclerosis
Malnutrition
Hypomobility
Small intestinal bacterial overgrowth
GI vascular ectasias

Table 7.2 Mimics of rheumatological autoimmune disorders

(1) Primary intestinal lymphangiectasias
(2) Celiac disease
(3) Extranodal non-Hodgkin lymphoma
(4) Carcinoid syndrome
(5) Crohn's disease
(6) Whipple's disease
(7) Small bowel tuberculosis

altered physiology, such as malnutrition, small intestinal bacterial overgrowth (SIBO), pseudo-obstruction, arteriovenous malformation (AVM) and bowel perforation can occur in these diseases. Primary small intestine conditions such as intestinal lymphangiectasia, celiac disease, Crohn's disease, small intestine lymphoma, and gastrointestinal tract infections, can have rheumatic manifestations, which highlight the value of careful patient assessment and proper use of diagnostics (Table 7.2).

7.2 Small Intestine Anatomy

The small intestine is a hollow viscus that is functionally delineated into three regions: the duodenum, jejunum, and ileum. Throughout its' length the wall of the small intestine is composed of mucosa, submucosa, muscularis propria, and serosa. Within these layers are an inner circular muscle layer and an outer longitudinal muscle layer along with the submucosal plexus and myenteric plexus which are important components of the enteric nervous system. The function of the small intestine varies along its' length and therefore so does its' cellular composition. The position within the abdominal cavity also varies by region. Villi are fingerlike projections of the mucosa that increase the absorptive surface area of the underlying mucosa and therefore are longest in the duodenum and proximal jejunum because these are the regions in which the greatest absorption occurs. Following this logic, villi are shortest in the distal ileum where very little absorption occurs. Most of the duodenum resides within the retroperitoneum, while the jejunum and ileum are positioned as intraperitoneal structures. An important distinguishing feature of the duodenum is the presence of Brunner's glands. These glands are located below the submucosa and are composed of endocrine cells and submucosal ramifying tubules lined principally by cells resembling the mucus-secreting cells of the gastric antral mucosa. They secrete an alkaline mucus-like substance that protects the duodenum from the acidic chyme produced by the stomach. The presence of these glands in the duodenum extend to approximately the sphincter of Oddi. The sphincter of Oddi functions to control the flow of digestive juices from the liver and pancreas into the small intestine to coincide with the arrival of chyme from the stomach. The proximal duodenum receives chyme from the stomach, bile from the liver, and pancreatic juice from the pancreas which assist in the macromolecular breakdown of ingested food to enhance absorption of nutrients. The absorption of iron from dietary sources takes place in the duodenum in the presence of bile. The ligament of Treitz is a thin band of muscle that supports the small intestine at the transition from the duodenum to the beginning of the jejunum. The jejunum is anatomically distinguished from the ileum by the presence of plicae circulares, also known as valvulae conniventes, in the mucosa, which contributes to a thicker wall in the jejunum. The mesentery contains less fat in the jejunum when compared to the ileum. The jejunum is responsible for absorbing fully digested carbohydrates, proteins, fats, and minerals (including passive calcium absorption) while the ileum is important for vitamin B12 and bile acid absorption. The ileum ends at the ileocecal valve. The specific changes to the mucosa, submucosa, muscularis propria, and serosa in the small intestine are important to consider when approaching a patient with rheumatic disease and gastrointestinal tract symptoms [1].

The first aspect of understanding small intestinal pathology is determining whether the pathology is related to luminal injury, peritoneal involvement, perfusion abnormalities, or nervous system dysfunction. The innermost layer of the lumen is the mucosa, which is composed of epithelium, lamina propria, and muscularis mucosae. Overlaying the mucosa on the luminal side is a thick mucin layer that adds another layer of barrier function for the gastrointestinal tract. There are four major luminal epithelial cells in the small intestine, including Paneth, enteroendocrine, goblet, and enterocyte. Paneth cells are crypt cells that secrete potent antibacterial granules, including lysozyme and α-defensin, which are critical for mucosal immunity. They originate from crypt stem cells and remain juxtaposed to the crypt maintaining the health of the stem cell niche. A single layer of columnar epithelial cells called enterocytes lines the mucosal villi. Between the enterocytes are goblet cells that secrete mucin to protect the intestinal wall as chyme and undigested food passes. At the base of each villus are intestinal crypt cells that secrete fluids, electrolytes, and contains a stem cell that can further differentiate into a goblet cell, an enterocyte, or an enteroendocrine cell. Enteroendocrine cells produce hormones that slow down the digestive process [1].

The mucosal immune system of the small intestine protects luminal surfaces against harmful microbes; provide a barrier to undigested foreign antigens; and prevents the development of immune responses to these antigens. In addition to Paneth cells, M cells are specialized cells that are in the follicle-associated epithelium surrounding Peyer patches, which are specialized aggregates of lymphoid follicles in the lamina propria that recognize and process antigen. The long-term effects of immunosuppression on mucosal immunity are not well-known in rheumatologic and vasculitic conditions [1].

The structure of the submucosa is important for understanding motility issues in rheumatic disease. Myogenic, neural, and hormonal factors regulate small intestinal motility. The submucosa is the strength layer of the bowel wall and is composed of dense connective tissue that includes blood vessels, lymphatics, nerve fibers, and immune cells. The Meissner, or submucosal plexus, is also positioned in the submucosa and is an important component of the enteric nervous system (ENS). The submucosal plexus provides innervation to intestinal glands, endocrine cells, and blood vessels in the mucosal layer. Below the submucosa, is the muscularis propria that is composed of both an outer longitudinal and an inner circular smooth muscle layer. Between these two muscle layers, is the myenteric, or Auerbach plexus that also composes the ENS and facilitates bowel motility. The ENS is an independently functioning system that can affect vascular tone motility, secretion, and hormone release in the small intestine. The ENS is innervated by the autonomic nervous system (ANS). The ANS also directly innervates many other structures and cells within the gastrointestinal system. The luminal microbiota, gastrointestinal tract, ENS, ANS, and central nervous system (CNS) are the major components of the microbiota-gut-brain axis. The serosa is the outermost layer of the bowel wall and is a single layer of mesothelial cell and an essential structure to understand in serositis [1].

7.3 Systemic Lupus Erythematosus

Small bowel involvement in SLE is an important cause of morbidity in this patient population, with vasculitis and thrombosis the most frequent pathological mechanism described [2, 3]. Lupus enteritis, pseudo-obstruction, and mesenteric thrombosis are important small intestinal considerations for a SLE patient presenting with acute abdominal pain. Lupus enteritis describes either serosal vasculitis or inflammation of the small bowel with supportive imaging and/or biopsy finding [4]. Imaging is most used for diagnosis since lupus enteritis is seldom confirmed on histology. Contrast enhanced computed tomography (CT) scanning is the gold standard for diagnosis of lupus enteritis and should demonstrate the presence of bowel wall thickening, dilatation of intestinal segments, mesenteric abnormalities (including engorgement of mesenteric vessels and/or increased attenuation of mesenteric fat without mesenteric thrombosis), ascites, peritoneal enhancement, retroperitoneal lymphadenopathy, and the "target sign" of submucosal edema [5, 6]. If thrombosis is suspected, angiography is an invasive diagnostic and therapeutic measure that is reserved for cases with high pretest probability and a non-diagnostic CT [7]. Early laparoscopy or laparotomy is reserved for perforation or concern for intestinal viability. Paracentesis is only useful if concern for etiology or therapeutic relief due to volume.

The most common clinical symptom of lupus enteritis is abdominal pain in almost all patients, however, there may be other nonspecific symptoms of dysmotility and peritoneal irritation, including vomiting, diarrhea, fever, and ascites [5]. No single biological finding can be considered pathognomonic for lupus enteritis, and laboratory studies mostly reflected SLE disease activity, including low complement levels and cytopenia. There is no higher prevalence of antiphospholipid antibodies in lupus enteritis, and CRO is not typically very elevated. An association with anti-endothelial cell antibodies is reported [8], but this laboratory cannot be considered a diagnostic tool is associated with disease activity in various systemic vasculitis diseases [9]. Endoscopic biopsies are not generally helpful unless ruling out alternatively diagnoses, but capsule endoscopy may reveal ulcerations [5, 10]. Corticosteroids are first-line therapy, with additional immunosuppressants, such as azathioprine, mycophenolate mofetil, cyclophosphamide, or rituximab, recommended in the case of relapse [5]. While responsiveness to steroids is well-reported, bowel rest and intravenous fluids may be necessary. If untreated, the disease may evolve to intestinal necrosis and perforation, thus heightened suspicion for enteritis is warranted in an SLE patients with gastrointestinal complaints.

Intestinal pseudo-obstruction (IPO) is considered rare and occasionally the presenting feature of SLE [11]. This severe form of gastrointestinal dysmotility with recurrent episodes of intestinal subocclusion mimics a mechanical obstruction and, like lupus enteritis, can present with abdominal pain, distention, nausea, and vomiting. In addition to distention of the small intestine, CT imaging can reveal pyeloureterectasis and biliary tract dilatation [12]. Patients that have this triad of features, also known as visceral muscle dysmotility syndrome, on CT imaging should carefully assessed for underlying SLE if they do not have this prior diagnosis [13]. Pathogenesis is suspected to be due to vasculitis of the visceral smooth muscles, thus leading to muscular damage and hypomotility of the submucosal muscles. Therapeutic management of IPO includes corticosteroid and immunosuppressants, as delayed treatment can be life-threatening [12].

7.4 Sarcoidosis

Encapsulating peritoneal sclerosis (EPS) can complicate both SLE and sarcoidosis independent of use of peritoneal dialysis [14, 15]. A fibro-collagenous membrane encasing the small intestine that results in recurrent small bowel obstructions characterizes EPS [16]. Immune dysregulation with pro-inflammatory, pro-angiogenic cytokine resulting mesothelial-to-mesenchymal transition with subsequent fibrosis is the proposed mechanism of this disease. Laboratory findings in EPS are non-specific and related to underlying infection, malnutrition, and inflammation, thus imaging is important for diagnosis. Abdominal plain films and cross-sectional imaging with CT of the abdomen may show peritoneal thickening with calcification as well as dilated loops of bowel with air-fluid levels and lymphadenopathy (Fig. 7.1). Small bowel follow-through may show delayed transit, distension proximal to small bowel adhesions. However, many patients undergo exploratory laparotomy for diagnosis. Histologic findings in EPS are non-specific and may overlap with findings in simple peritoneal sclerosis or infectious peritonitis, thus the occurrence in a patient with SLE or sarcoid often requires other diagnostic testing for these conditions. With the small bowel obstruction, TPN is required since enteral feeding is not often tolerated. Despite nutritional support, mortality is high.

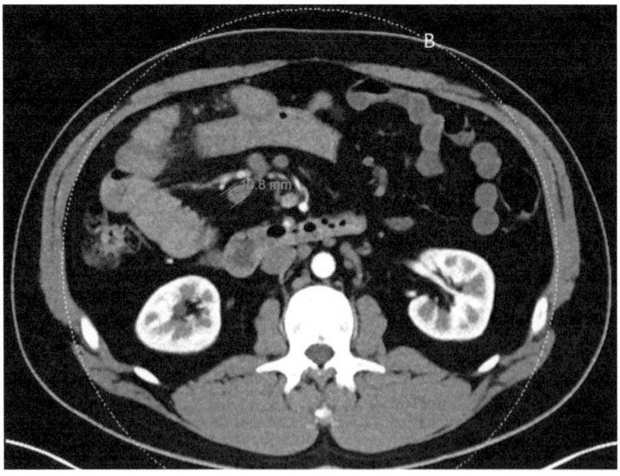

Fig. 7.1 GI manifestation of sarcoid: extensive small bowel lymphadenopathy seen on CT

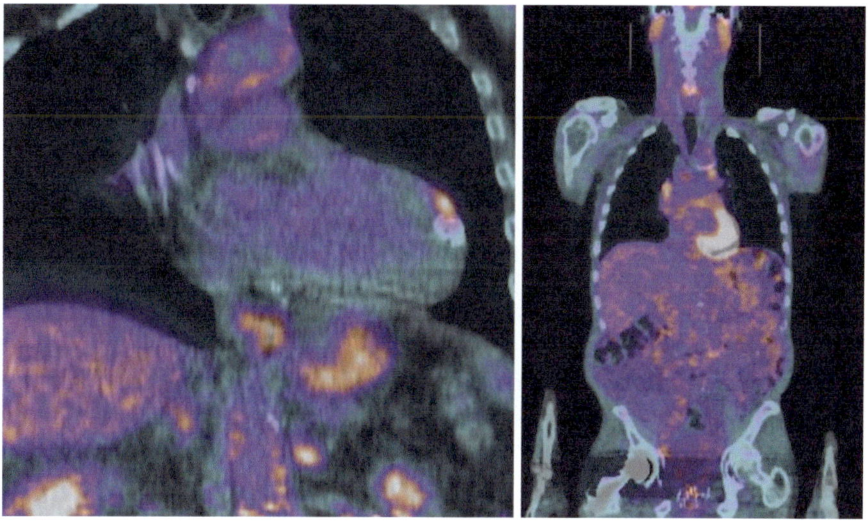

Fig. 7.2 PET-CT utilization—Sarcoid with PET active cardiac and esophageal involvement (Panel A), IgG4-related disease with PET Avidity in cervical, retroperitoneal, mediastinal, inguinal, lymphadenopathy (Panel B)

Immunosuppressive therapy is reserved for patients thought to have an active inflammatory component after excluding infection. The appropriate dosing and duration of corticosteroids are not established, but discontinuation after 1 month of inadequate treatment response is proposed. Surgical techniques are technically challenging thus reserved for patients that have failed medical therapy and include ablation of fibrotic tissue and lysis of adhesions (enterolysis) but may require resection of perforated or ischemic bowel.

In addition to involvement of the peritoneal cavity, gastrointestinal sarcoidosis is a rare manifestation of this disease. Diagnostic laparoscopy of non-caseating granulomas with exclusion of other causes of granulomatous disease, and evidence of sarcoidosis in at least one other organ system makes the diagnosis [17]. Other rare complications include megaloblastic anemia caused by terminal ileum infiltration, mesenteric venous insufficiency due to pressure from enlarged sarcoid lymphadenopathy (Fig. 7.2a), and protein-losing enteropathy.

Gastrointestinal sarcoidosis can occur in a patient with known diagnosis or as initial presentation. Treatment of gastrointestinal sarcoidosis depends on symptomatology and disease activity [18]. Gastrointestinal sarcoidosis monitoring of is accomplished by clinical symptoms and radiographic improvement, but there is no evidence for the role of serum angiotensin converting enzyme or serum interlukin-2 receptor in monitoring [17]. While the optimal duration of corticosteroid treatment for gastrointestinal sarcoidosis is not known, treatment for at least 1 year is proposed [17]. Surgical intervention may be necessary in patients with bowel obstruction, perforation, or massive hemorrhage. A high index of suspension is essential in patients presenting with small-bowel obstruction and previous history of sarcoidosis.

7.5 Systemic Sclerosis

The small bowel is the third most commonly affected organ in SSc [19]. Neuronal and myogenic abnormalities result from an initial vascular dysfunction causing endothelial cell injury followed by an inflammation with aggregation of perivascular mononuclear infiltrates with cytokine and growth factor upregulation, and subsequent deposition of extracellular matrix components in the mucosa and submucosa [20]. Malnutrition in SSc may result from small intestine involvement, thus is important to assess in all patients particularly in patients with low serum prealbumin [21]. Screening is especially important as malnutrition represents a potentially modifiable risk factor with nutritional intervention [22]. Abdominal imaging is also recommended in screening patients with an RNA polymerase III antibody with abdominal symptoms due to the increase in malignancy seen in these patients (Fig. 7.3) [23].

The small intestine manifestations can include hypomotility and bacterial overgrowth [24]. Intestinal pseudo-obstruction disorder can be indicated by crises of diffuse abdominal pain, constipation, bloating, and abdominal distention of variable intensity occurring intermittently, creating a picture of repetitive partial or complete bowel obstruction (Fig. 7.4) [25]. Opioids are a modifiable risk factor for this complication [26]. Management of pseudo-obstruction includes hospitalization to exclude mechanical causes, bowel rest, intravenous fluids, and nutritional support [27]. In SSc-associated small intestine dysmotility, surgical resection is discouraged and reserved for cases that have failed conservative therapies to exclude intestinal obstruction and provide decompression [27]

Imaging of small intestine involvement in SSc can reveal the hide-bound bowel sign, which describes the narrow separation between the valvulae conniventes, which are of normal thickness despite dilatation of the bowel lumen that appear on

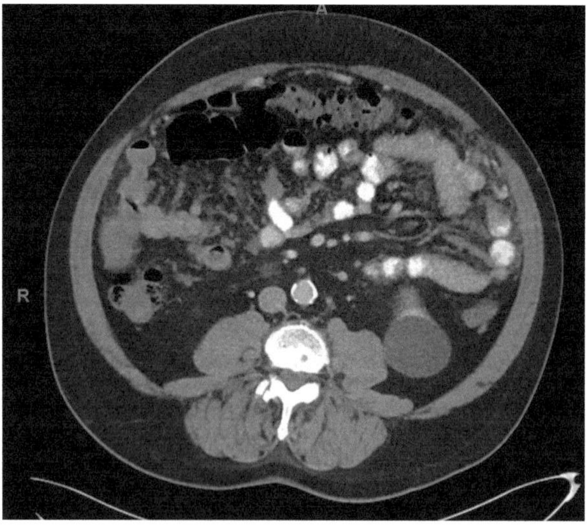

Fig. 7.3 Peritoneal carcinomatosis, compatible with malignant involvement in SSc patient with RNApol3 antibody

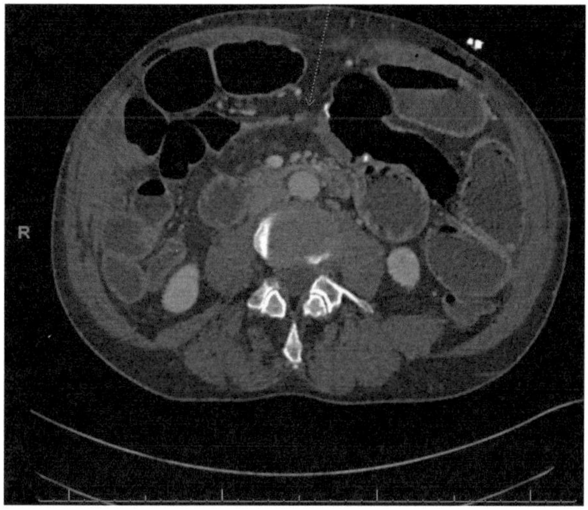

Fig. 7.4 Dilated small bowel loops measuring up to 5.4 cm with air-fluid levels. There is a short segment of decompressed small bowel proximal to a patent anastomosis site representing small bowel obstruction

a barium study of the small bowel in patients with SSc [22]. The cause of hidebound appearance is thought to be asymmetric smooth muscle atrophy of the inner circular muscularis layer relative to the outer longitudinal layer. Contraction of the longitudinal layer results in foreshortening of the bowel and close juxtaposition of the valvulae conniventes.

A decrease in the intestinal peristalsis can lead to stasis and dilatation causing bacterial overgrowth. An increase of the concentration of colonic-type bacteria in the small bowel is the hallmark of small intestinal bacterial overgrowth (SIBO) with a cut off of 10^5 CFU/mL considered as the optimal threshold for diagnosis [28]. A small study of 55 SSc patients diagnosed by lactulose breath test and treated with rifaximin demonstrated a significant reduction in intestinal symptoms [29]. However, accurate diagnosis of SIBO continues to pose a number of challenges in clinical practice and is often treated empirically [27]. While the prevalence of SIBO in SSc varies according to the SIBO diagnostic test performed, geographic area, and SSc diagnostic criteria, approximately one-third of SSc patients test positive for SIBO with a significantly increased risk over the controls [30]. A longer SSc disease duration is associated with a positive breath test for SIBO [31]. The most common clinical manifestations of SIBO are watery diarrhea, bloating, abdominal pain, and distension. Additionally, deficit of B12, D, A, and E vitamins as well as iron and calcium are possible. The presence of diarrhea may be a predictor of SIBO in SSc, thus should be considered diagnostically in SSc patients with this symptom. Antibiotic treatment can lead to eradication of SIBO and gastrointestinal symptomatic improvement in SSc patients. SIBO could even represent a pathogenetic link with SSc in which a perturbation of intestinal microbiota occurs [32]. Routine use of prokinetics and probiotics in SSc patients with SIBO requires further study [33, 34].

Gastrointestinal vascular ectasia comprises angiodysplasia, which are discrete, flat or slightly raised bright-red lesions and that occur in the small intestine of SSc

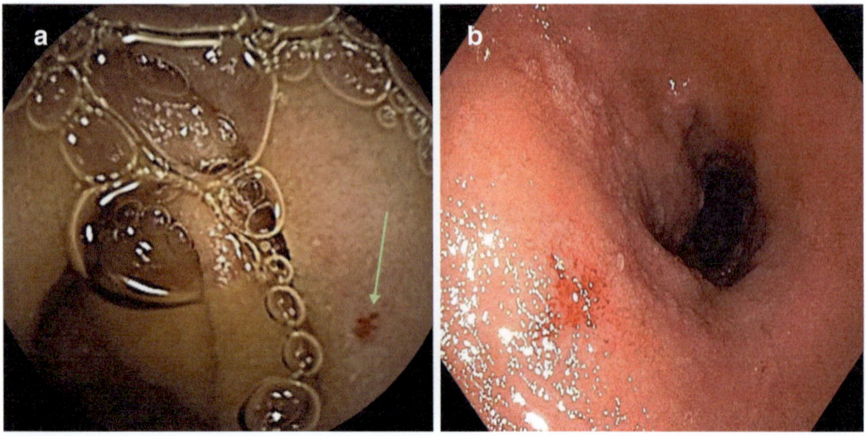

Fig. 7.5 Angiodysplasia seen on Wireless Capsule endoscopy (Panel A) and on endoscopy (Panel B)

patients that can be seen on direct visualization with endoscopy or on wireless capsule endoscopy (Fig. 7.5). The clinical presentation most commonly results chronic gastrointestinal blood loss that leads to chronic anemia. Diagnosis is most commonly made with double-balloon enteroscopy. Endoscopic hemostasis with argon plasma coagulation is a safe modality for treatment of both angiodysplasia and vascular ectasia bleeding [35].

7.6 Polyarteritis Nodosa and Vasculitis

Polyarteritis Nodosa (PAN) is a necrotizing, focal segmental vasculitis that affects small- and medium-sized arteries, without arteriolitis or capillaritis. Approximately 1% of patients with rheumatoid arthritis develop vasculitis, which clinically and histologically resembles classic PAN [36]. It may occur in various organs, but approximately half of cases have gastrointestinal involvement [37]. The small intestinal complications of PAN can present as an acute abdomen, including infarction and perforation [38]. Patients with PAN have constitutional symptoms, including fever, weight loss, malaise, arthralgia, and/or myalgia as well as gastrointestinal tract symptoms including abdominal pain, nausea, and/or diarrhea. Gastrointestinal tract involvement is the major cause of death in hepatitis B virus (HBV)-associated PAN [39]. In addition to acute surgical needs, treatment combines an antiviral drug with plasma-exchange.

In all necrotizing vasculitides, peritonitis, bowel perforation, gastrointestinal ischemia or infarctions and intestinal occlusion are associated with higher mortality in patients [40]. Churg-Strauss syndrome is a small and medium vessel vasculitis that is also known as allergic granulomatous angiitis with gastrointestinal events reported in one third of patients. Ulcerations of the small intestinal can result in perforation, ischemia, bleeding, or obstruction. Most macroscopic involvement are identified by conventional endoscopy, capsule endoscopy, and laparotomy or at autopsy [41]. Prompt surgical intervention when indicated and the combined use of steroids and immunosuppression is the standard of care, though outcomes of small intestinal involvement are poor [40].

Although rare, IgG4-related sclerosing disease of the small bowel can also present as necrotizing mesenteric arteritis. This is a biopsy diagnosis, which reveals transmural inflammatory infiltrate of IgG4 plasma cells in the wall of the bowel and mesenteric artery with a concurrent elevated serum IgG4 level [42] (Fig. 7.2b).

7.7 Degos

The small bowel is the most common internal organ involved in the malignant form of atrophic papulosis (Degos disease), which is a rare thrombo-occlusive vasculopathy [43]. Markers of inflammation, including ESR and CRP can be helpful for assessing for extra-cutaneous involvement [44]. Importantly, the bowel involvement in Degos is primarily serosal, with poor visualization on both magnetic resonance imaging (MRI) and endoscopic imaging, and often requiring laparoscopic visualization. Ischemic micro-perforations result in considerable morbidity and mortality, thus a heightened awareness and referral for laparotomy in patients with classic skin lesions of central porcelain-white atrophy and surrounding telangiectatic rim that have abdominal symptoms is imperative prior to bowel perforation and peritonitis. Treatment with eculizumab, a complement C5 inhibitor, has demonstrated some efficacy in delaying disease progression, with the addition of treprostinil becoming the mainstay of therapy for patients who develop small intestine disease [44].

7.8 Mimic of Rheumatologic Autoimmune Disease

Mimics of rheumatologic autoimmune disease can present with systemic features, but are defined by classic biopsy findings, which highlights the importance of tissue acquisition for diagnosis (Table 7.2) A rare disorder known as primary intestinal lymphangiectasia is characterized by dilated intestinal lacteals that results in lymph leakage into the small bowel lumen causing a protein-losing enteropathy characterized by lymphopenia, hypoalbuminemia and hypogammaglobulinemia. This entity is associated with bilateral lower limb edema, pleural effusion, pericarditis or chylous ascites, this can be mistaken for rheumatologic disease. Like autoimmune disease, fatigue, abdominal pain, weight loss, inability to gain weight, moderate diarrhea or fat-soluble vitamin deficiencies due to malabsorption may also be present. Exudative enteropathy is confirmed by the elevated 24-h stool alpha1-antitrypsin clearance, with diagnosis confirmed by endoscopic observation of intestinal lymphangiectasia with the corresponding histology of intestinal biopsy specimens. A permanent low-fat diet and medium-chain triglyceride (MCT) supplementation is the foundation of medical management since MCT are absorbed directly into the portal venous circulation and avoid lacteal overloading while the absence of fat prevents chylous engorgement of the intestinal lymphatic vessels thereby averting their rupture and lymph loss [45].

Patients with rheumatologic disease can have an overlap condition. Celiac disease is associated with other autoimmune diseases like Sjögren disease, and can present with musculoskeletal pain, skin manifestations, and fatigue [46]. Endoscopic features include duodenal blunting, scalloped or loss of folds, and mucosal mosaic pattern (Fig. 7.6). Highly sensitive and specific anti-endomysium and tissue transglutaminase serological tests assist in the diagnosis. Duodenal biopsies that demonstrate histological findings compatible with celiac sprue followed by a favorable clinical and serological response to gluten-free diet is now considered sufficient to confirm the diagnosis [47].

The small intestine is the second most common gastrointestinal location for extra-nodal non-Hodgkin lymphoma [48]. Primary small intestinal lymphoma is commonly of B-cell origin and consists of different subtypes with varying biologic behaviors. Diagnosis is supported on MR enterography and confirmed on biopsy [49]. *Campylobacter jejuni* is implicated in immunoproliferative small intestinal disease and highlights the importance of understanding the role of continuous immune stimulation (from either chronic infections or auto inflammatory diseases) in genetic aberrations resulting in lymphoid transformation [50].

Carcinoid syndrome is a paraneoplastic syndrome caused by the release of serotonin and other substances from well-differentiated neuroendocrine tumors of the small intestine. Classically, patients complain of flushing (90%), diarrhea (70%), and wheezing (15%) [51].The measurement of both serum and plasma 5-hydroxyindoleacetic acid can be used for the diagnosis and monitoring of patients. CT imaging is of poor utility in detecting primary carcinoid tumors but is helpful in

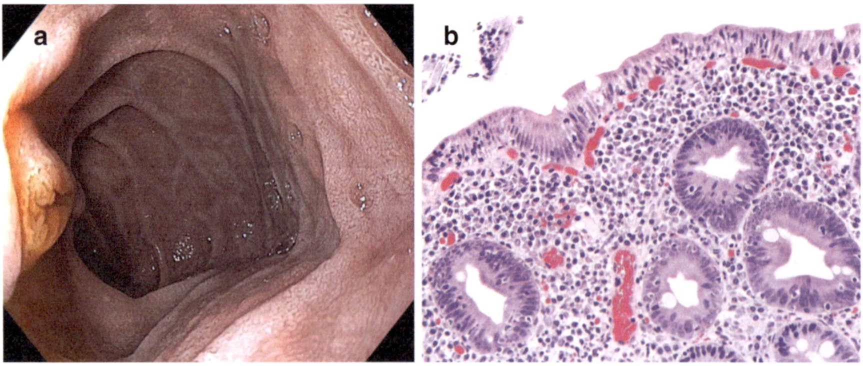

Fig. 7.6 Upper Endoscopy showing Celiac disease with duodenal blunting, atrophy, and loss of folds on endoscopy (Panel A), small bowel biopsy showing villous atrophy and lymphocytic infiltration

evaluating the extent of tumor spread before surgical exploration. An abdominal MRI scan can identify metastases of carcinoid syndrome to the liver and mesentery. Somatostatin scintigraphy may detect resectable tumors that would be unrecognized with regular imaging studies [51].

Common presenting symptoms of small intestinal involvement with Crohn's disease include diarrhea, cramping, abdominal pain, and weight loss. Fever and arthritis can occur. When the diagnosis of Crohn's disease is considered, stool studies for Clostridium difficile, ova and parasites, and culture may be useful [52]. Traditional and capsule endoscopy are essential for diagnosing and monitoring small intestinal Crohn's disease (Fig. 7.7). Cross-sectional imaging techniques, including CT, MRI, and ultrasonography are helpful for identifying complications that result from transmural involvement including fistula or abscess formation [53]. Fecal calprotectin can assess for inflammation in Crohn's disease but does not distinguish from infection.

Chronic infections of the small intestine cause significant morbidity and mortality. A rheumatologist should have a heightened awareness since immunodeficiency increase the susceptibility to many chronic intestinal infections. Specific, to patients on immunosuppression, MR enterography is helpful for evaluation of small bowel tuberculosis (TB). However, endoscopy and intestinal biopsies are critical for establishing a diagnosis. Whipple's disease due to the causative organism *Tropheryma whipplei* is rare, but extended treatment with broad-spectrum antibiotics is effective in most cases [54]. The mucosal immune responses in Whipple's elicit barrier dysfunction, and diarrhea is caused by loss of absorptive capacity and leak flux of ions and water [55]. An understanding of the assessment of mechanism of disease in chronic bowel infections offers the opportunity to better understand management in rheumatologic disease.

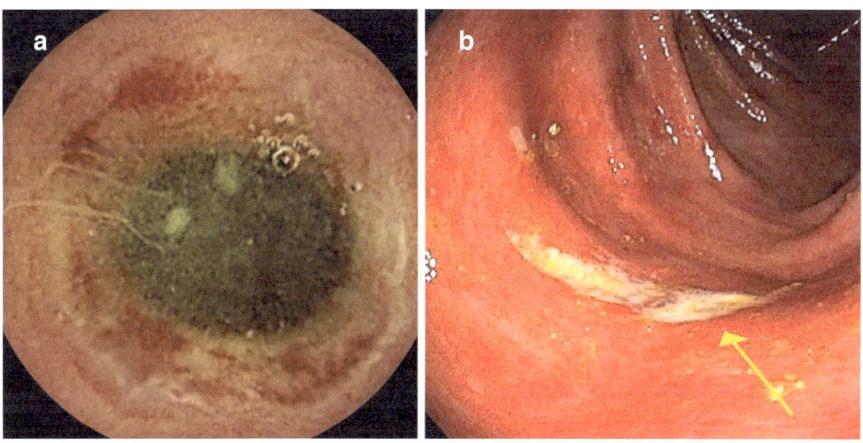

Fig. 7.7 Wireless Capsule endoscopy showing jejunal stricture from Crohn's (Panel A), cCrohn's disease with deep ulcer and surround erythema and inflammation (Panel B)

Nonsteroidal anti-inflammatory drug (NSAID) enteropathy is a concern for patients with rheumatic disease receiving this analgesic therapy for musculoskeletal complaints. Mucosal erosions and strictures, possibly exacerbated by concurrent therapies that alter intestinal microbiome composition, can complicate a rheumatic disease patients' course. NSAID-induced small intestinal enteropathy results from altered gastrointestinal cellular integrity with amplified inflammation from bile acids and gut microbiota [56]. To minimize adverse effect, patients using NSAID therapy should be advised to take the lowest effective dose for the minimum necessary duration. There should be a low threshold to hold NSAID therapy in a rheumatic disease patient with gastrointestinal complaints.

7.9 Diagnostic Considerations

The first aspect of understanding small intestinal pathology is determining which imaging modality provides information related to luminal injury, peritoneal involvement, perfusion abnormalities, or nervous system dysfunction. Laboratory testing can be helpful for diagnosis of celiac, carcinoid, malnutrition, and malabsorption, but in general is non-specific in rheumatologic patients with small bowel symptomatology, highlighting the need for imaging to understand pathogenesis.

The primary blood supply for the small bowel is the superior mesenteric artery (SMA) with some collateral flow from the celiac arterial system via the superior and inferior pancreaticoduodenal arteries, as well as from the inferior mesenteric artery [57]. Through enhanced oxygen extraction and perfusion due to vasodilation, the intestines can autoregulate oxygen availability. Thus, the splanchnic circulation must be reduced by more than 50% before the small intestine becomes ischemic. The four major causes of acute mesenteric ischemia are superior SMA embolus, SMA thrombosis, mesenteric venous thrombosis, and nonocclusive mesenteric vasoconstriction. Nonocclusive mesenteric ischemia can occur if excessive sympathetic activity results in secondary vasoconstriction of the mesenteric arteries [58].

Radiological small bowel imaging is considered as the primary imaging approach to diagnose pathological changes of the small bowel. Enterography includes timed intravenous contrast, is useful in the assessment of the solid organs, and provides detailed information on the small bowel. Enterography is useful for suspected small bowel bleeding, usually performed after negative endoscopy; suspected small bowel tumor (for example, carcinoid, polyposis syndromes, lymphoma), celiac disease; or suspected chronic mesenteric ischemia. Enteroclysis is the use of a contrast agent normally administered through a nasogastric tube and is valuable in detecting the presence of obstruction and in differentiating partial from complete small bowel blockages.

Small bowel radiographic imaging includes barium studies (small bowel follow-through), CT (multidetector CT, CT enterography, and CT enteroclysis), ultrasound (sonoenteroclysis), and magnetic resonance imaging (MRI; enterography and enteroclysis). CT angiography (CTA) and contrast-enhanced MR angiography

(MRA) are excellent noninvasive screening techniques for patients suspected of having mesenteric ischemia of all causes. CTA has higher spatial resolution and faster acquisition times, allowing assessment of the peripheral visceral branches and the inferior mesenteric artery with greater accuracy than contrast-enhanced MRA, and allows identification of calcified plaques [57]. Contrast-enhanced MRA lacks radiation and iodinated contrast agents make it the preferred imaging option for children and patients with azotemia [58].

Endoscopy-based imaging methods such as double-balloon endoscopy or wireless capsule endoscopy can visualize the complete small bowel but are invasive diagnostic methods [59]. Jejunal aspirate culture is the gold-standard for SIBO diagnosis, though breath testing non-invasive breath tests, namely lactulose breath tests and glucose breath tests are more commonly non-invasive tests used to assess for this condition [60]. In vitro modeling with enterocyte, goblet, and immune-like cells exposed to a synthetic microbial community representative of commensal inhabitants of the small intestine may offer improved insight [61].

Manometric investigations may also help to identify the presence of neuropathic or myopathic disorders that affect the small bowel, particularly chronic intestinal pseudo-obstruction. Manometric studies of small intestine motility should be preceded by an accurate exclusion of other organic and/or metabolic disorders by means of radiologic and endoscopic studies [62]. The availability of less invasive radioisotopic techniques may represent a reasonable alternative to manometric investigations, although these techniques are more expensive.

The use of ambulatory manometry together with impedance recordings provides data not only motor activity but on mucosal integrity. Structural/anatomical differences of intestinal villus and tight junctions from the proximal duodenum to jejunum may affect the baseline impedance values. Thus, mucosal status as expressed by the baseline impedance value may provide insight that is critical for understanding the lumen of small intestine [63].

7.10 Conclusion

The duodenum, jejunum, and ileum can be affected in rheumatologic and vasculitic conditions with resultant profound symptomatology. Laboratory tests are, in general, non-specific for diagnosis of rheumatologic small bowel involvement and imaging is imperative for diagnosis of peritoneal involvement, perfusion abnormalities, and nervous system dysfunction. Endoscopy provides information on luminal abnormalities and can help in assessment of rheumatologic mimics that require tissue diagnosis. High morbidity and mortality can result if there is a delay in diagnosis, thus abdominal symptoms in patients with known rheumatologic disease should always be assessed promptly. Advances in luminal assessments of host-microbiome interactions and mucosal impedance in the small intestine may offer new insights on pathogenesis. Longitudinal use of noninvasive diagnostics may help clarify the effect of long-term immunosuppression on small bowel health, though admittedly these are not yet available in the clinical setting [64].

References

1. Abbott AMAL, Jensen EH. Shackelford's surgery of the alimentary tract, 17th edn, vol 2. Elsevier; 2013.
2. Ebert EC, Hagspiel KD. Gastrointestinal and hepatic manifestations of systemic lupus erythematosus. J Clin Gastroenterol. 2011;45:436–41.
3. Frittoli RB, Vivaldo JF, Costallat LTL, Appenzeller S. Gastrointestinal involvement in systemic lupus erythematosus: a systematic review. J Transl Autoimmun. 2021;4:100106.
4. Isenberg DA, Rahman A, Allen E, Farewell V, Akil M, Bruce IN, D'Cruz D, Griffiths B, Khamashta M, Maddison P, et al. BILAG 2004. Development and initial validation of an updated version of the British Isles Lupus Assessment Group's disease activity index for patients with systemic lupus erythematosus. Rheumatology (Oxford). 2005;44:902–6.
5. Janssens P, Arnaud L, Galicier L, Mathian A, Hie M, Sene D, Haroche J, Veyssier-Belot C, Huynh-Charlier I, Grenier PA, et al. Lupus enteritis: from clinical findings to therapeutic management. Orphanet J Rare Dis. 2013;8:67.
6. Aiyappan SK, Suvindran A. Lupus enteritis. Pan Afr Med J. 2019;33:205.
7. Hmoud B, Singal AK, Kamath PS. Mesenteric venous thrombosis. J Clin Exp Hepatol. 2014;4:257–63.
8. Kwok SK, Seo SH, Ju JH, Park KS, Yoon CH, Kim WU, Min JK, Park SH, Cho CS, Kim HY. Lupus enteritis: clinical characteristics, risk factor for relapse and association with anti-endothelial cell antibody. Lupus. 2007;16:803–9.
9. Legendre P, Regent A, Thiebault M, Mouthon L. Anti-endothelial cell antibodies in vasculitis: a systematic review. Autoimmun Rev. 2017;16:146–53.
10. Endo H, Kondo Y, Kawagoe K, Ohya TR, Yanagawa T, Asayama M, Hisatomi K, Teratani T, Yoneda M, Inamori M, et al. Lupus enteritis detected by capsule endoscopy. Intern Med. 2007;46:1621–2.
11. Zhang FJ, Zhang J, Zhou LP, Wang AM, Li XM. Intestinal pseudo-obstruction as the initial manifestation of systemic lupus erythematosus. Am J Emerg Med. 2019;37:176 e171–176 e172.
12. Zhang L, Xu D, Yang H, Tian X, Wang Q, Hou Y, Gao N, Zhang L, Li M, Zeng X. Clinical features, morbidity, and risk factors of intestinal pseudo-obstruction in systemic lupus erythematosus: a retrospective case-control study. J Rheumatol. 2016;43:559–64.
13. Xu D, Yang H, Lai CC, Li P, Zhang X, Yang XO, Zhang FC, Qian JM. Clinical analysis of systemic lupus erythematosus with gastrointestinal manifestations. Lupus. 2010;19:866–9.
14. Pepels MJ, Peters FP, Mebis JJ, Ceelen TL, Hoofwijk AG, Erdkamp FL. Sclerosing peritonitis: an unusual cause of ascites in a patient with systemic lupus erythematosus. Neth J Med. 2006;64:346–9.
15. Ngo Y, Messing B, Marteau P, Nouel O, Pasquiou A, Lavergne A, Rambaud JC. Peritoneal sarcoidosis. An unrecognized cause of sclerosing peritonitis. Dig Dis Sci. 1992;37:1776–80.
16. Danford CJ, Lin SC, Smith MP, Wolf JL. Encapsulating peritoneal sclerosis. World J Gastroenterol. 2018;24:3101–11.
17. Zakaria A, Al Share B, Turk I, Ahsan S, Farra W. An uncommon cause of a small-bowel obstruction. Case Rep Gastrointest Med. 2017;2017:1628215.
18. Ebert EC, Kierson M, Hagspiel KD. Gastrointestinal and hepatic manifestations of sarcoidosis. Am J Gastroenterol. 2008;103:3184–92; quiz 3193
19. Chatzinikolaou SLQB, Murray C. Radiological findings in gastrointestinal scleroderma. JSRD. 2019;5:21–32.

20. Denton CP, Black CM. Scleroderma—clinical and pathological advances. Best Pract Res Clin Rheumatol. 2004;18:271–90.
21. Harrison E, Herrick AL, McLaughlin JT, Lal S. Malnutrition in systemic sclerosis. Rheumatology (Oxford). 2012;51:1747–56.
22. Xiang H, Han J, Ridley WE, Ridley LJ. Hidebound sign: small bowel in systemic sclerosis. J Med Imaging Radiat Oncol. 2018;62(Suppl 1):80.
23. Weeding E, Casciola-Rosen L, Shah AA. Cancer and scleroderma. Rheum Dis Clin N Am. 2020;46:551–64.
24. Sakkas LI, Simopoulou T, Daoussis D, Liossis SN, Potamianos S. Intestinal involvement in systemic sclerosis: a clinical review. Dig Dis Sci. 2018;63:834–44.
25. Hachulla E, Agard C, Allanore Y, Avouac J, Bader-Meunier B, Belot A, Berezne A, Bouthors AS, Condette-Wojtasik G, Constans J, et al. French recommendations for the management of systemic sclerosis. Orphanet J Rare Dis. 2021;16:322.
26. Dein E, Kuo PL, Hong YS, Hummers LK, Mecoli CA, McMahan ZH. Evaluation of risk factors for pseudo-obstruction in systemic sclerosis. Semin Arthritis Rheum. 2019;49:405–10.
27. Nagaraja V, McMahan ZH, Getzug T, Khanna D. Management of gastrointestinal involvement in scleroderma. Curr Treatm Opt Rheumatol. 2015;1:82–105.
28. Losurdo G, Salvatore D'Abramo F, Indellicati G, Lillo C, Ierardi E, Di Leo A. The influence of small intestinal bacterial overgrowth in digestive and extra-intestinal disorders. Int J Mol Sci. 2020:21.
29. Parodi A, Sessarego M, Greco A, Bazzica M, Filaci G, Setti M, Savarino E, Indiveri F, Savarino V, Ghio M. Small intestinal bacterial overgrowth in patients suffering from scleroderma: clinical effectiveness of its eradication. Am J Gastroenterol. 2008;103:1257–62.
30. Feng X, Li XQ, Jiang Z. Prevalence and predictors of small intestinal bacterial overgrowth in systemic sclerosis: a systematic review and meta-analysis. Clin Rheumatol. 2021;40:3039–51.
31. Sawadpanich K, Soison P, Chunlertrith K, Mairiang P, Sukeepaisarnjaroen W, Sangchan A, Suttichaimongkol T, Foocharoen C. Prevalence and associated factors of small intestinal bacterial overgrowth among systemic sclerosis patients. Int J Rheum Dis. 2019;22:695–9.
32. Gibiino G, Ianiro G, Cammarota G, Gasbarrini A. The gut microbiota: its anatomy and physiology over a lifetime. Minerva Gastroenterol Dietol. 2017;63:329–36.
33. Pittman N, Rawn SM, Wang M, Masetto A, Beattie KA, Larche M. Treatment of small intestinal bacterial overgrowth in systemic sclerosis: a systematic review. Rheumatology (Oxford). 2018;57:1802–11.
34. Garcia-Collinot G, Madrigal-Santillan EO, Martinez-Bencomo MA, Carranza-Muleiro RA, Jara LJ, Vera-Lastra O, Montes-Cortes DH, Medina G, Cruz-Dominguez MP. Effectiveness of Saccharomyces boulardii and metronidazole for small intestinal bacterial overgrowth in systemic sclerosis. Dig Dis Sci. 2020;65:1134–43.
35. Chiu YC, Lu LS, Wu KL, Tam W, Hu ML, Tai WC, Chiu KW, Chuah SK. Comparison of argon plasma coagulation in management of upper gastrointestinal angiodysplasia and gastric antral vascular ectasia hemorrhage. BMC Gastroenterol. 2012;12:67.
36. Babian M, Nasef S, Soloway G. Gastrointestinal infarction as a manifestation of rheumatoid vasculitis. Am J Gastroenterol. 1998;93:119–20.
37. Yajima S, Asano H, Fukano H, Ohara Y, Shinozuka N, Li CP, Yamada T. Necrosis of the small intestine leading to a diagnosis of polyarteritis nodosa: a case report. J Med Case Rep. 2019;13:55.
38. Isaia M, Christou D, Kallis P, Georgiou P, Nikolaou N, Hadjicostas P. Multiple small intestinal perforations in a patient with Hepatitis B Virus-associated Polyarteritis Nodosa. J Surg Case Rep. 2017;2017:rjx041.
39. Guillevin L, Mahr A, Callard P, Godmer P, Pagnoux C, Leray E, Cohen P. French Vasculitis Study G: Hepatitis B virus-associated polyarteritis nodosa: clinical characteristics, outcome, and impact of treatment in 115 patients. Medicine (Baltimore). 2005;84:313–22.
40. Pagnoux C, Mahr A, Cohen P, Guillevin L. Presentation and outcome of gastrointestinal involvement in systemic necrotizing vasculitides: analysis of 62 patients with polyarteritis

nodosa, microscopic polyangiitis, Wegener granulomatosis, Churg-Strauss syndrome, or rheumatoid arthritis-associated vasculitis. Medicine (Baltimore). 2005;84:115–28.
41. Beye B, Lesur G, Claude P, Martzolf L, Kieffer P, Sondag D. Small bowel involvement documented by capsule endoscopy in Churg-Strauss syndrome. Pan Afr Med J. 2015;22:41.
42. Wong DD, Pillai SR, Kumarasinghe MP, McGettigan B, Thin LW, Segarajasingam DS, Hollingsworth PN, Spagnolo DV. IgG4-related sclerosing disease of the small bowel presenting as necrotizing mesenteric arteritis and a solitary jejunal ulcer. Am J Surg Pathol. 2012;36:929–34.
43. Toledo AE, Shapiro LS, Farrell JF, Magro CM, Polito J. Laparoscopy shows superiority over endoscopy for early detection of malignant atrophic papulosis gastrointestinal complications: a case report and review of literature. BMC Gastroenterol. 2015;15:156.
44. Lu JD, Sachdeva M, Silverberg OM, Shapiro L, Croitoru D, Levy R. Clinical and laboratory prognosticators of atrophic papulosis (Degos disease): a systematic review. Orphanet J Rare Dis. 2021;16:203.
45. Vignes S, Bellanger J. Primary intestinal lymphangiectasia (Waldmann's disease). Orphanet J Rare Dis. 2008;3:5.
46. Fraser K, Robertson L. Chronic urticaria and autoimmunity. Skin Therapy Lett. 2013;18:5–9.
47. Farrell RJ, Kelly CP. Diagnosis of celiac sprue. Am J Gastroenterol. 2001;96:3237–46.
48. Kohno S, Ohshima K, Yoneda S, Kodama T, Shirakusa T, Kikuchi M. Clinicopathological analysis of 143 primary malignant lymphomas in the small and large intestines based on the new WHO classification. Histopathology. 2003;43:135–43.
49. Radmard AR, Amouei M, Kooraki S, Atashi SN, Montazeri SA, Vaezi M, Laghi A. Potential MR enterography features to differentiate primary small intestinal lymphoma from Crohn disease. AJR Am J Roentgenol. 2020;215:864–73.
50. Schreuder MI, van den Brand M, Hebeda KM, Groenen P, van Krieken JH, Scheijen B. Novel developments in the pathogenesis and diagnosis of extranodal marginal zone lymphoma. J Hematop. 2017;10:91–107.
51. Gade AK, Olariu E, Douthit NT. Carcinoid syndrome: a review. Cureus. 2020;12:e7186.
52. Veauthier B, Hornecker JR. Crohn's disease: diagnosis and management. Am Fam Physician. 2018;98:661–9.
53. Panes J, Bouzas R, Chaparro M, Garcia-Sanchez V, Gisbert JP, Martinez de Guerenu B, Mendoza JL, Paredes JM, Quiroga S, Ripolles T, et al. Systematic review: the use of ultrasonography, computed tomography and magnetic resonance imaging for the diagnosis, assessment of activity and abdominal complications of Crohn's disease. Aliment Pharmacol Ther. 2011;34:125–45.
54. Bourke B, Hussey S. Chronic infections of the small intestine. Curr Opin Gastroenterol. 2015;31:104–10.
55. Epple HJ, Friebel J, Moos V, Troeger H, Krug SM, Allers K, Schinnerling K, Fromm A, Siegmund B, Fromm M, et al. Architectural and functional alterations of the small intestinal mucosa in classical Whipple's disease. Mucosal Immunol. 2017;10:1542–52.
56. Bindu S, Mazumder S, Bandyopadhyay U. Non-steroidal anti-inflammatory drugs (NSAIDs) and organ damage: a current perspective. Biochem Pharmacol. 2020;180:114147.
57. Bala M, Kashuk J, Moore EE, Kluger Y, Biffl W, Gomes CA, Ben-Ishay O, Rubinstein C, Balogh ZJ, Civil I, et al. Acute mesenteric ischemia: guidelines of the World Society of Emergency Surgery. World J Emerg Surg. 2017;12:38.
58. Shih MC, Hagspiel KD. CTA and MRA in mesenteric ischemia: part 1, Role in diagnosis and differential diagnosis. AJR Am J Roentgenol. 2007;188:452–61.
59. Schreyer AG, Stroszczynski C. Radiological imaging of the small bowel. Dig Dis. 2011;29(Suppl 1):22–6.
60. Losurdo G, Leandro G, Ierardi E, Perri F, Barone M, Principi M, Leo AD. Breath tests for the non-invasive diagnosis of small intestinal bacterial overgrowth: a systematic review with meta-analysis. J Neurogastroenterol Motil. 2020;26:16–28.

61. Calatayud M, Dezutter O, Hernandez-Sanabria E, Hidalgo-Martinez S, Meysman FJR, Van de Wiele T. Development of a host-microbiome model of the small intestine. FASEB J. 2019;33:3985–96.
62. Bassotti G, Bologna S, Ottaviani L, Russo M, Dore MP. Intestinal manometry: who needs it? Gastroenterol Hepatol Bed Bench. 2015;8:246–52.
63. Nakagawa K, Hara K, Fikree A, Siddiqi S, Woodland P, Masamune A, Aziz Q, Sifrim D, Yazaki E. Patients with dyspepsia have impaired mucosal integrity both in the duodenum and jejunum: in vivo assessment of small bowel mucosal integrity using baseline impedance. J Gastroenterol. 2020;55:273–80.
64. Zhu J, Frech T. Gut disease in systemic sclerosis—new approaches to common problems. Curr Treatm Opt Rheumatol. 2019;5:11–9.

Chapter 8
Rheumatologic Diseases and GI Conditions: Colon Chapter

Promila Banerjee, Jake Jasurda, Paul Kalapala, Kajali Mishra, and Alice Van Pelt

8.1 Normal Physiology of Colon, Including Motility

The colon begins at the ileocecal valve and is comprised of several anatomically distinct portions, including the cecum, ascending colon, transverse colon, descending colon, and sigmoid colon. Similar to the small intestine, the colonic wall is composed of mucosa, submucosa, muscularis propria and serosa. However, while the small intestine functions to digest food and assimilate nutrients, the primary function of the colon is to regulate fluid, electrolytes and bacterial degradation products. Given this difference in function, there are several important differences in the composition of the colonic wall compared to that of the small intestine.

The most noticeable difference is the grossly smooth, flattened appearance of the colon due to the absence of villi which are abundantly seen in the small intestine. Instead, numerous invaginations called crypts are seen throughout the colon and primarily contain goblet cells, or mucus producing cells. The muscularis propria is composed of a continuous inner circular smooth muscle layer and a discontinuous

P. Banerjee (✉)
Loyola Stritch School of Medicine, Maywood, IL, USA

GI Division, Edward Hines VA Hospital, Hines, IL, USA

J. Jasurda
Loyola University Medical Center, Maywood, IL, USA

P. Kalapala
Creighton University School of Medicine, Omaha, NE, USA

K. Mishra
John H Stroger Jr, Hospital of Cook County, Chicago, IL, USA

A. Van Pelt
GI Division, Edward Hines VA Hospital, Hines, IL, USA

M. Tadros et al. (eds.), *GI Diseases Associated with Rheumatological and Vasculitic Conditions*, Clinical Gastroenterology,
https://doi.org/10.1007/978-3-032-07868-1_8

outer longitudinal layer consisting of 3 longitudinal smooth muscle bundles called tenia coli. This outer layer is shorter than the overall length of the colon resulting in the creation of a series of sacculations, or haustra, throughout the colon [1].

On average, about 9 L of fluid that enter the GI tract per day and 8 L of this is absorbed prior to reaching the colon. Typically, about 800 mL are resorbed in the colon per day, however absorption rates can reach up to 4 L per day depending on the fluid delivery rate from the small intestine, allowing the colon to compensate for malabsorptive states or small bowel disease [2, 3].

8.2 Constipation

Constipation is often thought to reflect less than three bowel movements per week; however, patients typically experience a wider range of symptoms including hard or firm stools, sensation of incomplete evacuation, abdominal discomfort, bloating, excessive straining, or the need for manual maneuvers to facilitate defecation [4]. It is prudent for physicians to be aware of these as patients may exhibit several of these symptoms while continuing to have daily bowel movements.

Constipation is extremely common in patients with systemic scleroderma, along with fecal incontinence. Other common colonic symptoms include diarrhea, rectal prolapse, spontaneous perforation, and colonic infarction. While extracolonic GI manifestations of scleroderma have been well described, 20–50% of patients with systemic scleroderma have been reported to have also been reported to have colonic involvement [5].

Colonic manifestations related to systemic scleroderma have been attributed to a combination of colonic dysmotility, decreased compliance and muscular atrophy [6]. Anti-myenteric antibodies have been linked to the pathogenesis of systemic scleroderma and disrupt the autoregulatory release of acetylcholine from myenteric neurons [7]. In severe cases of dysmotility, myoelectric activity has been demonstrated to be nearly absent on myoelectric recordings [8]. The chronic inflammatory changes seen in systemic scleroderma also contribute to progressive fibrosis and muscular atrophy, further disrupting normal colonic motility.

In patients with systemic scleroderma and constipation, colonic transit is prolonged in the right colon and in the entire colon leading to colonic inertia. In extreme cases, this can lead to colonic pseudo-obstruction. Intestinal pseudo-obstruction occurs in two phases: an early, neuropathic phase and a late, myopathic phase. Treatment of this early neuropathic phase involves use of prokinetic drugs such as erythromycin or neostigmine. If these fail, or in later myopathic phase, these drugs and dietary modifications may be ineffective, at which point endoscopic placement or surgical placement of a venting tube, or surgical resection, may be needed.

Rectosigmoid function is also altered in patients with systemic scleroderma. In normal patients, rectosigmoid motility increase after eating, which is mediated by a cholinergic pathway. However, patients with systemic scleroderma do not exhibit this postprandial increase in motility. There is an absence or decreased rectoanal inhibitory reflex on anorectal manometry.

Over time, the smooth muscle atrophy in the colonic wall can lead to a loss of haustra in the colon and predispose patients to the development of large diverticuli. The risk of further complications among these patients are compounded by fibrosis of the colonic wall and fecal impaction with slow transit[8]. In addition, patients with underlying rheumatic disease have been found to be 3.5 times more likely to develop sigmoid diverticular abscess perforation compared to patients without underlying rheumatic disease and 32 times more likely if concurrently on corticosteroid therapy [9].

8.3 Diarrhea

Diarrhea is commonly seen in conditions such as Ehlers Danlos syndrome, multiple connective tissue disease and scleroderma and may be attributed to several different etiologies. Non-infectious diarrhea in these conditions is most commonly due to intestinal hypomotility may induce colonic stasis and in turn potentiate bacteria overgrowth resulting in a malabsorptive diarrhea [10]. However, chronic intestinal ischemia and progressive fibrosis of the colonic wall leading to reduction in surface area available for absorption and intestinal permeability may also contribute to diarrhea in these conditions [11]. Treatment of small bowel bacterial overgrowth, and conservative measures such as a low-residue diet, anti-diarrheals (such as loperamide) and bile-acid binding resins (such as cholestyramine) can be helpful. If these measures fail, pelvic floor physical therapy with biofeedback is also an option. If rectoanal inhibitory reflex is absent on anorectal manometry, and anal sphincter pressures are decreased, then a posterior anal sphincter repair may be helpful.

8.4 Bowel Ischemia

Ischemic colitis is commonly due to low arterial flow states such as in atherosclerotic diseases or heart failure. However, in patients with rheumatologic conditions such as Behcet's disease, systemic lupus erythematosus, PAN or Churg-Strauss syndrome, veno-occlusive disease by systemic thrombosis is a more common cause of ischemic colitis. Another clinical spectrum is acute and chronic ischemia of the small bowel. Vasculitis when involving the mesentery presents as chronic mesenteric insufficiency, however, presentations can be acute if accompanied with acute thrombus. Extra intestinal manifestation correlate well with the chronicity and pattern of mesenteric involvement [12]. It can be clinically challenging to diagnose it in an acute setting with minimal information provided by imaging and endoscopy. While biopsy remains the gold standard, angiography can help in confirming the disease as well.With prompt initiation of immunosuppressive treatment, surgery may be avoided. In acute settings the mortality is as high as 50-75% even with surgical intervention. Prognosis is remarkably improved when there is minimal delay in surgical intervention [13].

8.5 Intestinal Pseudo-obstruction

Failure of the intestinal motility system causing obstructive symptoms without an obvious blockage, is a condition known as Chronic pseudo obstruction. The clinical spectrum can vary based on time and extent of intestinal involvement. Chronic pseudo obstruction, although rare, is a result of neuropathic (enteric nervous system), myopathic(smooth muscles) or interstitial cells of Cajal abnormalities. These abnormalities can be idiopathic or secondary to another disease process like autoimmune conditions.

Chronic pseudo obstruction can be the first presentation of Lupus in about 40% of patients. Lack of awareness can lead to delayed diagnosis, whereas prompt steroid treatment can prevent complications needing surgical intervention [14]. Similarly, studies have reported that around 9% of patients have GI involvement in patients with systemic sclerosis. It is unclear how many have CPO, however, high incidence of constipation needing pro motility agents have been noted in the majority of these patients [15, 16]. Acute hospitalization needing ICU management or surgical intervention is rare but has been reported as well.

8.6 Colonic Pneumatosis

Pneumatosis of the colon is commonly secondary to bacterial infections and defective mucosal healing, both of which are seen in patients with CTD or vasculitis like SLE. The disease process is often complicated with immunosuppression that is used to manage the primary pathology.

CTD , especially SSc, has been reported as an important underlying condition. The fibrosis of the smooth muscle cells in the GI tract leads to hypomotility inturn resulting in bacterial overgrowth. Bacterial overgrowth can further cause distention due to gas production and raise the intraluminal pressure leading to seepage of gas into the intestinal wall. Bacterial infection can also directly damage mucosa causing gas penetration into the intestinal wall [17, 18].

SLE is another rheumatological condition that can potentially get complicated with pneumatosis coli. However the proposed pathogenesis is via vasculitis rather than direct damage to the mucosal wall [19, 20].

Myositis associated with other rheumatological conditions like RA, ANCA vasculitis and MCTD has been reported. Histological findings were mostly consistent with microangiopathy [21, 22]. Pneumatosis can be fatal in juvenile conditions but in adults it is directly related to the disease activity of PM/DM and can be controlled with steroids [23, 24].

8.7 Incidence of Microscopic Colitis in Patients with Rheumatologic Disease

Mucosal level changes identified in random biopsy of normal endoscopic appearing colon in patients with diarrhea, establishes diagnosis of MC. Immune responses to changes in gut microbiota are responsible for microscopic findings seen in MC [25]. These changes can be associated with different rheumatological conditions or are the result of treatment options for rheumatological conditions.

Autoimmune diseases have been associated with MC in 30-50% of cases, mostly patients with IBD, celiac and rheumatoid arthritis, however, more recently Takayasu Arteritis has been reported in association with MC. TA is a large vessel vasculitis with unclear pathogenesis. Overlapping dysregulated immune responses may be contributing to this disease association [26].

A review of 460 patients who developed diarrhea after starting rituximab for hematologic or rheumatologic conditions found that 4.6% developed histologically confirmed colitis. In 57.1% of those who developed colitis, clinical and histologic findings were consistent with IBD (7 Crohn's disease, 5 ulcerative colitis), while 42.9% [9] were diagnosed with microscopic colitis. Patients who developed IBD had received a statistically significant higher number of doses before the onset of colitis than those who developed microscopic colitis [27].

8.8 Incidence of IBD in Patients with Rheumatologic Disease

Advances in diagnostics and the emergence of genome-wide association studies have allowed for the identification of genomic loci that are both unique to individual autoimmune disorders and those that are shared across of cluster of disorders. These findings serve not only to provide a better understanding of disease pathogenesis but may also provide insight into novel therapies to treat these diseases. In a study conducted by Zhernakova et al., 28 genome wide association studies, 28 replication meta-analyses investigating genetic overlap between several different immune and inflammatory mediated disorders (ankylosing spondylitis, asthma, auto-immune thyroid disease, celiac disease, multiple sclerosis, psoriasis, rheumatoid arthritis, systemic lupus erythematosus, type 1 diabetes mellitus, Crohn's disease and ulcerative colitis), 23 different genes overlapped between two or more diseases [28]. Subsequent studies have identified at least 51 genes associated with IBD that overlap with 23 different immune or inflammatory mediated disorders [29]. Additionally an increased prevalence of rheumatoid arthritis, psoriasis, ankylosing spondylitis, primary sclerosing cholangitis, atopic dermatitis and multiple sclerosis has been demonstrated among patients with underlying diagnosis of IBD [29–34].

Extraintestinal manifestations of Crohn's disease and ulcerative occur in 20–30% of patients and varies based on site, onset and activity of the underlying inflammatory bowel disease [35]. Patients with ulcerative pancolitis experience extraintestinal manifestations roughly twice and four times more frequently when compared to patients with isolated left sided colitis or proctitis respectively [36]. Similarly, patients with ileocolic Crohn's disease will experience extraintestinal symptoms 37% of the time compared to 25% among patients with ileal disease alone [37]. IBD-associated arthralgias are more commonly seen in patients with Crohn's disease compared to ulcerative colitis and are strongly associated with flares of their underlying IBD. Frequently, knee and ankle joint involvement will occur first, however involvement of other peripheral sites, such as elbows, wrists metacarpophalangeal, metatarsophalangeal and proximal interphalangeal joints, may follow [38].

Patients who develop a polyarticular arthritis, typically symmetrical and predominately affecting the upper extremities may be more less likely to correlate with IBD activity when compared to patients exhibiting pauci or oligoarticular arthritis of the large joints in the lower extremities [39]. Generally, IBD-related peripheral arthropathies are non-erosive and non-deforming and development of erosive arthritis should prompt investigation into other rheumatologic conditions [39].

8.9 NSAID Colopathy

Non-steroidal anti-inflammatory drugs (NSAIDs) are a mainstay therapy in the treatment of rheumatoid diseases owing to their analgesic and anti-inflammatory effects. Adverse GI effects of these medications has been well documented over the past 80 years [40]. Incidence of NSAID induced injury to the upper GI tract has been most evident. Cyclooxygenase (COX) inhibitors inhibit mucosal prostaglandins that in turn lead to disruption of the protective mucus layer, inhibition of protective bicarbonate secretion, and vasoconstriction resulting in mucosal injury and possible ulcer formation. Mucosal repair is also prostaglandin dependent and COX inhibitors may potentiate further injury [41].

NSAID induced injury in the small intestine and colon may follow a similar mechanism of injury to that of the upper GI tract, although precise mechanisms are still being examined. Symptoms in the lower GI tract range from silent injury, overt bleeding or perforation [42]. Patients may not exhibit overt symptoms and clinical suspicion is raised in the setting of unexplained anemia or hypoalbuminemia. Endoscopic findings, such as erosions and ulcers, may be consistent with NSAID colopathy in the appropriate clinical context. Strictures may also develop as a result of chronic inflammatory changes in the setting of mucosal injury. Distinct from this is the development of colonic diaphragm disease (CDD) which results in the development of diaphragm-like strictures in the colon with normal appearing mucsoa. This phenomenon has a greater association with use of oxicams, diclofenac or long-acting NSAID formulations and use of proton pump inhibitors does not appear to lessen the risk of stricture formation [43].

Treatment typically involves discontinuation of the offending NSAID. Use of COX-2 inhibitors and use of misoprostol cotherapy have been shown to have favorable outcomes with regard to NSAID enteropathy, however further management strategies for NSAID colopathy are still under investigation [38].

References

1. Reinus J, Simon D. Gastrointestinal anatomy and physiology the essentials [with Website]. Wiley Blackwell; 2014. http://doi.wiley.com/10.1002/9781118833001.ch8.
2. Rao SSC, Parkman HP, McCallum RW. Handbook of gastrointestinal motility and functional disorders. 348.
3. Loscalzo J, Fauci AS, Kasper DL, Hauser SL, Longo DL, Dan L, Jameson JL. Harrison's principles of internal medicine.
4. Bharucha A, Dorn S, Lembo A, Pressman A, Gastroenterological Association A. AGA American Gastroenterological Association Medical Position Statement on Constipation. 2013. https://doi.org/10.1053/j.gastro.2012.10.029.
5. McFarlane IM, Bhamra MS, Kreps A, et al. Gastrointestinal manifestations of systemic sclerosis. Rheumatology (Sunnyvale). 2018;8(1) https://doi.org/10.4172/2161-1149.1000235.
6. Battle WM, Snape WJ, Wright S, et al. Abnormal colonic motility in progressive systemic sclerosis. Ann Intern Med. 1981;94(6):749–52. https://doi.org/10.7326/0003-4819-94-6-749.
7. Howe S, Eaker EY, Sallustio JE, Peebles C, Tan EM, Williams RC. Antimyenteric neuronal antibodies in scleroderma. J Clin Invest. 1994;94(2):761–70. https://doi.org/10.1172/JCI117395.
8. Compton R. Scleroderma with diverticulosis and colonic obstruction. Am J Surg. 1969;118(4):602–6. https://doi.org/10.1016/0002-9610(69)90194-9.
9. Mpofu S, Mpofu CMA, Hutchinson D, Maier AE, Dodd SR, Moots RJ. Steroids, non-steroidal anti-inflammatory drugs, and sigmoid diverticular abscess perforation in rheumatic conditions. Ann Rheum Dis. 2004;63(5):588. https://doi.org/10.1136/ARD.2003.010355.
10. Bures J, Cyrany J, Kohoutova D, et al. Small intestinal bacterial overgrowth syndrome. World J Gastroenterol. 2010;16(24):2978–90. https://doi.org/10.3748/WJG.V16.I24.2978.
11. Sallam H, McNearney TA, Chen JDZ. Systematic review: pathophysiology and management of gastrointestinal dysmotility in systemic sclerosis (scleroderma). Aliment Pharmacol Ther. 2006;23(6):691–712. https://doi.org/10.1111/J.1365-2036.2006.02804.X.
12. Gaubitz M, Domschke W. Intestinale vaskulitiden—Eine diagnostischtherapeutische herausforderung. Z Gastroenterol. 2000;38(2):181–92. https://doi.org/10.1055/S-2000-14859.
13. Passam F, Diamantis I, GP-S in arthritis. Intestinal ischemia as the first manifestation of vasculitis. Elsevier; 2004. https://www.sciencedirect.com/science/article/pii/S0049017204001519.
14. Narváez J, Pérez-Vega C, Castro-Bohorquez FJ, Garcia-Quintana AM, Biosca M, Vilaseca-Momplet J. Intestinal pseudo-obstruction in systemic lupus erythematosus. Taylor Fr. 2003;32(3):191–5. https://doi.org/10.1080/03009740310002588.
15. Poirier T, GR-AJ. Gastrointestinal manifestations of progressive systemic scleroderma based on a review of 364 cases. search.ebscohost.com; 1972. http://search.ebscohost.com/login.aspx?direct=true&profile=ehost&scope=site&authtype=crawler&jrnl=00029270&AN=16439111&h=VJAfEVwr2M0%2BiBWXbZPvMYj%2BVJ1F%2Bfi3L%2B%2BY4bIagSMkDpIw9EjOd0dvq37Y7Gg6BR0j5z0yG6gNOzbUSuEeVg%3D%3D&crl=c.

16. Mecoli C, Purohit S, Sandorfi N, Rheumatology CD-TJ. Mortality, recurrence, and hospital course of patients with systemic sclerosis-related acute intestinal pseudo-obstruction. jrheum.org; 2014. https://www.jrheum.org/content/41/10/2049.short.
17. Honne K, Maruyama A, Onishi S, TN-TJ. Simultaneous pneumatosis cystoides intestinalis and pneumomediastinum in a patient with systemic sclerosis. jrheum.org; 2010. https://www.jrheum.org/content/37/10/2194.short.
18. Wilson F, Rheumatology KW-TJ. Pneumatosis intestinalis in limited scleroderma. jrheum.org; 2008. https://www.jrheum.org/content/35/2/352.short.
19. Yamaguchi Y, Ohno S, Yamazaki S, et al. A case of systemic lupus erythematosus complicated with pneumatosis cystoides intestinalis. academic.oup.com. 2005;15:440–4. https://doi.org/10.1007/s10165-005-0437-3.
20. Mizoguchi F, Nanki T, Medicine NM-I. Pneumatosis cystoides intestinalis following lupus enteritis and peritonitis. jstage.jst.go.jp; 2008. https://doi.org/10.2169/internalmedicine.47.0748.
21. Wada Y, Murayama N, Hirose S, et al. A case of pneumatosis cystoides intestinalis in a patient with polymyositis and interstitial pneumonia. Mod Rheumatol. 2004;14(3):260–3. https://doi.org/10.3109/S10165-004-0304-7.
22. Zarbalian Y, von Rosenvinge E, Reports WT. Recurrent pneumatosis intestinalis in a patient with dermatomyositis. casereports.bmj.com; 2013. https://casereports.bmj.com/content/2013/bcr-2013-200308.short.
23. Aoki Y, Nagashima T, Kamimura T, MI-J. Marked pneumatosis cystoides intestinalis in a patient with mixed connective tissue disease. jrheum.org; 2006. https://www.jrheum.org/content/jrheum/33/8/1705.full-text.pdf.
24. Nakagawa S, Akimoto T, Takeda SI, et al. Antineutrophil cytoplasmic antibody–associated glomerulonephritis complicated by pneumatosis intestinalis. Clin Med Insights Case Rep. 2015;8:65–70. https://doi.org/10.4137/CCREP.S26155.
25. Burke KE, D'Amato M, Ng SC, Pardi DS, Ludvigsson JF, Khalili H. Microscopic colitis. Nat Rev Dis Prim. 2021;7:1. https://doi.org/10.1038/S41572-021-00273-2.
26. Kanıtez NA, Toz B, Güllüoğlu M, et al. Microscopic colitis in patients with Takayasu's arteritis: a potential association between the two disease entities. Clin Rheumatol. 2016;35(10):2495–9. https://doi.org/10.1007/S10067-015-3149-X.
27. Eckmann JD, Chedid V, Quinn KP, Bonthu N, Nehra V, Raffals LE. De novo colitis associated with rituximab in 21 patients at a tertiary center. researchgate.net. 2020; https://doi.org/10.1016/j.cgh.2019.03.027.
28. Zhernakova A, Van Diemen CC, Wijmenga C. Detecting shared pathogenesis from the shared genetics of immune-related diseases. Nat Rev Genet. 2009;10(1):43–55. https://doi.org/10.1038/nrg2489.
29. Lees CW, Barrett JC, Parkes M, Satsangi J. New IBD genetics: common pathways with other diseases. https://doi.org/10.1136/gut.2009.199679.
30. Cohen R, Robinson D, Paramore C, Fraeman K, Renahan K, Bala M. Background: recent studies suggest that inflammatory bowel. 2001. https://doi.org/10.1002/ibd.20406.
31. Hammer B, Ashurst P, Naish J. Diseases associated with ulcerative colitis and Crohn's disease. Gut. 1968;9(1):17. https://doi.org/10.1136/GUT.9.1.17.
32. Bernstein CN, Wajda A, Blanchard JF. The clustering of other chronic inflammatory diseases in inflammatory bowel disease: a population-based study. Gastroenterology. 2005;129(3):827–36. https://doi.org/10.1053/J.GASTRO.2005.06.021.
33. Olsson R, Danielsson Å, Järnerot G, et al. Prevalence of primary sclerosing cholangitis in patients with ulcerative colitis. Gastroenterology. 1991;100(5):1319–23. https://doi.org/10.1016/0016-5085(91)70019-T.
34. Gupta G, Gelfand JM, Lewis JD. Increased risk for demyelinating diseases in patients with inflammatory bowel disease. Gastroenterology. 2005;129(3):819–26. https://doi.org/10.1053/J.GASTRO.2005.06.022.
35. National Cooperative Crohn's Disease Study: extraintestinal manifestations and perianal complications—PubMed. https://pubmed.ncbi.nlm.nih.gov/467943/.

36. Wright V, Watkinson G. The arthritis of ulcerative colitis. Br Med J. 1965;2(5463):670. https://doi.org/10.1136/BMJ.2.5463.670.
37. Greenstein AJ, Janowitz HD, Sachar DB. The extra-intestinal complications of Crohn's disease and ulcerative colitis: a study of 700 patients. Medicine (Baltimore). 1976;55(5):401–12. https://doi.org/10.1097/00005792-197609000-00004.
38. Lawrence MF, Lawrence JB. Sleisenger and Fordtran's gastrointestinal and liver disease: pathophysiology diagnosis management, vol 2, 11th edn. Philadelphia: Elsevier; 2021. https://www.mdconsult.internacional.edu.ec:2097/#!/content/book/3-s2.0-B9780323609623000746.
39. Arvikar SL, Fisher MC. Inflammatory bowel disease associated arthropathy. Curr Rev Musculoskelet Med. 2011;4(3):123–31. https://doi.org/10.1007/S12178-011-9085-8/TABLES/1.
40. Tachecí I, Bradna P, Douda T, et al. NSAID-induced enteropathy in rheumatoid arthritis patients with chronic occult gastrointestinal bleeding: a prospective capsule endoscopy study. Gastroenterol Res Pract. 2013; https://doi.org/10.1155/2013/268382.
41. Silverstein FE, Faich G, Goldstein JL, et al. Gastrointestinal toxicity with celecoxib vs nonsteroidal anti-inflammatory drugs for osteoarthritis and rheumatoid arthritis: the CLASS study: a randomized controlled trial. JAMA. 2000;284(10):1247–55. https://doi.org/10.1001/JAMA.284.10.1247.
42. Scheiman JM. NSAID-induced gastrointestinal injury: a focused update for clinicians. J Clin Gastroenterol. 2016;50(1):5–10. https://doi.org/10.1097/MCG.0000000000000432.
43. Farricielli L, Sanderson CDJ. Colonic diaphragm disease: an important NSAID complication to know. Fed Pract. 2017;34(3):38. /pmc/articles/PMC6370415/.

Chapter 9
Anorectal Diseases in Rheumatology

Muhammad Farhan Ashraf, Mary Strader, Ethan Pearlstein, Dharma Ayer, and Asra Batool

Rheumatic diseases (RD) can affect any part of the gastrointestinal (GI) system. GI involvement in RD may develop gradually and symptoms may vary in intensity, making the diagnosis of these clinical presentations challenging. While RD often present initially with GI symptoms, these are often non-specific, and include abdominal pain, diarrhea, bloating, fecal incontinence, nausea and dyspepsia [1]. It is imperative to recognize the early GI manifestations of RD as this may allow for more prompt diagnosis and treatment of the underlying disease. Further, it may prevent the misdiagnosis and mistreatment of these non-specific GI symptoms.

In this chapter, we will specifically discuss RD affecting the anorectal region, their pathophysiology and disease manifestations. Only a few RD affect the anorectal region. These include systemic sclerosis (SSc), sarcoidosis, systemic lupus erythematosus (SLE), and antiphospholipid syndrome (APS). These RD may present with fecal incontinence, rectal prolapse, GI bleeding, ulcers, anorectal pain, and hemorrhoids.

M. F. Ashraf
Department of Gastroenterology, Rochester General Hospital, Rochester, NY, USA

M. Strader
Gastroenterology Associates of Northern New York, Glens Falls, NY, USA

E. Pearlstein
Gastro Health, Miami, FL, USA

D. Ayer
Albany Medical College, Albany, NY, USA

A. Batool (✉)
Wellstar Gastroenterology, Marietta, GA, USA

M. Tadros et al. (eds.), *GI Diseases Associated with Rheumatological and Vasculitic Conditions*, Clinical Gastroenterology,
https://doi.org/10.1007/978-3-032-07868-1_9

9.1 Anatomy of the Anorectum

Four anatomic structures play an important role in the process of defecation and maintain fecal continence at rest. These anatomic structures are the rectum, internal anal sphincter, external anal sphincter, and the puborectalis muscle.

The rectum has three mucosal folds contributing to its capacity to hold stool. These folds are a continuation of the muscular colonic wall. The human rectum can accommodate up to 300 mL of stool without any significant increase in intraluminal pressure. Beyond this, the stretch receptors are activated resulting in the urge to defecate [2]. The contraction of the rectosigmoid junction in response to a sudden contraction of the sigmoid colon prevents rapid filling of the rectum. This reflex prevents fecal incontinence and is called the rectosigmoid junction guarding reflex [3].

The internal anal sphincter is a thickened layer of tonically contracted circular smooth muscle. The internal anal sphincter accounts for most of the resting tone in the anal canal. When stool enters the rectum, the internal anal sphincter relaxes for a short time by a reflex known as the recto anal inhibitory reflex (RAIR). This reflex allows anal stool sampling to differentiate between solids, liquids, and gas in the rectum [4, 5]. The RAIR is an intramural reflex independent of the spinal cord. Studies have shown that RAIR is preserved even in spinal cord injuries and cases of extrinsic denervation of the rectum [6, 7]. The internal anal sphincter is supplied by the enteric nervous system.

The external anal sphincter and puborectalis muscle are composed of striated muscle. The external anal sphincter and puborectalis muscles act as a functional unit and are responsible for the voluntary part of defecation. The external anal sphincter is innervated by the pudendal nerve, while the puborectalis is innervated by pelvic branches of S3 and S4. The puborectalis is one of a group of muscles comprising the pelvic diaphragm, and surrounds the anorectum like a sling, maintaining the anorectal angle and leading to fecal continence at rest.

9.2 Fecal Incontinence

Fecal incontinence is defined as the involuntary loss of feces. According to one population-based survey, the prevalence of fecal incontinence in the United States is 14.4% [8]. Etiologies include weakness of the internal and external anal sphincters, weakness of the puborectalis muscle, decreased perception of rectal sensation, and overflow of fecal material [9]. Among the RD, SSc is the most associated with fecal incontinence. In two studies, 40–71% of patients with SSc reported fecal incontinence [10, 11]. Fecal incontinence can have significant impact on daily functioning in work and social settings. Though fecal incontinence is more typically seen in the elderly, patients SSc at any age can suffer from fecal incontinence.

9.3 Physiology of Defecation and Continence

A carefully coordinated sequence of events is necessary for control of defecation. This sequence starts with stool entering the rectum and ends in the propulsion of fecal material through the anorectum. As stool enters the rectum, mechanoreceptors in the rectal wall sense its presence through rectal afferent nerves, prompting the urge to defecate through a sacral arc. Stool progressively distends the rectum, resulting in a reflexive relaxation of the internal anal sphincter (recto anal inhibitory reflex). Next, a phenomenon called "anal sampling" occurs where a small amount of stool passes through the anal canal after relaxation of the internal sphincter. Through the "anal sampling" process, the anal canal can differentiate between gaseous, liquid, and solid components of stool in the anorectum [12, 13]. At this point, if defecation is socially feasible, the anorectal angle is straightened by sitting or squatting, intra-abdominal pressure is increased via the Valsalva maneuver, the pelvic floor descends, the rectum contracts and voluntary relaxation of the external anal sphincter and puborectalis muscle occurs via the pudendal nerve. A pressure gradient created between the rectum and anal canal allows for stool to enter the lower rectum as the pelvic floor relaxes. Next, spontaneous rectosigmoid contractions begin to push stool through the now relaxed anal canal, resulting in defecation [14]. Propulsive rectosigmoid contractions continue until the rectum is fully emptied of stool. After defecation is complete, the external sphincter tone returns to normal [13]. If defecation is not possible after stool enters the rectum, the rectal wall relaxes, and the urge is suppressed for some time [3].

9.4 Pathophysiology of Fecal Incontinence

Several anorectal disorders can cause fecal incontinence, including anal trauma, neurologic disorders, childbirth, autonomic neuropathy in diabetes, overflow, infiltrative diseases, and idiopathic causes. In each of these diseases, one or more of the steps in the sequence of defecation is compromised and presents clinically with fecal incontinence.

9.4.1 Pathophysiology of Anorectal Involvement in Rheumatic Diseases (RD)

9.4.1.1 Anorectal Dysfunction in Systemic Sclerosis (SSc)

Among the RDs, SSc is most associated with fecal incontinence. Historically, it was believed that fecal incontinence was a late sequela of SSc, often after the manifestation of skin findings earlier in the disease course [15]. More recent studies suggest

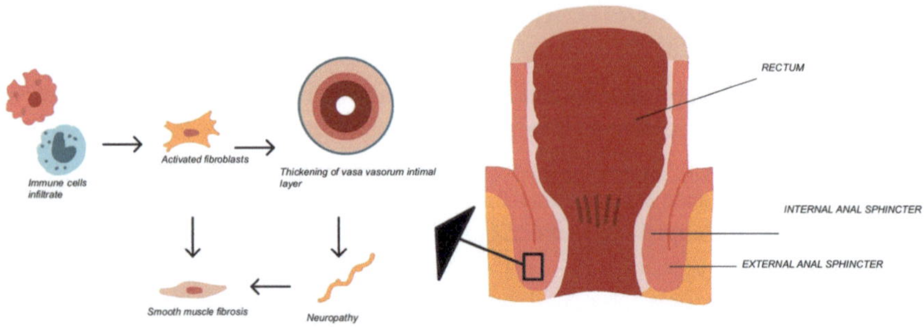

Fig. 9.1 Pathogenesis of Fecal Incontinence is Systemic Sclerosis (SSc)

that anorectal changes may occur before other clinical symptoms [16]. In one study including 96 patients with systemic sclerosis, 38% had fecal incontinence and 20% reported that colorectal symptoms caused social restrictions and poor quality of life [17].

The pathophysiology of fecal incontinence in SSc is complex and includes multiple mechanisms. The mechanisms include underlying neuropathy, smooth muscle dysfunction, smooth muscle atrophy and fibrosis, all of which affect the anorectum. The result is a reduction in mean resting pressure of the internal anal sphincter, dysfunction of the RAIR and thinning of the internal anal sphincter [18]. The pathogenesis is displayed on Fig. 9.1.

Anal resting pressure reflects the resting tone of the internal anal sphincter and is under the direct control of the adrenergic system [19]. At baseline, a high anal resting pressure in the lower internal sphincter allows for fecal continence. In SSc, the mean anal resting pressure is decreased as shown by multiple studies [10, 11, 20]. A loss of anal resting pressure contributes to fecal incontinence by loss of control over stool entering the rectum.

The second anorectal abnormality in SSc leading to fecal incontinence is a dysfunctional RAIR. Some studies have reported that this reflex is absent in 12–71% of patients with SSc [20]. RAIR is defined by reflexive relaxation of the internal anal sphincter in response to rectal distention. A successful RAIR requires a functional intramural nervous system and intact rectal sensation. It is proposed that in SSc, neuropathy causes loss of these uninterrupted intramural nerves and impairs rectal sensation, leading to loss of RAIR and ultimately fecal incontinence [21]. The intramural nervous system is essential to a normal RAIR and dysfunction at this level may be seen in SSc and has been shown in several histologic studies. One study involving deep rectal biopsies showed enteric neurons with abnormal axon terminals containing an exoplasm devoid of the cytoskeletal components [22].

The internal anal sphincter is a combination of circular and longitudinal smooth muscles. Research studies have shown that both symptomatic and asymptomatic patients with systemic sclerosis have thinning and atrophy of both the circular and

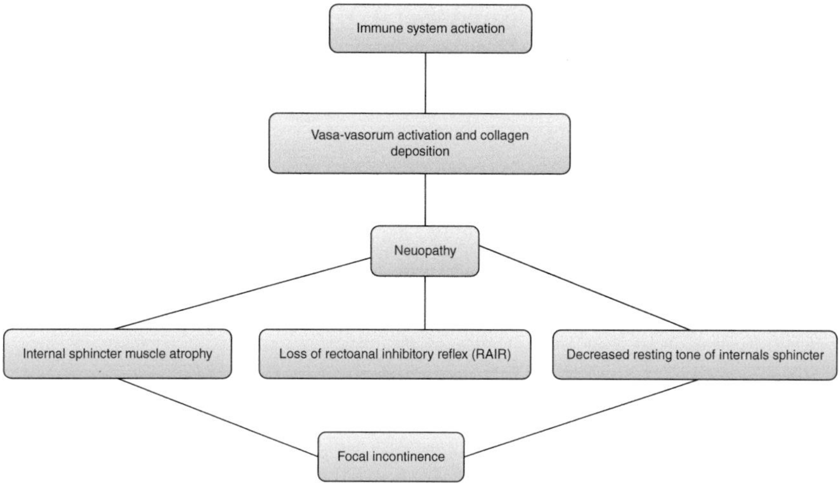

Fig. 9.2 Anorectal Abnormalities Associated with Fecal Incontinence in Systemic Sclerosis (SSc)

longitudinal smooth muscles of the internal anal sphincter [23]. Histologic studies have also shown thinning of the muscularis propria and fibrous replacement of both smooth muscle layers in SSc [24]. Neuropathy is again suggested to be the likely culprit of muscular atrophy. This can occur due to the involvement of vasa vasorum in neurons and excessive collagen deposition in SSc. Vascular involvement plays an important role in the pathogenesis of systemic sclerosis. Vascular intimal thickening and fibroblast activation are two important vascular phenomena in systemic sclerosis [25]. The enteric vessels of patients with SSc can show both duplication and partial obliteration of the basal lamina [22]. Due to underlying neuropathy, the circular and longitudinal smooth muscles of the internal anal sphincter begin to atrophy and eventually, the tissue is replaced by fibrosis [26] (Fig. 9.2).

Collagen deposition and ultimately fibrosis can be visualized with both endoanal ultrasonography and endoanal magnetic resonance imaging (MRI) [27]. The initial treatment for fecal incontinence in SSc is generally sphincter muscle training, however, its efficacy has been debated [28]. Antidiarrheal medications and biofeedback methods are often ineffective for the treatment of this disease. As suggested by several pilot studies, sacral nerve stimulation may be a more effective treatment modality [29].However, there is a lack of randomized controlled trials on anorectal disorders and GI disorders in general in patients suffering from SSc. In addition to fecal incontinence, atrophy of the internal anal sphincter in SSc may also cause rectal prolapse, but this is relatively rare. Reports of rectal prolapse in SSc are limited to a few case series [30].

9.5 Other Rheumatic Disorders (RD) with Anorectal Involvement

9.5.1 Sarcoidosis

Sarcoidosis is a multi-system disease and can involve any part of the body including the GI system. Although not common, sarcoidosis may affect the anorectum. Involvement of the anorectum in sarcoidosis can be further divided into perianal involvement of cutaneous sarcoidosis and a separate entity termed rectal sarcoidosis. Several case reports mention annular plaques in the perianal region, later confirmed to be cutaneous sarcoidosis on biopsy [31]. In other cases, biopsies of perianal ulcers are confirmed to be manifestations of cutaneous sarcoidosis [32]. Rectal involvement in sarcoidosis has also been reported in the literature as an incidental finding on rectal biopsy or via presentation as a polyp [33–35].

9.5.2 Systemic Lupus Erythematosus (SLE)

Systemic lupus erythematosus (SLE) is an autoimmune disease with several gastrointestinal manifestations, however anorectal involvement is rare. Only a few case reports in the literature mention anorectal involvement of SLE. A few cases of rectal stenosis and rectal ulcers, some complicated by perforation, were found to show pathologic features of SLE on biopsy [36–39]. SLE patients with anorectal involvement may present with rectal bleeding or pain. Interestingly, all cases of anorectal involvement with SLE were observed in patients less than 43 years of age. Although a rare complication of SLE, small vessel vasculitis is thought to play a role in the pathogenesis of these rectal findings. Treatment of these lesions is mainly with steroids.

9.5.3 Antiphospholipid Syndrome

Antiphospholipid syndrome (APS) is characterized by thrombosis and pregnancy-related complications including multiple spontaneous abortions. Since APS may lead to intra-abdominal thrombosis, it has been theorized that it may lead to an increased risk of hemorrhoidal disease. The prevalence of hemorrhoidal disease in the general population of the USA is 4.4% [40]. A recent cross-sectional study showed a 41.4% incidence of hemorrhoidal disease in patients with APS, with a majority of patients requiring surgical intervention [41]. More studies are needed to identify a significant relationship between hemorrhoidal disease and APS.

9.6 Conclusion

Anorectal involvement in RD, though relatively uncommon, can significantly affect patient quality of life. Among RD, SSc is most strongly associated with fecal incontinence due to multifactorial mechanisms, including neuropathy, smooth muscle atrophy, and fibrosis of the internal anal sphincter. Other conditions, including sarcoidosis, SLE, and APS, may present with a variety of anorectal manifestations such as perianal plaques, rectal stenosis, ulcers, or hemorrhoidal disease. Despite the clinical burden of these symptoms, therapeutic options remain limited, and high-quality evidence is lacking. Further research and RCTs are needed to guide management. Early identification of anorectal symptoms in patients with RD may facilitate earlier diagnosis, prevent complications, and improve outcomes through multidisciplinary care.

References

1. Kröner PT, Tolaymat OA, Bowman AW, Abril A, Lacy BE. Gastrointestinal manifestations of rheumatological diseases. Off J Am College Gastroenterol | ACG. 2019;114(9):1441–54. https://doi.org/10.14309/ajg.0000000000000260.
2. Sagar PM, Pemberton JH. Anorectal and pelvic floor function. Relevance of continence, incontinence, and constipation. Gastroenterol Clin N Am. 1996;25(1):163–82. https://doi.org/10.1016/s0889-8553(05)70370-8.
3. Shafik A, Shafik AA, El Sibai O, Ahmed I, Mostafa RM. Role of the rectosigmoidal junction in fecal continence: concept of the primary continent mechanism. Arch Surg. 2006;141(1):23–6. https://doi.org/10.1001/archsurg.141.1.23.
4. Lane RHS, Parks AG. Function of the anal sphincters following colo-anal anastomosis. Br J Surg. 2005;64(8):596–9. https://doi.org/10.1002/bjs.1800640820.
5. Sagar PM, Holdsworth PJ, Johnston D. Correlation between laboratory findings and clinical outcome after restorative proctocolectomy: serial studies in 20 patients with end-to-end pouch-anal anastomosis. Br J Surg. 2005;78(1):67–70. https://doi.org/10.1002/bjs.1800780121.
6. Lubowski DZ, Nicholls RJ, Swash M, Jordan MJ. Neural control of internal anal sphincter function. Br J Surg. 2005;74(8):668–70. https://doi.org/10.1002/bjs.1800740804.
7. Frenckner B. Function of the anal sphincters in spinal man. Gut. 1975;16(8):638–44. https://doi.org/10.1136/gut.16.8.638.
8. Menees SB, Almario CV, Spiegel BMR, Chey WD. Prevalence of and factors associated with fecal incontinence: results from a population-based survey. Gastroenterology. 2018;154(6):1672–81.e3. https://doi.org/10.1053/j.gastro.2018.01.062.
9. Wald A. Fecal incontinence in adults (Disease/Disorder overview). N Engl J Med. 2007;356(16):1648.
10. Chiou AW, Lin JK, Wang FM. Anorectal abnormalities in progressive systemic sclerosis. Dis Colon Rectum. 1989;32(5):417–21. https://doi.org/10.1007/bf02563695.
11. Leighton JA, Valdovinos MA, Pemberton JH, Rath DM, Camilleri M. Anorectal dysfunction and rectal prolapse in progressive systemic sclerosis. Dis Colon Rectum. 1993;36(2):182–5. https://doi.org/10.1007/bf02051176.
12. Palit S, Lunniss PJ, Scott SM. The physiology of human defecation. Dig Dis Sci. 2012;57(6):1445–64. https://doi.org/10.1007/s10620-012-2071-1.

13. Thiruppathy K, Mason J, Akbari K, Raeburn A, Emmanuel A. Physiological study of the anorectal reflex in patients with functional anorectal and defecation disorders. J Dig Dis. 2017;18(4):222–8. https://doi.org/10.1111/1751-2980.12462.
14. Bharucha AE. Pelvic floor: anatomy and function. Neurogastroenterol Motil. 2006;18(7):507–19. https://doi.org/10.1111/j.1365-2982.2006.00803.x.
15. Poirier TJ, Rankin GB. Gastrointestinal manifestations of progressive systemic scleroderma based on a review of 364 cases. Am J Gastroenterol. 1972;58(1):30–44.
16. Herrick AL, Barlow JD, Bowden A, Williams N, Hobson AR, Irving M, et al. Investigation of anal function in patients with systemic sclerosis. Ann Rheum Dis. 1996;55(6):370–4. https://doi.org/10.1136/ard.55.6.370.
17. Trezza M. Bowel problems in patients with systemic sclerosis. Scand J Gastroenterol. 1999;34(4):409–13. https://doi.org/10.1080/003655299750026434.
18. Thoua NM, Abdel-Halim M, Forbes A, Denton CP, Emmanuel AV. Fecal incontinence in systemic sclerosis is secondary to neuropathy. Off J Am College Gastroenterol | ACG. 2012;107(4):597–603. https://doi.org/10.1038/ajg.2011.399.
19. Bajwa A, Fellow R, Emmanuel A. The physiology of continence and evacuation. Best Pract Res Clin Gastroenterol. 2009;23(4):477–85. https://doi.org/10.1016/j.bpg.2009.06.002.
20. Basilisco G, Barbera R, Vanoli M, Bianchi P. Anorectal dysfunction and delayed colonic transit in patients with progressive systemic sclerosis. Dig Dis Sci. 1993;38(8):1525–9. https://doi.org/10.1007/bf01308615.
21. Heyt GJ, Oh MK, Alemzadeh N, Rivera S, Jimenez SA, Rattan S, et al. Impaired rectoanal inhibitory response in scleroderma (systemic sclerosis): an association with fecal incontinence. Dig Dis Sci. 2004;49(6):1040–5. https://doi.org/10.1023/b:ddas.0000034569.85066.69.
22. Malandrini A, Selvi E, Villanova M, Berti G, Sabadini L, Salvadori C, et al. Autonomic nervous system and smooth muscle cell involvement in systemic sclerosis: ultrastructural study of 3 cases. J Rheumatol. 2000;27(5):1203–6.
23. Thoua NM, Schizas A, Forbes A, Denton CP, Emmanuel AV. Internal anal sphincter atrophy in patients with systemic sclerosis. Rheumatology (Oxford). 2011;50(9):1596–602. https://doi.org/10.1093/rheumatology/ker153.
24. Engel AF, Kamm MA, Talbot IC. Progressive systemic sclerosis of the internal anal sphincter leading to passive faecal incontinence. Gut. 1994;35(6):857–9. https://doi.org/10.1136/gut.35.6.857.
25. Campbell PM, LeRoy EC. Pathogenesis of systemic sclerosis: a vascular hypothesis. Semin Arthritis Rheum. 1975;4(4):351–68. https://doi.org/10.1016/0049-0172(75)90017-7.
26. Sjogren RW. Gastrointestinal motility disorders in scleroderma. Arthritis Rheum. 1994;37(9):1265–82. https://doi.org/10.1002/art.1780370902.
27. Felt-Bersma RJ. Endoanal ultrasound in benign anorectal disorders: clinical relevance and possibilities. Expert Rev Gastroenterol Hepatol. 2008;2(4):587–606. https://doi.org/10.1586/17474124.2.4.587.
28. Omair MA, Lee P. Effect of gastrointestinal manifestations on quality of life in 87 consecutive patients with systemic sclerosis. J Rheumatol. 2012;39(5):992–6. https://doi.org/10.3899/jrheum.110826.
29. Kenefick NJ, Vaizey CJ, Nicholls RJ, Cohen R, Kamm MA. Sacral nerve stimulation for faecal incontinence due to systemic sclerosis. Gut. 2002;51(6):881–3. https://doi.org/10.1136/gut.51.6.881.
30. Petersen S, Tobisch A, Puhl G, Kötter I, Wollina U. Stubborn rectal prolapse in systemic sclerosis. Reumatologia. 2017;55(2):100–3. https://doi.org/10.5114/reum.2017.67606.
31. Chikeka I, Husain S, Grossman ME. Asymptomatic annular perianal sarcoidosis. JAAD Case Rep. 2020;6(12):1242–4. https://doi.org/10.1016/j.jdcr.2020.09.009.
32. Cohen GF, Wolfe CM. Recalcitrant diffuse cutaneous sarcoidosis with perianal involvement responding to adalimumab. J Drugs Dermatol. 2017;16(12):1305–6.
33. Gould SR, Handley AJ, Barnardo DE. Rectal and gastric involvement in a case of sarcoidosis. Gut. 1973;14(12):971–3. https://doi.org/10.1136/gut.14.12.971.

34. Tobi M, Kobrin I, Ariel I. Rectal involvement in sarcoidosis. Dis Colon Rectum. 1982;25(5).
35. A case of sarcoidosis presenting as a rectal polyp. Clin Endosc. 2008;36(4):238–41.
36. Yuasa S, Suwa A, Hirakata M, Hibi N, Iwao Y, Koizumi K, et al. A case of systemic lupus erythematosus presenting with rectal ulcers as the initial clinical manifestation of disease. Clin Exp Rheumatol. 2002;20(3):407–10.
37. Palvio DH, Christensen KS. Systemic lupus erythematosus with rectal stenosis simulating tumour or diverticulosis. Case report. Acta Chir Scand. 1987;153(1):63–5.
38. Teramoto J, Takahashi Y, Katsuki S, Sato T, Sakamaki S, Kobayashi D, et al. Systemic lupus erythematosus with a giant rectal ulcer and perforation. Intern Med. 1999;38(8):643–9. https://doi.org/10.2169/internalmedicine.38.643.
39. Mansoor AC, Jemshad A, Musambil M. Systemic lupus erythematosus presenting as rectal ulcer and longitudinal myelopathy. Int J Rheum Dis. 2017;20(11):1818–20. https://doi.org/10.1111/1756-185X.12654.
40. Johanson JF, Sonnenberg A. The prevalence of hemorrhoids and chronic constipation: an epidemiologic study. Gastroenterology. 1990;98(2):380–6. https://doi.org/10.1016/0016-5085(90)90828-O.
41. Cunha E, Guzela V, Balbi GGM, Sobrado C, Andrade D. Anorectal diseases in patients with Antiphospholipid syndrome: a cross-sectional study. Adv Rheumatol. 2020;60(1):51. https://doi.org/10.1186/s42358-020-00153-5.

Chapter 10
Liver Disease in Rheumatology

Bilal Ashraf, Dana Gornick, Wajeed Sumbal, Zainab Saeed, Ruben Peredo, and Micheal Tadros

10.1 Introduction

Rheumatic diseases can affect multiple organ systems, including the joints, eyes, heart, kidneys, skin, nails, and lungs. Their presentation can vary among different patients depending on the organ system involved. In this chapter, we will focus on the hepatic manifestations of various rheumatic diseases, which can range from asymptomatic, mild elevation of transaminases and cholestatic enzymes to jaundice and more severe manifestations such as hepatomegaly, hepatic cirrhosis, and acute liver failure. The causes of liver involvement can be broadly categorized as primary liver disease unrelated to rheumatic disease, hepatic manifestation of a primary rheumatic disease, or a hepatic side effect of the medications used to treat rheumatic diseases.

The most common autoimmune liver diseases (AILDs) include autoimmune hepatitis (AIH), primary biliary cholangitis (PBC), and primary sclerosing cholangitis (PSC). Miscellaneous diseases include systemic illnesses affecting the liver, like IgG4-related hepatopathy, sarcoidosis, common variable immune deficiency,

B. Ashraf · M. Tadros
Department of Medicine, Division of Gastroenterology, Albany Medical Center, Albany, NY, USA

D. Gornick
Department of Medicine, Cedars Sinai, Los Angeles, CA, USA

W. Sumbal · Z. Saeed
Department of Medicine, Albany Medical Center, Albany, NY, USA

R. Peredo (✉)
Department of Medicine, Division of Rheumatology, Stratton VA Medical Center, Albany, NY, USA
e-mail: ruben.peredo-wende@va.gov

M. Tadros et al. (eds.), *GI Diseases Associated with Rheumatological and Vasculitic Conditions*, Clinical Gastroenterology,
https://doi.org/10.1007/978-3-032-07868-1_10

and celiac disease. AILD coexists with rheumatic disease in approximately 30% of cases and may share common pathogenic mechanisms involving the development of autoimmunity. Rheumatic diseases that commonly co-occur with AIH include Sjögren's disease, rheumatoid arthritis (RA), and systemic lupus erythematosus (SLE). In contrast, rheumatic diseases associated with PBC include Sjögren's disease, RA, IgG4-related disease, and systemic sclerosis. It is imperative to differentiate primary rheumatic disease affecting the liver from rheumatic disease and overlapping AILD, as therapeutic options, potential complications, and overall prognosis differ.

In a study involving 306 patients with rheumatic disease, including SLE, Sjögren's syndrome, RA, scleroderma, polymyositis, and polyarteritis nodosa, 43% (133 patients) developed some liver disturbance. The leading cause of liver disturbance was liver disease associated with the primary rheumatic disease (37%). It was characterized by mild and transient elevation of alanine aminotransferase (ALT) and alkaline phosphatase (ALP) for 6 +/− 2 months. Liver histology was available for 15 of these patients, showing only minimal changes without the histologic findings of AIH. However, nine patients were categorized as "probable" to have AIH according to the AIH scoring system, and one patient with Scleroderma was classified as "definite" according to the AIH scoring system. Relying on the AIH scoring system without characteristic histological findings such as piecemeal necrosis, infiltration of plasma cells, and resetting of liver cells may result in AIH overdiagnosis. Liver biopsy and histology are key to the accurate diagnosis and differentiation of AIH in patients who happen to have rheumatic diseases versus liver disease associated with primary rheumatic disease (Table 10.1) [1, 22, 23, 28–31].

In the same study, histological analysis of the liver was performed in 51 patients with liver disturbances. Other than liver disease associated with rheumatic diseases, histological analysis showed that liver disturbances were a result of other underlying conditions such as drug-induced liver disease (17%), fatty liver (13%), viral

Table 10.1 Rheumatologic diseases, serologies, and associated liver diseases [1, 22, 23, 28–31]

Rheumatologic disease	Serology	Associated liver disease
SLE	ANA, dsDNA, Anti-Smith, Anti-Ro (SSA), Anti-La (SSB), RNP	ELE, PBC, AIH, PSC, OS
RA	RF, CCP	ELE, PBC, AIH, PSC, OS
Systemic sclerosis	Anti-centromere (Limited SSc); Scl-70, RNA Polymerase (Diffuse SSc)	ELE, PBC, AIH, PSC, cirrhosis
Sjogren's disease	Anti-Ro (SSA), Anti-La (SSB)	ELE, PBC, AIH, PSC
AAV	ANCA (PR3-ANCA, MPO-ANCA)	ELE, PBC, AIH,
IgG4-related disease	Elevated IgG4, IgG1, IgE; normal C3, C4	ELE, PSC, obstructive jaundice

Abbreviations: *AAV* ANCA-associated vasculitis, *AIH* autoimmune hepatitis, *ELE* elevated liver enzymes, *IgG4* immunoglobulin G4, *OS* overlap syndrome, *PBC* primary biliary cholangitis, *PSC* primary sclerosing cholangitis, *RA* rheumatoid arthritis, *SLE* systemic lupus erythematosus hepatitis, PBC, idiopathic portal hypertension, alcoholic liver injury, congestive hepatopathy, amyloidosis, cholelithiasis, and metastatic disease [1].

10.2 Pathogenesis of Autoimmune Liver Disease

The liver is exposed to a variety of antigens via the portal system and venous drainage of the digestive tract, ranging from harmless dietary antigens to more dangerous blood-borne pathogens like viruses, parasites, and bacteria, as well as cancer cells that metastasize from other parts of the body. The presence of immune-regulation and tolerance in the liver ensures that these regularly presented antigens do not result in an inappropriate immune response. Self-tolerance is maintained by cells like dendritic cells, Kupffer cells, hepatic sinusoidal endothelial cells, and hepatic stellate cells via the production of anti-inflammatory mediators. These include IL-10 and TGFβ, as well as inhibitory cell surface ligands, which prevent T cell activation, resulting in T cell apoptosis, anergy, or differentiation into regulatory T cells. [2] On the other hand, the liver also has innate lymphocytes, including $CD56^+$ T cells, natural killer T cells, γδ T cells, and mucosal-associated invariant T cells that recognize metabolites from microorganisms and promote targeted killing of cells and activation of other immune cells. In autoimmune liver diseases, as in any other autoimmune disease, immune tolerance to self-antigens is lost, and effector CD4+ and CD8+ T cells attack hepatic and biliary cells. The subsequent release of inflammatory cytokines like interferon-γ (IFN-γ) and interleukin-17 (IL-17) results in inflammation and liver injury. Regulatory T (Treg) cells normally regulate these effector T cells. Loss of this delicate balance of effector and regulatory T cells results in a loss of immune tolerance [3].

Additionally, genetic susceptibility plays a role in the development of autoimmune liver disease. MHC class II proteins present antigenic peptides to CD4+ T cells. The MHC class II allotypes DR3, DR4 and Dr52a predispose to AIH-1, DR7 predisposes to AIH-2, DR8 to PBC and DR52a to PSC [4–8]. Serum autoantibodies are present in AIH and PBS, but not in PSC, and may be positive in asymptomatic patients, or years before symptom onset or initial diagnosis [9, 10].

10.3 Pathogenesis of Systemic Rheumatic Diseases

Like AILDs, the pathogenesis of systemic rheumatic diseases involves the interplay of environmental and genetic factors, and the ultimate development of autoimmunity and resultant inflammation and injury to tissues [11]. Systemic rheumatic diseases are also known to have positive disease-associated biomarkers and autoantibodies during pre-clinical disease [12]. For example, in RA, rheumatoid factor and anti-citrullinated peptide proteins appear before the onset of inflammatory arthritis [13]. Similarly, antinuclear antibodies (ANA) in SLE are present before the onset of disease symptoms [14]. In one study, eleven asymptomatic mothers of children with neonatal lupus were found to be positive for Anti-Ro/SSA and anti-La/SSB antibodies, and eight of them developed Sjogren's disease within the next 4.75 years [15].

10.4 Autoimmune Hepatitis and Rheumatic Diseases

AIH is a chronic inflammatory disease characterized by failure of immune tolerance mechanisms and resultant T-cell-mediated destruction of hepatocytes. It commonly affects genetically predisposed individuals, more commonly affects women than men, with a female-to-male ratio of 4:1. It is thought to be precipitated by environmental triggers such as viral diseases [16, 17]. The global incidence of AIH is estimated to be 1 in 100,000 persons per year, with a higher incidence in Scandinavian countries [18, 19].

The International Autoimmune Hepatitis Group (IAIH-G) has devised diagnostic criteria based on multiple factors such as age, sex, ratio of liver enzymes, autoantibody titers, antimitochondrial antibodies, viral hepatitis markers, intravenous drug use, average alcohol consumption, presence of genetic factors (HLA, DR3, DR4), liver histology, response to therapy, and presence of other autoimmune disorders. Based on scoring, patients are categorized as "definite" or "probable" to have AIH [20, 21]. Given the co-occurrence between autoimmune disease and AIH, the IAH-G includes the presence of another autoimmune disorder in its diagnostic criteria for AIH.

AIH is associated with several extrahepatic manifestations. Non-specific joint pain has been reported in 10–60% of patients. A minority of patients with AIH also present with unexplained fevers and maculopapular rash, which often resolve upon the initiation of immunosuppressant therapy in the treatment of AIH. Concomitant autoimmune disorders have been reported in 20–50% of patients with AIH, including autoimmune thyroiditis (8–23%), diabetes (1–10%), RA (2–4%), mixed connective tissue disease (2–4%), inflammatory bowel disease (2–8%), Sjogren's disease (1–7%), systemic lupus erythematosus (1–3%) and glomerulonephritis (1%) [22, 23]. Infrequently, AIH is also associated with diseases like mononeuritis multiplex, multiple sclerosis, hemolytic anemia, and fibrosing alveolitis [19, 24–26].

Women with Type-1 AIH positive for HLA-DR4 are more likely to have other concurrent autoimmune disorders [25, 27]. Similarly, elderly patients with AIH have a higher frequency of rheumatic conditions like RA, Sjogren's disease, pericarditis, mononeuritis multiplex, and SLE as compared to young adults (13% versus 0%, $p = 0.02$) [22].

One study involving patients with Sjögren's syndrome showed that 47% of the patients had liver histology consistent with AIH [28]. AIH type 1 is predominantly characterized by antinuclear antibodies (ANA) and/or anti-smooth muscle antibodies (anti-SMA). In contrast, AIH type 2 typically presents with anti-liver kidney microsomal type 1 antibodies (anti-LKM1) and/or anti-liver cytosol type 1 antibodies (anti-LC1). In addition to these, other antibodies more specific to rheumatic diseases are also seen in AIH, which include anti-dsDNA, perinuclear anti-neutrophil cytoplasmic antibodies (pANCA), anti chromatin, rheumatoid factor, and anti-Ro/SSA [29]. Anti-cyclic citrullinated peptides (anti-CCP) were found in 9% of patients with AIH, independent of concurrent RA [29, 30]. In one study involving 179 patients with type 1 AIH, 11% (20 patients) were positive for anti-CCP antibodies. Those with seropositivity for anti-CCP had a higher frequency of RA (25% vs 0%, $p < 0.001$), higher occurrence of histologic cirrhosis on presentation (47% vs 20%, $p = 0.01$) and a higher chance of death due to hepatic failure (25% vs 9%, $p = 0.04$) compared to seronegative patients (Table 10.1) [28–31].

First-line treatment for AIH consists of corticosteroids alone or in combination with azathioprine. [32, 33]. Once remission is achieved, maintenance therapy includes azathioprine once steroids are successfully tapered off. In contrast to rheumatic disease, the dose of azathioprine needed in AIH is typically lower, requiring 50 mg/day, and should not exceed 150 mg/day [33, 34]. In patients with disease progression and/or intolerance to standard therapy, medications commonly prescribed to treat rheumatic diseases have been successfully used as alternative therapies for AIH. Methotrexate, mycophenolate mofetil, cyclosporin, tacrolimus, cyclophosphamide, and ursodeoxycholic acid have shown benefit in treating AIH [20, 35–38]. Other medications like infliximab, rituximab, sirolimus, and everolimus have been tried to treat refractory cases of AIH [39–41].

10.5 Primary Biliary Cholangitis (PBC) and Rheumatic Diseases

Primary biliary cholangitis (PBC) is characterized by auto-immune-mediated destruction of intrahepatic bile ducts, cholestasis, and in severe cases, liver cirrhosis [42]. High titers of antimitochondrial antibodies (AMA) are found in patients with PBC and are highly specific and sensitive for the diagnosis and prognosis of the disease [43, 44]. PBC predominantly affects females in the fifth or sixth decade of life, with a female-to-male ratio of 9:1 [42]. Diagnosis of PBC is based on the presence of two of the following three criteria:

1. Increase in ALP greater than 2 times the upper limit of normal, or GGT greater than 5 times the upper limit of normal
2. AMA positivity
3. Chronic granulomatous cholangitis and destruction of small or medium-sized bile ducts on liver biopsy

As in many rheumatic disorders, AMA can also be positive years before the onset of symptoms or diagnosis of PBC. One study found that 53% of patients with PBC had at least one additional autoimmune disease. The most prevalent was Sjogren's disease (25%), followed by Raynaud's phenomenon (24%), autoimmune thyroid disease (23%), RA (17%), systemic sclerosis (8%), and pernicious anemia (4%) [45]. In addition to AMA and ANA, 63% of patients with PBC were positive for other serum autoantibodies as well [45].

In another study involving 361 patients with PBC, 61.2% had at least one other extrahepatic autoimmune disorder. These included Hashimoto's thyroiditis (20.4%), Graves' thyroiditis (3.2%), Sjogren's disease (56.1%), Raynaud's disease (29.4%), RA (9.9%), systemic sclerosis (9.9%), cutaneous autoimmune disease (8.1%), SLE (3.6%), vasculitis (3.6%), celiac disease (1.4%) and other extrahepatic autoimmune conditions (13.2%) [46].

10.6 Primary Biliary Cirrhosis/Systemic Sclerosis Overlap Disease

Systemic sclerosis is a connective tissue disease characterized by autoimmunity and inflammation resulting in multisystem clinical manifestations, widespread vasculopathy, and progressive interstitial and perivascular fibrosis. Two major subgroups of systemic sclerosis are recognized based on LeRoy classification: limited cutaneous (lSSc) and diffuse cutaneous dSSc. Limited cutaneous systemic sclerosis, previously named CREST syndrome, involves fibrosis of the skin limited to the hands, forearms, and face only, along with Raynaud's phenomenon and less commonly, lung involvement. Diffuse cutaneous SSc, on the contrary, is a widespread, rapidly progressive disease involving the skin of the extremities and trunk, affects multiple organ systems, and has a less favorable prognosis [47–50]. LSSc has positive anti-centromere antibodies (ACA), anti-Th/To, anti-U1-RNP and PM/Scl. DSSc has positive anti-topoisomerase I antibodies (previously called anti-Scl-70), anti-RNA polymerase III, and anti-U3-RNP antibodies [51, 52].

Systemic sclerosis is one of the most common autoimmune rheumatic diseases associated with PBC, with 1% to 2% of patients with PBC having concomitant systemic sclerosis [53, 54]. 25% of the patients with SSc are positive for AMA, the pathognomonic autoantibody for PBC [55, 56]. In a study involving more than 800 patients with SSc, 2% were found to have PBC [57] [58]. Despite this link between PBC and SSc, the prevalence of PBC is still higher in the general population than in patients with SSc [58, 59]. In another study involving 43 patients with PBC/SSc overlap, 93% had limited systemic sclerosis, and interestingly, patients with PBC/SSc overlap had a slower rate of liver-disease progression compared to matched patients with PBC alone [60]. PBC patients should be carefully questioned regarding symptoms related to systemic sclerosis. For patients diagnosed with PBC/SSc overlap syndrome, further testing for additional organ involvement via spirometry or echocardiography may be warranted.

10.7 Primary Sclerosing Cholangitis and Rheumatic Diseases

PSC is a rare and chronic condition characterized by the development of small, bead-like protrusions and narrowing of the intrahepatic and extrahepatic biliary ducts, leading to cholestatic liver injury. While the disease often follows a prolonged asymptomatic period, it is progressive, resulting in complications such as strictures, recurrent episodes of cholangitis, and ultimately, end-stage liver disease.

In contrast to PBC, PSC affects both intra- and extrahepatic bile ducts [61]. Unlike PBC and AIH, which predominate in female patients, PSC more frequently affects men, with a 2:1 male/female ratio [62]. PSC also has a close association with inflammatory bowel disease. 7% of patients with IBD have PSC, and 70% of patients diagnosed with PSC show findings of IBD in some form [63, 64].

A small study in patients with generalized pustular psoriasis showed evidence of biliary involvement, with liver biopsy demonstrating neutrophilic cholangitis, and magnetic resonance cholangiopancreatography demonstrating features of PSC [65]. Even though many autoantibodies like anti-nuclear, anti-smooth muscle, and anti-mitochondrial antibodies are seen in PSC patients, they are highly nonspecific, and a precise autoantibody specific to PSC has yet to be identified [66]. In addition, up to 80% of PSC patients are P-ANCA positive, with higher rates seen in those with concurrent inflammatory bowel disease (IBD) [67].

10.8 Drug-Induced Liver Disease (DILI) in Rheumatic Diseases

Many drugs used to treat patients with rheumatic diseases can cause drug-induced liver injury, especially when they are used for a prolonged period or at a high dosage (Table 10.2) [69–85]. Acetaminophen is a readily available over-the-counter analgesic, is frequently used to treat arthritis, and is a first-line agent used to treat mild osteoarthritis. It can cause dose-dependent liver injury, especially when combined with alcohol. The recommended maximum dose of acetaminophen is 4 g in patients without pre-existing liver disease, and 2 g daily in elderly patients or patients with liver disease [69].

Non-steroidal anti-inflammatory drugs can also affect the liver, ranging from mild, temporary elevations in liver enzymes, which normalize after discontinuation, to severe liver injury, acute hepatitis, cholestatic disease, and acute liver failure. Diclofenac and sulindac are more hepatotoxic, whereas Ibuprofen and naproxen are less hepatotoxic compared to other NSAIDs. The combination of other antirheumatic medications with NSAIDs also increases the risk of hepatotoxicity [70–73].

Glucocorticoids are widely used to treat rheumatic diseases, and therefore are often used for prolonged periods. Glucocorticoid use can cause acute liver failure, and chronic usage is associated with fatty liver disease [74, 75]. There is also a risk of HBV reactivation depending upon the dosage and duration of therapy, and

Table 10.2 Rheumatologic disease therapies and associated liver toxicities [70–85]

Medication	Liver toxicity
Acetaminophen	ELE, liver failure
NSAIDs	ELE, acute hepatitis, cholestatic disease, acute liver failure
Glucocorticoids	ELE, NAFLD, HBV reactivation, acute liver failure
Methotrexate	ELE, NAFLD, fibrosis, acute necrosis
Thiopurines	ELE, cholestasis
Hydroxychloroquine	Acute hepatitis
Sulfasalazine	ELE, DRESS
Anti-TNFs	ELE, hepatitis B reactivation, AIH cholestasis, fulminant hepatitis
Rituximab	ELE, HBV reactivation
Tofacitinib	ELE

Abbreviations: *AIH*, autoimmune hepatitis; *DILI*, drug-induced liver injury; *DRESS*, drug reaction with eosinophilia and systemic symptoms; *ELE*, elevated liver enzymes; *HBV*, hepatitis B virus; *NAFLD*, non-alcoholic fatty liver disease; *NSAIDs*, nonsteroidal anti-inflammatory drugs; *TNF*, tumor necrosis factor.

hepatitis B surface antigen (HBsAg)/Hepatitis B core antibody (HBc) status of the patient. Those using 10 mg or more of prednisone or equivalent steroid for 4 or more weeks, and are HBsAg-positive/Anti-HBc positive, are considered high risk for reactivation of HBV. Patients with the same dose and duration, but who are HBsAg-negative/HBc-positive, are considered at moderate risk for HBV reactivation [76].

Synthetic Disease-Modifying antirheumatic drugs can also affect the liver. Sulfasalazine is commonly used to treat arthritis and IBD and can cause acute liver injury in 1 in 1000 users. Liver injury can also be part of DRESS syndrome [77, 78]. Leflunomide, another drug used for RA, can cause liver enzyme elevation in greater than 5% of patients, and in rare cases (0.02%), cause serious drug-induced hepatotoxicity and hospitalization [79, 80]. In rheumatoid arthritis patients using azathioprine, adverse hepatic reactions occurred in 2%. Another study showed that 1 in 1000 people receiving azathioprine developed liver injury requiring hospitalization [81, 82].

Methotrexate is another DMARD commonly used for RA and psoriatic arthritis. A meta-analysis showed that 11.2% of patients taking methotrexate developed liver-related adverse effects compared to 6.3% in the control group. 3.3% of patients on methotrexate had principal enzyme elevation, defined as more than 3 times above the upper limit of normal, compared to 1% in the control group. [83]

Biologics are another group of DMARDs that are increasingly used for the treatment of various rheumatic disorders. Anti-tumor necrosis factor (anti-TNF) drugs, such as infliximab, etanercept, adalimumab, and certolizumab, are one of the most prescribed classes of biologics. 37–42% of patients on these medications may develop asymptomatic liver enzyme elevations, 2–3 times the upper limit of normal. Immune-mediated hepatitis, cholestatic liver disease, and fulminant hepatitis secondary to hepatitis B reactivation have also been reported with the use of anti-TNF drugs [84].

Rituximab is an anti-CD20 antibody used to treat RA. It is associated with the reactivation of the B infection [85].

10.9 IGG4-Related Disease and IGG4-Related Hepatopathy

IgG4-related disease (IgG4-RD) is a chronic, fibroinflammatory multi organ disorder [68]. Clinical clues to diagnose IgG4-RD relate to any, but preferentially frequently affected organs (i.e., symmetrical swelling of salivary and/or lacrimal glands, lungs, kidneys, pancreas, and retroperitoneum [69], supported by high serum IgG4, polyclonal hypergammaglobulinemia, and in approximately 60% of patients, high serum IgE and peripheral eosinophilia [70]. In addition, the diagnosis is more likely when the radiographic findings favor IgG4-RD, showing diffuse organ enlargement, extensive ductal narrowing with potential for obstruction, and classical but not exclusively anterolateral fibrotic tissue surrounding the aorta, and in the retroperitoneal space (Table 10.4) [71, 72].

The histopathology of dense lymphoplasmacytic infiltrates rich in IgG4+ plasma cells, scattered eosinophils, fibrosis (in a storiform pattern), and obliterative phlebitis will confirm the disease [73] (Table 10.3). The favorable response to glucocorticoids in cases where the histopathology discloses no such clear-cut evidence due to fibrotic predominance or suboptimal tissue sampling will additionally support the diagnosis [74]. Placing all these features in perspective, the integrative approach for a definitive diagnosis of IgG4-RD includes the clinical, laboratory, radiographic, and histopathological findings, along with the favorable response to glucocorticoids (definition criteria) [74]. Different composite diagnostic criteria, like the HISORt (histology, imaging, serology, other organ involvement, and response to therapy) and the Japanese clinical diagnostic criteria, are excellent resources as guidance for the diagnosis of IgG4-sclerosing cholangitis (IgG4-SC) [75–77]. The diagnosis delay of months or years will find the affected organs/tissues in a state of irreversible damage and dysfunction, or presenting as a pseudotumor, at which point the pharmacologic intervention is questionable [76]. The transformation from lymphoplasmacytic to fibrotic tissue is assumed to depend on the time elapsed before any intervention, in addition to other unclear factors favoring fibrosis progression [73, 76, 78].

The etiology of IgG4-SC is not clear. Occupational hazards play a significant role, with higher rates reported in industry/mining workers [79]. Another vulnerable group with atopy in the background, identified by the elevated serum IgE and peripheral eosinophilia, reveals the allergic component participating in IgG4-RD, or coinciding simultaneously [70]. An overlap with autoimmune diseases reflects the intricate associations of these two inflammatory conditions, extending beyond

Table 10.3 Microscopic features for IgG4-SC

IgG4-hepatobiliary disease shares the same pathological lesion seen in almost all tissues affected by IgG4-related disease. Classic features include:
Lymphoplasmacytic infiltration
Storiform pattern of fibrosis
Obliterative phlebitis with a variable presence of eosinophils
Tissue IgG4 and IgG immunostaining on all specimens
A mean count of IgG4+ plasma cells in three high-power fields (HPF) and a ratio of IgG4: IgG plasma cells are calculated
Boston histological consensus criteria for bile duct and liver
>10 IgG4+ plasma cells per HPF in a biopsy specimen
>50 IgG4+ plasma cells per HPF in a resection specimen
Plus, an IgG4+: IgG+ plasma cell ratio of >40% in the context of two of three classic features

Adapted from Culver 2016 [72, 117]

coincidence. In patients with IgG4-hepatobiliary disease, half of the patients, for instance, will have positive antinuclear antibodies, and the rheumatoid factor in 20% [80], while a fraction might have an autoimmune disease [81].

IgG-RD preferentially affects the pancreas, and based on geo-epidemiological studies, it may be associated with variable frequencies of IgG4-hepatobiliary disease. The prevalence of AIP in Japanese patients was 4.6 per 100,000 in 2011, and the incidence was 1.4 per 100,000. In 1.5% of them, it was associated with IgG4-sclerosing cholangitis (IgG4-SC) [82, 83] and mainly with intrahepatic compromise [82]. This contrasted with an estimated prevalence of 8% in cohorts from Western countries (US and UK) [84, 85], a difference presumably linked to a different genetic background. HLA-DRB1*0405 and HLA-DRB1*0401 haplotypes have higher frequencies in AIP Japanese patients vs. the population without AIP [86]. In Western countries, patients with AIP are associated with HLA-DRB1*0301 and HLA-DQB1*0201, as compared with individuals without the disease [87].

The spectrum of IgG4-hepatopathy exhibits three prevailing phenotypes with superimposing features between them.

1. Autoimmune Hepatitis (AIH) pattern (IgG4-AIH), with analog features to AIH, presents with high alanine aminotransaminase, ALT, aspartate aminotransferase, AST, alkaline phosphatase, ALP, gamma-glutamyl transferase, GGT, IgG, IgG4, and a positive ANA test (in about half of them). Similarly, histopathology includes portal inflammation, interface hepatitis, lobular hepatitis, bile duct damage, canalicular cholestasis, and rosette formation [88]. The main difference in the proposed definition for IgG4-AIH vs. AIH relies on the presence of more than 5 IgG4-positive plasma cells per high-power field [89]. If AIP is associated with liver disease, the biopsies reveal IgG4-plasma cells in 47%, contrasting with AIH, primary sclerosing cholangitis, or primary biliary cholangitis [90], suggesting other organ involvement in IgG4-RD may favor IgG4-AIH. Conversely, authors debate whether this presentation is a variant of AIH [91, 92].

2. The nodular or pseudotumor presentation exhibits either a lymphoplasmacytic or fibrohistiocytic histopathologic pattern [93]. The former displays nodules or tumors of massive lymphoplasmacytic concentration, rich in IgG4-plasma cells, accompanied by obliterative phlebitis, while storiform fibrosis prevails in the latter [68]. Both should be screened to rule out potential malignancy, like the inflammatory myofibroblastic tumor [72].
3. Sclerosing cholangitis in IgG4-RD presents with four distinct features, with type 1,3–4 affecting the biliary extrahepatic and type 2 with diffuse intrahepatic cholangiopathy and lower common bile duct stricture, with (a) additional prestenotic dilatation, or (b) without prestenotic dilatation [94] (Table 10.4). Radiology will contribute to narrowing the diagnosis of IgG4-SC. The ultrasound might show

Table 10.4 Classification of IgG4-Sclerosing Cholangitis, based on cholangiography

Type	Site involved	Highlights	Differential diagnosis	Diagnostic/ evaluation approaches
Type 1	Distal common bile duct stricture	Associated with AIP	Pancreatic cancer Bile duct cancer Chronic pancreatitis	IDUS EUS-FNA Biopsy of bile duct
Type 2a	Diffuse intrahepatic cholangiopathy and a lower common bile duct stricture Pre-stenotic dilatation	May show extra-hepatic strictures	PSC SSC Pancreatic carcinoma Distal bile duct cancer	Liver biopsy Colonoscopy (to verify IBD)
Type 2b	Diffuse intrahepatic cholangiopathy and lower common bile duct stricture No pre-stenotic dilatation			
Type 3	Hilar and distal common bile duct stricture		Hilar bile duct cancer Pancreatic cancer Distal bile duct cancer Gallbladder cancer	EUS (bile duct, pancreas) IDUS (bile duct)
Type 4	Hilar stricture	Challenging to diagnose	Hilar bile duct cancer Gallbladder cancer	EUS (bile duct, pancreas) IDUS (bile duct)

Ancillary approaches for diagnosis and differentials. Adapted from Culver, 2016 [72] and Ohara, 2012 [77]

Abbreviations: *IBD* inflammatory bowel disease, *EUS* endoscopic ultrasound-guided fine needle aspiration, *IDUS* intraductal sonography, *AIP* autoimmune hepatitis, *PSC* primary sclerosing cholangitis, *SSC* secondary sclerosing cholangitis biliary duct dilatation, extrahepatic biliary stenosis, or a mass. Similarly, the CT scan will also show biliary tree dilatation, strictures, thickened gallbladder wall, masses, and compromise in other organs (i.e., the pancreas or retroperitoneum), raising further suspicion for this disorder. Magnetic resonance imaging (cholangiography) describing the biliary tree status will define the biliary duct wall more precisely (symmetry, smooth inner and outer margins, continuous vs skip lesions, and wall thickness). Other resources like PET CT and cholangiography, endoscopic retrograde cholangiopancreatography (for additional tissue, cell sampling), endoscopic and intraductal ultrasonography, and cholangioscopy [95] might contribute to additional supportive evidence and sampling collection. Cholangioscopy will enable the placement of stents to decompress the biliary tree when necessary [84]. Differentials in the assessment to consider are primary sclerosing cholangitis, secondary cholangitis, and cholangiocarcinoma. [96]. An oriented interview, specific physical clues on the exam, serology and biochemical profile, radiographic images, and, mainly, tissue sampling will define the specific disorder.

Even though the pathogenesis is quite complex, recent research has revealed key aspects within the major players in this disorder. Once active, the immune system develops a T-cell-mediated antigen-driven response, with the T cells orchestrating the central mediator (CD4, follicular regulatory, follicular helper), and effector functions (CD4 and CD8 cytotoxic cells) [97]. The interaction between T and B-cells, and via plasma cell immunoglobulin production, will promote the generation of particular antibodies (IgG4) to target the defined antigens. The specificity represents immunoglobulin editing and selection via class switching, reaching a point of clonality [98]. Confirmatory studies revealed circulating monoclonal premature B-cell subsets (plasmablasts) and identical IgG4, with the former correlating with disease activity, response to therapy, and relapses [98–100]. Several candidate antigens and their counterpart antibodies have been identified and considered to participate in the pathogenesis [101–106]. Nonetheless, reproducibility and external validity revealed weak results to generalize such findings [97]. The significance of IgG4 is translated by the chronicity of an antigen exposure with failure to clear it. Subsequently, IgG4 production runs unopposed. Additionally, the failed clearance following the initial stimulus relies in part on the IgG4 anti-inflammatory properties: in contrast to other IgG isotypes, IgG4 has bispecific variable regions (Fab-arm exchange); poor complement activation capabilities; and inadequate capacity to bind to Fc receptors [107]. Moreover, by raising the IgG4 pool under the stimulus of IL-10, a regulatory cytokine, combined with IL-4, the plasma cell will commit to producing IgG4 over IgE [108]. Serum IgG4 has weak diagnostic purposes but may acquire significance with higher concentrations [72]. On extreme elevations, for instance, or >5.6 g/l, it has a specificity and positive predictive value of 100% to differentiate between IgG4-SC from cholangiocarcinoma [109]. Elevated serum IgG4 levels also predict relapses (if >2.8 g/l at the diagnosis) and correlate with more organ involvement [84, 110, 111]. Conversely, lower serum IgG4 levels show lower sensitivity and specificity [112]. To define hepatobiliary disorder, diseases presenting with high IgG4 include those of an autoimmune nature and malignancy, and up to 5% of healthy individuals [107, 109, 112]. Elevated IgG4 may be present in PSC in a quarter of cases, with additional high plasma IgG4 cell counts on the biopsy in approximately 20%. This PSC subtype is more likely to be associated with IBD and to carry a more aggressive disease course. Proposed biomarkers like the serum IgG4: IgG1, IgG4: IgG RNA ratios, and IgG1: IgG4 ratio >0.24 might help distinguish from IgG4-SC [109, 113]. Conversely, normal serum IgG4 in IgG-SC poses more challenges in differentiation from cholangiocarcinoma and PSC. IgG4-RD seems to behave less aggressively in such cases and has lower relapse rates and number of affected organs [84, 114]. In this scenario, again, IgG4: IgG RNA ratio, and peripheral blood plasmablasts might help differentiate IgG4-SC, but more studies are required for validation [114–116]. Additional data to diagnose IgG4-SC relies on the biopsy (Boston histological consensus criteria) (Table 10.3) and tissue staining to calculate the IgG4: IgG ratio, over the classical findings of this disease [117] (Table 10.3).

Different from other fibrotic processes (i.e., systemic sclerosis), glucocorticoids may clear the tumor bulk, and to some extent, a vast majority of fibrotic deposits (i.e., retroperitoneum), highlighting the dynamic, reversible fibroinflammatory process underneath. On the other hand, failing to respond to glucocorticoids is a key criterion for excluding IgG-RD, and if so, other diagnoses might be considered [74]. In IgG4-SC on glucocorticoid therapy, remission is achieved faster [118], and clinical, laboratory, and cholestasis features will improve in about two-thirds of patients, in around 4–6 weeks [84]. Relapses ensue if glucocorticoids (in approximately half of patients) are discontinued without having started any steroid-sparing drug, and overall, at 1 year of glucocorticoid, an estimated 40% of patients may fail to achieve remission [118, 119]. On the flip side of the coin, drawbacks associated with glucocorticoid toxicity should be contemplated at the time of planning the pharmacologic therapy [120]. Azathioprine, mycophenolate mofetil, hydroxychloroquine, methotrexate, and tacrolimus are therapy options to consider, with mycophenolate mofetil being explored with more accuracy [85, 121–123]. Again, biliary stenting shows adjuvant therapy when necessary [84]. Specific B-cell targeting therapy (anti-CD20) is effective in IgG4-RD. Rituximab, a monoclonal antibody, has been shown to have a marked improvement in tumor reduction size, serum IgG4 reduction, plasmablast numbers, and circulating cytotoxic CD4 and markers of fibrosis [100, 116, 124, 125]. It has been reserved for incomplete remission, or glucocorticoid dependence, or glucocorticoid/immunosuppressor intolerance [122, 126]; however, the use of rituximab seems to be spreading for its benefits and efficacy, including IgG4-SC [127, 128]. Pharmacologic drug intervention will define prognosis and avoid potential biliary cirrhosis, potential malignancy, and mortality [84, 85, 129].

10.10 Celiac Disease and the Liver

Celiac disease (CD) is primarily recognized as a chronic immune-mediated enteropathy triggered by the ingestion of gluten [130]. Traditionally, its hallmark manifestation is malabsorption due to damage to the intestinal mucosa. However, emerging evidence has positioned CD as a multisystem disorder capable of affecting various organs, including the liver [131].

Liver involvement in CD can range from mild elevations in hepatic enzymes to celiac hepatitis and cirrhosis [132]. The underlying mechanism is poorly understood. One prevailing theory posits that increased intestinal permeability, a common feature of CD, facilitates the translocation of toxins, antigens, autoantibodies, and inflammatory cytokines into the portal circulation, subsequently leading to liver damage [133].

Most patients present without overt signs or symptoms of liver disease. Initial laboratory findings often reveal only mild elevations in serum aspartate aminotransferase (AST) and alanine aminotransferase (ALT), while alkaline phosphatase (ALP) and gamma-glutamyl transferase (GGT) levels typically remain within normal ranges [134]. Abdominal ultrasound is not routinely recommended during the initial work-up for liver involvement in CD. The introduction of a gluten-free diet (GFD) has been shown to elicit a favorable response in most patients, with normalization of liver enzyme levels occurring in approximately 75–95% of individuals within a year of strict adherence to the diet [134, 135].

Conversely, the presence of elevated alkaline phosphatase (ALP), low serum albumin, prolonged prothrombin time, and hyperbilirubinemia can indicate more severe liver disease or cirrhosis. In such scenarios, imaging studies may reveal a nodular echotexture on ultrasound [136, 137]. Although liver biopsy has limited utility in the assessment of liver involvement in celiac disease, it may be warranted in specific cases where patients are unresponsive to GFD or exhibit co-existing conditions [138]. Histologic findings from biopsy specimens are often nonspecific. They may include peri-portal inflammation, bile duct obstruction, increased Kupffer cells, mononuclear infiltration in the parenchyma, steatosis, and mild fibrosis [139, 140]. In rare instances, extensive fibrosis and cirrhosis have also been reported [136, 138].

Autoimmune liver diseases, including primary biliary cholangitis (PBC), primary sclerosing cholangitis (PSC), and autoimmune hepatitis (AIH), have been reported with CD in the literature [141–143]. This relationship may be attributed to shared autoimmune mechanisms, particularly evident in the case of PSC, where both conditions are linked to the at-risk HLA-DQ2 gene [144]. In the context of these concurrent autoimmune liver diseases, the efficacy of a gluten-free diet (GFD) appears to be limited [145].

10.11 Common Variable Immunodeficiency and Liver Disease

Common Variable Immunodeficiency (CVID) is the second most prevalent primary immunodeficiency disorder, primarily characterized by B-cell dysfunction, though defects in T-cells and antigen-presenting cells (APCs) are also noted [146]. A hallmark of CVID is primary hypogammaglobulinemia, with over 90% of patients experiencing recurrent infections [147]. Autoimmunity occurs in 20–30% of CVID patients, despite their immunodeficient status [148]. Additionally, these patients face increased risks of lymphoproliferation and malignancies, with benign lymphoproliferation affecting more than 20% [149] and lymphomas affecting 3–10% [150]. Non-caseating granulomas can develop in 8–22% of cases [151].

Liver disease is prevalent in CVID due to various factors, including infections, autoimmune processes, lymphoproliferation, and granulomatous reactions [147]. The manifestations of liver involvement can range from mild enzyme elevations to severe conditions like cirrhosis, portal hypertension, and liver cancer [149, 152, 153]. Common liver-related autoimmune conditions in CVID include autoimmune hepatitis (AIH), primary sclerosing cholangitis (PSC), and primary biliary cholangitis (PBC) [146, 154].

Patients with liver involvement may present asymptomatically or with symptoms such as fatigue, jaundice, edema, ascites, hepatomegaly, splenomegaly, or esophageal varices [152]. Laboratory findings often reveal liver enzyme abnormalities, particularly elevated alkaline phosphatase (ALP) [152]. Importantly, specific autoantibodies, like antimitochondrial antibodies (AMA) in PBC and anti-smooth muscle antibodies (ASMA) in PSC, may be low or undetectable in CVID patients [155]. Thus, regular biochemical (liver enzyme tests) and morphological assessments (ultrasound, MRI) are crucial for early detection of liver complications. This may help identify patients eligible for biopsy promptly. Considering the association of autoimmunity and CVID, data on genome-wide association studies on hepatic autoimmunity may shed light on potential genetic markers [156].

Nodular regenerative hyperplasia (NRH) is a typical hepatic lesion in CVID, reported in approximately 32% of patients in one study [149, 157]. It is believed to arise from intrahepatic vasculopathy, characterized by chronic cytotoxic T-cell infiltration of the sinusoidal endothelium, leading to hepatocyte nodules and increased portal pressure [158]. The predominant histopathological finding in NRH is an intrasinusoidal inflammatory infiltrate of CD3+ CD8+ T cells, often with colocalizing sinusoidal dilation and non-fibrosing granulomas [152].

Individuals carriers of CVID are also susceptible to liver infections, including historical cases of iatrogenic hepatitis C due to contaminated intravenous immunoglobulin [159]. It is essential to monitor viral loads, as serological tests may yield false negatives. Additionally, opportunistic pathogens or extraintestinal parasites, such as Giardia, can contribute to liver infections [160].

Malignancy is a significant cause of mortality in CVID, with the liver being a common site for metastasis, especially from gastric adenocarcinoma and extranodal non-Hodgkin lymphoma [161]. Primary liver cancer, while rare, can also occur [162].

The primary clinical interventions for CVID include immunoglobulin replacement therapy and anti-infection measures [163]. For autoimmune complications, corticosteroids or immunomodulators may be prescribed, generally at lower doses and for shorter durations [148, 164]. In select cases, splenectomy may be considered [24]. Currently, no specific treatments for CVID-related liver involvement exist. Despite optimal management of complications, chronic liver damage may progress to end-stage liver disease, where liver transplantation (LT) and hematopoietic stem cell transplantation represent the only potential curative options, albeit with significant risks [165, 166].

10.12 ANCA-Associated Vasculitis and the Liver

Anti-neutrophil cytoplasmic antibody (ANCA)-associated vasculitis (AAV) is a group of diseases characterized predominantly by small vessel necrotizing vasculitis. This includes granulomatosis with polyangiitis (GPA, Wegener), microscopic polyangiitis (MPA), and eosinophilic granulomatosis with polyangiitis (EGPA, Churg-Strauss) [167]. The three types of AAV are differentiated by their clinical features, eosinophils, and associated ANCA patterns, with specificity for proteinase-3 (PR3) or myeloperoxidase (MPO) [168]. Both the etiology and pathophysiology of AAV remain uncertain [168]. AAV can affect any organ, in a vasculitic or granulomatous disease pattern [169]. Although it has rarely been described, liver involvement can occur, and subclinical liver involvement is a frequent event in patients with active AAV [170, 171]. Hepatic involvement in patients with small vessel vasculitis has been associated with an adverse prognosis for survival [171].

In a retrospective study of 75 patients with small vessel vasculitis, 54 patients (49.4%) had LFT abnormalities during the active disease state [171]. This consisted of a cholestatic pattern (i.e., increased gamma-GT and ALP) and a hepatocellular pattern (with increased ALT and AST). Elevated liver enzymes were present in 2–25% of AAV patients at the time of diagnosis, and liver involvement was primarily observed in patients with GPA and not in MPA or EGPA, respectively [171].

Liver involvement in AAV has also previously been described in several case reports, specifically in cases of GPA, MPA, and EGPA [172–174].

10.13 Sarcoidosis and the Liver

Sarcoidosis is a chronic, multisystemic disease of unclear etiology, with non-caseating granulomas as the hallmark [175]. The diagnosis is sustained by clinical and radiographic features, and supported by histopathology and a biochemical

Table 10.5 Differential diagnosis of necrotizing and non-necrotizing granuloma in the assessment of sarcoidosis

Necrotizing granuloma		Non-necrotizing granuloma	
Infectious	Non-infectious	Infectious	Non-infectious
Mycobacteria	Vasculitis-associated	GLUS syndrome[c]	**Inflammatory**
M. tuberculosis	Granulomatosis with polyangiitis[a]	*M. tuberculosis*	Hypersensitivity
Non-tuberculous mycobacteria	Eosinophilic granulomatosis with polyangiitis		Sarcoidosis
Fungal	**Others**		Hot tub lung disease
Histoplasma	Rheumatoid nodule		Berylliosis
Coccidioides	Necrotizing sarcoidosis[b]		Foreign material-associated
Blastomyces	Aspiration pneumonia		Aspiration pneumonia
Aspergillus			Talc granulomatosis
Cryptococcus			Systemic immunological-associated
Parasites			Crohn's disease
Dirofilaria			Chronic granulomatous disease
Others			Granulomatous and lymphocytic interstitial lung disease
Francisella tularensis			Common Variable Immunodeficiency
Bartonella henselae			Sarcoid-like reaction of malignancy
Actinomyces			Drugs induced sarcoid-like reaction
			Granulomas of unknown etiology

Adapted from Chopra, et al. 2020 [176] and Rosen, 2007 [185]

[a]GPA shows rare epithelioid cells with poorly formed granulomas; additional large areas of basophilic necrosis will characterize this disease

[b]Necrotizing sarcoidosis, a variant of sarcoidosis

[c]GLUS syndrome: granulomatous lesions of unknown significance. Multiple organ involvement, including the liver (hepato-splenomegaly). The presence of B lymphocytes and NK cells distinguishes sarcoidosis. Viral origin is considered

profile [175]. The differential diagnoses of granuloma should exclude those of infectious origin, malignancy, drugs, vasculitis (i.e., granulomatosis with polyangiitis), beryllium exposure, steatosis, PSC, PBC, and others, before considering a definitive diagnosis [176] (Table 10.5). The angiotensin-converting enzyme (ACE) is not a diagnostic tool, and its utility is limited as a marker of disease activity and response to therapy in patients with initial high ACE levels. In addition, although not specific, a profile of low-normal parathyroid hormone, low 25-hydroxyvitamin D, high 1,25 1,25-dihydroxyvitamin D, low phosphorus, and hypercalcemia might support active sarcoidosis as the central orchestrator [177]. The disease is frequent in African Americans and individuals of Northern European ancestry [176, 178]. The incidence averages 6.1 per 100,000 individuals per year in the U.S. [179], with onset of the disease at a younger age in African Americans, and with a peak incidence ranging between 20 and 50 years of age [179–182]. Another peak incidence is seen in elderly patients [182, 183]. Prevalence varies between 1 and 40 per 100,000 individuals, with 35.5 per 100,000 for African-Americans and 10.9 per 100,000 for Caucasians [175]. African American men might carry extrapulmonary features [184].

Sarcoidosis preferentially affects the lungs, and the granuloma formation is thought to follow a failed process to clear a persistent and poorly degradable antigen [185]. This antigen is thought to be inhaled in aerosol particles. Several antigenic candidates are hypothesized to trigger the disease, including those associated with agriculture, insecticides, metal-related debris, and dust (World Trade Center in 2001) [186], Mycobacteria, *Propionibacterium acnes,* and others [187–190]. A genetic background could either determine spontaneous resolution (HLA-DRB1*03) or drive the inflammation into chronicity (HLA-DRB1*14 or HLA-DRB1*15) [191]. Additional loci outside the MHC II class participate in the disease course. A sarcoid granuloma consists of a confluence of modified macrophages, or epithelioid cells, encircling a center filled with giant cells [185]. These cells, derived from the fusion of macrophages, occasionally present with coexistent partial necrosis in the center. In the cytoplasm of giant cells, the presence of inclusion bodies, like the Schaumann's bodies, might support the diagnosis, but it may be seen in other conditions (i.e., hypersensitivity pneumonitis) [185]. The Caseum material (cheese-like appearance), or liquefaction, primarily excludes a sarcoid granuloma from Mycobacteria spp., fungi, and other etiologies. Surrounding the epithelioid cell layer lies a mantle rich in lymphocytes consisting of CD8 T and CD4 cells. The latter cell subset may also be found within the epithelioid layer [192]. The vascular involvement with vasculitic features involves arteries and veins of different sizes [193]. The Th1 type of immune response fuels the granuloma vitality and reproducibility, with IL-1, IL-6, and TNF-alpha cytokines playing the leading role [194]. The substitution of granuloma by fibrotic tissue, usually seen in chronic lesions, is driven by fibroblast growth factors, released from the homing epithelioid cells [194].

The lungs reveal early changes of hilar adenopathy, spreading to the parenchyma as the disease progresses, to finally transform into a fibrotic lung. In half of the patients, sarcoidosis affects extra-pulmonary organs. Following the lungs, peripheral lymph nodes, and skin, the affected liver runs silently primarily, with involvement reported in up to 90% of cases, verified in autopsies and biopsies [195], with a prevalence ranging between 20% and 30% [196]. The affected liver is highlighted by clinical and laboratory features, including a profile of transaminitis, with high ALT and AST, and mainly a cholestatic pattern (alkaline phosphatase and gamma glutamyl transferase might be several times (5–10 times) above the normal levels). Correlations of liver enzymes with inflammation and damage is controversial. However, patients with high liver tests, or 1.5 times above the ULN for over 3 months, should be tested every 3–6 months [196]. Recommended indications for a liver biopsy might center on patients with 1 or 2 abnormal liver tests, at ≥ x 3 times the UNL. In case 3–4 liver tests were abnormal, and running at ≥ x 3 times the UNL, a liver biopsy should be indicated. An estimate of 25% of liver biopsies showed proof of advanced fibrosis (stages 3 and 4) in such scenarios [196–198]. The liver synthesis capacity should be explored [196]. A biopsy might determine the progression of fibrosis, which is why the appropriate therapy should be practiced. It is rare to encounter jaundiced patients with sarcoidosis, for which other causes of hepatic harm should be looked for. Five to thirty percent of patients may carry nausea, vomiting, constitutional symptoms (fever and fatigue), abdominal pain, pruritus, features of portal hypertension with esophageal varices, hepatomegaly, and splenomegaly [197–202]. Intrahepatic or extrahepatic cholestasis is associated with biliary duct stenosis compressed by confluent granuloma or fibrosis in the former, and by obstructing lymphadenopathy in the latter. Micronodular cirrhosis might follow intrahepatic cholestasis in 6–8% of all patients [203, 204]; on the other hand, signs of portal hypertension and without full features of cirrhosis are frequent in up to 78% [205], in association with perisinusoidal obstruction [206]. Inflammation affects the periportal and portal tracts, sinusoidal dilatation, and nodular regenerative hyperplasia. Among the most relevant differentials, primary sclerosing cholangitis and primary biliary cholangitis should be considered, as well as all other relevant non-caseating granulomas found on biopsies. The ultrasonography might reveal a heterogeneous echogenicity, and a coarse pattern might reflect the diffuse hepatic involvement [207], while focal calcifications and contour irregularity reveal local lesions [208]. Nodular sarcoidosis might reveal focal lesions, and the intra- and extrahepatic biliary dilatation might be seen on the US, CT, and MRI. Radiographic images help establish differences between PSC; otherwise, most cases are within normal limits. Hepatic lesions on the CT might be seen in 5% of patients [209]. The specificity of an MRI will rely on the capabilities to differentiate sarcoidosis from malignancy [210], in addition to defining subcapsular and peripheral wedge-shaped atrophy, both patterns of advanced liver disease and/or cirrhosis [210].

Since most patients with hepatic sarcoidosis may be asymptomatic, treatment might focus on patient subgroups with active disease. The pharmacologic therapy based on retrospective data highlights the use of glucocorticoids. This drug has been effective for treating cholestasis, pruritus, transaminitis, and improving lesions on the biopsy (number of granulomas) [96, 211]. In patients with porta hepatis adenopathy, glucocorticoids play a crucial role in the outcome as the lymph nodes might shrink, thereby enabling the resolution of a proper biliary flow from a previously obstructed biliary duct [212]. Conventional glucocorticoid dosage, or prednisone 20–40 mg daily for 6–12 weeks, tapered by 5–10 mg every 4–8 weeks and maintained at a low dose to prevent relapses, is practiced regularly [211, 213]. The current practice to avoid glucocorticoid use as much as necessary prevents the array of setbacks the drug carries on comorbid disorders most patients may have [120]. Glucocorticoid-sparing drugs are aimed at preventing relapses while avoiding further cumulative glucocorticoid toxicity. The utility of azathioprine or methotrexate, although not fully evaluated in prospective, extensive, multicenter studies, has proven to normalize the transaminitis [214]. Close monitoring of the liver enzymes with any of the two drugs might suggest toxicity, for which interventions are recommended. Conventional alternative medicines have been tried, like mycophenolate mofetil, cyclophosphamide, cyclosporine, thalidomide, and pentoxifylline. Biologic monoclonal antibody therapy seems to be a promising alternative for severe cases. TNF-alpha antagonists such as infliximab, indicated with a concomitant immunosuppressant, maximize their efficacy while reducing the time of glucocorticoid use, normalizing transaminitis, lymphadenopathy, and reducing obstructive cholestasis [215]. Improving cholestasis features, fatigue, and pruritus sustains the utility of ursodeoxycholic acid. The best results are obtained when combined with prednisolone [216]. Ursodeoxycholic acid prevents the biliary tree from the toxic effects of bile acids. At the same time, it reverses cell inflammatory signals by decreasing the presence of MHC II and I on different cells (epithelial cells in the biliary tree) [216]. Liver transplantation is reserved for end-stage liver disease; cases are a small percentage of all liver transplants (0.012%) [217]. Outcomes seem to be comparable with other causes for liver transplant (cholestasis) in terms of patient and graft survival [217, 218].

10.14 Conclusions

The presence of an autoimmune disease, either vasculitis, sarcoidosis, connective tissue disease, or primary immune deficiency, should alert the clinician to look for possible liver involvement in the presence of clinical symptoms related to hepatopathy, or when the elevation of liver enzymes escapes the conventional explainable causes. In evaluating hepatopathies, it is essential to ascertain the underlying autoimmune/inflammatory process to tailor the therapy for each case. For instance, in the presence of PSC related to Sjogren's disease, the treatment might differ in part as compared to what the treatment of PSC related to systemic sclerosis might be, by precluding the use of glucocorticoids in the second scenario, which will avoid the potential to cause scleroderma renal crisis. In the initial assessment for an autoimmune/inflammatory process, the serology and an approach to the immune system are helpful to guide the potential underlying hepatic disorder. Additional supportive studies, including radiographic and tissue samples, will contribute to achieving an accurate diagnosis while excluding other differential causes, including malignancy, and staging the disease status. The wisdom to start pharmacologic therapy should rely on an integrative assessment of each case, the disease nature and prognosis, disease stage, and the comorbid disorders.

References

1. Kojima H, Uemura M, Sakurai S, Ann T, Ishii Y, Imazu H, et al. Clinical features of liver disturbance in rheumatoid diseases: clinicopathological study with special reference to the cause of liver disturbance. J Gastroenterol. 2002;37(8):617–25.
2. Doherty DG. Immunity, tolerance and autoimmunity in the liver: a comprehensive review. J Autoimmun. 2016;66:60–75.
3. Mills KH. Regulatory T cells: friend or foe in immunity to infection? Nat Rev Immunol. 2004;4(11):841–55.
4. Doherty DG, Donaldson PT, Underhill JA, Farrant JM, Duthie A, Mieli-Vergani G, et al. Allelic sequence variation in the HLA class II genes and proteins in patients with autoimmune hepatitis. Hepatology. 1994;19(3):609–15.
5. Coss Adame E, Granados J, Uribe M, Torre A. Does HLA-DR7 differentiate the overlap syndrome of auto-immune hepatitis-primary biliary cirrhosis (AIH-PBC) from those with auto-immune hepatitis type 1? Ann Hepatol. 2011;10(1):28–32.
6. Agarwal K, Jones DE, Bassendine MF. Genetic susceptibility to primary biliary cirrhosis. Eur J Gastroenterol Hepatol. 1999;11(6):603–6.
7. Farrant JM, Doherty DG, Donaldson PT, Vaughan RW, Hayllar KM, Welsh KI, et al. Amino acid substitutions at position 38 of the DR beta polypeptide confer susceptibility to and protection from primary sclerosing cholangitis. Hepatology. 1992;16(2):390–5.
8. Ma WT, Chang C, Gershwin ME, Lian ZX. Development of autoantibodies precedes clinical manifestations of autoimmune diseases: a comprehensive review. J Autoimmun. 2017;83:95–112.
9. Toh BH. Diagnostic autoantibodies for autoimmune liver diseases. Clin Transl Immunol. 2017;6(5):e139.
10. Rullo OJ, Tsao BP. Recent insights into the genetic basis of systemic lupus erythematosus. Ann Rheum Dis. 2013;72(Suppl 2):ii56–61.
11. Gerlag DM, Raza K, van Baarsen LG, Brouwer E, Buckley CD, Burmester GR, et al. EULAR recommendations for terminology and research in individuals at risk of rheumatoid arthritis: report from the Study Group for Risk Factors for Rheumatoid Arthritis. Ann Rheum Dis. 2012;71(5):638–41.
12. Aho K, Palosuo T, Heliovaara M. Predictive significance of rheumatoid factor. J Rheumatol. 1995;22(11):2186–7.
13. Majka DS, Deane KD, Parrish LA, Lazar AA, Baron AE, Walker CW, et al. Duration of preclinical rheumatoid arthritis-related autoantibody positivity increases in subjects with older age at time of disease diagnosis. Ann Rheum Dis. 2008;67(6):801–7.
14. Arbuckle MR, McClain MT, Rubertone MV, Scofield RH, Dennis GJ, James JA, et al. Development of autoantibodies before the clinical onset of systemic lupus erythematosus. N Engl J Med. 2003;349(16):1526–33.
15. McCune AB, Weston WL, Lee LA. Maternal and fetal outcome in neonatal lupus erythematosus. Ann Intern Med. 1987;106(4):518–23.
16. Liberal R, Krawitt EL, Vierling JM, Manns MP, Mieli-Vergani G, Vergani D. Cutting edge issues in autoimmune hepatitis. J Autoimmun. 2016;75:6–19.
17. Jepsen P, Gronbaek L, Vilstrup H. Worldwide incidence of autoimmune liver disease. Dig Dis. 2015;33(Suppl 2):2–12.
18. Alvarez F, Berg PA, Bianchi FB, Bianchi L, Burroughs AK, Cancado EL, et al. International Autoimmune Hepatitis Group Report: review of criteria for diagnosis of autoimmune hepatitis. J Hepatol. 1999;31(5):929–38.
19. Werner M, Prytz H, Ohlsson B, Almer S, Bjornsson E, Bergquist A, et al. Epidemiology and the initial presentation of autoimmune hepatitis in Sweden: a nationwide study. Scand J Gastroenterol. 2008;43(10):1232–40.
20. Manns MP, Czaja AJ, Gorham JD, Krawitt EL, Mieli-Vergani G, Vergani D, et al. Diagnosis and management of autoimmune hepatitis. Hepatology. 2010;51(6):2193–213.

21. Wong GW, Heneghan MA. Association of extrahepatic manifestations with autoimmune hepatitis. Dig Dis. 2015;33(Suppl 2):25–35.
22. Czaja AJ. Autoimmune liver disease and rheumatic manifestations. Curr Opin Rheumatol. 2007;19(1):74–80.
23. Abraham S, Begum S, Isenberg D. Hepatic manifestations of autoimmune rheumatic diseases. Ann Rheum Dis. 2004;63(2):123–9.
24. Wong GK, Goldacker S, Winterhalter C, Grimbacher B, Chapel H, Lucas M, et al. Outcomes of splenectomy in patients with common variable immunodeficiency (CVID): a survey of 45 patients. Clin Exp Immunol. 2013;172(1):63–72.
25. Muratori P, Granito A, Quarneti C, Ferri S, Menichella R, Cassani F, et al. Autoimmune hepatitis in Italy: the Bologna experience. J Hepatol. 2009;50(6):1210–8.
26. Perdigoto R, Carpenter HA, Czaja AJ. Frequency and significance of chronic ulcerative colitis in severe corticosteroid-treated autoimmune hepatitis. J Hepatol. 1992;14(2–3):325–31.
27. Muratori P, Lenzi M, Cassani F, Lalanne C, Muratori L. Diagnostic approach to autoimmune hepatitis. Expert Rev Clin Immunol. 2017;13(8):769–79.
28. Matsumoto T, Morizane T, Aoki Y, Yamasaki S, Nakajima M, Enomoto N, et al. Autoimmune hepatitis in primary Sjogren's syndrome: pathological study of the livers and labial salivary glands in 17 patients with primary Sjogren's syndrome. Pathol Int. 2005;55(2):70–6.
29. Czaja AJ. Autoantibodies in autoimmune liver disease. Adv Clin Chem. 2005;40:127–64.
30. Fusconi M, Vannini A, Dall'Aglio AC, Pappas G, Cassani F, Ballardini G, et al. Anti-cyclic citrullinated peptide antibodies in type 1 autoimmune hepatitis. Aliment Pharmacol Ther. 2005;22(10):951–5.
31. Montano-Loza A, Czaja AJ, Carpenter HA, Piette A, Murphy D, Shums Z, et al. Frequency and significance of antibodies to cyclic citrullinated peptide in type 1 autoimmune hepatitis. Autoimmunity. 2006;39(4):341–8.
32. Murray-Lyon IM, Stern RB, Williams R. Controlled trial of prednisone and azathioprine in active chronic hepatitis. Lancet. 1973;1(7806):735–7.
33. Cook GC, Mulligan R, Sherlock S. Controlled prospective trial of corticosteroid therapy in active chronic hepatitis. Q J Med. 1971;40(158):159–85.
34. Cropley A, Weltman M. The use of immunosuppression in autoimmune hepatitis: a current literature review. Clin Mol Hepatol. 2017;23(1):22–6.
35. Haridy J, Nicoll A, Sood S. Methotrexate therapy for autoimmune hepatitis. Clin Gastroenterol Hepatol. 2018;16(2):288–9.
36. Malekzadeh R, Nasseri-Moghaddam S, Kaviani MJ, Taheri H, Kamalian N, Sotoudeh M. Cyclosporin A is a promising alternative to corticosteroids in autoimmune hepatitis. Dig Dis Sci. 2001;46(6):1321–7.
37. Zachou K, Gatselis NK, Arvaniti P, Gabeta S, Rigopoulou EI, Koukoulis GK, et al. A real-world study focused on the long-term efficacy of mycophenolate mofetil as first-line treatment of autoimmune hepatitis. Aliment Pharmacol Ther. 2016;43(10):1035–47.
38. Czaja AJ, Carpenter HA, Lindor KD. Ursodeoxycholic acid as adjunctive therapy for problematic type 1 autoimmune hepatitis: a randomized placebo-controlled treatment trial. Hepatology. 1999;30(6):1381–6.
39. Weiler-Normann C, Schramm C, Quaas A, Wiegard C, Glaubke C, Pannicke N, et al. Infliximab as a rescue treatment in difficult-to-treat autoimmune hepatitis. J Hepatol. 2013;58(3):529–34.
40. Chatrath H, Allen L, Boyer TD. Use of sirolimus in the treatment of refractory autoimmune hepatitis. Am J Med. 2014;127(11):1128–31.
41. Ytting H, Larsen FS. Everolimus treatment for patients with autoimmune hepatitis and poor response to standard therapy and drug alternatives in use. Scand J Gastroenterol. 2015;50(8):1025–31.
42. Selmi C, Bowlus CL, Gershwin ME, Coppel RL. Primary biliary cirrhosis. Lancet. 2011;377(9777):1600–9.

43. Gershwin ME, Mackay IR, Sturgess A, Coppel RL. Identification and specificity of a cDNA encoding the 70 kd mitochondrial antigen recognized in primary biliary cirrhosis. J Immunol. 1987;138(10):3525–31.
44. Bogdanos DP, Komorowski L. Disease-specific autoantibodies in primary biliary cirrhosis. Clin Chim Acta. 2011;412(7-8):502–12.
45. Watt FE, James OF, Jones DE. Patterns of autoimmunity in primary biliary cirrhosis patients and their families: a population-based cohort study. QJM. 2004;97(7):397–406.
46. Floreani A, Franceschet I, Cazzagon N, Spinazze A, Buja A, Furlan P, et al. Extrahepatic autoimmune conditions associated with primary biliary cirrhosis. Clin Rev Allergy Immunol. 2015;48(2-3):192–7.
47. Gabrielli A, Avvedimento EV, Krieg T. Scleroderma. N Engl J Med. 2009;360(19):1989–2003.
48. Varga J, Abraham D. Systemic sclerosis: a prototypic multisystem fibrotic disorder. J Clin Invest. 2007;117(3):557–67.
49. LeRoy EC, Black C, Fleischmajer R, Jablonska S, Krieg T, Medsger TA Jr, et al. Scleroderma (systemic sclerosis): classification, subsets and pathogenesis. J Rheumatol. 1988;15(2):202–5.
50. Barnett AJ, Miller M, Littlejohn GO. The diagnosis and classification of scleroderma (systemic sclerosis). Postgrad Med J. 1988;64(748):121–5.
51. Steen VD. Autoantibodies in systemic sclerosis. Semin Arthritis Rheum. 2005;35(1):35–42.
52. Hamaguchi Y. Autoantibody profiles in systemic sclerosis: predictive value for clinical evaluation and prognosis. J Dermatol. 2010;37(1):42–53.
53. Corpechot C, Chretien Y, Chazouilleres O, Poupon R. Demographic, lifestyle, medical and familial factors associated with primary biliary cirrhosis. J Hepatol. 2010;53(1):162–9.
54. Gershwin ME, Selmi C, Worman HJ, Gold EB, Watnik M, Utts J, et al. Risk factors and comorbidities in primary biliary cirrhosis: a controlled interview-based study of 1032 patients. Hepatology. 2005;42(5):1194–202.
55. Gupta RC, Seibold JR, Krishnan MR, Steigerwald JC. Precipitating autoantibodies to mitochondrial proteins in progressive systemic sclerosis. Clin Exp Immunol. 1984;58(1):68–76.
56. Chou MJ, Lai MY, Lee SL, Tsay GJ. Reactivity of anti-mitochondrial antibodies in primary biliary cirrhosis and systemic sclerosis. J Formos Med Assoc. 1992;91(11):1075–80.
57. Gourh P, Agarwal SK, Divecha D, Assassi S, Paz G, Arora-Singh RK, et al. Polymorphisms in TBX21 and STAT4 increase the risk of systemic sclerosis: evidence of possible gene-gene interaction and alterations in Th1/Th2 cytokines. Arthritis Rheum. 2009;60(12):3794–806.
58. Tuffanelli DL, Winkelmann RK. Systemic scleroderma, a clinical study of 727 cases. Arch Dermatol. 1961;84:359–71.
59. D'Angelo WA, Fries JF, Masi AT, Shulman LE. Pathologic observations in systemic sclerosis (scleroderma). A study of fifty-eight autopsy cases and fifty-eight matched controls. Am J Med. 1969;46(3):428–40.
60. Rigamonti C, Shand LM, Feudjo M, Bunn CC, Black CM, Denton CP, et al. Clinical features and prognosis of primary biliary cirrhosis associated with systemic sclerosis. Gut. 2006;55(3):388–94.
61. Sarkar S, Bowlus CL. Primary sclerosing cholangitis: multiple phenotypes, multiple approaches. Clin Liver Dis. 2016;20(1):67–77.
62. Bowlus CL. Cutting edge issues in primary sclerosing cholangitis. Clin Rev Allergy Immunol. 2011;41(2):139–50.
63. Palmela C, Peerani F, Castaneda D, Torres J, Itzkowitz SH. Inflammatory bowel disease and primary sclerosing cholangitis: a review of the phenotype and associated specific features. Gut Liver. 2018;12(1):17–29.
64. Vavricka SR, Schoepfer A, Scharl M, Lakatos PL, Navarini A, Rogler G. Extraintestinal manifestations of inflammatory bowel disease. Inflamm Bowel Dis. 2015;21(8):1982–92.
65. Viguier M, Allez M, Zagdanski AM, Bertheau P, de Kerviler E, Rybojad M, et al. High frequency of cholestasis in generalized pustular psoriasis: Evidence for neutrophilic involvement of the biliary tract. Hepatology. 2004;40(2):452–8.

66. Hov JR, Boberg KM, Karlsen TH. Autoantibodies in primary sclerosing cholangitis. World J Gastroenterol. 2008;14(24):3781–91.
67. Terjung B, Worman HJ, Herzog V, Sauerbruch T, Spengler U. Differentiation of antineutrophil nuclear antibodies in inflammatory bowel and autoimmune liver diseases from antineutrophil cytoplasmic antibodies (p-ANCA) using immunofluorescence microscopy. Clin Exp Immunol. 2001;126(1):37–46.
68. Stone JH, Zen Y, Deshpande V. IgG4-related disease. N Engl J Med. 2012;366(6):539–51.
69. Brito-Zeron P, Ramos-Casals M, Bosch X, Stone JH. The clinical spectrum of IgG4-related disease. Autoimmun Rev. 2014;13(12):1203–10.
70. Della Torre E, Mattoo H, Mahajan VS, Carruthers M, Pillai S, Stone JH. Prevalence of atopy, eosinophilia, and IgE elevation in IgG4-related disease. Allergy. 2014;69(2):269–72.
71. Itoh S, Nagasaka T, Suzuki K, Satake H, Ota T, Naganawa S. Lymphoplasmacytic sclerosing cholangitis: assessment of clinical, CT, and pathological findings. Clin Radiol. 2009;64(11):1104–14.
72. Culver EL, Chapman RW. IgG4-related hepatobiliary disease: an overview. Nat Rev Gastroenterol Hepatol. 2016;13(10):601–12.
73. Deshpande V. The pathology of IgG4-related disease: critical issues and challenges. Semin Diagn Pathol. 2012;29(4):191–6.
74. Wallace ZS, Naden RP, Chari S, Choi HK, Della-Torre E, Dicaire JF, et al. The 2019 American College of Rheumatology/European League Against Rheumatism classification criteria for IgG4-related disease. Ann Rheum Dis. 2020;79(1):77–87.
75. Chari ST. Diagnosis of autoimmune pancreatitis using its five cardinal features: introducing the Mayo Clinic's HISORt criteria. J Gastroenterol. 2007;42(Suppl 18):39–41.
76. Khosroshahi A, Wallace ZS, Crowe JL, Akamizu T, Azumi A, Carruthers MN, et al. International consensus guidance statement on the management and treatment of IgG4-related disease. Arthritis Rheumatol. 2015;67(7):1688–99.
77. Ohara H, Okazaki K, Tsubouchi H, Inui K, Kawa S, Kamisawa T, et al. Clinical diagnostic criteria of IgG4-related sclerosing cholangitis 2012. J Hepatobiliary Pancreat Sci. 2012;19(5):536–42.
78. Lanzillotta M, Culver E, Sharma A, Zen Y, Zhang W, Stone JH, et al. Fibrotic phenotype of IgG4-related disease. Lancet Rheumatol. 2024;6(7):e469–e80.
79. de Buy Wenniger LJ, Culver EL, Beuers U. Exposure to occupational antigens might predispose to IgG4-related disease. Hepatology. 2014;60(4):1453–4.
80. Sah RP, Chari ST. Serologic issues in IgG4-related systemic disease and autoimmune pancreatitis. Curr Opin Rheumatol. 2011;23(1):108–13.
81. Riley M, Saad Shaukat MH, Bari M, Peredo-Wende R. Concomitant presentation of IgG(4)-negative idiopathic retroperitoneal fibrosis and Addison's disease. BMJ Case Rep 2019;12(10).
82. Kanno A, Masamune A, Okazaki K, Kamisawa T, Kawa S, Nishimori I, et al. Nationwide epidemiological survey of autoimmune pancreatitis in Japan in 2011. Pancreas. 2015;44(4):535–9.
83. Uchida K, Masamune A, Shimosegawa T, Okazaki K. Prevalence of IgG4-related disease in Japan based on nationwide survey in 2009. Int J Rheumatol. 2012;2012:358371.
84. Ghazale A, Chari ST, Zhang L, Smyrk TC, Takahashi N, Levy MJ, et al. Immunoglobulin G4-associated cholangitis: clinical profile and response to therapy. Gastroenterology. 2008;134(3):706–15.
85. Huggett MT, Culver EL, Kumar M, Hurst JM, Rodriguez-Justo M, Chapman MH, et al. Type 1 autoimmune pancreatitis and IgG4-related sclerosing cholangitis is associated with extrapancreatic organ failure, malignancy, and mortality in a prospective UK cohort. Am J Gastroenterol. 2014;109(10):1675–83.
86. Kawa S, Ota M, Yoshizawa K, Horiuchi A, Hamano H, Ochi Y, et al. HLA DRB10405-DQB10401 haplotype is associated with autoimmune pancreatitis in the Japanese population. Gastroenterology. 2002;122(5):1264–9.

87. Culver EL, et al. Human leucocyte antigen associations in IgG4-related disease and primary sclerosing cholangitis stratified by IgG4 levels, in a multicenter UK cohort. J Hepatol. 2016;64:S646.
88. Umemura T, Zen Y, Hamano H, Kawa S, Nakanuma Y, Kiyosawa K. Immunoglobin G4-hepatopathy: association of immunoglobin G4-bearing plasma cells in liver with autoimmune pancreatitis. Hepatology. 2007;46(2):463–71.
89. Chung H, Watanabe T, Kudo M, Maenishi O, Wakatsuki Y, Chiba T. Identification and characterization of IgG4-associated autoimmune hepatitis. Liver Int. 2010;30(2):222–31.
90. Krawitt EL. Autoimmune hepatitis. N Engl J Med. 1996;334(14):897–903.
91. Czaja AJ, Manns MP. Advances in the diagnosis, pathogenesis, and management of autoimmune hepatitis. Gastroenterology. 2010;139(1):58–72 e4.
92. Heneghan MA, Yeoman AD, Verma S, Smith AD, Longhi MS. Autoimmune hepatitis. Lancet. 2013;382(9902):1433–44.
93. Zen Y, Fujii T, Sato Y, Masuda S, Nakanuma Y. Pathological classification of hepatic inflammatory pseudotumor with respect to IgG4-related disease. Mod Pathol. 2007;20(8):884–94.
94. Stone JH, Khosroshahi A, Deshpande V, Chan JK, Heathcote JG, Aalberse R, et al. Recommendations for the nomenclature of IgG4-related disease and its individual organ system manifestations. Arthritis Rheum. 2012;64(10):3061–7.
95. Nakazawa T, Naitoh I, Hayashi K. Usefulness of intraductal ultrasonography in the diagnosis of cholangiocarcinoma and IgG4-related sclerosing cholangitis. Clin Endosc. 2012;45(3):331–6.
96. Moller K, Braden B, Culver EL, Jenssen C, Zadeh ES, Alhyari A, et al. Secondary sclerosing cholangitis and IgG4-sclerosing cholangitis - A review of cholangiographic and ultrasound imaging. Endosc Ultrasound. 2023;12(2):181–99.
97. Perugino CA, Stone JH. IgG4-related disease: an update on pathophysiology and implications for clinical care. Nat Rev Rheumatol. 2020;16(12):702–14.
98. Maillette de Buy Wenniger LJ, Doorenspleet ME, Klarenbeek PL, Verheij J, Baas F, Elferink RP, et al. Immunoglobulin G4+ clones identified by next-generation sequencing dominate the B cell receptor repertoire in immunoglobulin G4 associated cholangitis. Hepatology. 2013;57(6):2390–8.
99. Lin W, Zhang P, Chen H, Chen Y, Yang H, Zheng W, et al. Circulating plasmablasts/plasma cells: a potential biomarker for IgG4-related disease. Arthritis Res Ther. 2017;19(1):25.
100. Wallace ZS, Mattoo H, Carruthers M, Mahajan VS, Della Torre E, Lee H, et al. Plasmablasts as a biomarker for IgG4-related disease, independent of serum IgG4 concentrations. Ann Rheum Dis. 2015;74(1):190–5.
101. Lohr JM, Faissner R, Koczan D, Bewerunge P, Bassi C, Brors B, et al. Autoantibodies against the exocrine pancreas in autoimmune pancreatitis: gene and protein expression profiling and immunoassays identify pancreatic enzymes as a major target of the inflammatory process. Am J Gastroenterol. 2010;105(9):2060–71.
102. Hubers LM, Vos H, Schuurman AR, Erken R, Oude Elferink RP, Burgering B, et al. Annexin A11 is targeted by IgG4 and IgG1 autoantibodies in IgG4-related disease. Gut. 2018;67(4):728–35.
103. Frulloni L, Lunardi C, Simone R, Dolcino M, Scattolini C, Falconi M, et al. Identification of a novel antibody associated with autoimmune pancreatitis. N Engl J Med. 2009;361(22):2135–42.
104. Okazaki K, Uchida K, Ohana M, Nakase H, Uose S, Inai M, et al. Autoimmune-related pancreatitis is associated with autoantibodies and a Th1/Th2-type cellular immune response. Gastroenterology. 2000;118(3):573–81.
105. Asada M, Nishio A, Uchida K, Kido M, Ueno S, Uza N, et al. Identification of a novel autoantibody against pancreatic secretory trypsin inhibitor in patients with autoimmune pancreatitis. Pancreas. 2006;33(1):20–6.

106. Endo T, Takizawa S, Tanaka S, Takahashi M, Fujii H, Kamisawa T, et al. Amylase alpha-2A autoantibodies: novel marker of autoimmune pancreatitis and fulminant type 1 diabetes. Diabetes. 2009;58(3):732–7.
107. Carruthers MN, Khosroshahi A, Augustin T, Deshpande V, Stone JH. The diagnostic utility of serum IgG4 concentrations in IgG4-related disease. Ann Rheum Dis. 2015;74(1):14–8.
108. Della-Torre E, Bozzalla-Cassione E, Sciorati C, Ruggiero E, Lanzillotta M, Bonfiglio S, et al. A CD8alpha- subset of CD4+SLAMF7+ cytotoxic T cells is expanded in patients with IgG4-related disease and decreases following glucocorticoid treatment. Arthritis Rheumatol. 2018;70(7):1133–43.
109. Boonstra K, Culver EL, de Buy Wenniger LM, van Heerde MJ, van Erpecum KJ, Poen AC, et al. Serum immunoglobulin G4 and immunoglobulin G1 for distinguishing immunoglobulin G4-associated cholangitis from primary sclerosing cholangitis. Hepatology. 2014;59(5):1954–63.
110. Wallace ZS, Mattoo H, Mahajan VS, Kulikova M, Lu L, Deshpande V, et al. Predictors of disease relapse in IgG4-related disease following rituximab. Rheumatology (Oxford). 2016;55(6):1000–8.
111. Culver EL, Sadler R, Simpson D, Cargill T, Makuch M, Bateman AC, et al. Elevated serum IgG4 levels in diagnosis, treatment response, organ involvement, and relapse in a prospective IgG4-related disease UK cohort. Am J Gastroenterol. 2016;111(5):733–43.
112. Oseini AM, Chaiteerakij R, Shire AM, Ghazale A, Kaiya J, Moser CD, et al. Utility of serum immunoglobulin G4 in distinguishing immunoglobulin G4-associated cholangitis from cholangiocarcinoma. Hepatology. 2011;54(3):940–8.
113. Manganis CD, Chapman RW, Culver EL. Review of primary sclerosing cholangitis with increased IgG4 levels. World J Gastroenterol. 2020;26(23):3126–44.
114. Al-Soudi A, Doorenspleet ME, Esveldt RE, Burgemeister LT, Hak AE, van den Born BJH, et al. IgG4:IgG RNA ratio differentiates active disease from remission in granulomatosis with polyangiitis: a new disease activity marker? A cross-sectional and longitudinal study. Arthritis Res Ther. 2019;21(1):43.
115. Beuers U, Hubers LM, Doorenspleet M, Maillette de Buy Wenniger L, Klarenbeek PL, Boonstra K, et al. IgG4-associated cholangitis—a mimic of PSC. Dig Dis. 2015;33(Suppl 2):176–80.
116. Mattoo H, Mahajan VS, Della-Torre E, Sekigami Y, Carruthers M, Wallace ZS, et al. De novo oligoclonal expansions of circulating plasmablasts in active and relapsing IgG4-related disease. J Allergy Clin Immunol. 2014;134(3):679–87.
117. Deshpande V, Zen Y, Chan JK, Yi EE, Sato Y, Yoshino T, et al. Consensus statement on the pathology of IgG4-related disease. Mod Pathol. 2012;25(9):1181–92.
118. Kamisawa T, Shimosegawa T, Okazaki K, Nishino T, Watanabe H, Kanno A, et al. Standard steroid treatment for autoimmune pancreatitis. Gut. 2009;58(11):1504–7.
119. Inoue D, Yoshida K, Yoneda N, Ozaki K, Matsubara T, Nagai K, et al. IgG4-related disease: dataset of 235 consecutive patients. Medicine (Baltimore). 2015;94(15):e680.
120. Stone JH, McDowell PJ, Jayne DRW, Merkel PA, Robson J, Patel NJ, et al. The glucocorticoid toxicity index: measuring change in glucocorticoid toxicity over time. Semin Arthritis Rheum. 2022;55:152010.
121. Yunyun F, Yu P, Panpan Z, Xia Z, Linyi P, Jiaxin Z, et al. Efficacy and safety of low dose Mycophenolate mofetil treatment for immunoglobulin G4-related disease: a randomized clinical trial. Rheumatology (Oxford). 2019;58(1):52–60.
122. Hart PA, Topazian MD, Witzig TE, Clain JE, Gleeson FC, Klebig RR, et al. Treatment of relapsing autoimmune pancreatitis with immunomodulators and rituximab: the Mayo Clinic experience. Gut. 2013;62(11):1607–15.
123. Sandanayake NS, Church NI, Chapman MH, Johnson GJ, Dhar DK, Amin Z, et al. Presentation and management of post-treatment relapse in autoimmune pancreatitis/immunoglobulin G4-associated cholangitis. Clin Gastroenterol Hepatol. 2009;7(10):1089–96.

124. Khosroshahi A, Carruthers MN, Deshpande V, Unizony S, Bloch DB, Stone JH. Rituximab for the treatment of IgG4-related disease: lessons from 10 consecutive patients. Medicine (Baltimore). 2012;91(1):57–66.
125. Khosroshahi A, Bloch DB, Deshpande V, Stone JH. Rituximab therapy leads to rapid decline of serum IgG4 levels and prompt clinical improvement in IgG4-related systemic disease. Arthritis Rheum. 2010;62(6):1755–62.
126. Topazian M, Witzig TE, Smyrk TC, Pulido JS, Levy MJ, Kamath PS, et al. Rituximab therapy for refractory biliary strictures in immunoglobulin G4-associated cholangitis. Clin Gastroenterol Hepatol. 2008;6(3):364–6.
127. Carruthers MN, Topazian MD, Khosroshahi A, Witzig TE, Wallace ZS, Hart PA, et al. Rituximab for IgG4-related disease: a prospective, open-label trial. Ann Rheum Dis. 2015;74(6):1171–7.
128. Stone JH, Carruthers MN, Topazian MD, Khosroshahi A, Witzig TE, Wallace ZS, et al. Response to: 'Is rituximab effective for IgG4-related disease in the long term? Experience of cases treated with rituximab for 4 years' by Yamamoto et al. Ann Rheum Dis. 2015;74(8):e47.
129. Yamamoto M, Takahashi H, Tabeya T, Suzuki C, Naishiro Y, Ishigami K, et al. Risk of malignancies in IgG4-related disease. Mod Rheumatol. 2012;22(3):414–8.
130. Farrell RJ, Kelly CP. Celiac sprue. N Engl J Med. 2002;346(3):180–8.
131. Hu WT, Murray JA, Greenaway MC, Parisi JE, Josephs KA. Cognitive impairment and celiac disease. Arch Neurol. 2006;63(10):1440–6.
132. Rubio-Tapia A, Murray JA. The liver in celiac disease. Hepatology. 2007;46(5):1650–8.
133. Hagander B, Berg NO, Brandt L, Norden A, Sjolund K, Stenstam M. Hepatic injury in adult coeliac disease. Lancet. 1977;2(8032):270–2.
134. Bardella MT, Fraquelli M, Quatrini M, Molteni N, Bianchi P, Conte D. Prevalence of hypertransaminasemia in adult celiac patients and effect of gluten-free diet. Hepatology. 1995;22(3):833–6.
135. Novacek G, Miehsler W, Wrba F, Ferenci P, Penner E, Vogelsang H. Prevalence and clinical importance of hypertransaminasaemia in coeliac disease. Eur J Gastroenterol Hepatol. 1999;11(3):283–8.
136. Sharma BC, Bhasin DK, Nada R. Association of celiac disease with non-cirrhotic portal fibrosis. J Gastroenterol Hepatol. 2006;21(1 Pt 2):332–4.
137. Kaukinen K, Halme L, Collin P, Farkkila M, Maki M, Vehmanen P, et al. Celiac disease in patients with severe liver disease: gluten-free diet may reverse hepatic failure. Gastroenterology. 2002;122(4):881–8.
138. Green RM, Flamm S. AGA technical review on the evaluation of liver chemistry tests. Gastroenterology. 2002;123(4):1367–84.
139. Bonamico M, Pitzalis G, Culasso F, Vania A, Monti S, Benedetti C, et al. [Hepatic damage in celiac disease in children]. Minerva Pediatr. 1986;38(21):959–62.
140. Jacobsen MB, Fausa O, Elgjo K, Schrumpf E. Hepatic lesions in adult coeliac disease. Scand J Gastroenterol. 1990;25(7):656–62.
141. Logan RF, Ferguson A, Finlayson ND, Weir DG. Primary biliary cirrhosis and coeliac disease: an association? Lancet. 1978;1(8058):230–3.
142. Volta U, De Franceschi L, Molinaro N, Cassani F, Muratori L, Lenzi M, et al. Frequency and significance of anti-gliadin and anti-endomysial antibodies in autoimmune hepatitis. Dig Dis Sci. 1998;43(10):2190–5.
143. Hay JE, Wiesner RH, Shorter RG, LaRusso NF, Baldus WP. Primary sclerosing cholangitis and celiac disease. A novel association. Ann Intern Med. 1988;109(9):713–7.
144. Boberg KM, Spurkland A, Rocca G, Egeland T, Saarinen S, Mitchell S, et al. The HLA-DR3,DQ2 heterozygous genotype is associated with an accelerated progression of primary sclerosing cholangitis. Scand J Gastroenterol. 2001;36(8):886–90.
145. Dickey W, McMillan SA, Callender ME. High prevalence of celiac sprue among patients with primary biliary cirrhosis. J Clin Gastroenterol. 1997;25(1):328–9.

146. Xiao X, Miao Q, Chang C, Gershwin ME, Ma X. Common variable immunodeficiency and autoimmunity—an inconvenient truth. Autoimmun Rev. 2014;13(8):858–64.
147. Salzer U, Warnatz K, Peter HH. Common variable immunodeficiency: an update. Arthritis Res Ther. 2012;14(5):223.
148. Cunningham-Rundles C, Bodian C. Common variable immunodeficiency: clinical and immunological features of 248 patients. Clin Immunol. 1999;92(1):34–48.
149. Bonilla FA, Barlan I, Chapel H, Costa-Carvalho BT, Cunningham-Rundles C, de la Morena MT, et al. International Consensus Document (ICON): common variable immunodeficiency disorders. J Allergy Clin Immunol Pract. 2016;4(1):38–59.
150. Gathmann B, Mahlaoui N, Ceredih, Gerard L, Oksenhendler E, Warnatz K, et al. Clinical picture and treatment of 2212 patients with common variable immunodeficiency. J Allergy Clin Immunol. 2014;134(1):116–26.
151. Ardeniz O, Cunningham-Rundles C. Granulomatous disease in common variable immunodeficiency. Clin Immunol. 2009;133(2):198–207.
152. Ward C, Lucas M, Piris J, Collier J, Chapel H. Abnormal liver function in common variable immunodeficiency disorders due to nodular regenerative hyperplasia. Clin Exp Immunol. 2008;153(3):331–7.
153. Azizi G, Abolhassani H, Asgardoon MH, Alinia T, Yazdani R, Mohammadi J, et al. Autoimmunity in common variable immunodeficiency: epidemiology, pathophysiology and management. Expert Rev Clin Immunol. 2017;13(2):101–15.
154. Mahdavinia M, Mirsaeidi M, Bishehsari F, McGrath K. Primary sclerosing cholangitis in common variable immune deficiency. Allergol Int. 2015;64(2):187–9.
155. Song J, Lleo A, Yang GX, Zhang W, Bowlus CL, Gershwin ME, et al. Common variable immunodeficiency and liver involvement. Clin Rev Allergy Immunol. 2018;55(3):340–51.
156. Webb GJ, Hirschfield GM. Using GWAS to identify genetic predisposition in hepatic autoimmunity. J Autoimmun. 2016;66:25–39.
157. Azzu V, Fonseca M, Duckworth A, Kennard L, Moini N, Qurashi M, et al. Liver disease is common in patients with common variable immunodeficiency and predicts mortality in the presence of cirrhosis or portal hypertension. J Allergy Clin Immunol Pract. 2019;7(7):2484–6 e3.
158. Hartleb M, Gutkowski K, Milkiewicz P. Nodular regenerative hyperplasia: evolving concepts on underdiagnosed cause of portal hypertension. World J Gastroenterol. 2011;17(11):1400–9.
159. Jones TPW, Buckland M, Breuer J, Lowe DM. Viral infection in primary antibody deficiency syndromes. Rev Med Virol. 2019;29(4):e2049.
160. Uzzan M, Ko HM, Mehandru S, Cunningham-Rundles C. Gastrointestinal Disorders Associated with Common Variable Immune Deficiency (CVID) and Chronic Granulomatous Disease (CGD). Curr Gastroenterol Rep. 2016;18(4):17.
161. Gangemi S, Allegra A, Musolino C. Lymphoproliferative disease and cancer among patients with common variable immunodeficiency. Leuk Res. 2015;39(4):389–96.
162. Pulvirenti F, Pecoraro A, Cinetto F, Milito C, Valente M, Santangeli E, et al. Gastric Cancer is the leading cause of death in Italian adult patients with common variable immunodeficiency. Front Immunol. 2018;9:2546.
163. Kasztalska K, Ciebiada M, Cebula-Obrzut B, Gorski P. Intravenous immunoglobulin replacement therapy in the treatment of patients with common variable immunodeficiency disease: an open-label prospective study. Clin Drug Investig. 2011;31(5):299–307.
164. Cunningham-Rundles C. Autoimmune manifestations in common variable immunodeficiency. J Clin Immunol. 2008;28(Suppl 1):S42–5.
165. Montalti R, Mocchegiani F, Vincenzi P, Svegliati Baroni G, Nicolini D, Vivarelli M. Liver transplantation in patients with common variable immunodeficiency: a report of two cases. Ann Transplant. 2014;19:541–4.
166. Murakawa Y, Miyagawa-Hayashino A, Ogura Y, Egawa H, Okamoto S, Soejima Y, et al. Liver transplantation for severe hepatitis in patients with common variable immunodeficiency. Pediatr Transplant. 2012;16(6):E210–6.

167. Jennette JC, Falk RJ, Bacon PA, Basu N, Cid MC, Ferrario F, et al. 2012 revised International Chapel Hill Consensus Conference Nomenclature of Vasculitides. Arthritis Rheum. 2013;65(1):1–11.
168. Millet A, Pederzoli-Ribeil M, Guillevin L, Witko-Sarsat V, Mouthon L. Antineutrophil cytoplasmic antibody-associated vasculitides: is it time to split up the group? Ann Rheum Dis. 2013;72(8):1273–9.
169. Holl-Ulrich K, Klass M. Wegener's granulomatosis with granulomatous liver involvement. Clin Exp Rheumatol. 2010;28(1 Suppl 57):88–9.
170. Selmi C, De Santis M, Gershwin ME. Liver involvement in subjects with rheumatic disease. Arthritis Res Ther. 2011;13(3):226.
171. Pavone L, Grasselli C, Chierici E, Maggiore U, Garini G, Ronda N, et al. Outcome and prognostic factors during the course of primary small-vessel vasculitides. J Rheumatol. 2006;33(7):1299–306.
172. Ruiz-Ferreras E, Martin-Arribas A, Tabernero-Fernandez G, Lerma-Marquez JL, Fraile-Gomez P, Garcia-Cosmes P, et al. Microscopic polyangiitis in a patient with primary biliary cirrhosis: treatment complications. Nefrologia. 2016;36(1):78–80.
173. Tovoli F, Vannini A, Fusconi M, Frisoni M, Zauli D. Autoimmune liver disorders and small-vessel vasculitis: four case reports and review of the literature. Ann Hepatol. 2013;13(1):136–41.
174. Lohani S, Nazir S, Tachamo N, Pagolu P. Autoimmune hepatitis and eosinophilic granulomatosis with polyangiitis: a rare association. BMJ Case Rep. 2017:2017.
175. Statement on sarcoidosis. Joint Statement of the American Thoracic Society (ATS), the European Respiratory Society (ERS) and the World Association of Sarcoidosis and Other Granulomatous Disorders (WASOG) adopted by the ATS Board of Directors and by the ERS Executive Committee, February 1999. Am J Respir Crit Care Med. 1999;160(2):736–55.
176. Chopra A, Avadhani V, Tiwari A, Riemer EC, Sica G, Judson MA. Granulomatous lung disease: clinical aspects. Expert Rev Respir Med. 2020;14(10):1045–63.
177. Valeyre D, Prasse A, Nunes H, Uzunhan Y, Brillet PY, Muller-Quernheim J. Sarcoidosis. Lancet. 2014;383(9923):1155–67.
178. Pietinalho A, Hiraga Y, Hosoda Y, Lofroos AB, Yamaguchi M, Selroos O. The frequency of sarcoidosis in Finland and Hokkaido, Japan. A comparative epidemiological study. Sarcoidosis. 1995;12(1):61–7.
179. Henke CE, Henke G, Elveback LR, Beard CM, Ballard DJ, Kurland LT. The epidemiology of sarcoidosis in Rochester, Minnesota: a population-based study of incidence and survival. Am J Epidemiol. 1986;123(5):840–5.
180. Kowalska M, Niewiadomska E, Zejda JE. Epidemiology of sarcoidosis recorded in 2006–2010 in the Silesian voivodeship on the basis of routine medical reporting. Ann Agric Environ Med. 2014;21(1):55–8.
181. Hillerdal G, Nou E, Osterman K, Schmekel B. Sarcoidosis: epidemiology and prognosis. A 15-year European study. Am Rev Respir Dis. 1984;130(1):29–32.
182. Morimoto T, Azuma A, Abe S, Usuki J, Kudoh S, Sugisaki K, et al. Epidemiology of sarcoidosis in Japan. Eur Respir J. 2008;31(2):372–9.
183. Varron L, Cottin V, Schott AM, Broussolle C, Seve P. Late-onset sarcoidosis: a comparative study. Medicine (Baltimore). 2012;91(3):137–43.
184. Judson MA. Extrapulmonary sarcoidosis. Semin Respir Crit Care Med. 2007;28(1):83–101.
185. Rosen Y. Pathology of sarcoidosis. Semin Respir Crit Care Med. 2007;28(1):36–52.
186. Crowley LE, Herbert R, Moline JM, Wallenstein S, Shukla G, Schechter C, et al. "Sarcoid like" granulomatous pulmonary disease in World Trade Center disaster responders. Am J Ind Med. 2011;54(3):175–84.
187. Ishige I, Usui Y, Takemura T, Eishi Y. Quantitative PCR of mycobacterial and propionibacterial DNA in lymph nodes of Japanese patients with sarcoidosis. Lancet. 1999;354(9173):120–3.

188. Swaisgood CM, Oswald-Richter K, Moeller SD, Klemenc JM, Ruple LM, Farver CF, et al. Development of a sarcoidosis murine lung granuloma model using Mycobacterium superoxide dismutase A peptide. Am J Respir Cell Mol Biol. 2011;44(2):166–74.
189. Newman LS, Rose CS, Bresnitz EA, Rossman MD, Barnard J, Frederick M, et al. A case control etiologic study of sarcoidosis: environmental and occupational risk factors. Am J Respir Crit Care Med. 2004;170(12):1324–30.
190. Kalis C, Gumenscheimer M, Freudenberg N, Tchaptchet S, Fejer G, Heit A, et al. Requirement for TLR9 in the immunomodulatory activity of Propionibacterium acnes. J Immunol. 2005;174(7):4295–300.
191. Baughman RP, Teirstein AS, Judson MA, Rossman MD, Yeager H Jr, Bresnitz EA, et al. Clinical characteristics of patients in a case control study of sarcoidosis. Am J Respir Crit Care Med. 2001;164(10 Pt 1):1885–9.
192. Semenzato G, Pezzutto A, Chilosi M, Pizzolo G. Redistribution of T lymphocytes in the lymph nodes of patients with sarcoidosis. N Engl J Med. 1982;306(1):48–9.
193. Takemura T, Matsui Y, Saiki S, Mikami R. Pulmonary vascular involvement in sarcoidosis: a report of 40 autopsy cases. Hum Pathol. 1992;23(11):1216–23.
194. Zissel G, Prasse A, Muller-Quernheim J. Immunologic response of sarcoidosis. Semin Respir Crit Care Med. 2010;31(4):390–403.
195. Vatti R, Sharma OP. Course of asymptomatic liver involvement in sarcoidosis: role of therapy in selected cases. Sarcoidosis Vasculitis Diffuse Lung Dis. 1997;14(1):73–6.
196. Cremers J, Drent M, Driessen A, Nieman F, Wijnen P, Baughman R, et al. Liver-test abnormalities in sarcoidosis. Eur J Gastroenterol Hepatol. 2012;24(1):17–24.
197. Devaney K, Goodman ZD, Epstein MS, Zimmerman HJ, Ishak KG. Hepatic sarcoidosis. Clinicopathologic features in 100 patients. Am J Surg Pathol. 1993;17(12):1272–80.
198. Kahi CJ, Saxena R, Temkit M, Canlas K, Roberts S, Knox K, et al. Hepatobiliary disease in sarcoidosis. Sarcoidosis Vasculitis Diffuse Lung Dis. 2006;23(2):117–23.
199. Dulai PS, Rothstein RI. Disseminated sarcoidosis presenting as granulomatous gastritis: a clinical review of the gastrointestinal and hepatic manifestations of sarcoidosis. J Clin Gastroenterol. 2012;46(5):367–74.
200. Maddrey WC, Johns CJ, Boitnott JK, Iber FL. Sarcoidosis and chronic hepatic disease: a clinical and pathologic study of 20 patients. Medicine (Baltimore). 1970;49(5):375–95.
201. Judson MA. Hepatic, splenic, and gastrointestinal involvement with sarcoidosis. Semin Respir Crit Care Med. 2002;23(6):529–41.
202. Bilir M, Mert A, Ozaras R, Yanardag H, Karayel T, Senturk H, et al. Hepatic sarcoidosis: clinicopathologic features in thirty-seven patients. J Clin Gastroenterol. 2000;31(4):337–8.
203. Malhotra A, Naniwadekar A, Sood G. Hepatobiliary and pancreatic: cirrhosis secondary to hepatic sarcoidosis. J Gastroenterol Hepatol. 2008;23(12):1942.
204. Gupta S, Faughnan ME, Prud'homme GJ, Hwang DM, Munoz DG, Kopplin P. Sarcoidosis complicated by cirrhosis and hepatopulmonary syndrome. Can Respir J. 2008;15(3):124–6.
205. Moreno-Merlo F, Wanless IR, Shimamatsu K, Sherman M, Greig P, Chiasson D. The role of granulomatous phlebitis and thrombosis in the pathogenesis of cirrhosis and portal hypertension in sarcoidosis. Hepatology. 1997;26(3):554–60.
206. Valla DC, Benhamou JP. Hepatic granulomas and hepatic sarcoidosis. Clin Liver Dis. 2000;4(1):269–85, ix–x.
207. Karaosmanoglu AD, Onur MR, Saini S, Taberi A, Karcaaltincaba M. Imaging of hepatobiliary involvement in sarcoidosis. Abdom Imaging. 2015;40(8):3330–7.
208. Kessler A, Mitchell DG, Israel HL, Goldberg BB. Hepatic and splenic sarcoidosis: ultrasound and MR imaging. Abdom Imaging. 1993;18(2):159–63.
209. Dourakis SP, Cokkinos DD, Soultati AS, Alexopoulou A, Nezi V, Archimandritis AJ. A case of liver sarcoidosis mimicking cirrhosis. Clin Imaging. 2007;31(1):47–9.
210. Ferreira A, Ramalho M, de Campos RO, Heredia V, Roque A, Vaidean G, et al. Hepatic sarcoidosis: MR appearances in patients with chronic liver disease. Magn Reson Imaging. 2013;31(3):432–8.

211. Tadros M, Forouhar F, Wu GY. Hepatic sarcoidosis. J Clin Transl Hepatol. 2013;1(2):87–93.
212. Bloom R, Sybert A, Mascatello VJ. Granulomatous biliary tract obstruction due to sarcoidosis. Report of a case and review of the literature. Am Rev Respir Dis. 1978;117(4):783–7.
213. Judson MA. An approach to the treatment of pulmonary sarcoidosis with corticosteroids: the six phases of treatment. Chest. 1999;115(4):1158–65.
214. Kennedy PT, Zakaria N, Modawi SB, Papadopoulou AM, Murray-Lyon I, du Bois RM, et al. Natural history of hepatic sarcoidosis and its response to treatment. Eur J Gastroenterol Hepatol. 2006;18(7):721–6.
215. Riviere E, Jourde W, Gensous N, Demant X, Ribeiro E, Duffau P, et al. Efficacy and safety of Infliximab in systemic sarcoidosis according to GenPhenReSa organ-involvement phenotype: a retrospective study of 55 patients. Respir Res. 2024;25(1):124.
216. Bakker GJ, Haan YC, Maillette de Buy Wenniger LJ, Beuers U. Sarcoidosis of the liver: to treat or not to treat? Neth J Med. 2012;70(8):349–56.
217. Vanatta JM, Modanlou KA, Dean AG, Nezakatgoo N, Campos L, Nair S, et al. Outcomes of orthotopic liver transplantation for hepatic sarcoidosis: an analysis of the United Network for Organ Sharing/Organ Procurement and Transplantation Network data files for a comparative study with cholestatic liver diseases. Liver Transpl. 2011;17(9):1027–34.
218. Bilal M, Satapathy SK, Ismail MK, Vanatta JM. Long-term outcomes of liver transplantation for hepatic sarcoidosis: a single center experience. J Clin Exp Hepatol. 2016;6(2):94–9.

Chapter 11
Pancreatic Involvement in Rheumatologic Diseases

Promila Banerjee, Judy Trieu, and Joshua Kalapala

11.1 Anatomy and Physiology

The pancreas is a lobulated gland that is located at the level of L1 to L2 lumbar vertebrae. It is divided into the head, neck, body, and tail. The uncinate process is a projection of pancreatic tissue extending from the lower part of the head of the pancreas. The main pancreatic duct starts in the tail of the pancreas and courses towards the head of the pancreas, joining the cystic duct at the level of the major papilla. Most of the population also has an accessory duct that meets the duodenum via the minor papillae [1]. Although anatomic variations occur, this description is of the common anatomic ductal structures [2]. The pancreas receives a rich blood supply from branches of the celiac and superior mesenteric arteries [3].

The pancreas is comprised of an exocrine and endocrine component. The exocrine portion consists of acinar cells that secrete digestive enzymes into the lumen of ductules, where it mixes with the bicarbonate and water secreted by the duct cells to create the alkaline pancreatic juice. The endocrine portion consists of islet cells that primarily produce insulin and other hormones that aid in the regulation of digestion and hunger.

P. Banerjee (✉)
Loyola Stritch School of Medicine, Maywood, IL, USA

Edward Hines Jr VA Hospital, Hines, IL, USA
e-mail: Promila.Banerjee@va.gov

J. Trieu
Division of Gastroenterology, Washington University, St. Louis, MS, USA

J. Kalapala
University of Wisconsin, Madison, WI, USA

M. Tadros et al. (eds.), *GI Diseases Associated with Rheumatological and Vasculitic Conditions*, Clinical Gastroenterology,
https://doi.org/10.1007/978-3-032-07868-1_11

11.2 Pancreatic Involvement in Rheumatological Diseases

Involvement of the pancreas in rheumatologic diseases is fairly uncommon, most of which have only been reported in the form of cases or small observational cohorts. The etiology is typically associated with the underlying rheumatologic condition, but in many cases, the pathogenesis is unclear. However, it is, important to exclude drug-induced pancreatitis, such as with azathioprine, 6-mercaptopurine, and steroids, that have been named culprits of pancreatic injury in the past, as these may play a role in the treatment of pancreatic manifestations.

11.3 Acute Pancreatitis in Systemic Lupus Erythematosus

Patients with Systemic Lupus Erythematosus (SLE) have an increased risk of acute pancreatitis, with an estimated incidence of 0.4–1.1 per 1000 patients [4]. SLE-associated acute pancreatitis can be diagnosed once other common causes have been ruled out, including alcohol, biliary obstruction, and drugs/medications. The pathophysiology of SLE-associated acute pancreatitis is not clearly defined, but a possible mechanism involves the inflammatory process of vasculitis [5]. Another proposed mechanism is the presence of increased antiphospholipid antibodies because patients with SLE-associated acute pancreatitis experienced more hypercoagulable events, such as strokes and deep vein thromboses, and the presence of antiphospholipid antibodies was not increased [6]. Patients with SLE-associated acute pancreatitis also have an increased risk of disease severity during hospitalizations, including acute respiratory failure, acute renal failure, hypotensive shock, and sepsis [7]. Lower complement component 3 may predict disease severity [8]; however, there are several reports that active disease prior to presentation predicts mortality, which can be as high as 27% [7–9]. Although some observational studies have noted a decrease in mortality when patients with SLE-associated acute pancreatitis are treated with corticosteroids or other agents, such as azathioprine [4, 9], the data is still lacking, and the harmful effects of immunosuppression during critical illness must be weighed against the benefits [5].

11.4 Pancreatic Infarction and Acute Pancreatitis in Polyarteritis Nodosa

Polyarteritis nodosa (PAN) is a small and medium vessel vasculitis that affects multiple organ systems, involving the gastrointestinal tract in up to 53% of patients with PAN [10]. Pancreatic involvement is rare, described in cases within the literature. In a series of autopsies performed on patients with acute pancreatitis, only one patient was found to have associated PAN [11]. The clinical presentation of acute pancreatitis among patients with PAN can be difficult to discern, particularly if they have overlapping vasculitis entities ([12] Yokoi), including mesenteric vasculitis, which is high on the differential for a patient with a rheumatologic disorder presenting with abdominal pain ([13] Hatemi); however, in the other vasculitides, the pancreas is not involved. In PAN, the etiology of acute pancreatitis is presumed to be related to pancreatic thrombosis and infarction due to necrotizing vasculitis of vessels supplying the pancreas [14]. The affected vessels may develop areas of stenosis, leading to further ischemic damage [15]. Active vasculitis and stenosed vessels can result in recurrent pancreatitis with associated high morbidity and mortality [15–17]. Pancreatic fibrosis has also been seenin patients with PAN, possibly due to sequelae of repeated insult to the pancreas [18]. Reported cases of acute due to PAN were treated with corticosteroids and cyclophosphamide with some success [15–17, 19].

11.5 Pancreatic Atrophy in Systemic Sclerosis

Patients with Systemic sclerosis and scleroderma may develop pancreatic atrophy, and a percentage can result in exocrine pancreatic insufficiency (EPI). Pancreatic fibrosis can be seen in up to 17% of patients with scleroderma. However, it has been shown that it is not significantly higher than in the general population; the pathogenesis remains unknown [20, 21].EPI among patients with systemic sclerosis is still anecdotally common, with reports of secretory function of 33–61% among this patient population [22]. More recent studies demonstrated that diagnostic fecal elastase levels for EPI were not different among patients with systemic sclerosis and controls. However, there was an observed higher incidence of diagnostic EPI among patients with systemic sclerosis compared to controls [23]. Therefore, diagnosis of EPI with fecal elastase <200 ug/g is critical in order to appropriately treat with pancreatic enzyme replacement therapy. There is little to no data on the empiric use of pancreatic enzyme replacement therapy among patients with systemic sclerosis and scleroderma with chronic diarrhea, especially as small intestinal bacterial overgrowth (SIBO) is the more common etiology of chronic diarrhea in this population. Some suggest empiric treatment of SIBO first, and if there is no response, test for EPI as above to determine whether pancreatic enzyme replacement therapy is warranted [21].

11.6 Acute Pancreatitis in Behcet Disease

Gastrointestinal manifestations of Behcet Disease can be as high as 61%, but pancreatic involvement is rare [24]. Behcet Disease is a rare cause of acute pancreatitis, with only a handful of case reports in the literature. The first reported case was in 1992 of a young man who presented with acute pancreatitis and was diagnosed with

Behcet disease [25]. Again, vasculitis is the proposed etiology, causing inflammation of blood vessels supplying the pancreas, resulting in ischemic damage [25]. Recurrent acute pancreatitis can also occur [26]. Treatment with corticosteroids was used in some cases, although patients who had conservative management had similar outcomes [26].

11.7 Acute Pancreatitis in Rheumatoid Arthritis

The incidence of acute pancreatitis in patients with rheumatoid arthritis (RA) is unclear, but a national study in Taiwan calculated an incidence of 187.5 per 100,000 person-years, higher than that of the general population [27]. In fact, having RA may be predictive of not only developing acute pancreatitis but also chronic pancreatitis and primary pancreatic adenocarcinoma, despite limited evidence [28]. The leading theory behind the higher incidence of pancreatic involvement among patients with RA is arteritis of pancreatic vessels, leading to focal ischemia and necrosis [29]. There have been suggestions of overlap with autoimmune pancreatitis as well. There are two types of autoimmune pancreatitis—Type 1 and Type 2. Type 2 is associated with systemic inflammation and tends to overlap with another autoimmune disease; it may be the more common type of autoimmune pancreatitis among patients with RA [30]. The role of corticosteroids and disease-modifying anti-rheumatic drugs (DMARDs) is unclear in terms of whether they increase or decrease the risk of acute pancreatitis [27, 28].

11.8 Chronic Pancreatitis in Sjogren's syndrome

Sjogren's syndrome (SS) is an autoimmune disease that affects exocrine organs. Gastrointestinal clinical manifestations include salivary, esophageal, gastric, hepatobiliary, and pancreatic [31]. Chronic pancreatitis can be seen among patients with SS, although the incidence is unknown. Patients produce lower pancreatic secretions after stimulation, possibly due to hyposecretion of bicarbonate [32], and a percentage of these patients may develop exocrine pancreatic insufficiency [31]. The pathogenesis is unclear, but there may be a similar underlying mechanism in the disease process. Carbonic anhydrase II is an antigen in the duct cells of exocrine organs, including salivary glands and the pancreas. Patients with SS have higher serum antibodies to carbonic anhydrase II, which may lead to the destruction of salivary glands and the pancreas [33, 34]. Although chronic pancreatitis is more commonly seen in patients with SS, cases of acute pancreatitis have been reported in association with SS. However, this association needs to be substantiated [35].

11.9 Mesenteric Panniculitis

Mesenteric panniculitis is the inflammation of the mesenteric fat of unknown pathophysiology. Few reports have associated it with acute pancreatitis, proposing that the adjacent mesenteritis caused inflammation to the pancreatic parenchyma [36, 37]. However, mesenteric panniculitis is more often a great mimicker of acute pancreatitis [38–40], and even one report of mimicking pancreatic cancer [41]. Mesenteric panniculitis is exceedingly rare, but it should be a differential if acute pancreatitis with normal lipase levels is suspected. Of note, pancreatic fat necrosis can closely resemble lupus panniculitis. Given that individuals with lupus have a higher incidence of pancreatitis, it is essential to note this similarity. Therefore, lipase levels should be assessed in any patient with lupus suspected to have panniculitis.

11.10 Treatment and Management

Management of pancreatic involvement in rheumatologic diseases depends on the pancreatic manifestation, and even so, there is very little data. In the setting of acute pancreatitis in SLE, PAN, and Behcet disease, initial treatment is standard of care treatment for acute pancreatitis with intravenous fluids and supportive care. In a large observational study among patients with SLE who developed acute pancreatitis, mortality was higher among patients who did not receive immunosuppression. However, other small cohorts did not see a difference [4, 9]. Similarly, corticosteroids have been reported in PAN and Behcet disease, but there are too few cases to attempt to associate them with morbidity or mortality [15, 16, 26].

For patients who may develop true exocrine pancreatic insufficiency and resulting clinically significant nutritional deficiency, more so among patients with systemic sclerosis and Sjogren's syndrome, pancreatic enzyme replacement therapy can be used [21]. Modifying lifestyle, such as tobacco and alcohol cessation, can also prevent further insult to the pancreas, as practiced in the general population, but there is no data that is specific to patients with rheumatologic conditions.

Fortunately, there have not been any reports of increased incidence of pancreatic malignancy among these patients. Therefore, surveillance is not warranted.

11.11 Conclusion

Pancreatic manifestations among patients with rheumatologic diseases vary in their clinical presentation. Acute pancreatitis tends to be facilitated by vasculitis, resulting in ischemic injury to the pancreas, which can be associated with severe complications such as necrotizing pancreatitis and infection. Acute management of these patients is controversial, and there are unclear benefits to using corticosteroids or other immunosuppressive drugs. Chronic pancreatitis and pancreatic atrophy appear to be due to the "silent" destruction of pancreatic parenchyma through small vessel ischemia or immunogenic cross-reactivity and may result in exocrine pancreatic insufficiency. However, the overall pathogenesis and management of chronic manifestations of the pancreas remain unclear. Pancreatic involvement in rheumatologic diseases, although uncommon, is important to recognize, especially in its acute presentations.

References

1. Kleitsch WP. Anatomy of the pancreas: a study with special reference to the duct system. AMA Arch Surg. 1955;71:795–802.
2. Stamm BH. Incidence and diagnostic significance of minor pathologic changes in the adult pancreas at autopsy: a systematic study of 112 autopsies in patients without known pancreatic disease. Hum Pathol. 1984;15:677–83.
3. Rottenberg N. Macroscopic and microscopic vasculature of the duodenal-biliary-pancreatic complex. Morphol Embryol (Bucur). 1989;35:15–9.
4. Breuer GS, Baer A, Dahan D, Nesher G. Lupus-associated pancreatitis. Autoimmun Rev. 2006;5(5):314–8.
5. Dima A, Balaban DV, Jurcut C, Jinga M. Systemic lupus erythematosus-related acute pancreatitis. Lupus. 2021;30(1):5–14.
6. Makol A, Petri M. Pancreatitis in systemic lupus erythematosus: frequency and associated factors—a review of the Hopkins Lupus Cohort. J Rheumatol. 2010;37(2):341–5.
7. Rim D, Kaye A, Choi C, Ahlawat S. Inpatient outcomes of acute pancreatitis among patients with systemic lupus erythematosus: a nationwide analysis. Cureus. 2021;13(7):e16349.
8. Muhammed H, Jain A, Irfan M, Charles S, Dwivedi P, Chavan PP, Khubchandani R, Sharma A, Phatak S, Shukla AN, Shah R, Subramanian N, Pandya SC, Singh YP, Chengappa KG, Thabah M, Rajasekhar L, Shobha V, Negi VS, Dhir V, Sharma A, Misra R, Aggarwal A; SLE-SIG of IRA Clinical features, severity and outcome of acute pancreatitis in systemic lupus erythematosus. Rheumatol Int. 2021. https://doi.org/10.1007/s00296-021-04834-2. Epub ahead of print.
9. Nesher G, Breuer GS, Temprano K, Moore TL, Dahan D, Baer A, Alberton J, Izbicki G, Hersch M. Lupus-associated pancreatitis. Semin Arthritis Rheum. 2006;35(4):260–7.
10. Pagnoux C, Mahr A, Cohen P, Guillevin L. Presentation and outcome of gastrointestinal involvement in systemic necrotizing vasculitides: analysis of 62 patients with polyarteritis nodosa, microscopic polyangiitis, Wegener granulomatosis, Churg-Strauss syndrome, or rheumatoid arthritis-associated vasculitis. Medicine (Baltimore). 2005;84(2):115–28.
11. Pellegrini CA, Paloyan D, Acosta JM, Skinner DB. Acute pancreatitis of rare causation. Surg Gynecol Obstet. 1977;144(6):899–902.
12. Yokoi Y, Nakamura I, Kaneko T, Sawayanagi T, Watahiki Y, Kuroda M. Pancreatic mass as an initial manifestation of polyarteritis nodosa: a case report and review of the literature. World J Gastroenterol. 2015;21(3):1014–9.
13. Hatemi I, Hatemi G, Çelik AF. Systemic vasculitis and the gut. Curr Opin Rheumatol. 2017;29(1):33–8.
14. McKay JW, Baggenstoss AH, Wollaeger EE. Infarcts of the pancreas. Gastroenterology. 1958;35(3):256–64.
15. Flaherty J, Bradley EL 3rd. Acute pancreatitis as a complication of polyarteritis nodosa. Int J Pancreatol. 1999;25(1):53–7.

16. Ghosh AK, Sakhuja V, Malik N, Kathuria P, Chugh KS, Pancreatic pseudocyst. A rare complication of polyarteritis nodosa. Dig Dis Sci. 1993;38(7):1347–50.
17. Mowrey FH, Lundberg EA. The clinical manifestations of essential polyanglitis (periarteritis nodosa), with emphasis on the hepatic manifestations. Ann Intern Med. 1954;40(6):1145–64.
18. Suresh E, Beadles W, Welsby P, Luqmani R. Acute pancreatitis with pseudocyst formation in a patient with polyarteritis nodosa. J Rheumatol. 2005;32(2):386–8.
19. Bocanegra T, Vasey FB, Espinoza LR, Germain BF. Pancreatic pseudocyst: a complication of necrotizing vaculitis (polyarteritis nodosa). Arch Intern Med. 1980;140(10):1359–61.
20. D'Angelo WA, Fries JF, Masi AT, Shulman LE. Pathologic observations in systemic sclerosis (scleroderma). A study of fifty-eight autopsy cases and fifty-eight matched controls. Am J Med. 1969;46(3):428–40.
21. McFarlane IM, Bhamra MS, Kreps A, Iqbal S, Al-Ani F, Saladini-Aponte C, Grant C, Singh S, Awwal K, Koci K, Saperstein Y, Arroyo-Mercado FM, Laskar DB, Atluri P. Gastrointestinal manifestations of systemic sclerosis. Rheumatology (Sunnyvale). 2018;8(1):235.
22. Ebert EC. Gastric and enteric involvement in progressive systemic sclerosis. J Clin Gastroenterol. 2008;42(1):5–12.
23. Bozovic G, Pullerits R, Ståhl A, Ydström K, Wenger D, Marsal J, Thulin P, Andréasson K. Exocrine pancreatic function is preserved in systemic sclerosis. Arthritis Res Ther. 2019;21(1):52.
24. Lakhanpal S, Tani K, Lie JT, Katoh K, Ishigatsubo Y, Ohokubo T. Pathologic features of Behçet's syndrome: a review of Japanese autopsy registry data. Hum Pathol. 1985;16(8):790–5.
25. Le Thi Huong D, Wechsler B, Dell'Isola B, Lautier-Frau M, Palazzo L, Bletry O, Piette JC, Godeau P. Acute pancreatitis in Behçet's disease. Dig Dis Sci. 1992;37(9):1452–3.
26. Hum M, Mahmood MN, Huang V, Dytoc M. Pancreatitis as a rare manifestation of Behçet disease. JAAD Case Rep. 2017;3(6):470–3.
27. Chang CC, Chiou CS, Lin HL, Wang LH, Chang YS, Lin HC. Increased risk of acute pancreatitis in patients with rheumatoid arthritis: a population-based cohort study. PLoS One. 2015;10(8):e0135187.
28. Alkhayyat M, Abou Saleh M, Grewal MK, Abureesh M, Mansoor E, Simons-Linares CR, Abelson A, Chahal P. Pancreatic manifestations in rheumatoid arthritis: a national population-based study. Rheumatology (Oxford). 2021;60(5):2366–74.
29. Bély M, Apáthy A. Recurrent pancreatic arteritis and vasculogenic relapsing pancreatitis in rheumatoid arthritis—a retrospective clinicopathologic and immunohistochemical study of 161 autopsy patients. Pathol Oncol Res. 2008;14(4):473–80.
30. Ben Abdelghani K, Ben Tekaya A, Ennaifer R, Souabni L, Zakraoui L, Sibilia J. Acute pancreatitis in rheumatoid arthritis: causes. Joint Bone Spine. 2014;81(4):377–8.
31. Sheikh SH, Shaw-Stiffel TA. The gastrointestinal manifestations of Sjögren's syndrome. Am J Gastroenterol. 1995;90(1):9–14.
32. Sumii T, Ando B, Sakai K. [Chronic pancreatitis and pancreatic dysfunction associated with Sjögren's syndrome]. Nihon Rinsho. 1995;53(10):2525–9.
33. Nishimori I, Miyaji E, Morimoto K, Kohsaki T, Okamoto N, Onishi S. Diminished cellular immune response to carbonic anhydrase II in patients with Sjögren's syndrome and idiopathic chronic pancreatitis. JOP. 2004;5(4):186–92.
34. Kino-Ohsaki J, Nishimori I, Morita M, Okazaki K, Yamamoto Y, Onishi S, Hollingsworth MA. Serum antibodies to carbonic anhydrase I and II in patients with idiopathic chronic pancreatitis and Sjögren's syndrome. Gastroenterology. 1996;110(5):1579–86.
35. Chang CC, Chang YS, Wang SH, Lin SY, Chen YH, Chen JH. Primary Sjogren's syndrome and the risk of acute pancreatitis: a nationwide cohort study. BMJ Open. 2017;7(8):e014807.
36. Belabbes F, Cherkaoui R, Abdallaoui L, Lafhel R, Habi J, Nadi A, Delsa H, Rouibaa F. Mesenteric panniculitis associated with acute pancreatitis. J Pancreas (Online). 2021;S5:17–20.
37. Mohamed H, Mehdi C, Ikram M, Myriam M, Habib B, Adnene C. Mesenteric panniculitis associated with acute pancreatitis: about a case. Pan Afr Med J. 2016;24:206.

38. Jani PG, Jivanjee M. Mesenteric panniculitis mimicking acute pancreatitic: a case report and literature review. East Cent Afr J Surg. 2013;18(2).
39. Kingston T, Adham K, Harb R, Shakhatreh M. What lies beneath: a case of mesenteric panniculitis masquerading as recurrent acute pancreatitis. Am J Gastroenterol. 2016;111:S991.
40. McLaughlin PD, Filippone A, Maher MM. The "misty mesentery": mesenteric panniculitis and its mimics. AJR Am J Roentgenol. 2013;200(2):W116–23.
41. Scudiere JR, Shi C, Hruban RH, Herman JM, Fishman EK, Schulick RD, Wolfgang CL, Makary MA, Thornton K, Montgomery E, Horton KM. Sclerosing mesenteritis involving the pancreas: a mimicker of pancreatic cancer. Am J Surg Pathol. 2010;34(4):447–53.

Chapter 12
Autoimmune Cholangiopathies

Umer Malik, Bilal Ashraf, Sonia B. Samuel, and Stephen Hasak

12.1 Introduction

The biliary ductal system is a complex network of interconnected ducts that serves a vital role in the liver's functions of digestion, storage, and detoxification. These ducts originate within the liver as the canals of Hering, which converge to form bile ductules. These ductules combine to form a network of intra-hepatic ducts, which drain the right and left hepatic lobes and converge to form the common hepatic duct. Joined by the pancreatic duct and cystic duct originating from the gallbladder, these structures form a unified channel called the common bile duct. This duct opens into the duodenum, where the Sphincter of Oddi allows for the episodic release of bile and pancreatic content to aid in the digestion of carbohydrates, lipids, and proteins.

Intra-hepatic and extra-hepatic ducts are lined with biliary epithelial cells called cholangiocytes. These cells are adapted to withstand exposure to the high levels of chemicals and foreign antigens present in bile, allowing them to maintain immune tolerance, which is essential for their proper functioning without triggering immune responses. A breakdown of these defenses can lead to autoimmune cholangiopathies.

U. Malik
Gastroenterology, Marietta, GA, USA

B. Ashraf
Department of Medicine, Duke University School of Medicine, Durham, NC, USA

S. B. Samuel
Osteopathic Medicine, Albany Medical College, Albany, NY, USA

S. Hasak (✉)
Department of Gastroenterology, Albany Med Health System, Albany, NY, USA
e-mail: hasaks@amc.edu

M. Tadros et al. (eds.), *GI Diseases Associated with Rheumatological and Vasculitic Conditions*, Clinical Gastroenterology,
https://doi.org/10.1007/978-3-032-07868-1_12

12.2 Mechanisms of Immune Tolerance in Biliary Epithelial Cells

Biliary epithelial cells (BECs) are constantly exposed to a vast array of chemicals and pathogens. This is facilitated by IRAK receptors (IRAK-M), which are members of the TLR-IL-1R family of transmembrane receptors, as well as the production of defensins, secretory IgA, and various cytokines. These mechanisms enable the biliary system to maintain immune tolerance and protect the biliary tract from damage caused by infections and chemicals. Additionally, the lack of expression of MHC class II molecules under physiological conditions also contributes to immune tolerance. Over expression of HLA class II has been observed in graft versus host disease, primary sclerosing cholangitis and primary biliary cholangitis. The expression of PPAR-g leads to the production of NF-κB, which down regulates the production of pro-inflammatory cytokines, including TNF-α and IL-1β [1].

12.3 Sclerosing Cholangitis

Despite the body's adaptive measures, several conditions can result in inflammation of the biliary system at different levels, leading to progressive inflammation, fibrosis, and stenosis. These changes can be seen in the setting of primary sclerosis or secondary sclerosis. Regardless of the underlying inciting event, all cholangiopathies share the clinical feature of cholestasis, manifested by elevated cholestatic enzymes, jaundice, and pruritus. Among primary sclerosing cholangiopathies, they are further divided into primary sclerosing cholangitis and IgG4 related disease. While the clinical presentation of both conditions is similar, their treatment differs significantly, making an accurate diagnosis crucial. Secondary sclerosing cholangiopathies may occur in the setting of infections of the biliary tract, choledocholithiasis, or postoperative stenosis.

12.4 Primary Sclerosing Cholangitis

Primary sclerosing cholangitis (PSC) is a rare and chronic condition characterized by the development of small, bead-like protrusions and narrowing of the intrahepatic and extrahepatic biliary ducts, leading to cholestatic liver injury. The disease often follows a prolonged asymptomatic period, but it is progressive, resulting in complications such as stricturing, recurrent episodes of cholangitis, and ultimately, end-stage liver disease.

12.5 Epidemiology

PSC is a rare condition with a global prevalence of approximately 0.7 per 100,000 people, although this varies geographically. [2] The highest rates are seen in North America and Northern Europe [2], while significantly lower rates are observed in Asia [3]. PSC disproportionately affects males, accounting for 65–70% of cases, although there is a slight female predominance in cases of PSC without underlying inflammatory bowel disease (IBD) [3]. PSC and IBD have a close association, with an estimated 70% of patients with PSC also having IBD, most commonly ulcerative colitis [4]. PSC tends to affect a younger population, with the average age of diagnosis being between 30 and 40 years old [5]. Several studies have noted the incidence of PSC is increasing [6–8], although this could be, in part, a result of the utilization of magnetic resonance cholangiopancreatography (MRCP) as a diagnostic tool.

12.6 Pathophysiology

The mechanism behind primary sclerosing cholangitis (PSC) is not fully understood, but it is believed to involve a complex interplay between genetic, immunogenic, and environmental factors.

Primarily, PSC is thought to be caused by an autoimmune attack on the bile duct cells, either through the presence of autoantibodies or abnormally activated T lymphocytes. However, the specific antigen responsible for this attack has yet to be identified. Nonetheless, there is evidence to support the idea that PSC involves aberrant activation of both humoral and cellular immunity. Autoantibodies, particularly those that react with biliary or colonic epithelial antigens, are commonly found in patients with PSC [9]. Other antibodies detected in PSC include anti-nuclear, anti-smooth muscle, and anti-mitochondrial antibodies [9]. In addition, up to 80% of PSC patients have perinuclear anti-neutrophil cytoplasmic antibodies (P-ANCA), with higher rates seen in those with concurrent inflammatory bowel disease (IBD) [10]. While P-ANCA typically targets myeloperoxidase, the P-ANCA seen in PSC specifically targets a myeloid nuclear envelope protein. Elevated levels of IgM and occasionally IgG are also frequently observed in the blood of PSC patients [11]. While there is conflicting evidence on whether the number of T cells in the peripheral circulation increases or decreases in PSC, the number of CD4+ T cells in the liver has been found to be increased in these patients [12].

The genetic basis of PSC is supported by the finding that first-degree relatives of PSC patients have a fourfold increased risk of developing the condition [13]. Genome-wide association studies have identified several genes associated with PSC, the strongest being within the human leukocyte antigen (HLA) locus on chromosome 6 [14]. The HLA complex consists of a family of genes that encode major histocompatibility complex (MHC) proteins, which present foreign antigens to T cells in order to initiate an immune response. Certain HLA subgroups (HLA-B8, DR3, DR2, and A1) are more common in PSC patients, providing further evidence that PSC involves immune dysfunction [15]. Additionally, polymorphisms in the IL2RA gene, which codes for a receptor that is essential for regulatory T cell function and is constitutively expressed on these cells, have been linked to PSC [16].

Dysfunctional variants in genes that play a role in the protection of cholangiocytes against toxic bile acids via a mechanism called the "biliary HCO3' umbrella" have also been identified [17]. The TGR5 receptor, located on the apical surface of cholangiocytes, senses bile acid and stimulates the secretion of bicarbonate to protect these cells from injury. The enzyme fucosyltransferase 2 (FUT2) also plays a role in stabilizing the biliary epithelial glycocalyx and maintaining the bicarbonate umbrella [18, 19]. Dysfunctional variants in both of these genes have been proposed as potential contributing factors in the pathophysiology of PSC [17].

The "PSC-Microbiome Hypothesis" posits that primary sclerosing cholangitis (PSC) is the result of multiple pathogenic factors [20, 21]. One such factor is an increase in microbial antigens entering the liver through the enterohepatic circulation, potentially caused by a dysfunctional intestinal barrier [21]. Another factor is a change in gut microbiome diversity, with several studies showing decreased microbial diversity in PSC patients compared to healthy individuals. [22–24] A third factor is an abnormal response of cholangiocytes to microbial antigens, which may cause them to be over-sensitive and contribute to biliary damage [21]. Many studies suggest that the cholangiocytes are both the target and perpetrator of biliary damage [21, 25, 26]. Cholangiocyte cellular senescence, a state induced by chronic injury, has been observed even in the early stages of PSC, suggesting a possible link to the disease's pathogenesis [26].

12.7 Clinical Presentation

PSC has a highly variable natural history, with patients presenting with symptoms ranging from mild to severe. Many PSC patients are asymptomatic at the time of diagnosis and are only identified during routine lab work, which may reveal an obstructive cholestatic pattern of injury, including elevated alkaline phosphatase and gamma-glutamyl transferase levels with mildly increased aminotransferases [27, 28].

As the disease progresses, common symptoms may include right upper quadrant pain and fatigue [3, 29]. These symptoms often result from the progressive fibrosis and stricturing of the bile ducts, which eventually cause cholestatic injury. The obstruction of bile outflow can lead to conjugated hyperbilirubinemia, manifested as jaundice and pruritus. With less bile reaching the intestines, there is decreased stercobilinogen production, leading to the formation of clay-colored stools. Some patients may also notice dark-colored urine due to increased excretion of conjugated bilirubin. PSC may also cause deficiencies of fat-soluble vitamins, which require bile for absorption.

Inflammation and fibrosis of the biliary ducts can allow bacteria to accumulate upstream of any blockages, leading to ascending (acute) bacterial cholangitis. The risk of developing this condition increases even further in PSC patients who undergo endoscopic intervention of the biliary tract [30]. The hallmark symptoms of ascending cholangitis include Charcot's triad (right upper quadrant pain, jaundice, and fever), or Reynold's pentad, a more severe presentation that includes altered mental status and hypotension.

In a majority of patients with both PSC and inflammatory bowel disease (IBD) (PSC-IBD), IBD is recognized years before the diagnosis of PSC is made [6]. Only about 10% of patients are diagnosed with both conditions at the same time [31]. Therefore, many patients will present with signs and symptoms of IBD before PSC. While most patients with PSC-IBD are diagnosed with ulcerative colitis, about 20–30% are diagnosed with Crohn's or indeterminate colitis [32, 33]. In patients with PSC and ulcerative colitis, there is typically total colonic involvement, which is sometimes described as a separate phenotype [34, 35]. Patients with ulcerative colitis may complain of symptoms such as bloody diarrhea, rectal urgency, and tenesmus [36].

In most patients, the disease will inevitably progress to extensive liver damage and ultimately cirrhosis [37]. Portal hypertension sequelae are commonly seen, including variceal bleeding, ascites, and congestive splenomegaly. Rarely, portal hypertension can develop before cirrhosis due to nodular regenerative hyperplasia or obliterative venopathy [38].

A sudden worsening of jaundice, pruritus, weight loss, and a significant increase in liver enzymes should raise concern for cholangiocarcinoma, the most common malignancy in patients with PSC [39, 40]. Up to half of PSC patients with cholangiocarcinoma are identified within the first year of their diagnosis, and the cumulative lifetime incidence is 9–20% [40]. It is believed that chronic inflammation of the biliary tree, which progresses from low-grade to high-grade dysplasia and ultimately to carcinoma, is the underlying cause of cholangiocarcinoma in these patients [41, 42]. PSC also predisposes patients to other malignancies, including colorectal cancer, hepatocellular carcinoma, and gallbladder cancer [43]. Studies have shown a seven-fold increase in colorectal cancer in PSC patients compared to the general population [44], and PSC-IBD patients have a three-fold increased risk of developing colorectal cancer compared to those with IBD alone [45].

12.8 Diagnosis

PSC should be considered in a patient with persistently elevated cholestatic laboratory values, in particular, alkaline phosphatase and γ-glutamyl transpeptidase. Concern for PSC should be even greater in a patient who is already diagnosed with IBD. An elevated serum bilirubin is present in approximately 28–40% of patients and is associated with a poor prognosis [46]. While liver aminotransferases are usually only mildly elevated in PSC, an increase in the aspartate aminotransferase

(AST) relative to the alanine aminotransferase (ALT) may indicate the progression towards cirrhosis [46, 47]. Other laboratory values that may suggest this include low albumin, low platelets, and elevated prothrombin time. P-ANCA is detected in upwards of 80% of PSC cases, although it is not specific [46].

The next step in diagnosis is obtaining an magnetic resonance cholangiopancreatography (MRCP), which is currently considered the imaging standard for diagnosis [3]. This imaging modality is highly effective, with a sensitivity of 86% and specificity of 94% for detecting PSC [48]. In the early stages of the disease, MRCPs may show the classic "beaded" appearance, characterized by short, annular strictures alternating with normal or dilated segments within the extra- and/or intrahepatic ducts. [3, 49] In later stages, the "pruned tree" appearance may be observed, with proximal bile ducts becoming dilated and distal peripheral ducts becoming obliterated due to progressive fibrosis [48].

A percutaneous liver biopsy can help confirm a diagnosis of primary sclerosing cholangitis (PSC), although it is not always necessary. The biopsy may show the classic histological "onion-skin" appearance, characterized by concentric fibrosis that obliterates small bile ducts [50]. However, this finding is only present in less than a quarter of liver biopsies performed on patients with PSC, so the role of biopsy may be limited and reserved for cases where small duct PSC or a mixed variant of PSC and autoimmune hepatitis is suspected [50]. In cases where MRCP findings are negative but the liver biopsy is positive, this may indicate small duct PSC [51], which accounts for about 5% of all cases of PSC [28].

Excluding conditions that mimic PSC is an essential step in diagnosis, which can be achieved through various laboratory tests. Primary biliary sclerosis, an autoimmune disease characterized by destruction of bile ducts and a similar cholestatic lab pattern to PSC, should be considered if the patient tests positive for antimitochondrial antibodies [52]. Smooth muscle antibodies should also be measured, as they are elevated in many cases of autoimmune hepatitis and may present with similar symptoms of jaundice, abdominal pain, and fatigue. Other antibodies associated with autoimmune hepatitis include anti-liver/kidney microsomal type 1, anti-liver cytosol type 1, and anti-soluble liver antigen [53]. AIDs-cholangiopathy, a condition characterized by biliary obstruction due to infectious causes, can be investigated by measuring HIV antibodies [54]. While transabdominal ultrasound is rarely used in the diagnosis of PSC, it may be helpful if choledocholithiasis is being considered [46].

There is a subset of younger patients with PSC that exhibit features of autoimmune hepatitis, a condition known as "PSC-autoimmune hepatitis overlap syndrome". This condition should be suspected in patients with high levels of antinuclear antibodies, anti-smooth muscle antibodies, IgG, and liver aminotransferases [55]. To differentiate between the two conditions, a liver biopsy should be performed, as the mixed variant may respond to immunosuppressive therapy [55].

It is critical to differentiate IgG4-sclerosing cholangitis, a subtype of IgG4-related disease (IgG-RD), from PSC because the treatment differs. Two sets of criteria have been made to help identify IgG4-sclerosing cholangitis, the HISORt criteria and the Japanese Clinical Diagnostic Criteria, which will both be elaborated on in a later section [56].

12.9 Treatment/Management

At present, there are no medical treatment options for PSC. Studies examining the use of ursodeoxycholic acid (UDCA) have had mixed outcomes, and current guidelines recommend against its use [28]. Other immunosuppressive agents, including azathioprine, budesonide, methotrexate, mycophenolate mofetil, and tacrolimus, have also been studied with no evidence of clinical benefit for PSC [28].

Endoscopic interventions can be used to treat dominant strictures, which are defined as stenoses of less than 1.5 mm in diameter in the common bile duct or less than 1 mm in the left or right main hepatic ducts [51]. Dominant strictures have been reported to be found in about 45% of patients at the onset of diagnosis, with a lifetime prevalence of 10–62% [57, 58]. For patients experiencing persistent symptoms of pruritus or cholangitis, endoscopic dilation or stenting has been shown to provide some relief [28]. Stenting has been associated with increased risk of adverse events and cholangitis, so balloon dilation is generally the preferred initial treatment [59, 60]. Percutaneous cholangiography is reserved for treating strictures in patients with gastric bypass or those who have failed ERCP [28]. Pre-procedural antibiotics are currently recommended for patients with PSC due to their increased risk of post-ERCP cholangitis, although the optimal regimen has not been determined [28, 61].

Dominant strictures may be a sign of cholangiocarcinoma and should therefore be investigated through ERCP with cytology, biopsies, and fluorescence in-situ hybridization (FISH) to rule out malignancy [28, 51]. Cholangioscopy, an endoscopic technique that allows visualization of the bile and pancreatic ducts, may be used to guide biopsies and improve the sensitivity and specificity of testing, although data on its use in this context is limited [62].

Given the progressive nature of the disease, most patients will ultimately develop hepatic failure, and the only definitive treatment at this stage is an orthotopic liver transplant. After diagnosis of PSC, the median survival without a liver transplant has been reported to be 13–20 years [34, 63, 64]. Indications for a transplant are based on the Model for End Stage Liver Disease (MELD) score, which estimates survival among patients with advanced liver disease and helps to prioritize liver donations based on objective variables including the patient's international normalized ratio (INR), serum creatinine, and serum bilirubin, with a score ranging from 6 to 40. A MELD score greater than 15 indicates that a liver transplant would provide a survival benefit. Patients with PSC may receive additional points on their MELD score if they have recurrent episodes of cholangitis, cholangiocarcinoma without metastasis, or refractory pruritus [28]. Liver transplantation can provide significant benefits to patients with PSC, with 1- and 5-year survival rates of 90% and 85%, respectively [55]. However, recurrent or post-transplant PSC has been increasingly observed, with a recent meta-analysis reporting a 18% rate [65]. Risk factors for recurrent PSC include cholangiocarcinoma before transplant, acute cellular rejection of the transplant, diagnosis of inflammatory bowel disease (IBD), and a high MELD score [65].

12.10 IgG4-Related Sclerosing Cholangitis

IgG4-related disease, also known as IgG4-RD, is a slowly progressive disorder characterized by the infiltration of lymphocytes and IgG4-secreting plasma cells into various organs, resulting in fibro-inflammatory tissue changes and storiform fibrosis. It may present as inflammatory pseudotumors or diffuse organ enlargement and can affect multiple sites throughout the body, the most common of which are the lacrimal glands, salivary glands, pancreas, and retroperitoneum [66]. Other, less frequently affected sites include the bile ducts, lungs, kidneys, orbits, pachymeninges, thyroid gland, and aorta [66]. When involving the bile ducts, it is referred to as IgG4-related sclerosing cholangitis, a condition marked by infiltration and stenosis of the bile duct walls, leading to cholestasis [67]. While it is often seen in conjunction with autoimmune pancreatitis, it can also occur as a standalone condition.

12.11 Epidemiology

IgG4-sclerosing cholangitis is a condition that has been difficult to study epidemiologically due to its recent recognition as a distinct disease entity and the lack of consensus on diagnostic criteria. The term IgG4-RD now encompasses a number of previously separate conditions that had been based on organ involvement [68]. According to a nationwide survey in Japan, the incidence of IgG4-RD in 2009 ranged from 0.28 to 1.08 per 100,000 people, with 336 to 1300 new cases per year from 2003 to 2009 [69]. In 2020, another study conducted in Japan estimated the prevalence of the IgG4-sclerosing cholangitis subtype in 2018 to be 2.18 (95% confidence interval, 2.13–2.23) per 100,000 inhabitants [70]. The condition disproportionately affects males, with a male-to-female ratio of about 3.3:1, and is primarily diagnosed in individuals in their seventies or eighties [71, 72].

The percentage of patients with IgG4-RD who have biliary involvement has been estimated to range from 4% to 32%, although some of these studies were limited by small sample sizes [72–77] Patients with IgG4-sclerosing cholangitis often also have autoimmune pancreatitis, with one study reporting a prevalence of 83.7% in cases of IgG4-SC [78] Interestingly, cases of IgG4-sclerosing cholangitis without a diagnosis of autoimmune pancreatitis are more commonly seen in female patients [78].

12.12 Pathophysiology

The etiology of IgG4-RD is still a matter of debate, but the predominant theories emphasize genetic factors and aberrant interactions between the innate and adaptive immune systems.

A genome-wide association study of Japanese patients with IgG4-RD identified HLA-DRB1 and Fc Gamma Receptor 2 B (FCGR2B) regions as susceptibility loci [79]. These regions have both been associated with other autoimmune diseases, specifically FCGR2B with systemic lupus erythematosus [80]. It has also been suggested that decreased expression of genes involved in innate immunity, such as transcobalamin I and secretory leukocyte peptidase inhibitor, may play a role in the development of IgG4-RD [81].

Patients with IgG4-RD present with polyclonal hypergammaglobulinemia, with elevated concentrations of the IgG4 isotype seen in the blood and affected tissues [66, 82]. While elevated levels of IgG4 may occur in other disorders, concentrations greater than 5 g/L are almost exclusively seen in cases of IgG4-RD, highlighting the central role of this antibody in the etiology of the disease [82]. IgG4 antibodies possess several unique features that suggest they may have an anti-inflammatory effect on the body. For instance, they are capable of spontaneously exchanging one of their Fab fragments, a process known as "Fab-arm exchange," which generates asymmetrical, bispecific antibodies and contributes to their anti-inflammatory activity [83, 84]. Additionally, IgG4 molecules do not effectively bind the complement protein C1q, preventing the activation of the classical pathway of the complement system [83, 85]. Furthermore, these antibodies exhibit reduced binding affinity for Fc receptors, and therefore are less able to stimulate phagocytosis or cell-mediated toxicity [83, 86]. All of these characteristics support the hypothesis that IgG4 plays a role in mitigating inflammation, leading to ongoing debate over whether the elevated levels of IgG4 observed in IgG4-RD patients are a cause or a consequence of the disease.

Dysfunction of the innate immune system has also been suggested as a potential contributing factor in the development of IgG4-RD. Activation of toll-like receptors (TLRs) and nucleotide-binding oligomerization domain-containing protein 2 (NOD2) receptors on basophils and monocytes leads to the activation of B-cell activating factor (BAFF), which in turn increases IgG4 production by B cells in patients with IgG4-RD [87]. Additionally, affected tissues often have high levels of activated "M2" macrophages, which secrete fibrinogenic chemokines [88, 89].

The fact that multiple sites of the body are affected in IgG4-RD has led to the hypothesis that the immune system is targeting a common antigen. Several autoantigens have been identified as potential contributors to the formation of autoantibodies in IgG4-RD. For example, patients with IgG4-related autoimmune pancreatitis may produce autoantibodies against carbonic anhydrase, lactoferrin, and pancreatic secretory trypsin inhibitor [90–92]. Since these antigens are found in the biliary ducts, salivary glands, and pancreas, it is possible that they are common targets of the immune system in IgG4-RD. Other studies have identified autoantibodies against prohibitin, annexin A11, laminin 511-E8, and galectin-3 [93–96]. It has been observed that IgG4 responses against two or more of these antigens in a single patient with IgG4-RD are associated with a more severe disease phenotype [97].

Studies have suggested a potential role for B cells in the development of IgG4-RD. In patients with IgG4-sclerosing cholangitis, B cells in both the blood and duodenal papilla were found to have the same B-cell receptor (BCR) repertoire containing IgG4 clones. When these patients were treated with corticosteroids, their IgG4 levels and clinical symptoms declined, suggesting a role in pathogenesis [98]. Another study showed similar findings upon treatment with rituximab and also found that an expansion of activated B cells in the blood correlated with increased disease activity [99]. Certain populations of plasmablasts in IgG4-RD patients are positively correlated with IgG4 titers, the number of organs affected, and severity of the disease [100]. In particular, the CD19+CD24-CD38hi plasmablast subset has been found to secrete more IgG4 than other B cell populations [100].

At germinal centers within lymphoid organs, follicular helper T (Tfh) cells and B cells work together in the production of antibodies, isotype switching, and plasmablast genesis. Researchers found that specific subsets of circulating T follicular helper cells that produce IL-4, which promotes class switching to both IgE and IgG4, were present at higher levels in the blood of IgG4-RD patients than in healthy individuals [66]. In patients with IgG4-sclerosing cholangitis, a specific class of T regulatory (Treg) cells, FOXP3+CD4+CD25+ Tregs, is found infiltrating bile duct tissue [101, 102]. These Tregs secrete IL-10, which, in combination with IL-4, promotes class switching to IgG4 [103]. Tumor growth-factor-β (TGF-β), which stimulates fibrogenesis and is thought to contribute to the mass lesions and pseudotumors seen in IgG4-RD, is also secreted by the FOXP3+ Tregs [103].

12.13 Clinical Features

IgG-RD often has an insidious onset with a long latency period, making it difficult to detect. By the time it is diagnosed, about 60% of patients will have organ dysfunction [75]. The presentation of the disease varies depending on the affected organ, but many patients present with fibrotic, mass-like lesions that are often mistaken for malignancy [104]. The most common organ affected is the pancreas, with about 60% of patients with IgG4-RD having pancreatic involvement (Inoue 2015). Other commonly affected organs include the salivary glands, kidneys, lacrimal glands, and aorta [72]. Recently, four distinct phenotypes of IgG4-RD have been identified according to organ involvement: pancreato-hepato-biliary disease, retroperitoneal fibrosis and/or aortitis, head and neck-limited disease, and classic Mikulicz syndrome (head and neck disease) with systemic involvement [105].

In patients with bile duct involvement, or the pancreato-hepato-biliary subtype of IgG4-RD, the most common presenting symptoms are abdominal pain and recurrent jaundice [70, 106, 107]. These symptoms, similar to those seen in PSC, are a result of thickening of the bile duct walls, leading to cholestasis. Other potential presenting symptoms include pruritus, fatigue, conjugated hyperbilirubinemia, and fever from ascending cholangitis. Pancreatic insufficiency, manifesting as dramatic weight loss due to impaired digestion and absorption of nutrients, may also be present [66]. Among patients with the pancreatobiliary phenotype of IgG4-RD, diabetes mellitus is a common comorbidity [108].

Laboratory findings usually reflect a cholestatic pattern of injury, with elevated levels of serum bilirubin and alkaline phosphatase and mildly elevated aminotransferases [109]. Elevated levels of IgG4, often with a two-fold increase, may also be present [110].

Imaging can help identify patients with biliary involvement in IgG4-RD. Although ultrasound is often normal in the early stages of the disease, it may reveal circumferential bile duct wall thickening and dilation of intrahepatic bile ducts later on [111]. The bile duct lumen is usually narrowed but remains patent [109]. Ultrasound can also detect associated autoimmune pancreatitis, which is typically seen as a diffusely-enlarged pancreas with a surrounding hypoechoic halo, often described as "sausage-shaped" [66, 109]. While CT scans can also show bile duct wall thickening and dilation of proximal ducts, they are not the optimal choice for evaluating biliary disease [109]. However, CT scans can be used to differentiate between IgG4-sclerosing cholangitis and cholangiocarcinoma, with the former having significantly smaller stricture length, stricture wall thickness, and proximal duct diameter [112]. MRI is the preferred modality for visualizing the biliary system and pancreatic involvement in IgG4-RD. MRI will identify characteristic findings of the disease, including circular and symmetric thickening of the bile duct, smooth outer and inner margins, long segment strictures, and a retained lumen within the thickened segments [113].

12.14 Diagnosis

Accurate diagnosis of IgG4-sclerosing cholangitis requires a combination of clinical data, imaging, laboratory values, and histological findings. Currently, there are two sets of proposed diagnostic criteria for IgG4-related sclerosing cholangitis: the HISORt criteria and the Japanese Clinical Diagnostic Criteria [114, 115].

The HISORt criteria, which stands for histology, imaging, serology, other organ involvement, and response to therapy, were initially proposed from the Mayo Clinic to help diagnose autoimmune pancreatitis but can be used to identify IgG4-sclerosing cholangitis [114]. A characteristic histological finding in this condition is a lymphoplasmacytic infiltration greater than 10 IgG4+ plasma cells per high power field. Obliterative phlebitis can be seen with destruction of vessel walls, along with an irregular whorled pattern of fibrosis described as "storiform" [66, 109] more bile duct strictures will be identified along with duct wall thickening. Serological studies will include an IgG4 titer greater than 135 mg/dL. The presence of other organ involvement, particularly in the pancreas, kidneys, retroperitoneum, salivary glands, or lacrimal glands, supports the diagnosis of IgG4-SC. Finally, a clinical improvement upon treatment with corticosteroids is a hallmark feature of IgG4-SC.

The Japanese Clinical Diagnostic Criteria for IgG4-related sclerosing cholangitis were originally created in 2012 and were recently modified in 2020. These criteria incorporate guidelines similar to the HISORt criteria, but they also categorize IgG4-SC into four types based on stricture sites. Type 1 IgG4-SC is characterized by stenosis limited to the distal common bile duct, which can resemble pancreatic cancer, bile duct cancer, or chronic pancreatitis. An endoscopic ultrasound fine-needle aspiration (EUS-FNA) may be performed to exclude pancreatic cancer if there is a lesion in the pancreatic head, while a bile duct biopsy is recommended to rule out cholangiocarcinoma. In the second type of IgG4-SC, there is narrowing throughout the intra- and extrahepatic ducts, which may resemble PSC. Type 3 is marked by strictures in the lower bile duct and hilar region, while type 4 is characterized by stenoses localized to the hilar region only. Types 3 and 4 resemble cholangiocarcinoma and require a similar workup to type 1 (IDUS, EUS-FNA, bile duct biopsy) in order to rule out this diagnosis [115].

12.15 Treatment

After a diagnosis of IgG4-sclerosing cholangitis has been confirmed, the first-line treatment is glucocorticoids. The goal of treatment is to achieve and maintain remission, which is defined as the resolution of symptoms with decreased IgG4 levels and improvement of imaging findings [116]. To induce remission, treatment typically begins with a high-dose of glucocorticoids, followed by a gradual taper of the drug for about 4–6 weeks [116]. Once remission is achieved, a low maintenance dose is usually given for 1–3 years [116]. This treatment is remarkably effective, with approximately 97% of patients experiencing resolution of symptoms and improvement or complete normalization of biliary lesions [114]. However, around 30% of patients experience relapse of the condition after tapering or discontinuing their maintenance dose [117]. The negative effects of long-term glucocorticoids, including steroid-induced diabetes, osteoporosis, and infections, must be weighed against the benefits of treatment [116].

Other treatments may be considered in cases of corticosteroid resistance, relapses, or in patients with contraindications to steroids. Rituximab, a monoclonal antibody targeted against CD20, has been shown to be effective in treating both relapses and in inducing and maintaining remission. Rituximab targets and depletes B cells, which play a role in the pathogenesis of the disease, which may explain its effectiveness. While this treatment appears promising, no randomized control trial has been conducted yet. Other second-line treatment options include azathioprine, 6-mercaptopurine, mycophenolate mofetil, and methotrexate. Studies on the effectiveness of these drugs in IgG4-RD are sparse and are largely limited to autoimmune pancreatitis. One study showed no benefit of using immunomodulators over steroid treatment, with more than 50% of patients experiencing relapse on a maintenance dose [118].

Bile duct stenting is hardly ever performed in IgG4-sclerosing cholangitis because treatment with glucocorticoids is usually so successful. However, in the rare case that a patient has severe, refractory cholestatic jaundice or cholangitis, bile duct stenting may be used to alleviate symptoms [116].

References

1. Zhang H, Leung PSC, et al. How the biliary tree maintains immune tolerance? Biochim Biophys Acta (BBA) - Mol Basis Dis. 2018;1864(4, Part B):1367–73.
2. Trivedi PJ, et al. Epidemiology, natural history, and outcomes of primary sclerosing cholangitis: a systematic review of population-based studies. Clin Gastroenterol Hepatol. 2021.
3. Dyson JK, et al. Primary sclerosing cholangitis. Lancet (London, England). 2018;391(10139):2547–59. https://doi.org/10.1016/S0140-6736(18)30300-3.
4. de Vries AB, Janse M, Blokzijl H, Weersma RK. Distinctive inflammatory bowel disease phenotype in primary sclerosing cholangitis. World J Gastroenterol. 2015;21(6):1956–71. https://doi.org/10.3748/wjg.v21.i6.1956. PMID: 25684965; PMCID: PMC4323476
5. Hirschfield GM, et al. Primary sclerosing cholangitis. Lancet (London, England). 2013;382(9904):1587–99. https://doi.org/10.1016/S0140-6736(13)60096-3.
6. Bambha K, et al. Incidence, clinical spectrum, and outcomes of primary sclerosing cholangitis in a United States community. Gastroenterology. 2003;125(5):1364–9.
7. Escorsell A, et al. Epidemiology of primary sclerosing cholangitis in Spain. Spanish Association for the Study of the Liver. J Hepatol. 1994;21(5):787–91. https://doi.org/10.1016/s0168-8278(94)80240-8.
8. Lindkvist B, et al. Incidence and prevalence of primary sclerosing cholangitis in a defined adult population in Sweden. Hepatology (Baltimore, Md). 2010;52(2):571–7. https://doi.org/10.1002/hep.23678.
9. Hov JR, Boberg KM, Karlsen TH. Autoantibodies in primary sclerosing cholangitis. World J Gastroenterol: WJG. 2008;14(24):3781.
10. Terjung B, Worman HJ. Anti-neutrophil antibodies in primary sclerosing cholangitis. Best Pract Res Clin Gastroenterol. 2001;15(4):629–42.
11. Zauli D, et al. An autoantibody profile in primary sclerosing cholangitis. J Hepatol. 1987;5(1):14–8.
12. Poch T, et al. Single-cell atlas of hepatic T cells reveals expansion of liver-resident naive-like CD4+ T cells in primary sclerosing cholangitis. J Hepatol. 2021;75(2):414–23.
13. Bergquist A, et al. Increased risk of primary sclerosing cholangitis and ulcerative colitis in first-degree relatives of patients with primary sclerosing cholangitis. Clin Gastroenterol Hepatol. 2008;6(8):939–43.
14. Karlsen TH, et al. Primary sclerosing cholangitis–a comprehensive review. J Hepatol. 2017;67(6):1298–323.
15. Chapman RW, et al. Association of primary sclerosing cholangitis with HLA-B8. Gut. 1983;24(1):38–41. https://doi.org/10.1136/gut.24.1.38.
16. Sebode M, et al. Reduced FOXP3+ regulatory T cells in patients with primary sclerosing cholangitis are associated with IL2RA gene polymorphisms. J Hepatol. 2014;60(5):1010–6.
17. Maroni L, et al. Fucosyltransferase 2: a genetic risk factor for primary sclerosing cholangitis and Crohn's disease—a comprehensive review. Clin Rev Allergy Immunol. 2015;48(2):182–91.

18. Folseraas T, et al. Extended analysis of a genome-wide association study in primary sclerosing cholangitis detects multiple novel risk loci. J Hepatol. 2012;57(2):366–75.
19. de Buy Wenniger LJM, et al. The cholangiocyte glycocalyx stabilizes the 'biliary HCO3-umbrella': an integrated line of defense against toxic bile acids. Dig Dis. 2015;33(3):397–407.
20. Tabibian JH, et al. Primary sclerosing cholangitis and the microbiota: current knowledge and perspectives on etiopathogenesis and emerging therapies. Scand J Gastroenterol. 2014;49(8):901–8. https://doi.org/10.3109/00365521.2014.913189.
21. Tabibian JH, et al. Primary sclerosing cholangitis, part 1: epidemiology, etiopathogenesis, clinical features, and treatment. Gastroenterol Hepatol. 2018;14(5):293–304.
22. Rossen NG, et al. The mucosa-associated microbiota of PSC patients is characterized by low diversity and low abundance of uncultured Clostridiales II. J Crohn's Colitis. 2015;9(4):342–8.
23. Quraishi MN, et al. The gut-adherent microbiota of PSC-IBD is distinct to that of IBD. Gut. 2017;66(2):386–8. https://doi.org/10.1136/gutjnl-2016-311915.
24. Bajer L, et al. Distinct gut microbiota profiles in patients with primary sclerosing cholangitis and ulcerative colitis. World J Gastroenterol. 2017;23(25):4548–58. https://doi.org/10.3748/wjg.v23.i25.4548.
25. O'Hara SP, Karlsen TH, LaRusso NF. Cholangiocytes and the environment in primary sclerosing cholangitis: where is the link? Gut. 2017;66(11):1873–7.
26. Cazzagon N, et al. Cholangiocyte senescence in primary sclerosing cholangitis is associated with disease severity and prognosis. JHEP Rep. 2021;3(3):100286.
27. Broomé U, et al. Natural history and prognostic factors in 305 Swedish patients with primary sclerosing cholangitis. Gut. 1996;38(4):610–5. https://doi.org/10.1136/gut.38.4.610.
28. Lindor KD, Kowdley KV, Harrison EM. ACG clinical guideline: primary sclerosing cholangitis. Off J Am College Gastroenteroll ACG. 2015;110(5):646–59.
29. Kaplan GG, et al. The burden of large and small duct primary sclerosing cholangitis in adults and children: a population-based analysis. Am J Gastroenterol. 2007;102(5):1042–9. https://doi.org/10.1111/j.1572-0241.2007.01103.x.
30. Charatcharoenwitthaya P, Lindor KD. Primary sclerosing cholangitis: diagnosis and management. Curr Gastroenterol Rep. 2006;8(1):75–82. https://doi.org/10.1007/s11894-006-0067-8.
31. Yanai H, et al. Prognosis of primary sclerosing cholangitis in israel is independent of coexisting inflammatory bowel Disease. J Crohn's Colitis. 2015;9(2):177–84.
32. Tischendorf JJW, et al. Characterization, outcome, and prognosis in 273 patients with primary sclerosing cholangitis: a single center study. Off J Am College Gastroenteroll ACG. 2007;102(1):107–14.
33. Fevery J, et al. Patients with large-duct primary sclerosing cholangitis and Crohn's disease have a better outcome than those with ulcerative colitis, or without IBD. Aliment Pharmacol Ther. 2016;43(5):612–20.
34. Boonstra K, et al. Primary sclerosing cholangitis is associated with a distinct phenotype of inflammatory bowel disease. Inflamm Bowel Dis. 2012;18(12):2270–6.
35. O'Toole A, et al. Primary sclerosing cholangitis and disease distribution in inflammatory bowel disease. Clin Gastroenterol Hepatol. 2012;10(4):439–41.
36. Gajendran M, et al. A comprehensive review and update on ulcerative colitis. Dis Mon. 2019;65(12):100851.
37. Aadland E, et al. Primary sclerosing cholangitis: a long-term follow-up study. Scand J Gastroenterol. 1987;22(6):655–64.
38. Abraham SC, et al. Liver transplantation in precirrhotic biliary tract disease: portal hypertension is frequently associated with nodular regenerative hyperplasia and obliterative portal venopathy. Am J Surg Pathol. 2006;30(11):1454–61.
39. Trilianos P, et al. Greater biosynthetic liver dysfunction in primary sclerosing cholangitis suggests co-existent or impending cholangiocarcinoma. J Clin Transl Hepatol. 2016;4(1):1–4. https://doi.org/10.14218/JCTH.2015.00048.
40. Song J, et al. Cholangiocarcinoma in patients with primary sclerosing cholangitis (PSC): a comprehensive review. Clin Rev Allergy Immunol. 2020;58(1):134–49.

41. Boyd S, et al. Screening primary sclerosing cholangitis and biliary dysplasia with endoscopic retrograde cholangiography and brush cytology: risk factors for biliary neoplasia. Endoscopy. 2016;48(5):432–9.
42. Chung BK, Karlsen TH, Folseraas T. Cholangiocytes in the pathogenesis of primary sclerosing cholangitis and development of cholangiocarcinoma. Biochim Biophys Acta (BBA)-Mol Basis Dis. 2018;1864(4):1390–400.
43. Fevery J, et al. Malignancies and mortality in 200 patients with primary sclerosering cholangitis: a long-term single-centre study. Liver Int. 2012;32(2):214–22.
44. Lundberg Båve A, et al. Increased risk of cancer in patients with primary sclerosing cholangitis. Hepatol Int. 2021;15(5):1174–82.
45. Zheng H-H, Jiang X-L. Increased risk of colorectal neoplasia in patients with primary sclerosing cholangitis and inflammatory bowel disease: a meta-analysis of 16 observational studies. Eur J Gastroenterol Hepatol. 2016;28(4):383–90.
46. Chapman MH, et al. British Society of Gastroenterology and UK-PSC guidelines for the diagnosis and management of primary sclerosing cholangitis. Gut. 2019;68(8):1356–78.
47. Nyblom H, Nordlinder H, Olsson R. High aspartate to alanine aminotransferase ratio is an indicator of cirrhosis and poor outcome in patients with primary sclerosing cholangitis. Liver Int. 2007;27(5):694–9.
48. Khoshpouri P, et al. Imaging features of primary sclerosing cholangitis: from diagnosis to liver transplant follow-up. Radiographics. 2019;39(7):1938–64.
49. Vitellas KM, et al. Radiologic manifestations of sclerosing cholangitis with emphasis on MR cholangiopancreatography. Radiographics. 2000;20(4):959–75; quiz 1108–9, 1112. https://doi.org/10.1148/radiographics.20.4.g00jl04959
50. Sirpal S, Chandok N. Primary sclerosing cholangitis: diagnostic and management challenges. Clin Exp Gastroenterol. 2017;10:265–73. https://doi.org/10.2147/CEG.S105872.
51. European Association for the Study of the Liver. EASL Clinical Practice Guidelines: management of cholestatic liver diseases. J Hepatol. 2009;51(2):237–67.
52. Lleo A, et al. Primary biliary cholangitis. Lancet. 2020;396(10266):1915–26.
53. Muratori L, et al. Autoantibodies in autoimmune hepatitis. Dig Dis. 2015;33(Suppl. 2):65–9.
54. Naseer M, et al. Epidemiology, determinants, and management of AIDS cholangiopathy: a review. World J Gastroenterol. 2018;24(7):767–74. https://doi.org/10.3748/wjg.v24.i7.767.
55. Karlsen TH, Schrumpf E, Boberg KM. Update on primary sclerosing cholangitis. Dig Liver Dis. 2010;42(6):390–400.
56. Chari ST. Diagnosis of autoimmune pancreatitis using its five cardinal features: introducing the Mayo Clinic's HISORt criteria. J Gastroenterol. 2007;42(18):39–41.
57. Björnsson E, et al. Dominant strictures in patients with primary sclerosing cholangitis. Am J Gastroenterol. 2004;99(3):502–8. https://doi.org/10.1111/j.1572-0241.2004.04106.x.
58. Chapman RW, Williamson KD. Are dominant strictures in primary sclerosing cholangitis a risk factor for cholangiocarcinoma? Curr Hepatol Rep. 2017;16(2):124–9.
59. Chathadi KV, et al. The role of ERCP in benign diseases of the biliary tract. Gastrointest Endosc. 2015;81(4):795–803.
60. Ponsioen CY, et al. No superiority of stents vs balloon dilatation for dominant strictures in patients with primary sclerosing cholangitis. Gastroenterology. 2018;155(3):752–9.
61. Natt N, et al. ERCP-related adverse events in primary sclerosing cholangitis: a systematic review and meta-analysis Can J Gastroenterol Hepatol. 2022;2022.
62. Fung BM, et al. Cholangioscopy and its Role in Primary Sclerosing Cholangitis. Eur Med J Hepatol. 2020;8(1):42–53.
63. Weismüller TJ, et al. Patient age, sex, and inflammatory bowel disease phenotype associate with course of primary sclerosing cholangitis. Gastroenterology. 2017;152(8):1975–84.
64. Tan N, et al. Epidemiology and outcomes of primary sclerosing cholangitis: an Australian multicentre retrospective cohort study. Hepatol Int. 2022:1–11.

65. Steenstraten IC, et al. Systematic review with meta-analysis: risk factors for recurrent primary sclerosing cholangitis after liver transplantation. Aliment Pharmacol Ther. 2019;49(6):636–43.
66. Perugino CA, Stone JH. IgG4-related disease: an update on pathophysiology and implications for clinical care. Nat Rev Rheumatol. 2020;16(12):702–14. https://doi.org/10.1038/s41584-020-0500-7.
67. Stone JH, et al. IgG4-related disease: recommendations for the nomenclature of this condition and its individual organ system manifestations. Arthritis Rheum. 2012;64(10):3061.
68. Okazaki K, et al. IgG4 cholangiopathy: current concept, diagnosis, and pathogenesis. J Hepatol. 2014;61(3):690–5. https://doi.org/10.1016/j.jhep.2014.04.016.
69. Uchida K, et al. Prevalence of IgG4-related disease in Japan based on nationwide survey in 2009. Int J Rheumatol. 2012;2012:358371. https://doi.org/10.1155/2012/358371.
70. Tanaka A, et al. Epidemiological features of immunoglobulin G4-related sclerosing cholangitis in Japan. J Hepato-Biliary-Pancreatic Sci. 2020;27(9):598–603. https://doi.org/10.1002/jhbp.793.
71. Tanaka A, et al. Nationwide survey for primary sclerosing cholangitis and IgG4-related sclerosing cholangitis in Japan. J Hepato-Biliary-Pancreatic Sci. 2014;21(1):43–50. https://doi.org/10.1002/jhbp.50.
72. Inoue D, et al. IgG4-related disease: dataset of 235 consecutive patients. Medicine. 2015;94:15.
73. Lin W, et al. Clinical characteristics of immunoglobulin G4–related disease: a prospective study of 118 Chinese patients. Rheumatology. 2015;54(11):1982–90.
74. Chen Y, et al. Types of organ involvement in patients with immunoglobulin G4-related disease. Chin Med J. 2016;129(13):1525–32.
75. Wallace ZS, et al. IgG4-related disease: clinical and laboratory features in one hundred twenty-five patients. Arthritis Rheumatol. 2015;67(9):2466–75.
76. Campochiaro C, et al. IgG4-related disease in Italy: clinical features and outcomes of a large cohort of patients. Scand J Rheumatol. 2016;45(2):135–45.
77. Ebbo M, et al. IgG4-related systemic disease: features and treatment response in a French cohort: results of a multicenter registry. Medicine. 2012;91(1):49–56.
78. Naitoh I, et al. Clinical characteristics of immunoglobulin IgG4-related sclerosing cholangitis: comparison of cases with and without autoimmune pancreatitis in a large cohort. Dig Liver Dis. 2021;53(10):1308–14.
79. Terao C, et al. IgG4-related disease in the Japanese population: a genome-wide association study. Lancet Rheumatol. 2019;1(1):e14–22.
80. Verbeek JS, Hirose S, Nishimura H. The complex association of FcγRIIb with autoimmune susceptibility. Front Immunol. 2019;10:2061.
81. Nakamura T, et al. Impaired expression of innate immunity-related genes in IgG4-related disease: a possible mechanism in the pathogenesis of IgG4-RD. Mod Rheumatol. 2020;30(3):551–7.
82. Zhao EJ, et al. Polyclonal hypergammaglobulinaemia: assessment, clinical interpretation, and management. Lancet Haematol. 2021;8(5):e365–75.
83. Aalberse RC, et al. Immunoglobulin G4: an odd antibody. Clin Exp Allergy. 2009;39(4):469–77. https://doi.org/10.1111/j.1365-2222.2009.03207.x.
84. Rispens T, et al. Mechanism of immunoglobulin G4 Fab-arm exchange. J Am Chem Soc. 2011;133(26):10302–11. https://doi.org/10.1021/ja203638y.
85. Legatowicz-Koprowska M. IgG4-related disease: why is it so important? Centr-Eur J Immunol. 2018;43(2):204–8. https://doi.org/10.5114/ceji.2018.77391.
86. Nirula A, et al. What is IgG4? A review of the biology of a unique immunoglobulin subtype. Curr Opin Rheumatol. 2011;23(1):119–24. https://doi.org/10.1097/BOR.0b013e3283412fd4.
87. Watanabe T, et al. Toll-like receptor activation in basophils contributes to the development of IgG4-related disease. J Gastroenterol. 2013;48(2):247–53.

88. Furukawa S, et al. Preferential M2 macrophages contribute to fibrosis in IgG4-related dacryoadenitis and sialoadenitis, so-called Mikulicz's disease. Clin Immunol (Orlando, Fla). 2015;156(1):9–18. https://doi.org/10.1016/j.clim.2014.10.008.
89. Furukawa S, et al. Interleukin-33 produced by M2 macrophages and other immune cells contributes to Th2 immune reaction of IgG4-related disease. Sci Rep. 2017;7(1):1–10.
90. Kino-Ohsaki JUNKO, et al. Serum antibodies to carbonic anhydrase I and II in patients with idiopathic chronic pancreatitis and Sjogren's syndrome. Gastroenterology. 1996;110(5):1579–86.
91. Okazaki K, et al. Autoimmune-related pancreatitis is associated with autoantibodies and a Th1/Th2-type cellular immune response. Gastroenterology. 2000;118(3):573–81.
92. Asada M, et al. Identification of a novel autoantibody against pancreatic secretory trypsin inhibitor in patients with autoimmune pancreatitis. Pancreas. 2006;33(1):20–6. https://doi.org/10.1097/01.mpa.0000226881.48204.fd.
93. Du H, et al. Prohibitin is involved in patients with IgG4 related disease. PLoS One. 2015;10(5):e0125331.
94. Hubers LM, et al. Annexin A11 is targeted by IgG4 and IgG1 autoantibodies in IgG4-related disease. Gut. 2018;67(4):728–35.
95. Shiokawa M, et al. Laminin 511 is a target antigen in autoimmune pancreatitis. Sci Transl Med. 2018;10,453:eaaq0997. https://doi.org/10.1126/scitranslmed.aaq0997.
96. Perugino CA, et al. Identification of galectin-3 as an autoantigen in patients with IgG4-related disease. J Allergy Clin Immunol. 2019;143(2):736–745.e6. https://doi.org/10.1016/j.jaci.2018.05.011.
97. Liu H, et al. Disease severity linked to increase in autoantibody diversity in IgG4-related disease. Arthritis Rheumatol (Hoboken, NJ). 2020;72(4):687–93. https://doi.org/10.1002/art.41140.
98. Maillette de Buy Wenniger LJ, et al. Immunoglobulin G4+ clones identified by next-generation sequencing dominate the B cell receptor repertoire in immunoglobulin G4 associated cholangitis. Hepatology (Baltimore, Md). 2013;57(6):2390–8. https://doi.org/10.1002/hep.26232.
99. Mattoo H, et al. De novo oligoclonal expansions of circulating plasmablasts in active and relapsing IgG4-related disease. J Allergy Clin Immunol. 2014;134(3):679–87. https://doi.org/10.1016/j.jaci.2014.03.034.
100. Lin W, et al. Circulating plasmablasts/plasma cells: a potential biomarker for IgG4-related disease. Arthritis Res Ther. 2017;19(1):1–14.
101. Koyabu M, et al. Analysis of regulatory T cells and IgG4-positive plasma cells among patients of IgG4-related sclerosing cholangitis and autoimmune liver diseases. J Gastroenterol. 2010;45(7):732–41. https://doi.org/10.1007/s00535-010-0199-3.
102. Ito F, et al. IL-10+ T follicular regulatory cells are associated with the pathogenesis of IgG4-related disease. Immunol Lett. 2019;207:56–63.
103. Jeannin P, et al. IgE versus IgG4 production can be differentially regulated by IL-10. J Immunol. 1998;160(7):3555–61.
104. Cheuk W, Chan JKC. IgG4-related sclerosing disease: a critical appraisal of an evolving clinicopathologic entity. Adv Anat Pathol. 2010;17(5):303–32. https://doi.org/10.1097/PAP.0b013e3181ee63ce.
105. Wallace ZS, et al. Clinical phenotypes of IgG4-related disease: an analysis of two international cross-sectional cohorts. Ann Rheum Dis. 2019;78(3):406–12. https://doi.org/10.1136/annrheumdis-2018-214603.
106. Björnsson E, et al. Immunoglobulin G4 associated cholangitis: description of an emerging clinical entity based on review of the literature. Hepatology (Baltimore, Md). 2007;45(6):1547–54. https://doi.org/10.1002/hep.21685.
107. Tanaka A, et al. Clinical features, response to treatment, and outcomes of IgG4-related sclerosing cholangitis. Clin Gastroenterol Hepatol. 2017;15(6):920–6.

108. Lanzillotta M, et al. Clinical phenotypes of IgG4-related disease reflect different prognostic outcomes. Rheumatology. 2020;59(9):2435–42.
109. Madhusudhan KS, et al. IgG4-related sclerosing cholangitis: a clinical and imaging review. Am J Roentgenol. 2019;213(6):1221–31.
110. Oseini AM, et al. Utility of serum immunoglobulin G4 in distinguishing immunoglobulin G4-associated cholangitis from cholangiocarcinoma. Hepatology (Baltimore, Md). 2011;54(3):940–8. https://doi.org/10.1002/hep.24487.
111. Vlachou PA, et al. IgG4-related sclerosing disease: autoimmune pancreatitis and extrapancreatic manifestations. Radiographics. 2011;31(5):1379–402.
112. Arikawa S, et al. Comparison of sclerosing cholangitis with autoimmune pancreatitis and infiltrative extrahepatic cholangiocarcinoma: multidetector-row computed tomography findings. Jpn J Radiol. 2010;28(3):205–13.
113. Ohara H, et al. Clinical diagnostic criteria of IgG4-related sclerosing cholangitis 2012. J Hepato-Biliary-Pancreatic Sci. 2012;19(5):536–42.
114. Ghazale A, et al. Immunoglobulin G4-associated cholangitis: clinical profile and response to therapy. Gastroenterology. 2008;134(3):706–15. https://doi.org/10.1053/j.gastro.2007.12.009.
115. Nakazawa T, et al. Clinical diagnostic criteria for IgG4-related sclerosing cholangitis 2020:(Revision of the clinical diagnostic criteria for IgG4-related sclerosing cholangitis 2012). J Hepato—Biliary—Pancreatic Sci. 2021;28:3.
116. Drazilova S, et al. IgG4-related sclerosing cholangitis: rarely diagnosed, but not a rare disease. Can J Gastroenterol Hepatol. 2021;2021:1959832. https://doi.org/10.1155/2021/1959832.
117. Löhr J-M, et al. European Guideline on IgG4-related digestive disease–UEG and SGF evidence-based recommendations. United European Gastroenterol J. 2020;8(6):637–66.
118. Hart PA, et al. Treatment of relapsing autoimmune pancreatitis with immunomodulators and rituximab: the Mayo Clinic experience. Gut. 2013;62(11):1607–15.

Chapter 13
Peritoneal Diseases

Paul H. McClelland and Andrew M. Blakely

13.1 Introduction

Inflammatory disorders of the peritoneum and mesentery are rare and unique clinicopathological entities that represent a multitude of different presentations and disease processes. Broadly, these diseases can be divided into two major categories: inflammatory conditions that arise from multisystem rheumatologic or vasculitic disorders, or inflammatory conditions that arise intrinsically within the peritoneum. For the former, peritoneal inflammation often presents in the context of a broader syndrome and may be part of a constellation of symptoms, which can facilitate diagnosis and treatment. For the latter, inflammation arises within the peritoneum primarily without other characteristic features, which can hinder diagnosis and increase the likelihood of late-stage disease presentation. In either case, generalized peritoneal inflammation can have a broad impact on multiple organ systems, which underscores the importance of understanding the pathophysiology and treatment of diseases that cause this type of broad inflammatory process.

13.2 Multisystem Rheumatologic Disorders

To date, several multisystem inflammatory disorders have been described as having peritoneum-specific manifestations of disease (*see* Table 13.1). In these scenarios, peritoneal inflammation is rarely seen in isolation, and the presence of peritoneal

P. H. McClelland · A. M. Blakely (✉)
Center for Cancer Research, National Cancer Institute, National Institutes of Health, Bethesda, MD, USA
e-mail: andrew.blakely@nih.gov

M. Tadros et al. (eds.), *GI Diseases Associated with Rheumatological and Vasculitic Conditions*, Clinical Gastroenterology,
https://doi.org/10.1007/978-3-032-07868-1_13

Table 13.1 Comparison of peritoneal manifestations in multisystem rheumatologic disorders

Common characteristic: Found in the context of other nonperitoneal disease			
	Malignant Atrophic Papulosis (MAP)	Lupus Peritonitis (LP)	Systemic Sclerosis (SSc)
Defining characteristics	Unique skin lesions (umbilicated with central necrosis and surrounding telangiectasias) Serosal peritoneal lesions	Acute or chronic sterile ascites Systemic inflammatory signs (e.g., fever)	Sclerosis and dysmotility of the gastrointestinal tract SIBO PCI
Epidemiology	Very rare: fewer than 300 cases reported More MAP cases than BAP cases	Young to middle-aged females Occurs in 0.2–14.2% of SLE patients	Middle-aged females Diffuse vs. limited subtypes
Pathophysiology	Unknown Thrombotic vs. vasculitic vs. endothelial	Likely similar to lupus pericarditis/pleuritis B cell-mediated deposition of immune complexes in mesothelium	Can occur throughout the GI tract Limited direct involvement of the peritoneum
Diagnosis	Physical examination (skin lesions) Diagnostic laparoscopy with biopsy	Acute: rapid-onset ascites with signs of lupus flare Chronic: slow, insidious ascites	ANA, ACA Upper GI radiographic series Abdominal CT scan
Management	No universally effective treatment Possible efficacy with eculizumab with treprostinil	High-dose steroids, followed by taper Methylprednisolone with cyclophosphamide for refractory cases	Conservative management if possible Antibiotics for SIBO
Prognosis	Mortality 72–75% High rate of bowel perforation once serosal lesions emerge	Generally favorable prognosis	Associated with higher morbidity with other disorders

BAP benign atrophic papulosis, *SLE* systemic lupus erythematosus, *GI* gastrointestinal, *ANA* antinuclear antibodies, *ACA* anticentromere antibodies, *CT* computed tomography, *SIBO* small intestine bacterial overgrowth, *PCI* pneumatosis cystoides intestinalis

symptoms may be an indicator of progression or increased severity of the primary condition. Management of these cases typically revolves around treatment of the underlying disease, with peritonitis treated for symptomatic relief.

13.2.1 Malignant Atrophic Papulosis (Köhlmeier-Degos Disease)

Malignant atrophic papulosis (MAP) is a rare vasculopathy affecting small- and medium-sized blood vessels, primarily known for its characteristic dermatologic lesions. First described by Köhlmeier in 1941 [1], this disease was subsequently categorized as a separate disorder by Degos et al. the following year [2] and has since been discovered to have visceral and neurologic manifestations in addition to its classic epidermal form [3–6]. In all scenarios, characteristic lesions typically appear as small (2–5 mm), avascular, umbilicated porcelain-white papules with telangiectatic rims, although more complex lesions with additional features have also been described [4–7]. To date, relatively little is known about the pathogenesis and natural history of this disease, although there is growing evidence of a prognostic divide between skin-only benign atrophic papulosis (BAP) versus systemic malignant disease, for which peritoneal spread is the most common feature [6, 8, 9].

13.2.1.1 Epidemiology

MAP is a rare disease, with fewer than 300 cases reported in the literature [4, 8]. Most cases occur in adults aged 20–50 years, with approximately equal distribution between male and female sexes [4, 5, 8–10]. Rarely, MAP has also been described in young children, with anecdotal evidence of patients presenting with symptoms at 7 months [11] and 3 weeks [9]. Cases have been described in a wide variety of locales, without specific preponderance among racial or ethnic groups [4, 6, 12–17]. Historically, MAP has been more prevalent than its benign counterpart (64% of total cases) [4, 18], and conversion rates from BAP to MAP range between 29% and 60% [8]. Among patients with MAP, the most common sites of systemic spread are the abdominal viscera (73–100%), followed by the central nervous system (CNS, 22–64%). Additionally, there have been incidental findings of lesions located in the myocardium, pericardium, kidneys, bladder, lungs, pleura, liver, and pancreas, usually discovered during postmortem examination [5, 8].

13.2.1.2 Etiology and Pathophysiology

In general, histopathologic features seen on biopsy suggest localized ischemic necrosis to be a common feature of MAP-associated lesions. While findings vary between patients, characteristics of MAP at the cellular level generally include wedge-shaped central necrosis, arteriolar obliteration, increased mucin deposition, disarrangement of collagen fibers, and increased surrounding superficial vascularity [3, 5]. In skin lesions in particular, these features are typically accompanied by epidermal atrophy and hyperkeratosis [12–15, 17], whereas peritoneal lesions more commonly demonstrate serosal or subserosal involvement with mucosal sparing, often with endothelialitis, perivascular inflammation, microhemorrhages, fibro-obliterative healing, hyalinization, and macrophage-rich inflammatory infiltration (Figs. 13.1 and 13.2) [6]. These characteristic features are presumed to derive from autoimmune processes, although the exact pathophysiology behind these findings has yet to be determined.

To date, three primary mechanisms have been explored as possible drivers of MAP-associated localized ischemia: coagulopathy, vasculitis, and endothelial

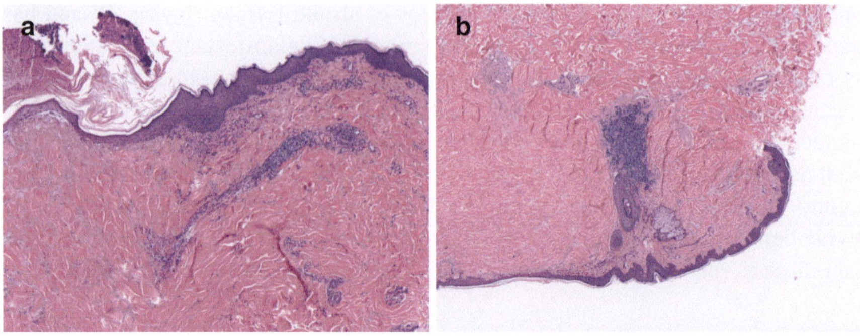

Fig. 13.1 Histopathologic slides from dermal punch biopsies of cutaneous MAP lesions. Characteristic findings include (**a**) irregularity of the basement membrane, type IV collagen and mucin deposition, and perivascular inflammation with $CD3^+$ lymphocytic infiltration [H&E, ×10], as well as (**b**) hyalinization of vessel walls with evidence of endothelial cell injury [H&E, ×10]

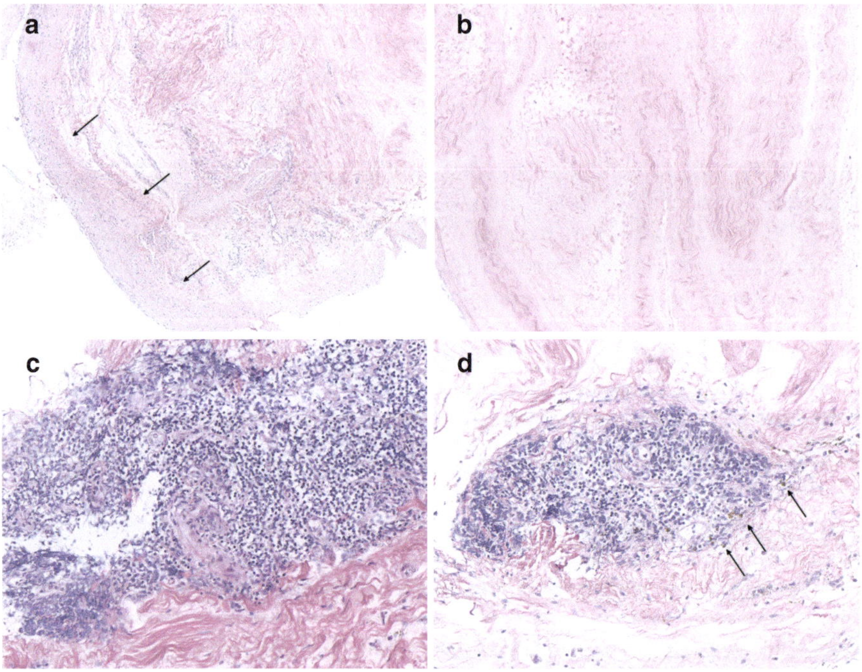

Fig. 13.2 Histopathologic slides from biopsies of peritoneal MAP lesions. Characteristic findings include (**a**) fibrotic thickening of the peritoneum (arrows) [H&E, ×10], (**b**) replacement of mesothelial tissue with hyalinized scarring [H&E, ×10], (**c**) perivascular lymphoid aggregates with small vessel wall thickening [H&E, ×40], and (**d**) vessel wall fibrosis and necrosis with stigmata of localized hemorrhage [H&E, ×40]

dysfunction [3, 5, 19, 20]. Evidence supporting all three of these theoretical models has been reported in the literature, but no consensus yet exists regarding a most likely cause of disease. Moreover, these proposed mechanisms are not mutually exclusive, and clinical signs and symptoms may arise from a combination of pathologic processes. This fact has led some investigators to classify MAP/BAP not as its own disease but rather as a complex and distinct manifestation of systemic lupus erythematosis (SLE), although this claim also has yet to be verified [5].

The evidence in support of a primary thrombo-occlusive etiology for MAP stems from systemic increases in fibrinogen and plasminogen activator inhibitor observed in select patients with the disease, as well as local loss of fibrinolytic activity observed within characteristic lesions. These findings have been pooled with additional evidence that patients with MAP occasionally have lower levels of systemic plasminogen and tissue plasminogen activator, while a small minority of patients have further been shown to express specific lupus anticoagulant and anticardiolipin antibodies, promoting a hypercoagulable state [3, 5]. More recently, a 2013 study demonstrated positive staining for stromal cell-derived factor (SDF)-1/CXCL12 in the perivascular, intravascular, and perineural areas of MAP lesions in two patients, which may indicate increased localized platelet activity due to stimulation of megakaryocyte precursors [21]. Moreover, regardless of precipitating factors, several patients have demonstrated symptomatic improvement after empiric treatment with antiplatelet therapy, which alludes to a thrombo-occlusive origin of disease [17]. However, despite these findings, the majority of patients with MAP present with a normal coagulation cascade and have no detectable platelet or fibrinolytic abnormalities, implying that coagulopathy alone cannot fully explain this disease process [3, 5].

Direct vasculitis has also been proposed as a possible cause of MAP, with several historical microscopy-based studies suggesting that autoimmune endothelial disruption drives thrombosis and subsequent ischemia in MAP-related lesions [22, 23]. This has since been corroborated in a 2011 study of 4 MAP patients that demonstrated increased C5b-9 deposits, interferon-α levels, and tubuloreticular inclusions in the vessel walls of cutaneous, gastrointestinal, and brain vessel lesions; these findings were discovered in the context of increased interferon gene signatures in peripheral blood mononuclear cells, suggesting a broad autoimmune reaction against small vessels in these tissues [20]. Further studies have shown SLE-like deposition of IgM on affected vessels in select patients with MAP, again suggesting that direct autoimmune injury to small vessels drives disease proliferation [19]. However, definitive classification of MAP as a primary vasculitis is undercut by the fact that the elastic lamina of affected small arteries typically remains intact, systemic autoimmune markers are generally low in patients presenting with MAP, and patents generally do not respond significantly to corticosteroid therapy [5].

Finally, intrinsic endothelial dysfunction has been linked to the centralized necrosis seen in MAP lesions, with endothelial swelling in particular considered to be a contributing factor [24]. This theory has primarily been supported by documented observation of tubuloreticular and intracytoplasmic inclusions within endothelial cells and small vessel walls, which have been hypothesized to arise from either primary autoimmune origins or secondary viral or bacterial causes [7]. To date, however, no viral DNA has been successfully isolated from MAP lesions [25], and the precise mechanism by which this type of endothelial swelling causes downstream necrosis in MAP remains unexplained [3, 5].

It has further been suggested that there may be a hereditary component to MAP, with limited data showing a possible pattern of autosomal dominant inheritance among patients with the disease [26, 27]. Currently, no genetic mutations have been linked to MAP, with inherited disease only appearing to occur in a minority of patients (9–23%) [4, 8, 18].

13.2.1.3 Clinical Description and Diagnosis

Grossly, MAP/BAP typically presents as multiple asymptomatic or pruritic lesions on the skin, with initial presence ranging from a few isolated lesions to hundreds emerging simultaneously (Fig. 13.3). Cutaneous involvement usually includes the trunk and/or the extremities, with characteristic sparing of the palms, soles, face, scalp, and genitalia. Lesions first appear as pink macules 2–5 mm in diameter, which gradually morph into erythematous, round, and firm papules within the first few days of symptoms [5, 12, 17, 28]. Over weeks, these papules eventually develop central necrosis and involute, resulting the emergence of a scaly white center with surrounding inflammation and hypervascularity around the papular rim, creating the pathognomonic umbilicated lesion for this disease [3–5, 16, 29]. Ultimately, this inflammation recedes, leaving a residual central white scar. Over the course of this evolution, lesions typically remain under 1 cm in size, with lesions greater than 2 cm only rarely described in the literature [30]. Diagnosis is generally made by gross examination of lesions, confirmed by punch biopsy.

Aside from rare exceptions [31], systemic disease only emerges after cutaneous involvement, and most patients presenting with MAP already have an established diagnosis of BAP from prior diagnostic workup. On presentation, these patients are

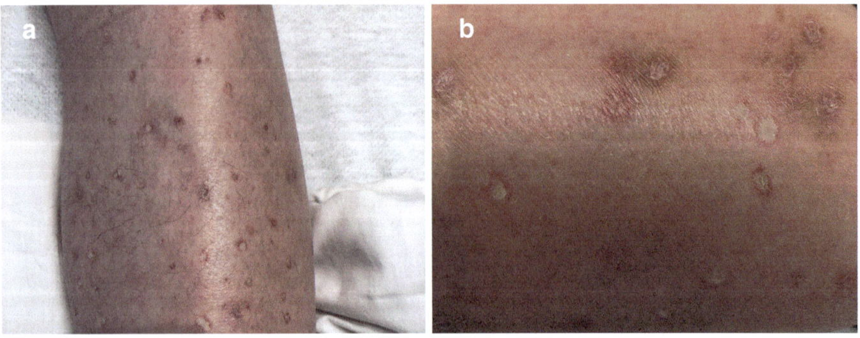

Fig. 13.3 Macroscopic examination of characteristic MAP-related cutaneous lesions. Lesions typically present as numerous small pruritic papules with central necrosis, surrounded by a telangiectatic rim. Pictured here, (**a**) lower extremity, and (**b**) closeup of upper extremity skin

usually asymptomatic, but since peritoneal spread occurs in more than 73% of patients with MAP, many experience nonspecific gastrointestinal symptoms such as abdominal pain, nausea, melena, and diarrhea [5, 8, 12–15]. In more severe cases, other symptoms such as pancreatitis, gastritis, peptic ulceration, ileus, and dysentery may also manifest, depending where symptomatic lesions are located [3–5].

If intraperitoneal involvement is suspected, diagnostic laparoscopy is the procedure of choice, allowing for visual assessment of serosal lesions, staging of peritoneal disease burden, and biopsy of suspect lesions if indicated. Much like cutaneous lesions, MAP-associated peritoneal lesions are characterized by an erythematous and hypervascular rim surrounding a central, white-colored infarct, which can potentially be found on any peritoneum-lined surface within the abdomen (Fig. 13.4). The evolution of serosal lesions from initial appearance up to the time of perforation is an area of ongoing investigation [3–5]. While biopsy of the parietal peritoneum confers minimal morbidity and is commonly performed, biopsy of serosal lesions

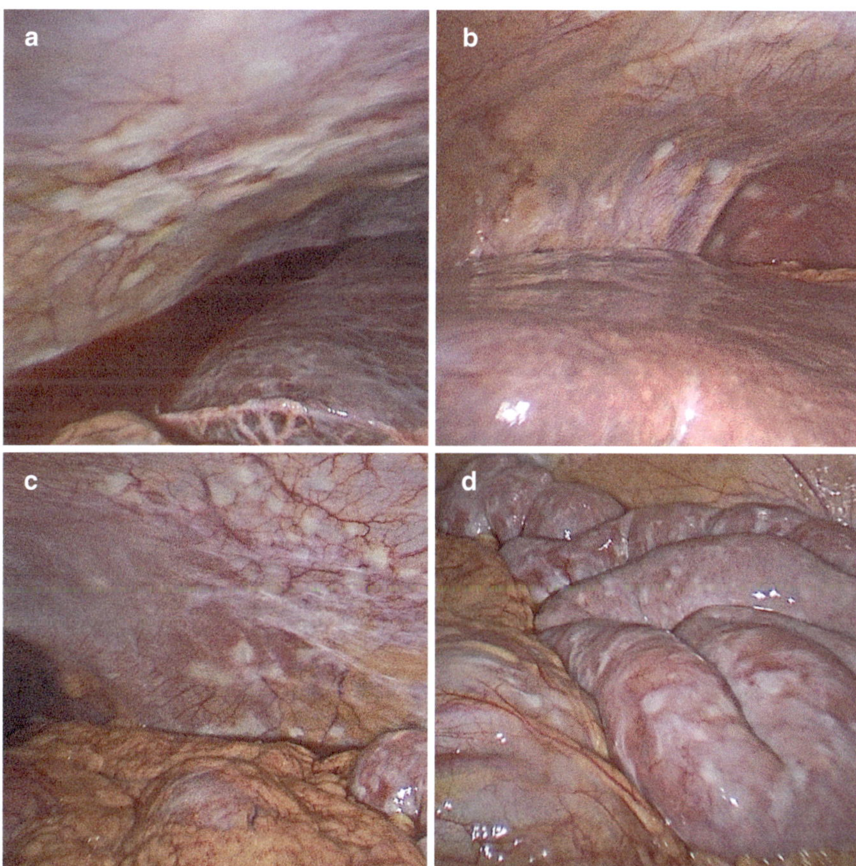

Fig. 13.4 Macroscopic examination of characteristic MAP-related lesions in the (**a**) parietal peritoneum, (**b**) subdiaphragmatic peritoneum, (**c**) omentum, and (**d**) small bowel serosa

compromises the bowel integrity and is thus generally avoided. Adjunctive evaluation with upper endoscopy, capsule endoscopy, and colonoscopy may provide an assessment from the mucosal perspective to identify transmural involvement, which is a putative precursor to bowel perforation; however, the value of endoscopic evaluation remains to be determined [6, 28]. If significant, serosal infarcts can lead to compromise and perforation of the bowel, which in turn can lead to peritonitis and death if left untreated [3, 5, 6, 8]. In these settings, clinical adjuncts such as computed tomography and serial blood draws can be useful to localize sites of inflammation and rule out intraabdominal collections or perforation, depending on patient stability [13]. The role of prophylactic formal bowel resection to avoid perforation remains unclear, particularly in multifocal serosal disease arising from a systemic disease process [3, 5, 6].

In patients with CNS manifestations of disease (22–64% of total MAP patients), infarcts generally occur in the brain and spinal cord, with symptoms corresponding to the location of neurovascular compromise [8, 32]. As a result, symptoms can vary widely among patients, with optic neuritis and its sequelae occurring most frequently [5]. Other neurologic deficits have also been reported, including hemiparesis, aphasia, monoplegia, and altered sensorium [32]. Like peritoneal disease, MAP-associated neurologic lesions rarely appear without initial cutaneous signs, with any definitive diagnosis of neural tissue infarction occurring in the postmortem setting [3, 8]. Prior to this, neurologic workup depends heavily on the location and severity of symptoms and can involve computed tomography, magnetic resonance imaging, optical examination, electroencephalogram, and electromyography, among other diagnostic tests [13]. In some cases, lumbar puncture with analysis of the cerebrospinal fluid (CSF) can be used to track progression of CNS disease, with early cases usually showing no abnormalities and more advanced cases demonstrating elevated CSF protein levels with increased total leukocyte counts [32, 33].

In rare cases of occult disease, it has been suggested that laboratory values may serve as a useful adjunct for diagnosis of MAP. In a 2021 systematic review of 105 patients with MAP or BAP diagnosis, Lu et al. found that combined elevated serum erythrocyte sedimentation rate and serum C-reactive protein were significantly elevated in MAP patients compared to BAP patients (27.1% vs. 3.6%), which was independently predictive of systemic involvement of disease [OR 21.3, 95% CI 2.62 to >100]. In contrast, antinuclear antibody and/or hypocomplementemia were similar between the two groups and did not yield a statistically significant correlation [4].

13.2.1.4 Management

To date, no universally effective treatment exists for MAP. Despite its presumed autoimmune origin, limited trials of immunosuppressive agents such as corticosteroids, methotrexate, tacrolimus, cyclosporine A, dapsone, azathioprine, aminosalicylates, thalidomide, and intravenous immunoglobulin have been largely ineffective [3, 4]. Moreover, immunosuppressive regimens have been found to worsen MAP symptoms in isolated cases [27]. Other treatments using combined antiplatelet therapy (e.g., aspirin and clopidogrel) have demonstrated limited efficacy in reducing and preventing skin lesions in some patients, but these treatments have not demonstrated similar efficacy in treating systemic lesions [3, 17].

More recently, biologic therapy with monoclonal antibodies has been trialed to treat MAP, with mixed success. Eculizumab, a complement inhibitor, was initially proposed as a potentially effective therapy after findings of extensive C5b-9 deposition in MAP lesions [20]. Patients subsequently undergoing treatment with eculizumab were found to have significant alleviation of symptoms, with several patients documented as no longer requiring intensive care within days after initiation of therapy. Moreover, one patient in particular has been reported to achieve durable 5-year survival after receiving 61 biweekly cycles of eculizumab monotherapy [34]. Despite this initial progress, later reports have indicated that eculizumab may only be effective if given to patients prior to the onset of significant complications (e.g., intestinal perforation), and eculizumab alone is unable to effect durable long-term survival, even if given early in disease course [35, 36]. Most recently, combination therapy with eculizumab and the prostacyclin vasodilator treprostinil has shown early promise as an effective, two-pronged therapy for treatment-refractory MAP, with Shapiro et al. describing rapid amelioration of progressive MAP in two patients when treprostinil was added to their existing eculizumab regimens [10]. In both cases, survival was extended to beyond 5 years despite having treatment-refractory and advanced disease, and both patients achieved good functional status at the time of publication [10, 36]. Despite these successes, a major barrier to the receipt of these biologic agents is their cost, as eculizumab is one of the most expensive therapeutic agents on the market and may be non-formulary for many health insurance plans.

Other biological agents such as infliximab, natalizumab, and rituximab have proven largely ineffective in treating MAP, although use of these medications has typically been limited to salvage scenarios in select patients [4, 33, 37, 38]. Unconventional therapies such as narrow-band ultraviolet light (UVB) have also been attempted in conjunction with systemic anticoagulation (aspirin, pentoxifylline, and warfarin), but this line of treatment has been similarly unsuccessful [14].

For patients presenting with significant sequelae of peritoneal disease such as gastrointestinal bleeding, bowel ischemia, bowel perforation, or peritonitis, standard endoscopic or surgical management is generally recommended. Low-level gastrointestinal bleeding without hemodynamic compromise can be managed endoscopically or with angioembolization, although these interventions have not been frequently reported in the literature [4]. Microperforation or contained collections without peritonitis can also be managed with systemic antibiotics as well as percutaneous or laparoscopic drainage; diagnostic laparoscopy is generally advised in this setting to assess the extent of bowel involvement, as well as to rule out occult lesions on other abdominal organs. Finally, frank perforation, free air on imaging, or peritonitis requires broad-spectrum antibiotic administration as well as emergent exploratory laparotomy, followed by bowel resection and possible ostomy creation to establish infectious source control [6, 8, 12–15, 17]. Ultimately, resection of all bowel with severe disease is generally recommended, with some studies advocating routine use of a second-look procedure for cases in which excessive ischemic damage has significantly compromised bowel wall integrity [39].

13.2.1.5 Prognosis

MAP is a highly lethal disease, with an overall mortality rate of 72–75% [4, 8, 18]. Long-term prognosis of atrophic papulosis is strongly linked to systemic disease, with approximately 62% of patients with MAP dying from intraperitoneal complications, 18% dying from CNS involvement, and 16% dying from pleuropericardial complications [5, 6, 12, 14, 15, 28, 40, 41]. In a 12-year, single-center prospective study of patients with atrophic papulosis, 8 of 11 patients (73%) with MAP experienced bowel perforation, contributing to a total mortality rate of 73% and a 5-year survival rate of 55% among this cohort; by contrast, there was no incidence of mortality among patients with exclusive skin disease. In this same study, patients with MAP were found to have a mean time of 0.9 years between onset of cutaneous symptoms and subsequent diagnosis of systemic disease, implying a rapidly degenerative clinical course among patients with more severe disease [8]. Similarly, a 2021 systematic review of 105 patients with atrophic papulosis found that 50% of patients with MAP had systemic involvement within 1 year after cutaneous onset, and median overall survival of MAP patients was 2.15 years (range 0.17–16.04 years). MAP patients in this study were found to have increased systemic inflammatory markers (ESR/CRP) and were less likely to have comorbid autoimmune connective tissue disease [4]. Despite these poor outcomes, early diagnosis and continuous monitoring can help extend survival by providing a longer window for supportive care, with additional time to trial potential therapeutic regimens.

13.2.2 Lupus Peritonitis

Systemic lupus erythematosis (SLE) is a complex autoimmune disorder affecting multiple organ systems. Serositis, in which mesothelial membranes become inflamed and produce effusions, is a diagnostic criterion of SLE and manifests in approximately 16% of total cases [42–44]. Among these cases, the pericardium and pleural membranes are the most common sites of disease, with primary lupus peritonitis (LP) only rarely described [44]. Despite this perceived infrequency, ascites occurs in 8–11% of SLE patients [45], and several autopsy studies have found stigmata of peritoneal inflammation in roughly 60–70% of SLE cases [46–48]. Moreover, while rare, LP can emerge as a presenting symptom of SLE, with symptoms manifesting either acutely in the form of rapid-onset peritonitis or chronically in the form of insidious massive ascites [49–57].

13.2.2.1 Epidemiology

SLE, and by extension LP, most commonly occurs in young women aged 25–44 years and is most frequently seen in individuals of African descent [58]. Clinically detectable LP occurs in relatively few patients (0.2–14.2% of cases) [59–61] and rarely manifests as a presenting symptom [52, 54, 59]. While data are limited, these rates of LP among SLE patients do not appear to vary significantly by race or ethnicity [59]. In a retrospective review of 67 SLE primary serositis cases among 37 patients, LP was responsible for 30% of episodes [62]. Due to the relative rarity of the condition, little data exist regarding prevalence of acute versus chronic LP, with most cases reported anecdotally [55, 63].

13.2.2.2 Etiology and Pathophysiology

Although the exact origin LP is unclear, it is thought to derive from similar processes as SLE-associated pericarditis or pleuritis. In particular, B cell-mediated deposition of autoantibodies has been proposed as a possible cause of this pathophysiology, with accumulation of immune complexes in mesothelial tissue subsequently driving complement activation and inflammation [63, 64]. Alternatively, direct vasculitis of small blood vessels in serous membranes has also been suggested as a possible cause of inflammation and subsequent symptomatology [52, 64]. In practice, empiric histopathological examination of inflamed peritoneal tissues has demonstrated perivascular aggregation of mononuclear and polynuclear leukocytes with apparent IgG and complement deposition, suggesting concomitant immune complex inflammation and vasculitis in this condition [51, 57, 63–68]. Therefore, these processes may work synergistically to weaken peritoneal integrity, induce adhesive disease, and produce inflammatory ascites.

In keeping with this model, direct analysis of LP-associated ascitic fluid has generally yielded high levels of leukocytes, anti-double-stranded DNA (anti-dsDNA) autoantibodies, and anti-nucleosome (anti-NCS) autoantibodies, as well as low complement levels [51, 63]. Cytokine profiling of LP-associated ascites has typically demonstrated high levels of IL-6 compared to other cytokines, which may be within normal limits or at elevated levels as well (IL-8, IL-10, TNF-α, IL-1β, MCP-1, and IGF-1) [63, 67].

Apolipoprotein A-1 has also been found to exist at high concentrations in LP-associated ascitic fluid, which is distinctive and may indicate an intrinsic anti-inflammatory response [67]. Together, these features are unique to LP-associated ascites and differentiate it from other potential causes of intraabdominal collections, such as SLE-associated nephrotic syndrome or bacterial peritonitis. Given that IL-6 is associated with endothelial cell permeability, this evidence may suggest a potential origin of the large effusions seen in these patients [69].

13.2.2.3 Clinical Description and Diagnosis

The most common symptom among all patients with LP is nonspecific abdominal pain, with some studies asserting that clinical or subclinical LP is a major contributor to abdominal pain complaints among SLE patients (35–79% of total cases) [59, 60]. Excluding this common symptom, clinical presentation of patients with LP varies substantially between individuals, with acute and chronic disease leading to significantly different presentations.

For patients suffering from acute LP, symptoms typically manifest as progressive, generalized, and severe abdominal pain over the course of 1–2 weeks, often accompanied by nausea/vomiting (82%) and diarrhea (65%) [59]. These symptoms usually coincide with abdominal distention due to rapid-onset accumulation of ascites, as well as diffuse tenderness to palpation [57, 70]. Patients may further present with signs and symptoms of systemic inflammation such as fever, chills, malaise, fatigue, myalgias, or arthralgias; other signs associated with SLE flare may also become apparent at this time (e.g., skin rashes) [53, 56, 57]. Due to the combination of fever, gastrointestinal upset, and acute abdominal pain with progressive distention, LP is easily mistaken for generalized peritonitis from appendicitis, bowel perforation/disruption, or other bacterial sources; however, vital signs are generally stable for these patients and leukocytosis is an uncommon feature [53, 59, 70].

By contrast, chronic LP most commonly manifests as the slow accumulation of intraabdominal ascites over months to years. These patients are typically asymptomatic aside from distention-related discomfort and have no concomitant systemic symptoms. Vital sign and basic laboratory findings are typically unremarkable for these patients, especially if receiving ongoing medical treatment for an established diagnosis of SLE [50–52, 55, 63].

Given the rarity of primary LP and the relatively higher prevalence of other sources of ascites, LP is typically a diagnosis of exclusion [51, 59, 63]. Moreover, the majority of patients presenting with LP have a preexisting diagnosis of SLE, which can aid in the subsequent diagnosis of LP [52, 53]. In both acute and chronic cases, routine laboratory workup with serum metabolic panels, complete blood counts, liver function tests, and urinalysis are indicated to rule out other potential sources of ascites. Similarly, while individual serum biomarkers have not been shown to correlate with presence of LP, biochemical workup with systemic lupus erythematosis disease activity index 2000 (SLEDAI-2K) scoring can also serve as a useful diagnostic adjunct since higher scores have been associated with active LP [59, 60, 63]. If findings are conflicting, further specialized laboratory testing can be performed to clarify diagnosis, such as serum CA-125 for pseudo-pseudo Meigs syndrome [54].

In addition to laboratory testing, imaging with abdominal ultrasound and computed tomography is essential to confirm ascites and rule out other possible disease processes. These modalities are also helpful in evaluating foci of disease and determining the need for more invasive intervention (e.g., surgery) [59]. Ascitic fluid sampling typically yields yellow/green, sterile, and thinly exudative ascites, which can further assist in diagnosis; however, routine diagnostic paracentesis is not generally indicated [53, 54, 57, 67].

13.2.2.4 Management

As with many SLE-related conditions, immunosuppression with corticosteroids remains a mainstay of therapy, particularly in the treatment of acute LP. Standard dosing typically includes an initial pulsing of intravenous methylprednisolone 1000 mg daily for up to 3 days, followed by prednisolone taper for 1–2 weeks afterwards [52, 54, 59]. Initial treatment with high-dose prednisolone (40 mg daily) has also been described, with mixed response rates [63, 70]. Adjunctive agents such as hydroxychloroquine have also been used in both the outpatient setting during steroid taper [52, 57] or as monotherapy [68], with good effect.

For treatment-refractory disease, combination therapies are recommended. The most common of these treatments involves the addition of cyclophosphamide to methylprednisolone therapy, although azathioprine has also proven effective in this context [71–73]. In these cases, temporizing measures such as diuresis and therapeutic paracentesis can be performed for supportive care or alleviation of symptoms [59]. For patients with deeply refractory disease, direct intraperitoneal injection of steroids has also been proposed as a possible strategy for treating LP, with one study reporting reduction of ascitic concentrations and complete remission of ascites in a single patient after receiving two doses of high-dose intraperitoneal dexamethasone (12 mg) [67]. Similarly, intraperitoneal injection of triamcinolone has also been shown to induce complete remission of refractory LP ascites in single-patient trials [74]. Outside of medical treatment, surgical intervention is rarely employed for LP and is only indicated in the context of severe vascular compromise or significant end-organ damage [59, 63].

13.2.2.5 Prognosis

Mortality from LP is uncommon, with most patients responding well to therapy [49–57, 59]. For patients who are unresponsive to therapy, cause of death usually occurs due to respiratory failure from increased intraabdominal pressure or prerenal failure from intravascular depletion [63]. In a single-center retrospective review of 16 patients with LP, Maruyama et al. were able to distinguish two LP subtypes based on radiologic involvement of the large or small intestine, with the aim of determining clinical predictors of morbidity and mortality: per this analysis, patients with large intestine LP were older, and had higher frequency of bowel wall thickening, and were more likely to present with features of intestinal pseudo-obstruction. However, patients with involvement of the small intestine were more likely to undergo treatment with corticosteroids, and complication and recurrence rates were comparable between the two groups [59].

13.2.3 Systemic Sclerosis

Systemic sclerosis (SSc) is a multisystem autoimmune disorder characterized by pervasive inflammation of connective tissues, excessive collagen deposition within the skin and internal organs, and vasculopathy with small-vessel proliferation. While the skin is the most commonly affected organ in SSc, gastrointestinal manifestations comprise a significant proportion of disease burden, with up to 90% of total cases involving some portion of the alimentary tract [75]. Within the abdomen, SSc is associated with decreased motility and chronic inflammation of the esophagus, stomach, small/large intestine, and anorectum, which can lead to widespread dysfunction and subsequent intraperitoneal complications [76]. In general, these complications do not involve the peritoneum directly but rather are either the direct sequelae of gastrointestinal pathology or the byproduct of long-term inflammatory processes within the intraabdominal space.

13.2.3.1 Epidemiology

SSc is a rare disease, with a historical prevalence of 38–443 total cases per million individuals and an incidence of 0.27–23 new cases per million per year [77]. The typical age of diagnosis is between 33 and 60 years, and there is significant female preponderance (7:1 F:M sex ratio), as well as increased representation among patients of African or indigenous descent in Western countries [77–79]. SSc is typically categorized by diffuse and limited subtypes, with gastrointestinal involvement occurring with equal frequency between these two groups [80]. While any part of the alimentary tract can be affected by SSc, the esophagus is the most commonly involved organ in presenting cases, followed by the stomach and small/large intestine [76, 81]. Peritoneal involvement is usually linked to gastrointestinal disease course and thus has a similar epidemiologic profile [82].

13.2.3.2 Etiology and Pathophysiology

Direct involvement of SSc in peritoneal mesothelial tissue is uncommon, and consistent histopathological peritoneal findings have yet to be established for the disease [82–84]. In a 1969 autopsy-based study of 58 SSc patients matched with equal controls, no significant difference was found in rates of gross peritonitis or peritoneal adhesions between SSc patients and their normal counterparts (7% vs. 9% and 23% vs. 28%, respectively), and histopathologic peritoneal findings were comparable between groups. In contrast, rates of pleural and pericardial involvement were consistently higher among SSc patients in this study, with increased evidence of fibrosis and adhesive disease observed during gross and histopathologic evaluation [85]

Because of this limited direct involvement, the majority of peritoneal pathology seen in SSc occurs indirectly via primary gastrointestinal pathophysiology. Like skin manifestations in SSc, the exact mechanism of SSc-related gastroenteritis is unknown, although current evidence suggests that anti-kinetochore autoimmune activity and vasculopathy are likely drivers of disease [86–88]. This autoimmune activity manifests in the gut as CD4+ T cell-mediated inflammation of the bowel wall, with infiltration of the lamina propria, vasculopathy and telangiectatic proliferation, mucosal atrophy and erosion, myenteric denervation, and replacement of smooth muscle cells in the muscularis with collagenous fibrous deposits [75]. If allowed to progress, these pathologic changes can manifest extraluminally and affect the greater intraperitoneal space.

A common effect of gastrointestinal SSc is bacterial overgrowth, which predominantly occurs in the small intestine and affects 12–56% of SSc patients [75, 89, 90]. As a primary disorder, bacterial overgrowth can cause abdominal pain, nausea/vomiting, diarrhea, and bloating, with advanced cases associated with malabsorptive signs such as weight loss, steatorrhea, and nutritional deficiencies [89, 91]. Extraluminally, bacterial overgrowth combined with ischemic damage and atrophy of the bowel wall can lead to pneumatosis cystoides intestinalis (PCI), which involves the formation of air-filled cysts within the intestinal wall that may rupture and cause benign pneumoperitoneum [82, 90, 92–96]. On rare occasions, this benign pneumoperitoneum can occur without any predisposing signs of PCI [97]. Increased bacterial burden within the gut can also increase the risk of spontaneous bacterial peritonitis (SBP), the likelihood of which is increased further by concomitant inflammatory disorders associated with SSc such as primary biliary cirrhosis (PBC) [98]. Finally, gastrointestinal SSc increases the risk of perforated viscus, which can also lead to significant bacterial peritonitis; this complication is much rarer than PCI and is associated with clear signs of peritoneal irritation such as fever, leukocytosis, abdominal guarding, rebound tenderness, and sepsis [96, 99–101].

Despite the apparent lack of direct involvement in the peritoneum, some studies have suggested that SSc may also play an indirect role in peritonitis by potentiating extraluminal intraabdominal inflammatory processes. This effect is suggested by the upregulation of SSc-associated pro-fibrotic growth factors such as transforming growth factor-β (TGF-β), connective tissue growth factor (CTGF), and insulin-like growth factor 1 (IGF-1) throughout the abdomen [90, 93], as well as the increased expression of other molecules known to promote peritoneal fibrosis specifically. These additional molecules include signaling molecules (e.g., lysophosphatidic acid, LPA), transcription factors (e.g., MKL/myocardin-like protein 1, MKL-1), cytoskeleton modulators (e.g., rho-associated protein kinase, rho-ROCK), and collagen chaperones (e.g., heat shock protein 47, HSP47), among other factors [102, 103]. Together, these molecules create a pro-inflammatory, pro-fibrotic environment in the abdominal cavity, which may prime tissues for additional inflammation after insult or complicate ongoing chronic inflammatory processes (*see* "Primary Peritoneal Inflammatory Disorders"). This environment may also exacerbate fibrosis attributable to iatrogenic causes, such as abdominopelvic radiation therapy [104].

In addition to inflammatory peritoneal conditions originating from the gastrointestinal tract, SSc has also been associated with accumulation of intraabdominal ascites, albeit by indirect pathology. For example, a potential link between SSc and portal hypertension-related ascites has been described in select cases, although a clear relationship between the two disorders has not been established [105, 106]. Similarly, SSc has been known to cause ascites secondary to nephrotic syndrome from renal failure [107].

13.2.3.3 Clinical Description and Diagnosis

Approximately one-half of SSc-associated gastrointestinal cases are symptomatic [108, 109], and intraperitoneal signs and symptoms vary significantly depending on which gastrointestinal organs are involved. For symptomatic patients, most complaints stem from long-term dysmotility and chronic inflammation of the gut, which classically manifest as dysphagia, symptomatic reflux, generalized abdominal pain, nausea/vomiting, malabsorption, poor nutrition, or obstructive symptoms. Due to the chronic nature of SSc, the majority of cases present non-emergently. Moreover, gastrointestinal symptoms may present in the broader context of multisystem disease, so characteristic signs in other organs such as the skin, lungs, heart, and kidneys may help to narrow diagnosis [81, 90, 110].

Abdominal imaging plays a major role in the assessment of intraperitoneal SSc. Contrast-enhanced radiographic studies including upper gastrointestinal imaging series with small bowel follow-through are commonly used to assess bowel motility, and esophagogastroduodenoscopy and manometry studies are further used to investigate the location and extent of gastrointestinal involvement. For generalized intraperitoneal signs, cross-sectional imaging such as computed tomography scans can help detect the presence of pneumoperitoneum or ascites, as well as bowel wall thickening and signs of fibrosis. In cases of SSc-related pneumoperitoneum, benign versus fulminant peritonitis is difficult to distinguish on imaging alone, and clinical correlation is often necessary [82, 92, 93]. Diagnostic paracentesis and peritoneal fluid analysis can be used to confirm the presence of SBP, with bacterial colonization in the absence of an obvious source as a defining characteristic [90].

Other imaging findings related to SSc-related peritoneal inflammation include calcification of abdominal lymph nodes and occasionally the peritoneum itself [111], as well as low-grade ^{18}F-fluorodeoxyglucose (^{18}F-FDG) uptake on positron emission tomography [84]. When combined with SSc-related fibrosis and bowel wall thickening, these findings can sometimes give a similar appearance to peritoneal carcinomatosis, which may merit further investigation with diagnostic laparoscopy and peritoneal biopsy [82, 84, 92].

Laboratory tests can further serve as an adjunct to clarify diagnosis and monitor long-term progress. Serum antinuclear antibodies (ANA) and anticentromere antibodies (ACA) are commonly associated with SSc, and anti-topoisomerase I antibodies (anti-Scl-70) and anti-RNA polymerase III antibodies in particular are associated with diffuse SSc [112]. In addition, markers of systemic inflammation are generally elevated in patients experience SSc symptoms (e.g., rheumatoid factor, CRP, ESR) [113]. Furthermore, serum protein electrophoresis will typically reveal elevated levels of γ-globulins in these patients [114].

13.2.3.4 Management

Treatment of SSc-related peritoneal manifestations depends on underlying gastrointestinal involvement. Invasive or surgical interventions are typically not required except in cases of significant pathology, such as massive ascites (paracentesis) or perforated viscus (exploratory laparotomy) [75, 90]. Specialized surgical interventions have been described for peritoneum-specific inflammation in select cases, usually involving resection of problematic portions of bowel causing recurrent peritoneal irritation [92]. However, these scenarios are extremely rare and the majority of cases respond well to conservative management.

For bacterial overgrowth-related conditions, antibiotics and prokinetics are mainstays of therapy and help clear accumulated intraluminal bacteria. In SSc-related SBP, antibiotics are generally narrowed based on pathogen sensitivities derived from diagnostic paracentesis, and repeat paracentesis to determine antibiotic efficacy is sometimes but not routinely performed [115, 116]. For cases of SSc-associated PCI and spontaneous pneumoperitoneum, empiric broad-spectrum antibiotics and prokinetics are used in tandem with bowel rest, nasogastric decompression (if vomiting), and supplemental/hyperbaric oxygen to facilitate reabsorption of intraperitoneal air. These interventions generally have good effect, with resolution of symptoms within 1–2 weeks [82, 92, 94, 97].

To date, data are limited regarding treatment of SSc-related fibrotic changes in the peritoneum and gut wall. Several anti-fibrotic agents have been trialed to alleviate cutaneous disease, although the effect of these medications on gastrointestinal disease is largely unknown. As a result, management of gastrointestinal SSc largely revolves around supportive care, with no clear target to combat fibrosis in the intraperitoneal space [117].

13.2.3.5 Prognosis

Intraperitoneal SSc involvement is rarely a direct cause of mortality. Longitudinally, however, the presence of gastrointestinal SSc has been associated with increased complication rates and worse overall survival. Chronic abdominal pain, esophageal dysfunction, gastroparesis, small intestinal bacterial overgrowth, pseudo-obstruction, colonic dysmotility, chronic constipation, and fecal incontinence all have a significant effect on patient morbidity and can potentiate concomitant disease processes, increase hospitalization rates, and produce worse outcomes [75, 118]. Moreover, patients with intraperitoneal manifestations of SSc have been found to have decreased wound healing and increased failure rates in select gastrointestinal surgeries [119]. Due to high variability in disease burden among patients, prognostic factors are often highly individualized and depend on multiple variables at the time of diagnosis.

13.3 Primary Peritoneal Inflammatory Disorders

Primary peritoneal inflammatory disorders often have complex etiologies, with multiple potential causative and instigating factors (*see* Table 13.2). Because they typically arise in isolation, the disease courses for these conditions are often slow and insidious, with many patients presenting at advanced stages of disease. As a result, these conditions can often be difficult to diagnose, monitor, and treat, and morbidity and mortality rates are high for patients presenting with significant symptomatology.

Table 13.2 Comparison of primary peritoneal inflammatory disorders

Common characteristic: Primary pathology is in the peritoneal space			
	Encapsulating Peritoneal Sclerosis (EPS)	Retroperitoneal Fibrosis (RPF)	Sclerosing Mesenteritis (SM)
Defining Characteristics	Inflammatory fibrocollagenous change of the peritoneum GI constriction and obstruction	Fibrosis around the abdominal aorta Obstructive uropathy	Inflammatory mesenteric mass Incidental finding on CT
Epidemiology	Primary: middle-aged males in tropical/subtropical countries Secondary: strongly associated with peritoneal dialysis	Middle-aged males Linked to cigarette and asbestos exposure	Middle-aged males Likely underreported due to occult disease
Pathophysiology	Follows a "two-hit" model of inflammation Multiple environmental triggers	Primary: IgG4-RD vs. non-IgG4-RD; $CD4^+$ T cell-mediated Secondary: multifactorial	Associated with abdominal trauma Possible association with malignancy
Diagnosis	Abdominal CT scan Thickened peritoneum Small bowel "cauliflower" sign	Abdominal CT scan ^{18}F-FDG PET scan Retroperitoneal biopsy	Abdominal CT scan "Fat halo" and "misty mesentery" signs
Management	Corticosteroids Tamoxifen Complete peritonectomy	Corticosteroids Methotrexate Rituximab Mycophenolate mofetil	Avoid treatment unless symptomatic Corticosteroids Tamoxifen
Prognosis	High perioperative complication rate Prolonged TPN use Mortality 25–88% within 1–2 years	Generally responds to therapy 72% relapse rate Mortality 10%	Spontaneous resolution in 8–27% of patients Treatment efficacy of 34% for advanced or refractory disease

CT computed tomography, *IgG4-RD* immunoglobulin G 4-related disease

13.3.1 *Encapsulating Peritoneal Sclerosis*

Encapsulating peritoneal sclerosis (EPS), or abdominal cocoon syndrome, is a rare but disabling condition in which the peritoneum experiences diffuse fibrocollagenous inflammation and thickening, resulting in encasement of the intraabdominal organs and obstruction of the gastrointestinal tract. First described in 1907 by Owtschinnikow ("*peritonitis chronica fibrosa incapsulata*") [120], EPS can be divided into two main categories: primary (idiopathic) EPS caused by intrinsic factors or secondary EPS triggered by external influences or other pathologic sources. Between these two subtypes, secondary EPS is much more common and has been linked to multiple different conditions, including peritoneal dialysis (PD), medication use, intraperitoneal infections, malignancy or intraperitoneal treatment of the same, trauma, environmental exposures, and systemic rheumatologic disorders [121–128]. To date, there is no established treatment for this disease, although strategies including immunosuppression with corticosteroids with or without surgical adhesiolysis and peritonectomy are commonly employed methods for mitigating symptoms [122, 129, 130]. Despite these measures, EPS remains a highly morbid condition, with a survival rate of 50% one year after diagnosis [131–133].

13.3.1.1 Epidemiology

Primary EPS is rare, and little epidemiological data are available for this condition. One systematic review of 73 studies performed in 23 countries demonstrated higher rates of reporting in tropical and subtropical countries (China 54%, India 18%, Turkey 9%, Nigeria 3%), with most diagnoses occurring in young to middle-age males (34.7 ± 19.2 years, 2:1 male-to-female ratio) [134]. However, reporting on this condition has been sporadic, with most available data limited to individual case reports [126, 135].

By contrast, secondary EPS occurs more frequently and is often a consequence of prolonged PD use, with the majority of available epidemiological statistics addressing this population specifically. Among patients undergoing PD, the prevalence of EPS is between 0.5% and 8.9% globally [124, 133], with an annual incidence of 0.14–2.5% [132, 136]. Duration of PD is one of the strongest risk factors for developing the disease, with prevalence rising from 0.5% to 6.6% [133] after 5 years of PD to 6–8% after 9 years of PD [137, 138] and 17.2% after 15 or more years of PD [137, 139]. The risk of developing EPS has been shown to be persistent even after PD cessation, with a variable but significant proportion of EPS cases being diagnosed after PD has been stopped (0–71%) [133].

13.3.1.2 Etiology and Pathophysiology

Due to its rarity, no clear underlying cause has been established for primary EPS. Among patients with this disease, broad inflammatory response within the peritoneal membrane with cytokine production, fibroblast proliferation, and stripping of the mesothelial layer are all common features, but triggering mechanisms for this immune response have yet to be determined [126, 134, 135]. Several theoretical models involving gynecologic pathology have been proposed, which typically include retrograde menses or anatomical variation of the uterus or fallopian tubes; however, women of child-bearing age only account for approximately 25% of patients with primary EPS, so these explanations are not comprehensive [140, 141]. Other hypotheses involving association with developmental disorders, vascular anomalies, and omental hypoplasia have also been conjectured, although none of these models have been demonstrated empirically [141–143].

In contrast, the pathogenesis of secondary EPS is multifactorial and is thought to follow a "two-hit" model, in which patients with various congenital or acquired predisposing factors experience pathologic triggers that instigate progression of disease [121, 123, 124, 126]. The predisposing factors within this model are generally thought to originate from underlying genetic susceptibilities or long-term peritoneal damage, although specific genes or mechanisms have yet to be identified. PD in particular is thought to predispose patients towards EPS via progressive erosion of the peritoneal mesothelium, which occurs not only through a mechanical washing effect but also through prolonged exposure to dialysate contents. These contents generally give the dialysate an acidic pH and have been shown to cause osmotic damage via deposition of glucose degradation products (GDP) as well as advanced glycation end products (AGE) within the mesothelium, which is exacerbated in uremic patients with high levels of oxidative stress [124, 144, 145]. Genetic variation in the receptor for AGEs may cause increased susceptibility to this type of damage, thereby worsening inflammatory response [146]. Moreover, systemic rheumatologic disorders such as sarcoidosis, SLE, and familial Mediterranean fever may further prime the peritoneum for EPS [147–149].

Following these pro-inflammatory factors, a number of intrinsic and external triggers have been hypothesized to instigate and potentiate EPS-related fibrocollagenous change. Infections from a wide variety of sources including bacteria, cytomegalovirus, fungi, tuberculous/nontuberculous mycobacteria, and some parasites have all been associated with precipitation of EPS, with *Staphylococcus aureus*, *Pseudomonas*, and fungi species as the most commonly involved pathogens [123, 124, 150, 151]. Medications have also been thought to induce EPS, with methotrexate, calcineurin inhibitors, antiepileptics, and β-blockers (e.g., practolol, propranolol, timolol, etc.) implicated as well [126, 134, 152–157]. Mechanical peritoneal irritation such as that from PD, abdominal surgeries (both standard surgeries and transplantation procedures), abdominal trauma, and ventriculoperitoneal/peritoneovenous shunt placement have further been associated with EPS, as has inflammation from chemical irritants such as foreign bodies, intraperitoneal chemotherapy, intraperitoneal iodine, talcum powder, asbestos, and silica [123, 124, 127, 128]. More rarely, internal or neoplastic disease can also induce secondary EPS, such as endometriosis, dermoid cysts, and luteinizing gynecologic tumors [123, 158, 159].

Regardless of etiology, primary and secondary EPS share a common pathway of disease progression. In both conditions, denudation of the peritoneal mesothelial layer results in the exposure of the submesothelial compact zone of the peritoneal wall, which subsequently undergoes mesothelial-to-mesenchymal transition (MMT) [121, 124]. This process involves dissociation of the cytoskeletal structure and cell-to-cell connections within the layers of mesothelium, phenotypic change of epithelial cells to myofibroblast-like cells with increased collagen IV production, and increased secretion of proinflammatory and angiogenic cytokines [160–163]. At the same time, this process coincides with increased mononuclear cell infiltration, peritoneal calcification, and hyaluronic acid deposition, with loss of embedded tryptase and mast cells implying decreased fibrinolytic capacity [124, 164]. To date, key mediators identified in EPS progression have included fibrogenic cytokines such as TGF-β1 and SMAD, as well as angiogenic factors such as vascular endothelial growth factor (VEGF) and endothelial nitric oxide synthase (eNOS) [121, 124, 165]. Other potential implicated factors include CTGF, fibroblast growth factor (FGF), platelet-derived growth factor (PDGF), hepatocyte growth factor (HGF), plasminogen activator inhibitor (PAI1), matrix metalloproteinases (MMPs), tumor necrosis factor (TNF), and mast cells [121]. Furthermore, the mucoprotein podoplanin (D2-40) as well as connective tissue growth factor 2 (CCN2) have further been noted to stain abundantly on histopathological slides, which not only aids diagnosis but also may provide potential therapeutic targets [124, 166, 167].

13.3.1.3 Clinical Description and Diagnosis

For primary EPS, disease course is usually slow and insidious, with most patients reporting a delay time of 3–4 years from symptom onset to presentation [123, 126, 134, 140]. Given the constrictive nature of EPS on the gastrointestinal tract, many patients initially experience anorexia and weight loss, and the majority of patients are malnourished by the time they seek medical care (75%, mean BMI 17.5 kg/m^2) [140]. Despite this gradual progression, up to 29.2% of patients with primary EPS ultimately require emergent corrective surgical procedures, suggesting a crescendo of symptoms and a more rapid disease course in the late stages of primary EPS [123, 134, 140]. Like primary EPS, secondary EPS symptoms typically emerge over a similar time frame, with the majority of patients with PD-associated secondary EPS becoming symptomatic within 5 years after stopping PD [133]. More rapid-onset scenarios have been described for this condition as well, with reports of some cases presenting within 12 weeks from the onset of symptoms [168, 169].

Acutely, the most common symptom for both primary and secondary EPS is bowel obstruction, typically seen in the form of nausea/vomiting, abdominal pain, constipation/obstipation, anorexia, and weight loss. These symptoms are often episodic in nature, with increasing frequency over time as intraabdominal organs become progressively constricted [123, 124, 126, 134]. Physical examination is characterized by visible signs of malnutrition and abdominal distention, usually with diffuse, nonspecific visceral abdominal pain [168, 170, 171]. In rare cases, a palpable and semi-firm abdominal mass representing peritoneal encasement can also be appreciated on physical examination, with or without ascites [134, 135, 140, 172, 173]. Laboratory tests, while useful for correcting electrolyte derangement or tracking inflammatory markers, are typically nondiagnostic in late stages of the disease when fibrosis of the peritoneum is complete [174].

Imaging is commonly used in the diagnosis of EPS and can help to differentiate EPS from other sources of obstruction. While plain abdominal films and contrast-enhanced radiography can shed light on obstructive symptoms, abdominal computed tomography is the preferred noninvasive test for diagnosis of EPS. Typical findings on imaging include thickened peritoneum with calcifications, encapsulated or tethered clusters of small bowel loops ("cauliflower sign"), obstructed or dilated bowel loops with one or more transition points, complex loculated ascites, and dense mesenteric fat [123, 126, 134, 161, 168, 169, 173, 175, 176]. In cases for which surgery is required, definitive diagnosis can be made via exploratory laparotomy, which allows direct assessment of fibrotic peritoneal thickening and organ encasement; these findings can then be confirmed with peritoneal biopsy [123, 126, 134].

13.3.1.4 Management

To guide management of EPS, a four-step staging model has been proposed, ordered by pre-EPS (stage I), inflammatory (stage II), progressive/encapsulating (stage III), and fibrotic/ileus (stage IV) phases [123, 126, 134, 168, 169]. In the pre-EPS stage, patients may have subtle clinical findings such as calcification of the peritoneum on imaging, as well as bloody dialysate or loss of ultrafiltration if undergoing PD. During the inflammatory stage, signs of systemic inflammation such as fever, leukocytosis, elevated serum CRP, anorexia, and diarrhea may be present. These symptoms eventually give way to signs of obstruction or ileus, with nausea/vomiting, abdominal pain, and constipation in the encapsulating stage. Finally, the fibrotic stage is typified by total obstruction, obstipation, and complete peritoneal encasement [123, 126, 134, 176]. Due to the evolving and insidious nature of inflammatory changes in EPS, there is currently no clear consensus on preferred treatment of this disease, with proposed therapies changing depending on current disease status [124].

In the more active inflammatory stages of EPS without complete obstruction, immunosuppression has commonly been used to attenuate fibrocollagenous change and reduce symptoms. So far, limited trials have been performed for several agents, including corticosteroids, colchicine, azathioprine, cyclosporine, mycophenolate mofetil, and mammalian target of rapamycin (mTOR) inhibitors [122, 123, 125, 126, 129, 137, 139, 168]. Among these medications, corticosteroids have been most extensively tested due to their broad immunosuppressive effect, inhibition of collagen synthesis pathways, and prevention of ascites, while other medications have either been used in conjunction with corticosteroids or have only been trialed in individual cases [121, 124]. Despite the proposed benefits of corticosteroids, evidence of overall therapeutic efficacy has been mixed, with some studies reporting isolated cases of near-complete regression and others reporting only limited effect with corticosteroid use. In a 2004 prospective Japanese multicenter trial including 39 EPS patients treated with prednisolone 10–40 mg daily, a subset of patients

(38.5%) were able to recover from symptomatic EPS on corticosteroids alone, with remaining patients either requiring surgery (total enterolysis) or dying from their disease [137]. By contrast, in a large retrospective cohort study addressing EPS-related outcomes in the United Kingdom in 2009, corticosteroid use was not significantly associated with any extension of median survival [131]. Most tellingly, in a meta-analysis of Japanese studies addressing use of corticosteroids in EPS, treatment with corticosteroids resulted in the return of bowel function in 79% of stage II cases, 57% of stage III cases, and 50% of stage IV cases, indicating that the early, pro-inflammatory stages of EPS may be most susceptible to corticosteroid therapy, with efficacy decreasing in later stages of disease [177].

Since immunosuppressive therapies may have limited benefit in patients with completed fibrosis of the peritoneum, anti-fibrotic therapy has also been employed as a means to treat EPS. The most common of these therapies is the selective estrogen receptor modulator (SERM) tamoxifen, which is known to have anti-fibrotic properties related to inhibition of TGF-β [123, 124, 126]. Like corticosteroids, evidence for the therapeutic efficacy of tamoxifen has been mixed, with anecdotal reports describing clinical regression of EPS but large-scale studies showing a more muted effect. In a 2011 Dutch multicenter retrospective study comparing 24 patients receiving tamoxifen with 39 not on tamoxifen therapy, overall mortality was observed to be significantly lower of the tamoxifen-receiving cohort (45.8% vs. 74.4%, $p = 0.03$), with improved albeit nonsignificant longitudinal survival also observed in this group (HR 0.39, $p = 0.056$) [178]. However, similar retrospective multicenter studies have demonstrated no survival benefit from tamoxifen, and few studies have analyzed the use of tamoxifen in isolation without concurrent therapy with corticosteroids [124, 131]. Therefore, much like corticosteroids, tamoxifen may in fact have greatest efficacy when given during the early stages of disease: in a prospective study of 23 patients with early signs of peritoneal sclerosis, none among the 9 patients given tamoxifen developed EPS, whereas 4/14 patients not taking tamoxifen eventually developed the disease [179].

In addition to tamoxifen, multiple other treatments have been proposed for EPS. Early inhibition of the renin-angiotensin-aldosterone system with angiotensin converting enzyme (ACE) inhibitors or angiotensin II receptor blockers (ARBs) has been associated with decreased intraperitoneal inflammation from angiotensin II mediated TGF-β1 upregulation, which has been associated with some degree of efficacy when used in tandem with corticosteroids [124, 125, 180]. Other medications, including mucolytic alkaloids (N-acetylcysteine), anti-inflammatory drugs (colchicine), xanthine derivatives (pentoxifylline), anti-diabetic drugs (rosiglitazone), growth factor inhibitors (pirfenidone), immunomodulators (thalidomide), and antifungals (itraconazole) have also been proposed as possible therapeutic agents but have largely been restricted to in vitro trials [124]. Furthermore, abrasive therapies such as dissolved molecular hydrogen or regenerative therapies such as peritoneal stem cell transplantation have also been conceptualized, although these treatments remain largely theoretical [124].

Regardless of staging, all patients with EPS should be evaluated for signs of malnutrition at the time of presentation, with correction of electrolytes and administration of nutritional support as needed. In practice, patients with severe or obstructive disease are often unable to tolerate enteral feeds and should instead be offered total parenteral nutrition (TPN), which has been associated with improved outcomes in the acute setting [140]. If complete obstruction is suspected, nasogastric decompression can help temporarily relieve symptoms and may in some cases resolve obstruction, although recurrence is likely. Given the extensive intraabdominal fibrosis in many of these patients, surgical intervention is often hazardous and should generally be reserved as a last-resort method of relieving obstructive symptoms, especially since surgical trauma can counterproductively trigger further inflammation and fibrosis. For this reason, typical procedures include simple lysis of adhesions to limit surgery-related inflammation, enterolysis with or without Noble plication to ensure obstructive relief, and complete peritonectomy for curative intent [122–124, 126]. In a 24-year summary analysis of 243 EPS patients undergoing surgery at a single center in Japan, perioperative mortality occurred in 6.2% of patients, with 25.1% eventually dying from EPS despite surgery; reoperative rates were also high in this group (23.8%), with survival at 1, 2, 3, 5, and 8 years after surgery noted to be 91%, 83%, 77%, 66%, and 53%, respectively [130]. Other studies have demonstrated acceptable morbidity and mortality with decreased recurrence rates in more complete surgical procedures (e.g., curative-intent complete peritonectomy), suggesting that more aggressive initial surgery may have greater therapeutic benefit and decrease the risk of relapse in patients with advanced EPS [123, 181].

13.3.1.5 Prognosis

EPS-related mortality is high, with reported rates varying between 25% and 58% and most deaths occurring within 1–2 years after diagnosis [122, 124, 130, 131, 136, 137]. The most common causes of death are typically bowel perforation with corresponding peritonitis and sepsis (60%), followed by malnutrition (10%) and pneumonia (10%) [124, 182]. While disease course varies between individuals, several predictive factors have been noted to indicate increased risk of mortality, including EPS onset after PD withdrawal, bloody ascites, bowel tethering, and elevated serum intact parathyroid hormone levels (>384 pg/mL) [182]. Even in surviving patients, EPS is a highly morbid condition, with many patients requiring TPN for months after therapy while waiting for symptoms to resolve [123, 183]. Early diagnosis of EPS is therefore critical to improving outcomes since low presenting stage, cessation of inflammatory triggers, and prompt immunosuppression have all been associated with improved overall survival [123, 124].

13.3.2 Retroperitoneal Fibrosis

Retroperitoneal fibrosis (RPF) is a rare inflammatory disease involving the insidious onset of fibrocollagenous change around the infrarenal abdominal aorta and iliac arteries. In most cases, this fibrosis originates over the anterior surface of the fourth and fifth lumbar vertebrae and extends beyond the abdominal great vessels to encase other organs, most commonly the ureters, kidneys, and retroperitoneal portions of the colon. First described by Ormond in 1948 [184], approximately 70% of RPF cases are idiopathic (primary), while the remainder are caused by a variety of conditions including infections, malignancy, medications, hemorrhage, radiotherapy, and other sources of inflammation [185, 186]. Regardless of origin, ureteral obstruction is the most common presenting symptom, with more advanced cases leading to obstructive hydroureteronephrosis, flank and abdominal pain, gonadal venous stasis, severe constipation, lower extremity edema, and renal failure [186–189]. Diagnosis is usually made through a combination of laboratory investigations, abdominal computed tomography, ^{18}F-FDG positron emission tomography (PET), and retroperitoneal biopsy [190, 191]. For secondary RPF in particular, management usually involves treatment of underlying disease; however, anti-inflammatory therapy for both primary and secondary RPF typically includes immunosuppression with corticosteroids, although fibrinolysis via tamoxifen has been proposed as well. In most cases, good clinical response to immunosuppression is usually seen in the first 6–9 months, although relapse occurs in up to 72% of patients, and multiple relapses are relatively common [192]. Despite this tendency for recurrence, RPF generally has low morbidity and mortality, and most patients experience good recovery with proper long-term management [187].

13.3.2.1 Epidemiology

Idiopathic RPF is a rare disorder, with a reported annual incidence of 0.1–1.3 cases per 100,000 individuals per year [186, 193, 194]. Most studies describe a 2–3:1 male-to-female ratio, with the majority of cases occurring between 40 and 60 years of age [186, 195–197]. While no racial predilection has been determined for this disease, several environmental factors have been linked to increased risk of developing RPF, most notably cigarette smoking and asbestos exposure. Taken separately, these two factors each confer a three- to four-fold increase in lifetime risk of developing RPF; when combined, this increases to an eight- to twelve-fold lifetime risk [198, 199].

Since secondary RPF originates from a variety of different sources, its incidence is often tied to that of the underlying disorder. Given this variability in occurrence, the incidence and prevalence of this condition have yet to be thoroughly described [200, 201].

13.3.2.2 Etiology and Pathophysiology

The etiology of idiopathic RPF is complex and largely unknown, although current evidence suggests that this condition can either arise as an immunoglobulin G4-related disease (IgG4-RD) or originate from other indeterminate causes [187]. At present, current evidence suggests that the majority of RPF cases are IgG4-related, which may shed light on disease pathogenesis and possible therapeutic targets. By contrast, the origin of non-IgG4-related primary RPF is likely multifactorial, and the inflammatory pathways leading to this condition are poorly understood [202–204].

IgG4-related primary RPF, which is defined by an $IgG4^+$/total IgG^+ plasma cell ratio of >40% on histopathological analysis, belongs to the IgG4-RD group of autoimmune disorders. These disorders share a common phenotype of gradual fibroinflammatory change and include diseases such as autoimmune pancreatitis (AIP) type 1, IgG4-related sclerosing cholangitis, sclerosing sialadenitis, and fibrosing orbital disease with proptosis. Broadly, these diseases are characterized by multiorgan involvement, slow-onset fibrosis, storiform lesions, and association with other autoimmune disorders [187, 204–206]. On the cellular level, the pathognomonic infiltration of tissues by $IgG4^+$ plasma cells is thought not to be a driver of pathology but instead to represent the end result of a primarily $CD4^+$ T cell-mediated inflammatory process. In currently proposed models, antigens of unknown origin are continuously presented by B lymphocyte lineage cells to nearby $CD4^+$ T cells, which in turn elaborate multiple proinflammatory and profibrotic compounds such as granzyme B, perforin, IL-1, interferon-γ, and TGF-β [187, 207, 208]. Concurrently, activated T follicular helper (Tfh) cells in nearby lymph node germinal centers are thought to become simultaneously activated via this process, facilitating B-cell class switching to the $IgG4^+$ plasma cells commonly seen on histopathologic analysis [209, 210]. In cases of idiopathic RPF, much of this pathophysiology is thought to occur multifocally in the adventitial walls of retroperitoneal great vessels and eventually in the broader paraaortic space, resulting in the classic clinical presentation of disease. Moreover, while cases of non-IgG4-related RPF lack the telltale sign of $IgG4^+$ plasma cell infiltration, they are theorized to undergo a similar $CD4^+$ T cell-mediated inflammatory process, although exact factors provoking this T-cell response are unclear [211, 212].

Further investigation has determined that certain genetic determinants may increase susceptibility to idiopathic RPF, which may help explain the relationship between RPF and various autoimmune disorders. Most notably, these factors include mutated HLA-DRB1*03 (associated with SLE and type 1 diabetes mellitus), polymorphism Δ32 on *CCR5* (a chemokine receptor), and the TTCCAT haplotype of the gene encoding CCL11/eotaxin-1 [187]. While the evidence linking these genes to RPF is still preliminary, these factors may assist in the prediction of idiopathic RPF in certain cohorts and further help elucidate the underlying pathology in this disease process.

For secondary RPF, a number of conditions have been implicated as potential drivers of disease, although there is varying evidence describing the exact pathologic mechanisms for each. Certain medications such as ergot alkaloids and dopamine agonists have been thought to induce secondary RPF through the upregulation of serotonin, which has been shown to promote myofibroblast proliferation and subsequent extracellular matrix expansion [193]. By this same token, carcinoid tumors have also been associated with increased likelihood of secondary RPF, although multiple malignancies including lymphomas (both Hodgkin and non-Hodgkin), sarcomas, and carcinomas (colorectal, breast, prostate, and bladder) have all been linked to RPF as well [186, 187, 195, 213]. Abdominal surgery, retroperitoneal hemorrhage, and intraabdominal radiation have further been shown to cause secondary RPF, likely through stimulation of inflammatory processes typically used for wound healing [187, 195, 200]. Other causes of secondary RPF include infectious sources (particularly tuberculosis, histoplasmosis, and actinomycosis) as well as biological agents such as etanercept and infliximab, although the mechanisms behind these causative factors are mostly unknown [187, 201].

13.3.2.3 Clinical Description and Diagnosis

The most common symptom of RPF is visceral pain, which accounts for over 90% of presenting cases. This pain is usually located in the abdomen, lower back, and flanks, with testicular pain in particular being a common feature in male patients [186, 189]. Chronic constipation (12–30%) and lower extremity edema (8–23%) are also common presenting symptoms, which may indicate involvement of the colon or inferior vena cava, respectively [188, 190, 213]. Furthermore, symptoms related to progressive kidney involvement may also be apparent, with increased urinary frequency, urgency, and dysuria as the most commonly reported complaints [197]. Other associated symptoms among presenting patients include fever, malaise, nausea/vomiting, constipation, anorexia, and weight loss; for secondary RPF in particular, symptoms associated with causal diseases may also be apparent [187].

Physical examination typically reveals nonspecific findings, although several subtle signs of RPF may manifest depending on extent of disease. For patients with arterial involvement, lower extremity claudication may be present (2–12%), whereas patients with venous or lymphatic involvement may have congestive signs such as lower extremity edema, lymphedema, deep vein thrombosis, and varicoceles [186, 189, 192, 196]. Moreover, fibrotic restriction of one or both of the renal arteries can manifest as new-onset hypertension, which has been noted to occur in 30–60% of presenting patients [186, 189].

Laboratory testing is similarly nondiagnostic in patients with RPF, although systemic inflammatory markers such as serum CRP and ESR are commonly elevated, and increased levels of serum IgG4 can be found in IgG4-related disease [187, 214]. Moreover, up to 60% of RPF patients present with elevated serum ANA, and patients with suspected concomitant autoimmune disorders will also have increased levels of various autoantibodies [215]. In patients with urinary involvement, eGFR is typically decreased, with high but normal-ratio blood urea nitrogen and serum creatinine consistent with urinary obstruction and postrenal azotemia [186, 197].

Diagnosis is typically performed via abdominal computed tomography or magnetic resonance imaging, which are not only helpful in confirming the existence of RPF but are also necessary to rule out other sources of disease [186, 187, 189]. On imaging, classic findings for RPF include a large, confluent mass in the retroperitoneum originating in the paraaortic space, with possible encasement of posterior abdominal structures and occasional signs of prior or ongoing inflammation (e.g., calcifications, lymphadenopathy, and fat stranding) [186]. Further evaluation with

^{18}F-FDG PET scan can confirm the inflammatory nature of a suspicious retroperitoneal mass and may also help determine the current level of inflammatory activity, although this test is not in itself diagnostic [187, 216]. Additional organ system-specific tests can also be useful in determining the severity of symptoms: for example, renal ultrasound, intravenous urography, and retrograde pyelography are essential for evaluating hydronephrosis and other RPF-associated urinary tract disorders [186, 187]. To confirm diagnosis, core-needle biopsy can either be performed percutaneously with imaging guidance or via surgical sampling, although direct tissue analysis is typically reserved for cases in which underlying malignancy is suspected or surgery is already indicated for other reasons (e.g., aortic aneurysm repair or ureterolysis for ureteral obstruction) [186, 201, 213].

13.3.2.4 Management

The first priority of RPF management is prompt correction of acute problems, followed by treatment of underlying disease. As a result, the majority of invasive procedures for RPF center around the management of ureteral obstruction, which is the most common cause of acute presentation in patients with this condition [186, 187, 200]. In recent years, surgical ureterolysis with intraperitonealization and omental wrapping has largely been replaced with minimally invasive cystoscopy-based measures (e.g., double-J stent placement), which have been shown to be highly effective in treating RPF-related urinary obstruction [217]. For patients who are poor surgical candidates or who cannot undergo cystoscopy, temporary or permanent percutaneous nephrostomy tubes offer another means to safely decompress the urinary tract and improve outcomes [187]. In patients with vascular involvement, medical treatment alone is often enough to relieve symptoms in sufficiently mild cases, although minimally invasive approaches such as intravascular stenting can be used in patients requiring more aggressive management [214, 215]. Gastrointestinal symptoms rarely progress past chronic constipation, which can usually be managed exclusively through medical therapy without surgical intervention [187].

For idiopathic RPF, high-dose glucocorticoids are the most frequently recommended therapy and are usually given empirically upon diagnosis. While dosing regimens vary between clinical practices, common protocols such as prednisone 1 mg/kg per day for 3–4 weeks are often recommended, followed by gradual taper in the following weeks and months. This management strategy is highly effective in the treatment of RPF, with the majority of patients showing improvement within the first few weeks after treatment, and up to 75–90% of patients experiencing clinical remission of disease on steroid therapy alone [192, 197, 218–221]. Despite these benefits, steroids occasionally fail to induce mass regression in RPF, which can result in residual fibrosis and persistent symptoms [187]. Moreover, patients unable to tolerate high doses of steroids may be forced to use low-dose steroid regimens, which may have decreased efficacy in some scenarios [192, 197].

To avoid steroid-related side effects, several other agents have been proposed for treatment of RPF, although these agents have primarily been studied as a way to reduce steroid dosing rather than replace steroid therapy altogether. In a limited trial of 28 treatment-naive RPF patients, mycophenolate mofetil used in conjunction with lower-dose prednisone (40 mg/day) was shown to elicit comparable responses to high-dose prednisone therapy alone, with 89% of patients demonstrating improvement over a mean follow-up interval of 2 years [222]. Similarly, another small-volume trial of 16 relapsing RPF patients over a 2-year follow-up period demonstrated a response rate of 79% on combined low-dose methotrexate and prednisone therapy [223]. Most recently, the anti-CD20 monoclonal antibody rituximab has also been trialed for the treatment of RPF, with several limited case series demonstrating remission rates of up to 75% in patients receiving this medication with or without steroids [224–226]. For IgG4-related RPF in particular, the anti-IL-6 receptor monoclonal antibody tocilizumab may also be used, although clinical data for this treatment are lacking [223]. Finally, despite being frequently used in the treatment of other fibrinogenic disorders, tamoxifen has been shown to have poor efficacy in RPF, with one trial demonstrating a substantially higher 26-month relapse probability among RPF patients placed on maintenance tamoxifen compared to those kept on a prednisone taper only (difference −33%, 95% CI −62 to −3, $p = 0.0372$) [197].

In secondary RPF, management is typically targeted at the underlying cause of disease, and this condition is rarely treated directly. Occasionally, prednisone therapy may be considered for refractory or highly symptomatic presentations of RPF, albeit only if allowable in the context of other concomitant disorders [187, 221].

13.3.2.5 Prognosis

Idiopathic RPF is a chronic relapsing disorder, with a recurrence rate of up to 72% regardless of treatment received [192]. As a result, longitudinal follow-up including serial abdominal imaging and repeat serum inflammatory marker testing is generally recommended, with repeat flares of disease treated with either retrial of high-dose prednisolone or steroid-sparing combined therapy [186, 187]. Due to the side effects of long-term steroid use, steroid treatments are generally limited to a maximum duration of 1–2 years and are tapered when possible; lifelong steroid use is not recommended for this disease [192, 197]. Ultimately, despite this potential for steroid-related morbidity, prognosis is generally favorable in patients with RPF, with an overall mortality rate of 10% among patients responsive to initial glucocorticoid therapy [218, 221].

13.3.3 Sclerosing Mesenteritis

Sclerosing mesenteritis (SM) is a comprehensive term referring to any benign chronic inflammatory condition involving fibrosis and fat necrosis within the abdominal mesentery. It is categorized into three main subtypes, which differ histologically but are otherwise clinically identical: mesenteric lipodystrophy (predominant fat necrosis), mesenteric panniculitis (predominant chronic inflammation), and retractile mesenteritis (predominant fibrosis) [227–229]. Initially described by Jura in 1924 [230], SM is an uncommon and poorly understood clinical entity, with an estimated prevalence of approximately 1% in the general adult population and no clear consensus on pathologic origin [228, 229, 231]. Moreover, it is often underdiagnosed, with 15% of cases producing no symptoms and up to 92% of cases being either diagnosed incidentally on imaging or presenting with symptoms attributable to another cause [232]. In symptomatic cases, patients typically present with nonspecific gastrointestinal complaints such as abdominal pain, nausea/vomiting, weight loss, and fever, with few cases presenting with signs of obstruction. Management of this condition typically involves immunosuppression with corticosteroids as well as fibrinolysis with tamoxifen, although up to 82.4% of patients report spontaneous resolution of symptoms and thus do not receive treatment [233]. As a result, this condition generally carries a favorable prognosis, with progression of disease only occurring in a minority of patients (2.3–16%) [228].

13.3.3.1 Epidemiology

SM is a rare disease, with varying reports on incidence and prevalence depending on method of diagnosis. In a 1985 analysis of 712 autopsies performed over a period of 6 months, SM was histopathologically confirmed in the mesenteric tissue of 9 patients, corresponding with a prevalence of 1.26% [231]. More recent analyses using large radiologic databases have yielded prevalence rates between 0.16% and 2.5%, depending on search criteria [228]. Still other prospective radiologic studies have estimated a prevalence of SM up to 7.8%, although this rate is possibly overestimated from the unintentional inclusion of secondary SM cases caused by occult malignancy [229, 234].

For confirmed cases of SM, diagnosis most commonly occurs between 40 and 70 years of age, with a mean age of 55 ± 19.2 years [228, 229, 235]. There is a roughly 2:1 male-to-female predominance, and there is an approximately equal distribution of cases among racial and ethnic groups [233, 235–239]. Since most studies analyzing SM have been performed in Western countries, limited data exist regarding geographic distribution of the disease [228].

13.3.3.2 Etiology and Pathophysiology

To date, the etiology of SM is largely unknown. Due to its nonspecific symptoms, SM has been linked to a variety of different conditions, including but not limited to abdominal trauma, autoimmune conditions, malignancy, and infection [228]. Each of these four proposed models has varying levels of supportive data, although any direct causal relationship between SM and other disorders has yet to be established.

At present, abdominal trauma is the most well-established precursor to SM, with abdominal surgery in particular having the strongest association with SM pathogenesis [228, 229]. In a 2017 systematic review of 192 SM cases between 1960 and 2015, prior abdominal trauma or surgery was the most commonly documented etiology of disease (28.6%), followed by malignancy (8.9%) and autoimmune conditions (5.7%) [235]. Similarly, in a single-center combined retrospective-prospective analysis of 92 SM cases, a prior history of abdominal surgery was noted in 35% of patients, which primarily consisted of cholecystectomies (18%) and appendectomies (13%) [240]. Further studies have suggested that the introduction of foreign bodies into the abdominal cavity may induce intraperitoneal fibrosis, with powdered surgical gloves implicated as a potential source of occult inflammation, although this has not been demonstrated empirically [227, 240]. Despite this perceived association, however, recent case-control studies have found no significant correlation between SM and past abdominal trauma or surgery, casting some doubt on this hypothesis [241, 242].

Autoimmunity has similarly been suggested as a possible predisposing factor for SM, although there is still limited evidence supporting this theory. In select studies, rheumatologic conditions have been observed in up to 10% of patients presenting with SM, with RPF as the most commonly represented concomitant disease [240]. Similarly, histopathologic analysis of SM-affected tissue has demonstrated infiltration with IgG4-positive plasma cells, suggesting a potential IgG4-mediated sclerosing inflammatory process (*see* "Retroperitoneal Fibrosis") [233]. However, this association is still largely speculative, and a mechanism by which autoimmune disorders could potentiate or precipitate SM has yet to be proposed [228, 229]. Furthermore, no statistically significant difference in autoimmune disorder prevalence among SM patients has been noted in recent case-control studies [241].

As for malignancy, SM has long been suspected of being a paraneoplastic process, but more recent data regarding this association are conflicting. Historically, higher rates of occult lymphoma have been found in patients with SM, with one seminal case series in 1974 noting that 8/53 (15.1%) patients presenting with SM were later diagnosed with lymphoma, and 16/53 (30.2%) were later diagnosed with other neoplasms [227]. Similarly, in a large retrospective radiologic study of 7620 abdominal computed tomography scans in 2000, 49 patients were found to have SM, of whom 34 (69.4%) had a coexisting malignancy [232]. This association is further corroborated in a 2014 case-control analysis of 94 SM patients and 188 controls, in which a higher rate of malignancy was found in SM patients in matched-pair analysis (48.9% vs. 46.3%, $p < 0.05$) as well as over a 5-year follow-up from initial diagnosis (14.6% vs. 6.9%, $p < 0.05$) [233]. At the same time, however, three other recent case-control studies have demonstrated no correlation between SM and malignancy [242, 243], with the exception of one study in which a higher prevalence of lymphoma was noted when comparing oncologic diagnoses among SM patients with malignancy specifically [241].

While SM has been linked to a multitude of infectious etiologies, most of these associations have been described anecdotally in case reports without more substantial supportive evidence. In light of this, SM has been associated with tuberculosis, Whipple disease, typhoid fever, cryptococcus, histoplasmosis, schistosomiasis, HIV, cholera, and syphilis, although further evidence is needed to clarify these potential relationships [228, 229, 244].

Regardless of etiology, SM is thought to follow a similar pattern as other inflammatory intraperitoneal disorders, with the three subtypes of SM representing a continuum of progressive disease. For SM in particular, this pattern is thought to be initial fat necrosis, followed by chronic inflammation, and ending with fibrosis. While this theory has not been independently verified via serial biopsy analysis, it appears likely based on pooled evidence from published pathology reports and gross descriptions of disease. The driving process behind this inflammatory change, however, is yet to be determined [244, 245].

13.3.3.3 Clinical Description and Diagnosis

Patients presenting with clinical SM often experience nonspecific abdominal symptoms, including abdominal pain (75%), constipation/diarrhea (30–40%), weight loss (25%), nausea/vomiting (20%), anorexia (15%), and occasionally signs of systemic inflammation such as fever (5–20%) [235, 240]. In rare cases typically involving a large inflammatory mass, clinical signs of obstruction may be apparent [229]. Among patients with an incidental finding of SM on imaging, between 16–40% are asymptomatic at the time of diagnosis [227, 239, 246]. Approximately 50% of patients present with a normal physical exam, with 20–30% endorsing tenderness to palpation and up to a third of patients presenting with a palpable abdominal mass. Laboratory findings in SM are typically nondescript, although inflammatory markers such as CRP and ESR are elevated in up to 80% of patients [235, 240, 247]. Additionally, leukocytosis is present in a minority of patients (16%), with some patients presenting with anemia (25%) and/or hypoalbuminemia (22%) [228, 235].

Abdominal computed tomography is the primary method of diagnosis, with many diagnoses made incidentally on imaging when searching for other disease processes. Since imaging findings are not always clear, an informal 5-point set of diagnostic criteria has been proposed to aid in diagnosis, in which 3 out of 5 points confirms SM: (1) mesenteric mass with clear mass effect on neighboring structures without invasion, (2) mesenteric mass with high attenuation (−50 to −70 Hounsfield units), (3) mesenteric fat containing small soft tissue nodes (<10 mm), (4) fat surrounding intraabdominal lymph nodes ("fat halo" sign), and (5) hyperattenuating pseudocapsule surrounding the mass without signs of concomitant ascites or malignancy [234]. Terms such as "misty mesentery" have also been used on computed tomography to further indicate diagnosis of SM, describing an increase in mesenteric fat density around the primary inflammation site. Moreover, other imaging modalities such as abdominal ultrasound and magnetic resonance imaging also have demonstrated efficacy in SM diagnosis, although findings in these studies are generally less standardized since they are less widely used [228, 229]. In most cases, a percutaneous stereotactic core needle biopsy is performed to confirm diagnosis [229].

Gross pathological findings during surgical exploration typically fall into three subtypes. Type I (42%) is identified as diffuse mesenteric thickening up to 10 cm in width with dirty yellow-orange appearance and demarcation within 3–5 cm of the mesenteric border. Type II (32%) involves the formation of a single, discrete inflammatory tumor, most typically located in the jejunal mesentery, with rubbery or firm consistency. Type III (26%) entails multiple discrete inflammatory tumors distributed throughout the mesentery [227, 239]. So far, these morphologies have not been shown to have significant prognostic value, although this classification can be useful to inform planning for future interventions [229].

13.3.3.4 Management

Because a sizable fraction of SM cases are asymptomatic and spontaneously resolve, observation with serial computed tomography is often sufficient for mild cases, without need for further intervention. In large radiologic series, only 1.1–6.1% of patients were documented to have undergone any therapy directed at SM [232, 233], although other single-center studies have reported treatment in up to 48% of patients [240]. Given the rarity of this diagnosis, there is no set protocol for continued monitoring of disease if no therapy is pursued, although follow-up to 5 years after initial diagnosis is commonly reported in the literature [228, 233].

For symptomatic patients requiring treatment beyond analgesics, corticosteroids and tamoxifen have often been employed as first-line therapy, offering a combined immunosuppressive and fibrinolytic mechanism of action. In a limited trial of twice-daily tamoxifen with a prednisone taper in 20 patients with significant symptomatic SM, 60% of patients experienced regression of disease at 12–16 weeks, with 30% maintaining stable disease and 10% experiencing progression. By comparison, only 1 of 12 patients (8.3%) receiving non-tamoxifen therapy (prednisone, azathioprine, and colchicine) was found to have improvement, and no other medical treatment modalities were successful [240]. Additionally, the angiogenesis inhibitor thalidomide has also shown some efficacy in treating SM, with one limited trial of 5 SM patients demonstrating a clinical response in 4 patients at 12 weeks and subsequent complete remission in 1 patient [247]. Other therapeutic trials have included tamoxifen monotherapy, colchicine, 6-mercaptopurine (6-MP), antibiotics, azathioprine, methotrexate, infliximab, cyclophosphamide, intravenous immunoglobulin, D-penicillamine, and tacrolimus, which have all shown varying levels of success in isolated cases [229, 235, 247].

Surgical intervention is typically reserved for refractory or fulminant cases of SM, with the goal of inflammatory mass removal and bowel resection if needed. Because patients with SM often have high mesenteric vascularity and fibrosis due to chronic inflammation, surgery is often technically difficult and complete removal of the offending mass is not always possible. In a limited report of 20 patients undergoing surgery for SM, complete or partial resection of SM masses was only achievable in 30% of patients, with the remainder of patients undergoing alternative procedures to mitigate symptoms: among these patients, 57% underwent bowel resection, 21% underwent palliative enteric bypass, and 21% underwent adhesiolysis only. Moreover, intervention with surgery only was associated with the lowest disease remission rates compared to medical-only therapy or combined medical/surgical treatments (17% vs. 38% vs. 50%, respectively) [240]. As a result, while surgery is essential for mitigating acute abdominal symptoms such as gastrointestinal obstruction or peritonitis, its role in the treatment of SM is largely adjunctive, and its use as a primary therapeutic option may best be reserved for cases in which medical therapy has proven ineffective [228, 229].

13.3.3.5 Prognosis

Given its frequently subclinical or self-limited disease course, SM generally carries a favorable prognosis. As demonstrated in several large retrospective radiological studies, diagnosed SM typically remains stable on imaging for the majority of patients for at least 5 years after diagnosis (70.2–96.5%), with spontaneous resolution occurring in 8–27% of patients and progression occurring in 2.3–16% of individuals [228]. In contrast, patients presenting with advanced disease are more likely to have a complex clinical course requiring weeks to months of medical treatment and possible surgical intervention, with an overall treatment efficacy of 34% [240]. Therefore, while careful monitoring alone is generally indicated in asymptomatic patients, prompt treatment with corticosteroids and tamoxifen is often recommended for patients presenting with more significant abdominal symptoms, with surgery generally reserved for select cases [228, 229].

13.4 Mesenteric Sequelae of Vasculitides

Vasculitides are a diverse group of generalized disorders characterized by inflammation of the vessel walls in various organ systems. They are typically categorized by large-, medium-, or small-vessel disease and can manifest anywhere in the body, depending on the condition. The abdominal mesentery is a complex vascular structure involving all three vessel types and thus is a common site for vasculitic disease, emerging either in synchrony with systemic disease or in isolation as a primary site of inflammation.

Because the mesentery acts as the primary blood supply for the abdominal visceral organs, disruption of blood flow via vasculitis, thrombosis, or obliteration of mesenteric arteries and veins can cause significant ischemic damage and may in some cases become life-threatening if left untreated. Therefore, management of mesenteric vasculitis generally focuses on two main objectives: initial acute management of vascular compromise, followed by treatment of the underlying disease process. Between these two objectives, management of acute intra-abdominal ischemia tends to follow similar endoscopic, intravascular, or surgical pathways regardless of disease origin, combining the therapeutic aims of minimizing bleeding, restoring blood flow where possible, and removing necrotic tissue. Long-term therapy, however, varies significantly based on diagnosis, and understanding fundamental pathophysiology and available treatment modalities is essential to optimizing outcomes.

13.4.1 General Clinical Description and Diagnosis

In most patients with mesenteric vasculitis, the majority of presenting signs and symptoms derive from downstream bowel ischemia and infarction. These symptoms generally include visceral abdominal pain, diffuse tenderness, and hematochezia, although other symptoms such as nausea/vomiting and diarrhea may also be present. Vasculitis-related thrombus formation generally results in acute mesenteric ischemia, in which patients experience sudden-onset diffuse abdominal pain lower gastrointestinal bleeding, with the classic finding of pain out of proportion to physical examination. In contrast, vasculitis causing chronic blood vessel stenosis and/or capillary destruction typically results in more insidious symptoms such as postprandial pain, anorexia, and weight loss. In severe cases, profound ischemia from vasculitis can cause necrosis of the bowel wall, which can result in intraluminal bleeding, intestinal gangrene, and perforation; patients in these scenarios typically present with peritonitis, abdominal guarding, altered mental status, hemodynamic instability, and sepsis [248].

Due to the wide variety of potential clinical manifestations, thorough workup is required when mesenteric vasculitis is suspected. Laboratory testing including basic metabolic panel, complete blood count, liver function tests, and urinalysis can help to determine baseline clinical status and the severity of current disease. During this initial survey, serum lactate can be particularly useful in assessing the presence of bowel ischemia when considered in the context of the clinical scenario. To establish a diagnosis of underlying vasculitis, nonspecific serum inflammatory markers such as CRP and ESR can be ordered first to determine the presence of inflammation, followed by more specific markers such as serum ANA, rheumatoid factor (RF), anti-neutrophilic cytoplasmic antibody (ANCA), and immunoglobulins [249].

Prompt imaging is essential to establishing a diagnosis, with abdominal computed tomography with intravenous contrast as the most widely used modality. On imaging, mesenteric inflammation with vascular compromise are often apparent, and signs of bowel ischemia may also be present, including bowel wall thickening, submucosal thumbprinting, dilated bowel loops, intramural pneumatosis, free fluid, and mesenteric or portal venous gas. In some cases, triple-phase computed tomographic angiography (CTA) can also be useful in pinpointing sites of vascular stenosis or occlusion, which may guide subsequent intervention. If intraluminal bleeding is apparent or suspected, endoscopic evaluation with esophagogastroduodenoscopy (EGD) or colonoscopy can also be performed [248].

13.4.2 Acute-Phase Management

Severe mesenteric ischemia with necrosis or bowel perforation is an indication for immediate surgical intervention, usually consisting of exploratory laparotomy with bowel resection and possible ostomy creation. For patients with acute onset of occlusion with non-necrotic bowel, less invasive revascularization techniques such as angiographic thrombectomy or stenting may be possible, although the therapeutic window for these is short in this context and combined approach with bowel resection may be indicated. Similarly, percutaneous transluminal angioplasty (PTA) may be useful in patients with a more chronic disease course, which can be performed with stenting to restore blood flow to poorly vascularized portions of the mesentery and bowel. In patients for whom angioplasty is not possible, autologous or synthetic mesenteric bypass grafting may provide therapeutic benefit [248, 249].

Intraluminal bleeding without bowel necrosis, if accessible by EGD or colonoscopy, can usually be treated with these interventions. However, refractory cases of gastrointestinal bleeding may require angiographic embolization or surgical intervention.

13.4.3 Disease-Specific Management

13.4.3.1 Lupus Mesenteric Vasculitis

Lupus mesenteric vasculitis (LMV) refers to specific SLE-related inflammation of the intraabdominal mesentery, which occurs in 0.2–9.7% of patients with the disease [250]. It is most commonly diagnosed in Asian countries, with Western countries having seemingly lower prevalence [251]. Between 8% and 40% of SLE patients have abdominal pain during the active stage of LMV, and LMV accounts for a significant portion of abdominal pain cases among SLE patients (29–65%) [250]. While the exact etiology of this condition is unknown, it is thought to either be a product of inflammatory vasculitis caused by immune complex deposition or anti-phospholipid antibody-mediated thrombosis of the mesenteric vessels [252–254]. In either case, the deposition of immune complexes in both the arterioles and venules of the mesentery cause widespread ulceration of the surrounding tissues, with additional risk of thrombosis due to the proliferation of antiphospholipid antibodies [251]. Due to widespread involvement of the mesentery and significant ischemic potential, clinical cases can vary widely on presentation, with symptoms ranging from nonspecific abdominal pain, bloating, and loose stool, to significant bowel ischemia, perforation, and peritonitis [250, 251].

Diagnosis of LMV is typically made via clinical correlation between evident SLE flare, acute abdominal pain, and imaging findings. Aside from classic signs of bowel ischemia and ascites on computed tomography, LMV often presents with a characteristic "comb sign," which represents engorgement of the mesenteric vessels against a backdrop of mesenteric edema. Typical management of this disease involves the use of high-dose corticosteroids (e.g., intravenous methylprednisolone) as well as intravenous cyclophosphamide in steroid-refractory cases, with aggressive and early surgical management indicated if bowel necrosis or perforation are suspected [251, 255]. Prognosis is generally poor, with some studies reporting a mortality of up to 50% of patients, although this risk is partially mitigated by early intervention [256] .

13.4.3.2 Polyarteritis Nodosa

Polyarteritis nodosa (PAN) is a necrotizing medium- and small-vessel vasculitis strongly associated with hepatitis B virus (HBV) infection, which accounts for approximately one-third of cases. Hepatitis C virus (HCV) infection is also associated with PAN, although the majority of cases are idiopathic; overall prevalence is 31 per million individuals. The male-to-female ratio of PAN is approximately 1.5:1, with most individuals diagnosed between 40 and 60 years [257]. The most frequently involved organ systems in PAN include the skin, peripheral nerves, muscles, joints, kidneys, and gastrointestinal tract. While the cutaneous and renal manifestations of PAN are most classically associated with the disease, gastrointestinal symptoms are present in more than 50% of patients, with abdominal pain being the most common presenting symptom [258]. In these patients, transmural inflammation of blood vessel walls can cause significant vascular compromise and ischemia of multiple organs associated with the gastrointestinal tract, including the gallbladder, liver, spleen, and mesenteric distribution. This inflammation further causes the formation of numerous aneurysms within involved vessels, which are interspersed with areas of stenosis, which increases the risk of thrombosis or bleeding [258, 259].

Clinical suspicion of gastrointestinal PAN is usually high among patients with characteristic skin lesions and abdominal pain, with more definitive diagnosis being made via abdominal CTA or catheter-based angiography. In these studies, blood vessels are found to have a beaded appearance, which is representative of the alternating aneurysm-stenosis pattern commonly seen in this disease process. Once bowel necrosis and severe ischemia have been treated or ruled out, treatment of PAN usually involves immunosuppression with pulse doses of corticosteroids with cyclophosphamide [260, 261]. For patients with underlying HBV or HCV, antiviral therapy is also indicated. Outcomes from this treatment are highly variable and depend on the extent of disease [257, 258, 260, 261].

13.4.3.3 ANCA Vasculitis

Anti-neutrophilic cytoplasmic autoantibody (ANCA) vasculitis is an umbrella term referring to three different necrotizing vasculitic diseases that primary involve small arteries: granulomatosis with polyangiitis (GPA, formerly Wegener granulomatosis), eosinophilic granulomatosis with polyangiitis (EGPA, also known as Churg-Strauss syndrome), and microscopic polyangiitis. These vasculitides are typically associated with male sex (1.5:1 male-to-female ratio), and an age of onset between 65 and 75 years [257]. GPA is associated with cytoplasmic ANCA (c-ANCA) seropositivity and typically involves the upper respiratory mucosae, lungs, and kidneys. EGPA is associated with perinuclear ANCA (p-ANCA) seropositivity and typically involves the upper respiratory mucosae, lungs, peripheral neurons, and skin. Microscopic polyangiitis is also associated with p-ANCA and typically involves the lungs, kidneys, and skin. As such, these three conditions typically involve the gastrointestinal tract only in late stages of disease, when other clinicopathological signs are usually already apparent [262].

Diagnosis of these diseases is usually accomplished via a combination of physical examination and serum ANCA testing, which is positive in over 80% of patients. Imaging can then be performed to evaluate the extent of disease. Mesenteric involvement is usually a sign of advanced disease; as such, it usually portends poor outcome. Treatment usually entails combination glucocorticoids and cyclophosphamide for induction, followed by long-term immunosuppression with either continued cyclophosphamide or newer agents such as rituximab [262].

13.4.3.4 Immunoglobulin-A Vasculitis

Immunoglobulin A (IgA) vasculitis, also known as Henoch-Schönlein purpura (HSP), is a small-vessel vasculitis that most frequently affects the skin, joints, gastrointestinal tract, and kidneys, among other organs. It predominantly occurs in children, with approximately 90% of cases manifesting in individuals under 10 years of age and peak incidence occurring at 6 years [263, 264]. However, it is still a rare condition with an overall annual incidence of 13–20 out of 100,000 individuals per year in children and 0.8–1.8 out of 100,000 individuals per year in adults [265]. The condition is best known for its palpable purpuric rash that occurs in the bilateral lower extremities after a triggering event (e.g., infection), which is usually accompanied by joint pain and hematuria [263]. In total, gastrointestinal symptoms occur in over 50% of patients, which typically manifest as acute-onset colicky abdominal pain (99%), intestinal bleeding (31%), diarrhea (26%), and rarely acute surgical abdomen (4%). These symptoms correlate with a wide variety of disorders, including intestinal obstruction, bowel wall ischemia, intussusception, and perforation [266].

The diagnosis for IgA vasculitis is usually straightforward due to the presence of a pathognomonic rash, and gastrointestinal involvement is usually easily deduced from concurrent abdominal pain and the timing of symptoms. However, given the potential severity of underlying pathology, evaluation with abdominal computed tomography is merited to rule out more serious bowel disease. Upper and lower gastrointestinal endoscopy can also be performed in patients with significant bleeding, which can be both diagnostic and therapeutic [263, 266, 267]. Approximately 50% of IgA vasculitis cases resolve spontaneously and therefore only require supportive care; other cases requiring therapy are typically treated with combination corticosteroids and adjunctive immunosuppressants (e.g., azathioprine, mycophenolate mofetil, or cyclophosphamide), with more severe presentations requiring intravenous formulations of these medications. Even among patients with more significant disease, prognosis is generally favorable, with 94% of children making a complete recovery by 2 years, although there are lingering risks of relapse and lifelong renal complications [267].

13.4.3.5 Takayasu Arteritis

Takayasu arteritis is a large-vessel granulomatous vasculitis that primarily affects the aortic arch, with extension to the subclavian and carotid arteries as well as the abdominal aorta. It is a rare disease, with an annual incidence of 0.3–3.3 new cases per million per year [268]. It primarily occurs in women (9:1 female-to-male ratio), with the majority of cases diagnosed between 15 and 45 years of age [269]. Inflammatory lesions are identified by stenosis of the affected vessel, which is caused by granulomatous and fibrotic thickening of the arterial media and adventitia with additional infiltration by plasma cells and lymphocytes. Due to the presence of stenotic lesions in high-pressure systems, claudication of the upper and lower extremities is common, and an audible bruit can sometimes be heard over the subclavian vessels or aorta on physical examination [268, 269].

Since it is primarily a large vessel disease, mesenteric involvement is not a typical presentation of this condition. However, involvement of the celiac axis or superior mesenteric artery has been known to occur, which is usually circumvented via the establishment of collaterals. In patients with insufficient collateral blood flow, symptoms manifest that are akin to chronic mesenteric ischemia [270]. Treatment for these patients typically involves glucocorticoids, although additional immunosuppression is required in some patients. In cases of refractory disease, percutaneous transluminal angioplasty (PTA) with or without stenting may be helpful in restoring blood supply and reducing symptoms [271].

13.4.3.6 Behçet Disease

Behçet disease is a variable-vessel vasculitis that is most commonly associated with ulceration of the eyes, oral mucosa, and genitals. It has an annual incidence of approximately 0.05–600 new cases per 100,000 individuals per year, with highest concentrations in Mediterranean countries and the Middle East. It mostly affects individuals aged 20–40 years and has no sex predominance. In addition to its characteristic eye, oral, and genital lesions, this disease is also associated with erythema nodosum-like skin lesions, uveitis, arthritis, arterial aneurysms, arterial and venous thrombosis, and intestinal ulceration [257]. This ulceration of the alimentary tract is most commonly seen in the terminal ileum, cecum, and ascending colon, which can produce symptoms such as recurrent abdominal pain, diarrhea, and hematochezia much like inflammatory bowel disease [272]. Treatment of this condition is usually accomplished via glucocorticoids, azathioprine, and infliximab, which have all been shown to improve symptoms in patients with mesenteric involvement [273].

13.4.3.7 Rheumatoid Arthritis

Patients with severe or refractory rheumatoid arthritis can occasionally present with an associated medium- and small-vessel vasculitis. While this vasculitis has been known to occur in the mesentery, gastrointestinal involvement is very rare and little is known about this disease process. Clinically, the medium-vessel phenotype of this disease typically presents as bowel ischemia, whereas the small-vessel phenotype presents as intestinal ulceration. Treatment for this condition is the same as that of standard rheumatoid arthritis, which includes glucocorticoids, other immunosuppressants, and biologic agents [274].

13.4.3.8 Single-Organ Vasculitis

Idiopathic localized vasculitis can occasionally occur in individual organs of the gastrointestinal tract, which often involves the appendix or select foregut organs, such as the gallbladder or the stomach. This condition usually manifests as abdominal pain, nausea/vomiting, and anorexia. Treatment involves either immunosuppression or excision of the affected organ, with varying clinical outcomes depending on the organ involved [275].

13.4.3.9 Other Vasculitides

Mesenteric vasculitis can also manifest in the context of other multisystem vasculitides, such as giant cell arteritis, Kawasaki disease, relapsing polychondritis, and cryoglobulinemic vasculitis. However, incidence of this phenomenon is rare, with only isolated cases reported in the literature [249].

Acknowledgments The authors wish to thank Billel Gasmi, MD and David E. Kleiner, MD PhD of the National Cancer Institute Center for Cancer Research for their assistance with slide procurement and histopathological analysis. The authors also wish to thank Cornelia Cudrici, MD of the National Heart, Lung, and Blood Institute for her clinical expertise and contributions to the figures in this chapter.

References

1. Köhlmeier W. Multiple Hautnekrosen bei Thrombangiitis obliterans. Arch f Dermat. 1941;181:783–92. https://doi.org/10.1007/BF01828450.
2. Degos R, Delort J, Tricot R. Dermatite papulosqameuse atrophiante. Bulletin de la Societe francaise de dermatologie et de syphiligraphie. 1942;49:148–50.
3. Theodoridis A, Makrantonaki E, Zouboulis CC. Malignant Atrophic Papulosis (Köhlmeier-Degos disease)—a review. Orphanet J Rare Dis. 2013;8:10–5. https://doi.org/10.1186/1750-1172-8-10.
4. Lu JD, Sachdeva M, Silverberg OM, Shapiro L, Croitoru D, Levy R. Clinical and laboratory prognosticators of atrophic papulosis (Degos disease): a systematic review. Orphanet J Rare Dis. 2021;16:203. https://doi.org/10.1186/s13023-021-01819-z.
5. Ball E, Newburger A, Ackerman AB. Degos' disease: a distinctive pattern of disease, chiefly of lupus erythematosus, and not a specific disease per se. Am J Dermatopathol. 2003;25:308–20. https://doi.org/10.1097/00000372-200308000-00005.
6. Toledo AE, Shapiro LS, Farrell JF, Magro CM, Polito J. Laparoscopy shows superiority over endoscopy for early detection of Malignant Atrophic Papulosis gastrointestinal complications: a case report and review of literature. BMC Gastroenterol. 2015;15:156. https://doi.org/10.1186/s12876-015-0387-y.
7. Nishida S, Howard RO. Is Degos' disease of viral origin? Lancet. 1968;291:1200–1. https://doi.org/10.1016/S0140-6736(68)91900-4.
8. Theodoridis A, Konstantinidou A, Makrantonaki E, Zouboulis C. Malignant and benign forms of atrophic papulosis (Köhlmeier-Degos disease): systemic involvement determines the prognosis. Br J Dermatol. 2014;170:110–5. https://doi.org/10.1111/bjd.12642.
9. Magrinat G, Kerwin KS, Gabriel DA. The clinical manifestations of Degos' syndrome. Arch Pathol Lab Med. 1989;113:354–62.
10. Shapiro LS, Toledo-Garcia AE, Farrell JF. Effective treatment of Malignant Atrophic Papulosis (Köhlmeier-Degos disease) with treprostinil—early experience. Orphanet J Rare Dis. 2013;8:52–6. https://doi.org/10.1186/1750-1172-8-52.
11. Torrelo A, Sevilla J, Mediero I, Candelas D, Zambrano A. Malignant Atrophic Papulosis in an infant. Br J Dermatol. 2002;146:916–8. https://doi.org/10.1046/j.1365-2133.2002.04677.x.
12. Ahmadi M, Rafi SA, Faham Z, Azhough R, Rooy SB, Rahmani O. A fatal case of Degos' disease which presented with recurrent intestinal perforation. WJGS. 2011;3:156–8. https://doi.org/10.4240/wjgs.v3.i10.156.
13. Fernandez-Perez ER, Grabscheid E, Scheinfeld NS. A case of systemic Malignant Atrophic Papulosis (Kohlmeier-Degos' disease). J Natl Med Assoc. 2005;97:421–5.
14. Hohwy T, Jensen M, Tøttrup A, Steiniche T, Fogh K. A fatal case of Malignant Atrophic Papulosis (Degos' disease) in a man with factor V Leiden mutation and Lupus anticoagulant. Acta Derm Venereol. 2006;86:245–7. https://doi.org/10.2340/00015555-0068.
15. Kim DW, Kang SB, Lee KH, Choe GY, Park SY, Nicholay M. Degos' disease (Malignant Atrophic Papulosis) as a fatal cause of acute abdomen: report of a case. Surg Today. 2008;38:866–70. https://doi.org/10.1007/s00595-007-3728-9.
16. Mareschal A, Razanamahery J, Aubin F. Malignant Atrophic Papulosis. 2020;156:204. https://doi.org/10.1001/jamadermatol.2019.3726.
17. Tummidi S, Nagendran P, Gedela S, Ramani JR, Shankaralingappa A. Degos disease: a case report and review of the literature. J Med Case Rep. 2020;14:204–8. https://doi.org/10.1186/s13256-020-02514-6.
18. Burg G, Vieluf D, Stolz W, Landthaler M, Braun-Falco O. Maligne atrophische papulose (Morbus Köhlmeier-Degos). Hautarzt. 1989;40:480–5.
19. Pukhalskaya T, Stiegler J, Scott G, Richardson CT, Smoller B. Degos disease (Malignant Atrophic Papulosis) with granular IgM on direct immunofluorescence. Cureus. 2021;13:e12677. https://doi.org/10.7759/cureus.12677.

20. Magro CM, Poe JC, Kim C, Shapiro L, Nuovo G, Crow MK, Crow YJ. Degos disease: A C5b-9/interferon—Mediated Endotheliopathy syndrome. Am J Clin Pathol. 2011;135:599–610. https://doi.org/10.1309/AJCP66QIMFARLZKI.
21. Meephansan J, Komine M, Hosoda S, Tsuda H, Karakawa M, Murata S, Demitsu T, Ohtsuki M. Possible involvement of SDF-1/CXCL12 in the pathogenesis of Degos disease. J Am Acad Dermatol. 2013;68:138–43. https://doi.org/10.1016/j.jaad.2012.06.031.
22. Soter NA, Murphy GF, Mihm MC. Lymphocytes and necrosis of the cutaneous microvasculature in malignant atrophic papulosis: a refined light microscope study. J Am Acad Dermatol. 1982;7:620–30. https://doi.org/10.1016/s0190-9622(82)70142-2.
23. Su WP, Schroeter AL, Lee DA, Hsu T, Muller SA. Clinical and histologic findings in Degos' syndrome (Malignant Atrophic Papulosis). Cutis. 1985;35:131–8.
24. Tribble K, Archer ME, Jorizzo JL, Sanchez R, Solomon AR, Gardner FH, Cavallo T. Malignant atrophic papulosis: absence of circulating immune complexes or vasculitis. J Am Acad Dermatol. 1986;2(Pt 2):365–9. https://doi.org/10.1016/s0190-9622(86)70180-1.
25. Páramo JA, Rocha E, Cuesta B, Arejola JM, Montejo M, Aguirre J, Prieto J, Rocha Hernando E. Fibrinolysis in Degos' disease. Thromb Haemost. 1985;54:730.
26. Katz SK, Mudd LJ, Roenigk HH. Malignant atrophic papulosis (Degos' disease) involving three generations of a family. 1997;37:5.
27. Powell B, Wojnarowska F, Morris. Benign familial Degos disease worsening during immunosuppression. Br J Dermatol. 1999;141:524–7. https://doi.org/10.1046/j.1365-2133.1999.03050.x.
28. Amaravadi RR, Tran TM, Altman R, Scheirey CD. Small bowel infarcts in Degos disease. Abdom Imaging. 2008;33:196–9. https://doi.org/10.1007/s00261-007-9225-1.
29. Chave T, Varma S, Patel G, Knight A. Malignant atrophic papulosis (Degos' disease): clinicopathological correlations. J Eur Acad Dermatol Venerol. 2001;15:43–5. https://doi.org/10.1046/j.1468-3083.2001.00216.x.
30. Degos R. Malignant atrophic papulosis. Br J Dermatol. 1979;100:21–35. https://doi.org/10.1111/j.1365-2133.1979.tb03566.x.
31. Fruhwirth J, Mischinger HJ, Werkgartner G, Beham A, Pfaffenthaller EC. Köhlmeier-Degos's disease with primary intestinal manifestation. Scand J Gastroenterol. 1997;32:1066–70. https://doi.org/10.3109/00365529709011226.
32. Subbiah P, Wijdicks E, Muenter M, Carter J, Connolly S. Skin lesion with a fatal neurologic outcome (Degos' disease). Neurology. 1996;46:636–40. https://doi.org/10.1212/wnl.46.3.636.
33. Goswami A, Lal S, Singhal K, Lal S, Batrani M. Skin, gut and nervous system—Think Degos Disease (P1.2-036). Neurology. 2019;15(Supplement):92.
34. Magro CM, Wang X, Garrett-Bakelman F, Laurence J, Shapiro LS, DeSancho MT. The effects of eculizumab on the pathology of malignant atrophic papulosis. Orphanet J Rare Dis. 2013;8:185. https://doi.org/10.1186/1750-1172-8-185.
35. Burgin S, Stone JH, Shenoy-Bhangle AS, McGuone D. Case 18-2014: a 32-year-old man with a rash, myalgia, and weakness. N Engl J Med 2014;370. Ed. by Cabot RC, Rosenberg ES, Harris NL, Shepard JAO, Cort AM, Ebeling SH, McDonald EK:2327–37. https://doi.org/10.1056/NEJMcpc1304161.
36. Shapiro L, Whelan P, Magro G. Correspondence, case 18-2014: a man with a rash, myalgia, and weakness. N Engl J Med. 2014;371:1361–2. https://doi.org/10.1056/NEJMc1408861.
37. De Breucker S, Vandergheynst F, Decaux G. Inefficacy of intravenous immunoglobulins and infliximab in Degos' disease. Acta Clin Belg. 2008;63:99–102. https://doi.org/10.1179/acb.2008.63.2.007.
38. Gmuca S, Boos MD, Treece A, Narula S, Billinghurst L, Bhatti T, Laje P, Perman MJ, Vossough A, Harding B, Burnham J, Banwell B. Degos disease mimicking primary vasculitis of the CNS. Neurol Neuroimmunol Neuroinflamm. 2016;3:e206. https://doi.org/10.1212/NXI.0000000000000206.

39. Pirolla E, Fregni F, Miura I, Misiara A, Almeida F, Zanoni E. Degos disease malignant atrophic papulosis or cutaneointestinal lethal syndrome: rarity of the disease. CEG. 2015;8:141–7. https://doi.org/10.2147/CEG.S59794.
40. Casparie MK, Meyer JW, van Huystee BE, Kneppelhout J, Mulder CJ. Endoscopic and histopathologic features of Degos' disease. Endoscopy. 1991;23:231–3. https://doi.org/10.1055/s-2007-1010665.
41. Lankisch MR, Johst P, Scolapio JS, Fleming CR. Acute abdominal pain as a leading symptom for Degos' disease (Malignant Atrophic Papulosis). Am J Gastroenterol. 1999;94:2.
42. Aringer M, Costenbader K, Daikh D, Brinks R, Mosca M, Ramsey-Goldman R, Smolen JS, Wofsy D, Boumpas DT, Kamen DL, Jayne D, Cervera R, Costedoat-Chalumeau N, Diamond B, Gladman DD, Hahn B, Hiepe F, Jacobsen S, Khanna D, Lerstrøm K, Massarotti E, McCune J, Ruiz-Irastorza G, Sanchez-Guerrero J, Schneider M, Urowitz M, Bertsias G, Hoyer BF, Leuchten N, Tani C, Tedeschi SK, Touma Z, Schmajuk G, Anic B, Assan F, Chan TM, Clarke AE, Crow MK, Czirják L, Doria A, Graninger W, Halda-Kiss B, Hasni S, Izmirly PM, Jung M, Kumánovics G, Mariette X, Padjen I, Pego-Reigosa JM, Romero-Diaz J, Rúa-Figueroa Fernández Í, Seror R, Stummvoll GH, Tanaka Y, Tektonidou MG, Vasconcelos C, Vital EM, Wallace DJ, Yavuz S, Meroni PL, Fritzler MJ, Naden R, Dörner T, Johnson SR. 2019 European League against Rheumatism/American College of Rheumatology classification criteria for systemic lupus erythematosus. Arthritis Rheumatol. 2019;71:1400–12. https://doi.org/10.1002/art.40930.
43. Kaklamanis P, Vayopoulos G, Stamatelos G, Dadinas G, Tsokos GC. Chronic lupus peritonitis with ascites. Ann Rheum Dis. 1991;50:176–7. https://doi.org/10.1136/ard.50.3.176.
44. Cervera R, Khamashta MA, Font J, Sebastiani GD, Gil A, Lavilla P, Mejía JC, Aydintug AO, Chwalinska-Sadowska H, de Ramón E, Fernández-Nebro A, Galeazzi M, Valen M, Mathieu A, Houssiau F, Caro N, Alba P, Ramos-Casals M, Ingelmo M, Hughes GR. Morbidity and mortality in systemic lupus erythematosus during a 10-year period: a comparison of early and late manifestations in a cohort of 1,000 patients. Medicine. 2003;82:299–308. https://doi.org/10.1097/01.md.0000091181.93122.55.
45. Salomon P, Mayer L. Nonhepatic gastrointestinal manifestations of systemic lupus erythematosus. In: Systemic lupus erythematosus. 2nd ed. New York: Churchill Livingstone; 1987.
46. Ropes MW. Systemic lupus erythematosus. Cambridge, MA: Harvard University Press; 1976.
47. Takeno M, Ishigatsubo Y. Intestinal manifestations in systemic lupus erythematosus. Intern Med. 2006;45:41–2. https://doi.org/10.2169/internalmedicine.45.0136.
48. Hoffman BI, Katz WA. The gastrointestinal manifestations of systemic lupus erythematosus: a review of the literature. Semin Arthritis Rheum. 1980;9:237–47. https://doi.org/10.1016/0049-0172(80)90016-5.
49. Alesaeidi S, Daraei M, Salami Khanshan A, Zainaldain H. A multisystem syndrome compatible with systemic lupus erythematosus: case report and review of literature. Casp J Intern Med. 2021;2021(Supplement 2):12. https://doi.org/10.22088/cjim.12.0.482.
50. Ishiguro N, Tomino Y, Fujito K, Nakayama S, Koide H. A case of massive ascites due to lupus peritonitis with a dramatic response to steroid pulse therapy. Jpn J Med. 1989;28:608–11. https://doi.org/10.2169/internalmedicine1962.28.608.
51. Ito H, Nanamiya W, Kuroda N, Inoue M, Sasaoka A, Chijiwa T, Nishiya K, Hashimoto K, Nakagawa O. Chronic lupus peritonitis with massive ascites at elderly onset: case report and review of the literature. Intern Med. 2002;41:1056–61. https://doi.org/10.2169/internalmedicine.41.1056.
52. Kheyri Z, Laripour A, Ala M. Peritonitis as the first presentation of systemic lupus erythematous: a case report. J Med Case Rep. 2021;15:611. https://doi.org/10.1186/s13256-021-03216-3.
53. Kiriakopoulos E, Perez V, Hoelle R. The great imitator strikes again: a case of a lupus flare-up presenting like an acute abdomen. HCA Healthc J Med. 2020:1. https://doi.org/10.36518/2689-0216.1012.

54. McVorran S, Song J, Pochineni V, Abrudescu-Opran A. Systemic lupus erythematosus presenting with massive ascites: a case of pseudo-pseudo Meigs syndrome. Case Rep Rheumatol. 2016;2016:1–5. https://doi.org/10.1155/2016/8701763.
55. Schousboe JT, Koch AE, Chang RW. Chronic lupus peritonitis with ascites: review of the literature with a case report. Semin Arthritis Rheum. 1988;18:121–6. https://doi.org/10.1016/0049-0172(88)90004-2.
56. Sugai S, Suda K, Tamegai K, Haino K, Nakatsue T, Narita I, Enomoto T, Nishijima K. Massive ascites due to lupus peritonitis in a patient with pre-eclampsia and systemic lupus erythematosus: a case report. BMC Pregn Childbirth. 2022;22:203. https://doi.org/10.1186/s12884-022-04550-0.
57. Zhou L, Ming Sun C, Li Chen W, Zhang H, Wang P, Wu J. Massive and painful ascites as a presenting manifestation of systemic lupus erythematosus flare: a case report and literature review. Rev Méd Chile. 2014;142:255–60. https://doi.org/10.4067/S0034-98872014000200016.
58. Pons-Estel GJ, Alarcón GS, Scofield L, Reinlib L, Cooper GS. Understanding the epidemiology and progression of systemic lupus erythematosus. Semin Arthritis Rheum. 2010;39:257–68. https://doi.org/10.1016/j.semarthrit.2008.10.007.
59. Maruyama A, Nagashima T, Iwamoto M, Minota S. Clinical characteristics of lupus enteritis in Japanese patients: the large intestine-dominant type has features of intestinal pseudo-obstruction. Lupus. 2018;27:1661–9. https://doi.org/10.1177/0961203318785770.
60. Lee CK. Acute abdominal pain in systemic lupus erythematosus: focus on lupus enteritis (Gastrointestinal Vasculitis). Ann Rheum Dis. 2002;61:547–50. https://doi.org/10.1136/ard.61.6.547.
61. Frittoli RB, Vivaldo JF, Costallat LTL, Appenzeller S. Gastrointestinal involvement in systemic lupus erythematosus: a systematic review. J Transl Autoimmun. 2021;4:100106. https://doi.org/10.1016/j.jtauto.2021.100106.
62. Man BL, Mok CC. Serositis related to systemic lupus erythematosus: prevalence and outcome. Lupus. 2005;14:822–6. https://doi.org/10.1191/0961203305lu2187oa.
63. Watanabe R, Fujii H, Kamogawa Y, Nakamura K, Shirai T, Ishii T, Harigae H. Chronic lupus peritonitis is characterized by the ascites with a large content of interleukin-6. Tohoku J Exp Med. 2015;235:289–94. https://doi.org/10.1620/tjem.235.289.
64. Pott Júnior H, Amate Neto A, Teixeira MAB, Provenza JR. Ascites due to lupus peritonitis: a rare form of onset of systemic lupus erythematosus. Rev Bras Reumatol. 2012;52:116–9.
65. Schocket AL, Lain D, Kohler PF, Steigerwald J. Immune complex vasculitis as a cause of ascites and pleural effusions in systemic lupus erythematosus. J Rheumatol. 1978;5:33–8.
66. Okamoto T, Okano Y, Kawagoe M, Hara M. Two cases of ascites due to lupus peritonitis. Ryumachi. 1981;21(Suppl):189–94.
67. Atisha-Fregoso Y, Hernández-Ramírez DF, Olivares-Martínez E, Núñez-Alvarez CA, Llorente L, Hernández-Molina G. Refractory ascites in systemic lupus erythematosus: further biological support of intraperitoneal steroid treatment as a suitable therapeutical option. Clin Rheumatol. 2017;36:707–11. https://doi.org/10.1007/s10067-016-3473-9.
68. Hammami S, Bdioui F, Ouaz A, Loghmari H, Mahjoub S, Saffar H. Successful treatment of massive ascites due to lupus peritonitis with hydroxychloroquine in old- onset lupus erythematosus. Pan Afr Med J. 2014:18. https://doi.org/10.11604/pamj.2014.18.165.2080.
69. Barnes TC, Anderson ME, Moots RJ. The many faces of interleukin-6: the role of IL-6 in inflammation, vasculopathy, and fibrosis in systemic sclerosis. Int J Rheumatol. 2011;2011:1–6. https://doi.org/10.1155/2011/721608.
70. Uzu T, Chikamori Y, Yamato M, Iwatani H, Kakihara M, Yamauchi A. Acute lupus peritonitis during treatment oflupus nephritis: successful treatment with methylprednisolone pulse therapy. Nephron. 2000;86:511–2. https://doi.org/10.1159/000045846.
71. Provenzano G, Rinaldi F, Le Moli S, Pagliaro L. Chronic lupus peritonitis responsive to treatment with cyclophosphamide. Br J Rheumatol. 1993;32:1116. https://doi.org/10.1093/rheumatology/32.12.1116.

72. Kawashiri S, Nishino A, Sueyoshi E, Okada A, Koga T, Yamasaki S, Nakamura H, Origuchi T, Kawakami A. A patient with systemic lupus erythematosus who developed massive small intestinal hemorrhaging during treatment for chronic lupus peritonitis. Mod Rheumatol. 2012;22:312–5. https://doi.org/10.3109/s10165-011-0499-3.
73. Kirshy DM, Gordon DH, Atweh NA. Abdominal computed tomography in lupus mesenteric arteritis. Comput Med Imaging Graph. 1991;15:369–72. https://doi.org/10.1016/0895-6111(91)90147-n.
74. Zhou QG, Yang XB, Hou FF, Zhang X. Successful treatment of massive ascites with intraperitoneal administration of a steroid in a case of systemic lupus erythematosus. Lupus. 2009;18:740–2. https://doi.org/10.1177/0961203308099709.
75. Shreiner AB, Murray C, Denton C, Khanna D. Gastrointestinal manifestations of systemic sclerosis. J Scleroderma Related Disord. 2016;1:247–56. https://doi.org/10.5301/jsrd.5000214.
76. Sallam H, Mcnearney TA, Chen JDZ. Systematic review: pathophysiology and management of gastrointestinal dysmotility in systemic sclerosis (Scleroderma). Aliment Pharmacol Ther. 2006;23:691–712. https://doi.org/10.1111/j.1365-2036.2006.02804.x.
77. Nikpour M, Stevens WM, Herrick AL, Proudman SM. Epidemiology of systemic sclerosis. Best Pract Res Clin Rheumatol. 2010;24:857–69.
78. Bergamasco A, Hartmann N, Wallace L, Verpillat P. Epidemiology of systemic sclerosis and systemic sclerosis-associated interstitial lung disease. CLEP. 2019;11:257–73. https://doi.org/10.2147/CLEP.S191418.
79. Bairkdar M, Rossides M, Westerlind H, Hesselstrand R, Arkema EV, Holmqvist M. Incidence and prevalence of systemic sclerosis globally: a comprehensive systematic review and meta-analysis. Rheumatology. 2021;60:3121–33. https://doi.org/10.1093/rheumatology/keab190.
80. Furst DE, Clements PJ, Saab M, Sterz MG, Paulus HE. Clinical and serological comparison of 17 chronic progressive systemic sclerosis (PSS) and 17 CREST syndrome patients matched for sex, age, and disease duration. Ann Rheum Dis. 1984;43:794–801. https://doi.org/10.1136/ard.43.6.794.
81. Hunzelmann N, Genth E, Krieg T, Lehmacher W, Melchers I, Meurer M, Moinzadeh P, Muller-Ladner U, Pfeiffer C, Riemekasten G, Schulze-Lohoff E, Sunderkoetter C, Weber M, Worm M, Klaus P, Rubbert A, Steinbrink K, Grundt B, Hein R, Scharffetter-Kochanek K, Hinrichs R, Walker K, Szeimies RM, Karrer S, Muller A, Seitz C, Schmidt E, Lehmann P, Foeldvari I, Reichenberger F, Gross W, Kuhn A, Haust M, Reich K, Bohm M, Saar P, Fierlbeck G, Kotter I, Lorenz HM, Blank N, Grafenstein K, Juche A, Aberer E, Bali G, Fiehn C, Stadler R, Bartels V. The registry of the German network for systemic scleroderma: frequency of disease subsets and patterns of organ involvement. Rheumatology. 2008;47:1185–92. https://doi.org/10.1093/rheumatology/ken179.
82. Vischio J, Matlyuk-Urman Z, Lakshminarayanan S. Benign spontaneous pneumoperitoneum in systemic sclerosis. JCR J Clin Rheumatol. 2010;16:379–81. https://doi.org/10.1097/RHU.0b013e3181ffeb49.
83. Cullinan DER. Discussion on scleroderma. Proc R Soc Med. 1952:17–32.
84. Saigusa S, Inoue Y, Ohi M, Imaoka H, Uratani R, Kobayashi M, Kusunoki M. Distinguishing between limited systemic scleroderma-associated pseudo-obstruction and peritoneal dissemination. Surg Case Rep. 2015;1:21. https://doi.org/10.1186/s40792-014-0010-4.
85. D'Angelo WA, Fries JF, Masi AT, Shulman LE. Pathologic observations in systemic sclerosis (Scleroderma). Am J Med. 1969;46:428–40. https://doi.org/10.1016/0002-9343(69)90044-8.
86. Steen VD, Powell DL, Medsger TA. Clinical correlations and prognosis based on serum autoantibodies in patients with systemic sclerosis. Arthritis Rheum. 1988;31:196–203. https://doi.org/10.1002/art.1780310207.
87. Van den Hoogen F, Khanna D, Fransen J, Johnson SR, Baron M, Tyndall A, Matucci-Cerinic M, Naden RP, Medsger TA, Carreira PE, Riemekasten G, Clements PJ, Denton CP, Distler O, Allanore Y, Furst DE, Gabrielli A, Mayes MD, van Laar JM, Seibold JR, Czirjak L, Steen VD, Inanc M, Kowal-Bielecka O, Müller-Ladner U, Valentini G, Veale DJ, Vonk

MC, Walker UA, Chung L, Collier DH, Ellen Csuka M, Fessler BJ, Guiducci S, Herrick A, Hsu VM, Jimenez S, Kahaleh B, Merkel PA, Sierakowski S, Silver RM, Simms RW, Varga J, Pope JE. 2013 classification criteria for systemic sclerosis: An American College of Rheumatology/European League against Rheumatism Collaborative Initiative. Ann Rheum Dis. 2013;72:1747–55. https://doi.org/10.1136/annrheumdis-2013-204424.

88. Tuffanelli DL, McKeon F, Kleinsmith DM, Burnham TK, Kirschner M. Anticentromere and anticentriole antibodies in the scleroderma spectrum. Arch Dermatol. 1983;119:560–6.
89. Bures J. Small intestinal bacterial overgrowth syndrome. WJG. 2010;16:2978. https://doi.org/10.3748/wjg.v16.i24.2978.
90. McFarlane IM, Bhamra MS, Kreps A, Iqbal S, Ani FA, Aponte CS, Grant C, Singh S, Awwal K, Do KK, Saperstein Y, Mercado FMA, Laskar DB, Atluri P. Gastrointestinal manifestations of systemic sclerosis. Rheumatology. 2018;8. https://doi.org/10.4172/2161-1149.1000235.
91. Dukowicz AC, Lacy BE, Levine GM. Small intestinal bacterial overgrowth: a comprehensive review. Gastroenterol Hepatol (N Y). 2007;3:112–22.
92. Kaneko M, Sasaki S, Teruya S, Ozaki K, Ishimaru K, Terai E, Nakayama H, Watanabe T. Pneumatosis cystoides intestinalis in patients with systemic sclerosis: a case report and review of 39 Japanese cases. Case Rep Gastrointest Med. 2016;2016:1–5. https://doi.org/10.1155/2016/2474515.
93. Kumar S, Singh J, Rattan S, DiMarino AJ, Cohen S, Jimenez SA. Review article: pathogenesis and clinical manifestations of gastrointestinal involvement in systemic sclerosis. Aliment Pharmacol Ther. 2017;45:883–98. https://doi.org/10.1111/apt.13963.
94. Koysombat K, Capanna MV, Stafford N, and Orchard T. Combination therapy for systemic sclerosis-associated pneumatosis intestinalis. BMJ Case Rep. 2018:bcr-2018–225068. https://doi.org/10.1136/bcr-2018-225068.
95. Sequeira W. Pneumatosis cystoides intestinalis in systemic sclerosis and other diseases. Sem Arthritis Rheumat. 1990;19:269–77. https://doi.org/10.1016/0049-0172(90)90049-L.
96. Medsger TA. Treatment of systemic sclerosis. Ann Rheum Dis Suppl. 1991;4(50):877–86. https://doi.org/10.1136/ard.50.Suppl_4.877.
97. Heil R, Schairer J, and Warren B. A case report of spontaneous pneumoperitoneum related to scleroderma without evidence of pneumatosis cystoides intestinalis. Pract Gastroenterol. 2016:4.
98. Rigamonti C. Clinical features and prognosis of primary biliary cirrhosis associated with systemic sclerosis. Gut. 2006;55:388–94. https://doi.org/10.1136/gut.2005.075002.
99. Jayson MI, Salmon PR, Gough J, Poliness T, Bishton RL. Spontaneous bowel perforation in intestinal scleroderma: first report of a non-fatal case. Postgrad Med J. 1972;48:56–8.
100. Guan J, Munaf A, Simmonds AV, Inayat I. When the benign pneumatosis intestinalis becomes no longer benign: a rare case of bowel perforation in a patient with systemic sclerosis. Case Rep Gastrointest Med. 2018;2018:1–4. https://doi.org/10.1155/2018/5124145.
101. Robinson JC. stercoral ulceration and perforation of the sclerodermatous colon: report of two cases and review of the literature. 1974:11.
102. Ho YY, Lagares D, Tager AM, Kapoor M. Fibrosis—a lethal component of systemic sclerosis. Nat Rev Rheumatol. 2014;10:390–402. https://doi.org/10.1038/nrrheum.2014.53.
103. Chu H, Wu T, Wu W, Tu W, Jiang S, Chen S, Ma Y, Liu Q, Zhou X, Jin L, Wang J. Involvement of collagen-binding heat shock protein 47 in scleroderma-associated fibrosis. Protein Cell. 2015;6:589–98. https://doi.org/10.1007/s13238-015-0171-3.
104. Varga J, Haustein UF, Creech RH, Dwyer JP, Jimenez SA. Exaggerated radiation-induced fibrosis in patients with systemic sclerosis. JAMA. 1991;265:3292–5.
105. Moschos J, Leontiadis GI, Kelly C, Henry J, Kadis S. Idiopathic portal hypertension complicating systemic sclerosis: a case report. BMC Gastroenterol. 2005;5:16. https://doi.org/10.1186/1471-230X-5-16.
106. Ishii M, Katada Y. Idiopathic portal hypertension in a systemic sclerosis patient heterozygous for factor V Leiden mutation. Rheumatol Int. 2003;23:44–6. https://doi.org/10.1007/s00296-002-0259-y.

107. Palma A, Sanchez-Palencia A, Armas JR, Milan JA, Fernandez-Sanz J, Llach F. Progressive systemic sclerosis and nephrotic syndrome. an unusual association resulting in postpartum acute renal failure. Arch Intern Med. 1981;141:520–1.
108. Turner R, Lipshutz W, Miller W, Rittenberg G, Schumacher HR, Cohen S. Esophageal dysfunction in collagen disease. Am J Med Sci. 1973;265:191–9. https://doi.org/10.1097/00000441-197303000-00002.
109. Akesson A, Wollheim FA. Organ manifestations in 100 patients with progressive systemic sclerosis: a comparison between the CREST syndrome and diffuse scleroderma. Br J Rheumatol. 1989;28:281–6. https://doi.org/10.1093/rheumatology/28.4.281.
110. Bassel M, Hudson M, Taillefer SS, Schieir O, Baron M, Thombs BD. Frequency and impact of symptoms experienced by patients with systemic sclerosis: results from a Canadian National Survey. Rheumatology. 2011;50:762–7. https://doi.org/10.1093/rheumatology/keq310.
111. Agarwal A, Yeh BM, Breiman RS, Qayyum A, Coakley FV. Peritoneal calcification: causes and distinguishing features on CT. Am J Roentgenol. 2004;182:441–5. https://doi.org/10.2214/ajr.182.2.1820441.
112. Ho KT, Reveille JD. The clinical relevance of autoantibodies in scleroderma. Arthritis Res Ther. 2003;5:80–93. https://doi.org/10.1186/ar628.
113. Ross L, Stevens W, Rabusa C, Wilson M, Ferdowsi N, Walker J, Sahhar J, Ngian GS, Zochling J, Roddy J, Tymms K, Major G, Strickland G, Proudman SM, Nikpour M. The role of inflammatory markers in assessment of disease activity in systemic sclerosis. Clin Exp Rheumatol. 2018;36(Suppl 113):126–34.
114. White B. Immunopathogenesis of systemic sclerosis. Rheum Dis Clin N Am. 1996;22:695–708. https://doi.org/10.1016/s0889-857x(05)70296-9.
115. Angeli P, Bernardi M, Villanueva C, Francoz C, Mookerjee RP, Trebicka J, Krag A, Laleman W, Gines P. EASL clinical practice guidelines for the management of patients with decompensated cirrhosis. J Hepatol. 2018;69:406–60. https://doi.org/10.1016/j.jhep.2018.03.024.
116. Runyon BA. Introduction to the Revised American Association for the study of liver diseases practice guideline management of adult patients with ascites due to cirrhosis 2012. Hepatology. 2013;57:1651–3. https://doi.org/10.1002/hep.26359.
117. Gyger G, Baron M. Systemic sclerosis: gastrointestinal disease and its management. Rheum Dis Clin N Am. 2015;41:459–73. https://doi.org/10.1016/j.rdc.2015.04.007.
118. Miller JB, Gandhi N, Clarke J, McMahan Z. Gastrointestinal involvement in systemic sclerosis: an update. J Clin Rheumatol. 2018;24:328–37. https://doi.org/10.1097/RHU.0000000000000626.
119. Kahana N, Freund MR, Koslowsky B, Blich O, Reissman P, Yellinek S. High failure rate following restorative surgery for rectal prolapse in systemic sclerosis patients. Am Surg. 2021:31348211047487. https://doi.org/10.1177/00031348211047487.
120. Owtschinnikow PJ. Peritonitis chronica fibrosa incapsulata. Arch Klin Chir. 1907;83:623–34.
121. Korte MR, Sampimon DE, Betjes MGH, Krediet RT. Encapsulating peritoneal sclerosis: the state of affairs. Nat Rev Nephrol. 2011;7:528–38. https://doi.org/10.1038/nrneph.2011.93.
122. Moinuddin Z, Summers A, Van Dellen D, Augustine T, Herrick SE. Encapsulating peritoneal sclerosis—a rare but devastating peritoneal disease. Front Physiol. 2015;5:470. https://doi.org/10.3389/fphys.2014.00470.
123. Danford CJ, Lin SC, Smith MP, Wolf JL. Encapsulating peritoneal sclerosis. World J Gastroenterol. 2018;24:3101–11. https://doi.org/10.3748/wjg.v24.i28.3101.
124. Jagirdar RM, Bozikas A, Zarogiannis SG, Bartosova M, Schmitt CP, Liakopoulos V. Encapsulating peritoneal sclerosis: pathophysiology and current treatment options. Int J Mol Sci. 2019;20:5765. https://doi.org/10.3390/ijms20225765.
125. Singhal M, Krishna S, Lal A, Narayanasamy S, Bal A, Yadav TD, Kochhar R, Sinha SK, Khandelwal N, Sheikh AM. Encapsulating peritoneal sclerosis: the abdominal cocoon. RadioGraphics. 2019;39:62–77. https://doi.org/10.1148/rg.2019180108.
126. Machado NO. Sclerosing encapsulating peritonitis. Sultan Qaboos Univ Med J. 2016;16:e142–51. https://doi.org/10.18295/squmj.2016.16.02.003.

127. Mangan C, Moinuddin Z, Summers A, de Reuver P, van Dellen D, Augustine T. Encapsulating peritoneal sclerosis following hyperthermic intraperitoneal chemotherapy. ANZ J Surg. 2019;89:E468–9. https://doi.org/10.1111/ans.14770.
128. Takebayashi K, Sonoda H, Shimizu T, Ohta H, Ishida M, Mekata E, Endo Y, Tani T, Tani M. Successful surgical approach for a patient with encapsulating peritoneal sclerosis after hyperthermic intraperitoneal chemotherapy: a case report and literature review. BMC Surg. 2014;14:57. https://doi.org/10.1186/1471-2482-14-57.
129. Habib SM, Betjes MGH, Fieren MWJA, Boeschoten EW, Abrahams AC, Boer WH, Struijk DG, Ruger W, Krikke C, Westerhuis R, de Sévaux RGL, van der Sande FM, Gaasbeek A, Korte MR, Eps Registry. Management of encapsulating peritoneal sclerosis: a guideline on optimal and uniform treatment. Neth J Med. 2011;69:500–7.
130. Kawanishi H, Banshodani M, Yamashita M, Shintaku S, Dohi K. Surgical treatment for encapsulating peritoneal sclerosis: 24 years' experience. Perit Dial Int. 2019;39:169–74. https://doi.org/10.3747/pdi.2018.00042.
131. Balasubramaniam G, Brown EA, Davenport A, Cairns H, Cooper B, Fan SLS, Farrington K, Gallagher H, Harnett P, Krausze S, Steddon S. The Pan-Thames EPS Study: treatment and outcomes of encapsulating peritoneal sclerosis. Nephrol Dial Transplant. 2009;24:3209–15. https://doi.org/10.1093/ndt/gfp008.
132. Betjes MGH, Habib SM, Boeschoten EW, Hemke AC, Struijk DG, Westerhuis R, Abrahams AC, Korte MR. Significant decreasing incidence of encapsulating peritoneal sclerosis in the Dutch population of peritoneal dialysis patients. Perit Dial Int. 2017;37:230–4. https://doi.org/10.3747/pdi.2016.00109.
133. Brown EA, Bargman J, van Biesen W, Chang MY, Finkelstein FO, Hurst H, Johnson DW, Kawanishi H, Lambie M, de Moraes TP, Morelle J, Woodrow G. Length of time on peritoneal dialysis and encapsulating peritoneal sclerosis—position paper for ISPD: 2017 update. Perit Dial Int. 2017;37:362–74. https://doi.org/10.3747/pdi.2017.00018.
134. Akbulut S. Accurate definition and management of idiopathic sclerosing encapsulating peritonitis. World J Gastroenterol. 2015;21:675–87. https://doi.org/10.3748/wjg.v21.i2.675.
135. Singh O, Gupta S, Shukla S, Mathur RK. Idiopathic sclerosing encapsulating peritonitis; rare cause of intestinal obstruction. Internet J Surg. 2008:20.
136. Kawanishi H, Moriishi M. Epidemiology of encapsulating peritoneal sclerosis in Japan. Perit Dial Int. 2005;25(Suppl 4):S14–8.
137. Kawanishi H, Kawaguchi Y, Fukui H, Hara S, Imada A, Kubo H, Kin M, Nakamoto M, Ohira S, Shoji T. Encapsulating peritoneal sclerosis in Japan: a prospective, controlled, multicenter study. Am J Kidney Dis. 2004;44:729–37. https://doi.org/10.1016/S0272-6386(04)00953-9.
138. Lambie M, Teece L, Johnson DW, Petrie M, Mactier R, Solis-Trapala I, Belcher J, Bekker HL, Wilkie M, Tupling K, Phillips-Darby L, Davies SJ. Estimating risk of encapsulating peritoneal sclerosis accounting for the competing risk of death. Nephrol Dial Transplant. 2019;34:1585–91. https://doi.org/10.1093/ndt/gfz034.
139. Johnson DW, Cho Y, Livingston BER, Hawley CM, McDonald SP, Brown FG, Rosman JB, Bannister KM, Wiggins KJ. Encapsulating peritoneal sclerosis: incidence, predictors, and outcomes. Kidney Int. 2010;77:904–12. https://doi.org/10.1038/ki.2010.16.
140. Li N, Zhu W, Li Y, Gong J, Gu L, Li M, Cao L, Li J. Surgical treatment and perioperative management of idiopathic abdominal cocoon: single-center review of 65 cases. World J Surg. 2014;38:1860–7. https://doi.org/10.1007/s00268-014-2458-6.
141. Wei B, Wei HB, Guo WP, Zheng ZH, Huang Y, Hu BG, Huang JL. Diagnosis and treatment of abdominal cocoon: a report of 24 cases. Am J Surg. 2009;198:348–53. https://doi.org/10.1016/j.amjsurg.2008.07.054.
142. Xu P, Chen LH, Li YM. Idiopathic sclerosing encapsulating peritonitis (or abdominal cocoon): a report of 5 cases. World J Gastroenterol. 2007;13:3649–51. https://doi.org/10.3748/wjg.v13.i26.3649.

143. Clement PB, Young RH, Hanna W, Scully RE. Sclerosing peritonitis associated with luteinized thecomas of the ovary. A clinicopathological analysis of six cases. Am J Surg Pathol. 1994;18:1–13. https://doi.org/10.1097/00000478-199401000-00001.
144. Schwenger V, Morath C, Salava A, Amann K, Seregin Y, Deppisch R, Ritz E, Bierhaus A, Nawroth PP, Zeier M. Damage to the peritoneal membrane by glucose degradation products is mediated by the receptor for advanced glycation end-products. J Am Soc Nephrol. 2006;17:199–207. https://doi.org/10.1681/ASN.2005020155.
145. Nakamura S, Niwa T. Advanced glycation end-products and peritoneal sclerosis. Semin Nephrol. 2004;24:502–5. https://doi.org/10.1016/j.semnephrol.2004.06.027.
146. Maruyama Y, Numata M, Nakayama M, Matsuo N, Nordfors L, Hosoya T, Lindholm B. Relationship between the -374T/A receptor of advanced glycation end products gene polymorphism and peritoneal solute transport status at the initiation of peritoneal dialysis. Ther Apher Dial. 2007;11:301–5. https://doi.org/10.1111/j.1744-9987.2007.00473.x.
147. Ngô Y, Messing B, Marteau P, Nouël O, Pasquiou A, Lavergne A, Rambaud JC. Peritoneal sarcoidosis. an unrecognized cause of sclerosing peritonitis. Dig Dis Sci. 1992;37:1776–80. https://doi.org/10.1007/BF01299875.
148. Pepels MJE, Peters FPJ, Mebis JJIR, Ceelen TL, Hoofwijk AGM, Erdkamp FLG. Sclerosing peritonitis: an unusual cause of ascites in a patient with systemic lupus erythematosus. Neth J Med. 2006;64:346–9.
149. Dabak R, Uygur-Bayramiçli O, Aydln DK, Dolapçloglu C, Gemici C, Erginel T, Turan C, Karadayl N. Encapsulating peritonitis and familial Mediterranean fever. World J Gastroenterol. 2005;11:2844–6. https://doi.org/10.3748/wjg.v11.i18.2844.
150. Slingeneyer A. Preliminary report on a cooperative international study on sclerosing encapsulating peritonitis. Contrib Nephrol. 1987;57:239–47. https://doi.org/10.1159/000414288.
151. Nomoto Y, Kawaguchi Y, Kubo H, Hirano H, Sakai S, Kurokawa K. Sclerosing encapsulating peritonitis in patients undergoing continuous ambulatory peritoneal dialysis: a report of the Japanese Sclerosing Encapsulating Peritonitis Study Group. Am J Kidney Dis. 1996;28:420–7. https://doi.org/10.1016/s0272-6386(96)90501-6.
152. Sachdev A, Usatoff V, Thaow C. Sclerosing encapsulating peritonitis and methotrexate. Aust NZ J Obstet Gynaecol. 2006;46:58–9. https://doi.org/10.1111/j.1479-828X.2006.00517.x.
153. Spanos G, Harissis HV, Dounousi E, Mitsis M, Pappas H, Georgiou GK, Siamopoulos KC, Fatouros M. A case of encapsulating peritoneal sclerosis presented shortly after renal transplantation. CEN Case Rep. 2013;3:40–3. https://doi.org/10.1007/s13730-013-0079-9.
154. Khanna A, Plummer M, Bromberek C, Bresnahan B, Hariharan S. Expression of TGF-beta and fibrogenic genes in transplant recipients with tacrolimus and cyclosporine nephrotoxicity. Kidney Int. 2002;62:2257–63. https://doi.org/10.1046/j.1523-1755.2002.00668.x.
155. Nauen DW, Martin A, Katz A, Cohen D, Ranganathan S. A case of luteinizing thecoma with sclerosing peritonitis: revisiting a link with anti-epileptic drugs. Pediatr Blood Cancer. 2010;54:470–2. https://doi.org/10.1002/pbc.22325.
156. Marigold JH, Pounder RE, Pemberton J, Thompson RP. Propranolol, oxprenolol, and sclerosing peritonitis. Br Med J (Clin Res Ed). 1982;284:870.
157. Liappas G, González-Mateo G, Aguirre AR, Abensur H, Albar-Vizcaino P, Parra EG, Sandoval P, Ramírez LG, del Peso G, Acedo JM, Bajo MA, Selgas R, Tomero JAS, López-Cabrera M, Aguilera A. Nebivolol, a B1-adrenergic blocker, protects from peritoneal membrane damage induced during peritoneal dialysis. Oncotarget. 2016;7:30133–46. https://doi.org/10.18632/oncotarget.8780.
158. Bahar B, Hu Z, Szpaderska A, Liotta M, Potkul RK, Smith D, Erşahin Ç. Fatal case of luteinized thecoma with sclerosing peritonitis in a 40-year-old woman. Int J Gynecol Pathol. 2014;33:30–4. https://doi.org/10.1097/PGP.0b013e31827d1a65.
159. Walker J, Moss EL, Ganesan R, Hirschowitz L. Sclerosing peritonitis associated with a luteinized adult granulosa cell tumor. Int J Gynecol Pathol. 2012;31:141–4. https://doi.org/10.1097/PGP.0b013e3182307b28.

160. Yang YM, Yang WX. Epithelial-to-mesenchymal transition in the development of endometriosis. Oncotarget. 2017;8:41679–89. https://doi.org/10.18632/oncotarget.16472.
161. Augustine T, Brown PW, Davies SD, Summers AM, Wilkie ME. Encapsulating peritoneal sclerosis: clinical significance and implications. NEC. 2009;111:c149–54. https://doi.org/10.1159/000191214.
162. Bozkurt D, Cetin P, Sipahi S, Hur E, Nar H, Ertilav M, Sezak M, Duman S. The effects of renin-angiotensin system inhibition on regression of encapsulating peritoneal sclerosis. Perit Dial Int. 2008;28(Suppl 5):S38–42.
163. Honda K, Oda H. Pathology of encapsulating peritoneal sclerosis. Perit Dial Int. 2005;25(Suppl 4):S19–29.
164. Alscher DM, Braun N, Biegger D, Fritz P. Peritoneal mast cells in peritoneal dialysis patients, particularly in encapsulating peritoneal sclerosis patients. Am J Kidney Dis. 2007;49:452–61. https://doi.org/10.1053/j.ajkd.2006.11.040.
165. Reimann D, Dachs D, Meye C, Gross P. Amino acid-based peritoneal dialysis solution stimulates mesothelial nitric oxide production. Perit Dial Int. 2004;24:378–84.
166. Braun N, Alscher MD, Fritz P, Latus J, Edenhofer I, Reimold F, Alper SL, Kimmel M, Biegger D, Lindenmeyer M, Cohen CD, Wüthrich RP, Segerer S. The spectrum of podoplanin expression in encapsulating peritoneal sclerosis. PLoS One. 2012;7:e53382. https://doi.org/10.1371/journal.pone.0053382.
167. Abrahams AC, Habib SM, Dendooven A, Riser BL, van der Veer JW, Toorop RJ, Betjes MGH, Verhaar MC, Watson CJE, Nguyen TQ, Boer WH. Patients with encapsulating peritoneal sclerosis have increased peritoneal expression of connective tissue growth factor (CCN2), transforming growth factor- 1, and vascular endothelial growth factor. PLoS One. 2014;9:e112050. https://doi.org/10.1371/journal.pone.0112050.
168. Kawanishi H, Moriishi M. Encapsulating peritoneal sclerosis: prevention and treatment. Perit Dial Int. 2007;27(Suppl 2):S289–92.
169. Candido PCM, Werner AF, Pereira IMF, Matos BA, Pfeilsticker RM, Silva R. Sclerosing encapsulating peritonitis: a case report, vol. 48. Radiol Bras; 2015. p. 56–8. https://doi.org/10.1590/0100-3984.2013.1909.
170. Akbulut S, Yagmur Y, Babur M. Coexistence of abdominal cocoon, intestinal perforation and incarcerated Meckel's diverticulum in an inguinal hernia: a troublesome condition. World J Gastrointest Surg. 2014;6:51–4. https://doi.org/10.4240/wjgs.v6.i3.51.
171. Kawanishi H, Shintaku S, Moriishi M, Dohi K, Tsuchiya S. Seventeen years' experience of surgical options for encapsulating peritoneal sclerosis. Adv Perit Dial. 2011;27:53–8.
172. Tannoury JN, Abboud BN. Idiopathic sclerosing encapsulating peritonitis: abdominal cocoon. World J Gastroenterol. 2012;18:1999–2004. https://doi.org/10.3748/wjg.v18.i17.1999.
173. Araújo JAB, Martines JAS, Martines BMR, da Silva AF, Lovisolo SM, de Castro CC. Idiopathic sclerosing encapsulating peritonitis: an uncommon cause of intestinal obstruction. Autops Case Rep. 2012;2:51–6. https://doi.org/10.4322/acr.2012.026.
174. Alston H, Fan S, Nakayama M. Encapsulating peritoneal sclerosis. Semin Nephrol. 2017;37:93–102. https://doi.org/10.1016/j.semnephrol.2016.10.010.
175. Hsu YH, Hsia CC, Tsai DM, Tu HY, Hung KY, Huang JW. Development of encapsulating peritoneal sclerosis following bacterial peritonitis in a peritoneal dialysis patient. Am J Kidney Dis. 2010;55:198–202. https://doi.org/10.1053/j.ajkd.2009.06.043.
176. Nakamoto H. Encapsulating peritoneal sclerosis–a clinician's approach to diagnosis and medical treatment. Perit Dial Int. 2005;25(Suppl 4):S30–8.
177. Maruyama Y, Nakayama M. Encapsulating peritoneal sclerosis in Japan. Perit Dial Int. 2008;28(Suppl 3):S201–4.
178. Korte MR, Fieren MW, Sampimon DE, Lingsma HF, Weimar W, Betjes MGH, Investigators of the Dutch Multicentre EPS Study. Tamoxifen is associated with lower mortality of encapsulating peritoneal sclerosis: results of the dutch multicentre EPS study. Nephrol Dial Transplant. 2011;26:691–7. https://doi.org/10.1093/ndt/gfq362.

179. Del Peso G, Bajo MA, Gil F, Aguilera A, Ros S, Costero O, Castro MJ, Selgas R. Clinical experience with tamoxifen in peritoneal fibrosing syndromes. Adv Perit Dial. 2003;19:32–5.
180. Lafrance JP, Létourneau I, Ouimet D, Bonnardeaux A, Leblanc M, Mathieu N, Pichette V. Successful treatment of encapsulating peritoneal sclerosis with immunosuppressive therapy. Am J Kidney Dis. 2008;51:e7–e10. https://doi.org/10.1053/j.ajkd.2007.07.036.
181. Ulmer C, Braun N, Rieber F, Latus J, Hirschburger S, Emmel J, Alscher MD, Steurer W, Thon KP. Efficacy and morbidity of surgical therapy in late-stage encapsulating peritoneal sclerosis. Surgery. 2013;153:219–24. https://doi.org/10.1016/j.surg.2012.07.033.
182. Tseng CC, Chen JB, Wang IK, Liao SC, Cheng BC, Ab W, Chang YT, Hung SY, Huang CC. Incidence and outcomes of encapsulating peritoneal sclerosis (EPS) and factors associated with severe EPS. PLoS ONE. 2018;13:e0190079. https://doi.org/10.1371/journal.pone.0190079.
183. AlZabali SM, AlAnazi A, Rahim KA, Faqeehi HY. Clinical improvement of encapsulating peritoneal sclerosis after challenging course and 6 months of total parenteral nutrition in child with nephronophthisis: a case report. J Med Case Rep. 2021;15:366. https://doi.org/10.1186/s13256-021-02905-3.
184. Ormond JK. Bilateral ureteral obstruction due to envelopment and compression by an inflammatory retroperitoneal process. J Urol. 1948;59:1072–9. https://doi.org/10.1016/s0022-5347(17)69482-5.
185. Stone JH. IgG4-related disease. In: Jameson JL, Fauci AS, Kasper DL, Hauser SL, Longo DL, Loscalzo J, editors. Harrison's principles of internal medicine. 20th ed. New York: McGraw-Hill Education; 2018.
186. Van Bommel EFH, Jansen I, Hendriksz TR, Aarnoudse ALHJ. Idiopathic retroperitoneal fibrosis: prospective evaluation of incidence and clinicoradiologic presentation. Medicine (Baltimore). 2009;88:193–201. https://doi.org/10.1097/MD.0b013e3181afc420.
187. Vaglio A, Maritati F. Idiopathic retroperitoneal fibrosis. J Am Soc Nephrol. 2016;27:1880–9. https://doi.org/10.1681/ASN.2015101110.
188. Kermani TA, Crowson CS, Achenbach SJ, Luthra HS. Idiopathic retroperitoneal fibrosis: a retrospective review of clinical presentation, treatment, and outcomes. Mayo Clin Proc. 2011;86:297–303. https://doi.org/10.4065/mcp.2010.0663.
189. Scheel PJ, Feeley N. Retroperitoneal fibrosis: the clinical, laboratory, and radiographic presentation. Medicine (Baltimore). 2009;88:202–7. https://doi.org/10.1097/MD.0b013e3181afc439.
190. Cronin CG, Lohan DG, Blake MA, Roche C, McCarthy P, Murphy JM. Retroperitoneal fibrosis: review of clinical features and imaging findings. AJR Am J Roentgenol. 2008;191:423–31. https://doi.org/10.2214/AJR.07.3629.
191. Vaglio A, Versari A, Fraternali A, Ferrozzi F, Salvarani C, Buzio C. (18)F-fluorodeoxyglucose positron emission tomography in the diagnosis and followup of idiopathic retroperitoneal fibrosis. Arthritis Rheum. 2005;53:122–5. https://doi.org/10.1002/art.20914.
192. Van Bommel EFH, Siemes C, Hak LE, van der Veer SJ, Hendriksz TR. Long-term renal and patient outcome in idiopathic retroperitoneal fibrosis treated with prednisone. Am J Kidney Dis. 2007;49:615–25. https://doi.org/10.1053/j.ajkd.2007.02.268.
193. Uibu T, Oksa P, Auvinen A, Honkanen E, Metsärinne K, Saha H, Uitti J, Roto P. Asbestos exposure as a risk factor for retroperitoneal fibrosis. Lancet. 2004;363:1422–6. https://doi.org/10.1016/S0140-6736(04)16100-X.
194. Vaglio A. Retroperitoneal fibrosis: new insights into clinical presentation and diagnosis. Medicine (Baltimore). 2009;88:208–10. https://doi.org/10.1097/MD.0b013e3181afc4d1.
195. Koep L, Zuidema GD. The clinical significance of retroperitoneal fibrosis. Surgery. 1977;81:250–7.
196. Kasales CJ, Hartman DS. Genitourinary case of the day. Retroperitoneal fibrosis. Am J Roentgenol. 1994;162:1454–6. https://doi.org/10.2214/ajr.162.6.8192023.
197. Vaglio A, Palmisano A, Alberici F, Maggiore U, Ferretti S, Cobelli R, Ferrozzi F, Corradi D, Salvarani C, Buzio C. Prednisone versus tamoxifen in patients with idiopathic retroperito-

neal fibrosis: an open-label randomised controlled trial. Lancet. 2011;378:338–46. https://doi.org/10.1016/S0140-6736(11)60934-3.

198. Goldoni M, Bonini S, Urban ML, Palmisano A, De Palma G, Galletti E, Coggiola M, Buzio C, Mutti A, Vaglio A. Asbestos and smoking as risk factors for idiopathic retroperitoneal fibrosis: a case-control study. Ann Intern Med. 2014;161:181–8. https://doi.org/10.7326/M13-2648.
199. Nesti M, Marinaccio A, Chellini E, Centers RO. Malignant Mesothelioma in Italy, 1997. Am J Ind Med. 2004;45:55–62. https://doi.org/10.1002/ajim.10313.
200. Vaglio A, Palmisano A, Corradi D, Salvarani C, Buzio C. Retroperitoneal fibrosis: evolving concepts. Rheumatic disease clinics of North America. Vasculitis. 2007;33:803–17. https://doi.org/10.1016/j.rdc.2007.07.013.
201. Urban ML, Palmisano A, Nicastro M, Corradi D, Buzio C, Vaglio A. Idiopathic and secondary forms of retroperitoneal fibrosis: a diagnostic approach. La Revue de Médecine Interne. 2015;36:15–21. https://doi.org/10.1016/j.revmed.2014.10.008.
202. Zen Y, Onodera M, Inoue D, Kitao A, Matsui O, Nohara T, Namiki M, Kasashima S, Kawashima A, Matsumoto Y, Katayanagi K, Murata T, Ishizawa S, Hosaka N, Kuriki K, Nakanuma Y. Retroperitoneal fibrosis: a clinicopathologic study with respect to immunoglobulin G4. Am J Surg Pathol. 2009;33:1833–9. https://doi.org/10.1097/pas.0b013e3181b72882.
203. Stone JR. Aortitis, periaortitis, and retroperitoneal fibrosis, as manifestations of IgG4-related systemic disease. Curr Opin Rheumatol. 2011;23:88–94. https://doi.org/10.1097/BOR.0b013e3283412f7c.
204. Khosroshahi A, Carruthers MN, Stone JH, Shinagare S, Sainani N, Hasserjian RP, Deshpande V. Rethinking Ormond's disease. Medicine (Baltimore). 2013;92:82–91. https://doi.org/10.1097/MD.0b013e318289610f.
205. Al-Mujaini A, Al-Khabori M, Shenoy K, Wali U. Immunoglobulin G4-related disease: an update. Oman Med J. 2018;33:97–103. https://doi.org/10.5001/omj.2018.20.
206. Mahajan VS, Mattoo H, Deshpande V, Pillai SS, Stone JH. IgG4-related disease. Annu Rev Pathol. 2014;9:315–47. https://doi.org/10.1146/annurev-pathol-012513-104708.
207. Mattoo H, Mahajan VS, Maehara T, Deshpande V, Della-Torre E, Wallace ZS, Kulikova M, Drijvers JM, Daccache J, Carruthers MN, Castelino FV, Stone JR, Stone JH, Pillai S. Clonal expansion of CD4(+) cytotoxic T lymphocytes in patients with IgG4-related disease. J Allergy Clin Immunol. 2016;138:825–38. https://doi.org/10.1016/j.jaci.2015.12.1330.
208. Della-Torre E, Bozzalla-Cassione E, Sciorati C, Ruggiero E, Lanzillotta M, Bonfiglio S, Mattoo H, Perugino CA, Bozzolo E, Rovati L, Arcidiacono PG, Balzano G, Lazarevic D, Bonini C, Falconi M, Stone JH, Dagna L, Pillai S, Manfredi AA. A CD8—subset of CD4+SLAMF7+ cytotoxic T cells is expanded in patients with IgG4-related disease and decreases following glucocorticoid treatment. Arthritis Rheumatol. 2018;70:1133–43. https://doi.org/10.1002/art.40469.
209. Chen Y, Lin W, Yang H, Wang M, Zhang P, Feng R, Chen H, Peng L, Zhang X, Zhao Y, Zeng X, Zhang F, Zhang W, Lipsky PE. Aberrant expansion and function of follicular helper T cell subsets in IgG4-related disease. Arthritis Rheumatol. 2018;70:1853–65. https://doi.org/10.1002/art.40556.
210. Ito F, Kamekura R, Yamamoto M, Takano K, Takaki H, Yabe H, Ikegami I, Shigehara K, Himi T, Takahashi H, Ichimiya S. IL-10+ T follicular regulatory cells are associated with the pathogenesis of IgG4-related disease. Immunol Lett. 2019;207:56–63. https://doi.org/10.1016/j.imlet.2019.01.008.
211. Vaglio A, Catanoso MG, Spaggiari L, Magnani L, Pipitone N, Macchioni P, Pulsatelli L, Nicastro M, Becchi G, Corradi D, Versari A, Boiardi L, Salvarani C. Interleukin-6 as an inflammatory mediator and target of therapy in chronic periaortitis. Arthritis Rheum. 2013;65:2469–75. https://doi.org/10.1002/art.38032.
212. Nicastro M, Vescovini R, Maritati F, Palmisano A, Urban ML, Incerti M, Fenaroli P, Peyronel F, Benigno GD, Mangieri D, Volpi R, Becchi G, Romagnani P, Corradi D, Vaglio

A. Fibrocytes in chronic periaortitis: a novel mechanism linking inflammation and fibrosis. Arthritis Rheumatol. 2019;71:1913–22. https://doi.org/10.1002/art.41024.
213. Vaglio A, Salvarani C, Buzio C. Retroperitoneal fibrosis. Lancet. 2006;367:241–51. https://doi.org/10.1016/S0140-6736(06)68035-5.
214. Maritati F, Rocco R, Buttini EA, Marvisi C, Nicastro M, Urban ML, Fenaroli P, Peyronel F, Benigno GD, Palumbo AA, Corradi D, Emmi G, Nicolograve P, Palmisano A, Vaglio A. Clinical and prognostic significance of serum IgG4 in chronic periaortitis. an analysis of 113 patients. Front Immunol. 2019:NA–NA.
215. Vaglio A, Corradi D, Manenti L, Ferretti S, Garini G, Buzio C. Evidence of autoimmunity in chronic periaortitis: a prospective study. Am J Med. 2003;114:454–62. https://doi.org/10.1016/S0002-9343(03)00056-1.
216. Moroni G, Castellani M, Balzani A, Dore R, Bonelli N, Longhi S, Martinelli I, Messa P, Gerundini P. The value of (18)F-FDG PET/CT in the assessment of active idiopathic retroperitoneal fibrosis. Eur J Nucl Med Mol Imaging. 2012;39:1635–42. https://doi.org/10.1007/s00259-012-2144-6.
217. Mertens S, Zeegers AGM, Wertheimer PA, Hendriksz TR, van Bommel EFH. Efficacy and complications of urinary drainage procedures in idiopathic retroperitoneal fibrosis complicated by extrinsic ureteral obstruction. Int J Urol. 2014;21:283–8. https://doi.org/10.1111/iju.12234.
218. Baker LR, Mallinson WJ, Gregory MC, Menzies EA, Cattell WR, Whitfield HN, Hendry WF, Wickham JE, Joekes AM. Idiopathic retroperitoneal fibrosis. A retrospective analysis of 60 cases. Br J Urol. 1987;60:497–503. https://doi.org/10.1111/j.1464-410x.1987.tb05028.x.
219. Alexopoulos E, Memmos D, Bakatselos S, Rombis V, Sakellariou G, Gaganakis J, Hadjidimitriou C, Papadimitriou M. Idiopathic retroperitoneal fibrosis: a long-term follow-up study. Eur Urol. 1987;13:313–7. https://doi.org/10.1159/000472808.
220. Kardar AH, Kattan S, Lindstedt E, Hanash K. Steroid therapy for idiopathic retroperitoneal fibrosis: dose and duration. J Urol. 2002;168:550–5.
221. Van Bommel EFH. Retroperitoneal fibrosis. Neth J Med. 2002;60:231–42.
222. Scheel PJ, Feeley N, Sozio SM. Combined prednisone and mycophenolate mofetil treatment for retroperitoneal fibrosis: a case series. Ann Intern Med. 2011;154:31–6. https://doi.org/10.7326/0003-4819-154-1-201101040-00005.
223. Alberici F, Palmisano A, Urban ML, Maritati F, Oliva E, Manenti L, Ferretti S, Cobelli R, Buzio C, Vaglio A. Methotrexate plus prednisone in patients with relapsing idiopathic retroperitoneal fibrosis. Ann Rheum Dis. 2013;72:1584–6. https://doi.org/10.1136/annrheumdis-2013-203267.
224. Urban ML, Maritati F, Palmisano A, Fenaroli P, Peyronel F, Trivioli G, Ferretti S, De Biase C, Grayson PC, Pegoraro F, Prisco D, Romagnani P, Emmi G, Vaglio A. Rituximab for chronic periaortitis without evidence of IgG4-related disease: a long-term follow-up study of 20 patients. Ann Rheum Dis. 2020;79:433–4. https://doi.org/10.1136/annrheumdis-2019-216258.
225. Maritati F, Corradi D, Versari A, Casali M, Urban ML, Buzio C, Vaglio A. Rituximab therapy for chronic periaortitis. Ann Rheum Dis. 2012;71:1262–4. https://doi.org/10.1136/annrheumdis-2011-201166.
226. Boyeva V, Alabsi H, Seidman MA, Paterson R, Kur J, Chen LYC, Chang SD, Carruthers M. Use of rituximab in idiopathic retroperitoneal fibrosis. BMC Rheumatol. 2020;4:40. https://doi.org/10.1186/s41927-020-00140-9.
227. Kipfer RE, Moertel CG, Dahlin DC. Mesenteric lipodystrophy. Ann Intern Med. 1974;80:582–8. https://doi.org/10.7326/0003-4819-80-5-582.
228. Danford CJ, Lin SC, Wolf JL. Sclerosing mesenteritis. Am J Gastroenterol. 2019;114:867–73. https://doi.org/10.14309/ajg.0000000000000167.
229. Green MS, Chhabra R, Goyal H. Sclerosing mesenteritis: a comprehensive clinical review. Ann Transl Med. 2018;6:336. https://doi.org/10.21037/atm.2018.07.01.
230. Jura V. Sulla mesenterite retractile esclerosante. Policlinica. 1924;31:575–81.

231. Kuhrmeier A. [Mesenteric lipodystrophy]. Schweiz Med Wochenschr. 1985;115:1218–24.
232. Daskalogiannaki M, Voloudaki A, Prassopoulos P, Magkanas E, Stefanaki K, Apostolaki E, Gourtsoyiannis N. CT evaluation of mesenteric panniculitis: prevalence and associated diseases. AJR Am J Roentgenol. 2000;174:427–31. https://doi.org/10.2214/ajr.174.2.1740427.
233. Van Putte-Katier N, van Bommel EFH, Elgersma OE, Hendriksz TR. Mesenteric panniculitis: prevalence, clinicoradiological presentation and 5-year follow-up. Br J Radiol. 2014;87:20140451. https://doi.org/10.1259/bjr.20140451.
234. Coulier B. Mesenteric panniculitis. Part 2: prevalence and natural course: MDCT prospective study. JBR-BTR. 2011;94:241–6. https://doi.org/10.5334/jbr-btr.659.
235. Sharma P, Yadav S, Needham CM, Feuerstadt P. Sclerosing mesenteritis: a systematic review of 192 cases. Clin J Gastroenterol. 2017;10:103–11. https://doi.org/10.1007/s12328-017-0716-5.
236. Buchwald P, Diesing L, Dixon L, Wakeman C, Eglinton T, Dobbs B, Frizelle F. Cohort study of mesenteric panniculitis and its relationship to malignancy. Br J Surg. 2016;103:1727–30. https://doi.org/10.1002/bjs.10229.
237. Scheer F, Spunar P, Wiggermann P, Wissgott C, Andresen R. Mesenteric panniculitis (MP) in CT—a predictor of malignancy? RöFo. 2016;188:926–32. https://doi.org/10.1055/s-0042-110100.
238. Badet N, Sailley N, Briquez C, Paquette B, Vuitton L, Delabrousse É. Mesenteric panniculitis: still an ambiguous condition. Diagn Interv Imaging. 2015;96:251–7. https://doi.org/10.1016/j.diii.2014.12.002.
239. Emory TS, Monihan JM, Carr NJ, Sobin LH. Sclerosing mesenteritis, mesenteric panniculitis and mesenteric lipodystrophy: a single entity? Am J Surg Pathol. 1997;21:392–8.
240. Akram S, Pardi DS, Schaffner JA, Smyrk TC. Sclerosing mesenteritis: clinical features, treatment, and outcome in ninety-two patients. Clin Gastroenterol Hepatol. 2007;5:589–96. https://doi.org/10.1016/j.cgh.2007.02.032.
241. Protin-Catteau L, Thiéfin G, Barbe C, Jolly D, Soyer P, Hoeffel C. Mesenteric panniculitis: review of consecutive abdominal MDCT examinations with a matched-pair analysis. Acta Radiol. 2016;57:1438–44. https://doi.org/10.1177/0284185116629829.
242. Gögebakan Ö, Albrecht T, Osterhoff MA, Reimann A. Is mesenteric panniculitis truely a paraneoplastic phenomenon? A matched pair analysis. Eur J Radiol. 2013;82:1853–9. https://doi.org/10.1016/j.ejrad.2013.06.023.
243. Khasminsky V, Ram E, Atar E, Steinminz A, Issa N, Bachar GN. Is there an association between mesenteric panniculitis and lymphoma? A case control analysis. Clin Radiol. 2017;72:844–9. https://doi.org/10.1016/j.crad.2017.05.008.
244. Vlachos K, Archontovasilis F, Falidas E, Mathioulakis S, Konstandoudakis S, Villias C. Sclerosing mesenteritis: diverse clinical presentations and dissimilar treatment options. a case series and review of the literature. Int Arch Med. 2011;4:17. https://doi.org/10.1186/1755-7682-4-17.
245. Endo K, Moroi R, Sugimura M, Fujishima F, Naitoh T, Tanaka N, Shiga H, Kakuta Y, Takahashi S, Kinouchi Y, Shimosegawa T. Refractory sclerosing mesenteritis involving the small intestinal mesentery: a case report and literature review. Intern Med. 2014;53:1419–27. https://doi.org/10.2169/internalmedicine.53.1813.
246. Canyigit M, Koksal A, Akgoz A, Kara T, Sarisahin M, Akhan O. Multidetector-row computed tomography findings of sclerosing mesenteritis with associated diseases and its prevalence. Jpn J Radiol. 2011;29:495–502. https://doi.org/10.1007/s11604-011-0587-5.
247. Ginsburg PM, Ehrenpreis ED. A pilot study of thalidomide for patients with symptomatic mesenteric panniculitis. Aliment Pharmacol Ther. 2002;16:2115–22. https://doi.org/10.1046/j.1365-2036.2002.01383.x.
248. Okazaki T, Shinagawa S, Mikage H. Vasculitis syndrome—diagnosis and therapy. J Gen Fam Med. 2017;18:72–8. https://doi.org/10.1002/jgf2.4.
249. Gnanapandithan K, Sharma A. Mesenteric vasculitis. In: StatPearls. Treasure Island: StatPearls Publishing; 2022.

250. Ju JH, Min JK, Jung CK, Oh SN, Kwok SK, Kang KY, Park KS, Ko HJ, Yoon CH, Park SH, Cho CS, Kim HY. Lupus mesenteric vasculitis can cause acute abdominal pain in patients with SLE. Nat Rev Rheumatol. 2009;5:273–81. https://doi.org/10.1038/nrrheum.2009.53.
251. Tian XP, Zhang X. Gastrointestinal involvement in systemic lupus erythematosus: insight into pathogenesis, diagnosis and treatment. World J Gastroenterol. 2010;16:2971–7. https://doi.org/10.3748/wjg.v16.i24.2971.
252. Helliwell TR, Flook D, Whitworth J, Day DW. Arteritis and venulitis in systemic lupus erythematosus resulting in massive lower intestinal haemorrhage. Histopathology. 1985;9:1103–13. https://doi.org/10.1111/j.1365-2559.1985.tb02788.x.
253. Del Papa N, Guidali L, Sala A, Buccellati C, Khamashta MA, Ichikawa K, Koike T, Balestrieri G, Tincani A, Hughes GR, Meroni PL. Endothelial cells as target for antiphospholipid antibodies. human polyclonal and monoclonal anti-beta 2-glycoprotein I antibodies react in vitro with endothelial cells through adherent beta 2-glycoprotein I and induce endothelial activation. Arthritis Rheum. 1997;40:551–61. https://doi.org/10.1002/art.1780400322.
254. Cervera R, Espinosa G, Cordero A, Oltra MR, Unzurrunzaga A, Rossiñol T, Plaza J, Bucciarelli S, Ramos-Casals M, Ingelmo M, Asherson RA, Font J, Catastrophic Antiphospholipid Syndrome (CAPS) Registry Project Group. Intestinal involvement secondary to the antiphospholipid syndrome (APS): clinical and immunologic characteristics of 97 patients: comparison of classic and catastrophic APS. Semin Arthritis Rheum. 2007;36:287–96. https://doi.org/10.1016/j.semarthrit.2006.09.003.
255. Medina F, Ayala A, Jara LJ, Becerra M, Miranda JM, Fraga A. Acute abdomen in systemic lupus erythematosus: the importance of early laparotomy. Am J Med. 1997;103:100–5. https://doi.org/10.1016/s0002-9343(97)80020-4.
256. Kwok SK, Seo SH, Ju JH, Park KS, Yoon CH, Kim WU, Min JK, Park SH, Cho CS, Kim HY. Lupus enteritis: clinical characteristics, risk factor for relapse and association with anti-endothelial cell antibody. Lupus. 2007;16:803–9. https://doi.org/10.1177/0961203307082383.
257. Watts RA, Hatemi G, Burns JC, Mohammad AJ. Global epidemiology of vasculitis. Nat Rev Rheumatol. 2022;18:22–34. https://doi.org/10.1038/s41584-021-00718-8.
258. Pagnoux C, Seror R, Henegar C, Mahr A, Cohen P, Le Guern V, Bienvenu B, Mouthon L, Guillevin L, French Vasculitis Study Group. Clinical features and outcomes in 348 patients with polyarteritis nodosa: a systematic retrospective study of patients diagnosed between 1963 and 2005 and entered into the French Vasculitis Study Group Database. Arthritis Rheum. 2010;62:616–26. https://doi.org/10.1002/art.27240.
259. Stanson AW, Friese JL, Johnson CM, McKusick MA, Breen JF, Sabater EA, Andrews JC. Polyarteritis nodosa: spectrum of angiographic findings. Radiographics. 2001;21:151–9. https://doi.org/10.1148/radiographics.21.1.g01ja16151.
260. Gayraud M, Guillevin L, le Toumelin P, Cohen P, Lhote F, Casassus P, Jarrousse B, French Vasculitis Study Group. Long-term followup of polyarteritis nodosa, microscopic polyangiitis, and Churg-Strauss Syndrome: analysis of four prospective trials including 278 patients. Arthritis Rheum. 2001;44:666–75. https://doi.org/10.1002/1529-0131(200103)44:3<666::AID-ANR116>3.0.CO;2-A.
261. Bourgarit A, Toumelin PL, Pagnoux C, Cohen P, Mahr A, Guern VL, Mouthon L, Guillevin L, French Vasculitis Study Group. Deaths occurring during the first year after treatment onset for polyarteritis nodosa, microscopic polyangiitis, and Churg-Strauss Syndrome: a retrospective analysis of causes and factors predictive of mortality based on 595 patients. Medicine (Baltimore). 2005;84:323–30. https://doi.org/10.1097/01.md.0000180793.80212.17.
262. Stone JH, Merkel PA, Spiera R, Seo P, Langford CA, Hoffman GS, Kallenberg CG, St. Clair EW, Turkiewicz A, Tchao NK, Webber L, Ding L, Sejismundo LP, Mieras K, Weitzenkamp D, Ikle D, Seyfert-Margolis V, Mueller M, Brunetta P, Allen NB, Fervenza FC, Geetha D, Keogh KA, Kissin EY, Monach PA, Peikert T, Stegeman C, Ytterberg SR, Specks U. Rituximab versus cyclophosphamide for ANCA-associated vasculitis. N Engl J Med. 2010;363:221–32. https://doi.org/10.1056/NEJMoa0909905.

263. Reamy BV, Williams PM, Lindsay TJ. Henoch-Schönlein Purpura. Am Fam Physician. 2009;80:697–704.
264. Gardner-Medwin JMM, Dolezalova P, Cummins C, Southwood TR. Incidence of Henoch-Schönlein Purpura, Kawasaki disease, and rare vasculitides in children of different ethnic origins. Lancet. 2002;360:1197–202. https://doi.org/10.1016/S0140-6736(02)11279-7.
265. Cojocariu C, Singeap AM, Chiriac S, Sfarti C, Girleanu I, Petrea O, Trifan A, Stanciu C. Gastrointestinal manifestations of IgA vasculitis-Henoch-Schönlein Purpura. IntechOpen; 2019. https://doi.org/10.5772/intechopen.86966.
266. Audemard-Verger A, Pillebout E, Amoura Z, Cacoub P, Jourde-Chiche N, Lioger B, Martis N, Moulis G, Rivière E, Baldolli A, Girard C, Goutte J, Gouellec NL, Raffray L, Urbanski G, Sanges S, Maurier F, Thervet E, Aouba A, Guillevin L, Maillot F, Terrier B, French Vasculitis Study Group (FVSG). Gastrointestinal involvement in adult IgA vasculitis (Henoch-Schönlein Purpura): updated picture from a French Multicentre and Retrospective Series of 260 cases. Rheumatology (Oxford). 2020;59:3050–7. https://doi.org/10.1093/rheumatology/keaa104.
267. Oni L, Sampath S. Childhood IgA vasculitis (Henoch Schonlein Purpura)-advances and knowledge gaps. Front Pediatr. 2019;7:257. https://doi.org/10.3389/fped.2019.00257.
268. Sanchez-Alvarez C, Crowson CS, Koster MJ, Warrington KJ. Prevalence of Takayasu arteritis: a population-based study. J Rheumatol. 2021;48:952. https://doi.org/10.3899/jrheum.201463.
269. Tomelleri A, Campochiaro C, Sartorelli S, Cavalli G, Luca GD, Baldissera E, Dagna L. Ab0621 gender differences in clinical presentation and vascular pattern in patients with Takayasu arteritis. Ann Rheum Dis. 2019;78(Suppl 2):1771–2. https://doi.org/10.1136/annrheumdis-2019-eular.2407.
270. Mehta R, Deepak N, John A, Shine N, Raj N, Balakrishnan N. Takayasu arteritis presenting as chronic mesenteric ischemia. Indian J Gastroenterol. 2004;23:73–4.
271. Setty HSN, Rao M, Srinivas KH, Srinivas BC, Usha MK, Jayaranganath M, Patil SS, Manjunath CN. Clinical, angiographic profile and percutaneous endovascular management of Takayasu's arteritis—a single centre experience. Int J Cardiol. 2016;220:924–8. https://doi.org/10.1016/j.ijcard.2016.06.194.
272. Koster MJ, Warrington KJ. Vasculitis of the mesenteric circulation. Best Pract Res Clin Gastroenterol. 2017;31:85–96. https://doi.org/10.1016/j.bpg.2016.12.003.
273. Hisamatsu T, Ueno F, Matsumoto T, Kobayashi K, Koganei K, Kunisaki R, Hirai F, Nagahori M, Matsushita M, Kobayashi K, Kishimoto M, Takeno M, Tanaka M, Inoue N, Hibi T. The 2nd edition of consensus statements for the diagnosis and management of intestinal Behçet's disease: indication of anti-TNF monoclonal antibodies. J Gastroenterol. 2014;49:156–62. https://doi.org/10.1007/s00535-013-0872-4.
274. Puéchal X, Gottenberg JE, Berthelot JM, Gossec L, Meyer O, Morel J, Wendling D, de Bandt M, Houvenagel E, Jamard B, Lequerré T, Morel G, Richette P, Sellam J, Guillevin L, Mariette X, Investigators of the AutoImmunity Rituximab Registry. Rituximab therapy for systemic vasculitis associated with rheumatoid arthritis: results from the autoimmunity and rituximab registry. Arthritis Care Res. 2012;64:331–9. https://doi.org/10.1002/acr.20689.
275. Salvarani C, Calamia KT, Crowson CS, Miller DV, Broadwell AW, Hunder GG, Matteson EL, Warrington KJ. Localized vasculitis of the gastrointestinal tract: a case series. Rheumatology (Oxford). 2010;49:1326–35. https://doi.org/10.1093/rheumatology/keq093.

Part II
Special Consideration

Chapter 14
Malnutrition and Weight Loss

Katherine L. White, John McLaughlin, Ariane L. Herrick, Kirstine Farrer, Simon Lal, and Michael Hughes

K. L. White
Department of Gastroenterology, Stockport NHS Foundation Trust, Stockport, UK

Department of Gastroenterology, Northern Care Alliance NHS Foundation Trust, Salford Royal, UK

J. McLaughlin
Department of Gastroenterology, Northern Care Alliance NHS Foundation Trust, Salford Royal, UK

Division of Diabetes, Endocrinology and Gastroenterology, Faculty of Biology, Medicine and Health, The University of Manchester, Manchester, UK

A. L. Herrick
Centre for Musculoskeletal Research, Division of Musculoskeletal and Dermatological Sciences, The University of Manchester, Northern Care Alliance NHS Foundation Trust, Manchester Academic Health Science Centre, Manchester, UK

National Institute for Health and Care Research (NIHR) Manchester Biomedical Research Centre (BRC), Manchester, UK

K. Farrer · S. Lal
Division of Diabetes, Endocrinology and Gastroenterology, Faculty of Biology, Medicine and Health, The University of Manchester, Manchester, UK

Intestinal Failure Unit, Northern Care Alliance, Salford, UK

M. Hughes (✉)
Centre for Musculoskeletal Research, Division of Musculoskeletal and Dermatological Sciences, The University of Manchester, Northern Care Alliance NHS Foundation Trust, Manchester Academic Health Science Centre, Manchester, UK

National Institute for Health and Care Research (NIHR) Manchester Biomedical Research Centre (BRC), Manchester, UK

Department of Rheumatology, Salford Royal, Northern Care Alliance NHS Foundation Trust, Salford, UK
e-mail: Michael.hughes-6@postgrad.manchester.ac.uk

M. Tadros et al. (eds.), *GI Diseases Associated with Rheumatological and Vasculitic Conditions*, Clinical Gastroenterology,
https://doi.org/10.1007/978-3-032-07868-1_14

14.1 Causes

14.1.1 Definitions and Epidemiology

The term malnutrition can be used to describe undernutrition and usually refers to deficiency of calories to meet energy requirement [1]. This can occur through decreased oral intake or can be an effect of acute disease through increased energy requirement or can be multifactorial. The word malnutrition can also refer to specific micro- and macronutrient deficiencies [2]. Conversely it may describe overweight and obese states which can result in other illnesses such as cardiovascular disease. Obesity will not be described further in this chapter. Weight loss is generally described as a percentage loss over a specified time period. Finally, sarcopenia is a newer term which refers specifically to loss of muscle mass and function [3]. This can be a more sensitive measure of nutritional status than weight or body mass index (BMI) as patients can be sarcopenic and maintain a normal or even a high BMI.

In many rheumatological and vasculitic conditions the prevalence of malnutrition is not known. Furthermore, it can be difficult to detect due to the different definitions which are used and the different ways in which it may be measured. In a large Canadian study of 586 patients with systemic sclerosis (SSc), 18% of patients were found to be at risk of malnutrition and this was influenced by factors such as the number of gastrointestinal (GI) complaints, shorter disease duration and diffuse disease [4]. In another study within the multinational, longitudinal European League Against Rheumatism (EULAR) Scleroderma Trials and Research (EUSTAR) database 438 patients had significant weight loss versus 3169 patients who did not (defined as weight loss of 4.5 kg or at least 5% body weight at 5 months onwards) [5]. After multiple testing this study found that shorter disease duration, raised erythrocyte sedimentation rate, raised creatinine kinase, pulmonary hypertension and interstitial lung disease were associated with weight loss. Interestingly, GI symptoms were not associated with weight loss. This finding was replicated in a study of 69 patients with SSc [6]. In a separate study measurement of bioelectrical impedance analysis (BIA) in patients with SSc demonstrated that 56% had evidence of malnutrition [7].

In a small recent study sarcopenia (detected by BIA and hand-grip strength) was detected in 31.5% of patients at time of diagnosis of rheumatoid arthritis (RA) and 8.7% after 3 months of disease modifying treatment of RA [8]. Weight loss can also occur in patients with rheumatoid vasculitis either as a constitutional symptom or rarely by affecting the GI tract directly [9].

Arthropathy is the most frequent extra-intestinal manifestation of inflammatory bowel disease (IBD) [10]. Peripheral arthropathies often correlate with active bowel inflammation and may improve with treatment of gastrointestinal inflammation [11]. Axial arthropathies often have an independent disease course and may not improve with treatment of underlying IBD. Several studies have found a high rate of subclinical IBD in patients with ankylosing spondylitis [12–14]. These patients are frequently prescribed non-steroidal anti-inflammatory drugs which can exacerbate potential underlying IBD. Malnutrition and weight loss is common in patients with IBD with rates of 65–75% in patients with Crohn's disease and 18–62% in patients with ulcerative colitis [15]. There are no available data on whether the presence of arthropathy in patients with IBD impacts on nutrition.

Patients with vasculitides often report weight loss among other 'B symptoms' such as fever at diagnosis [16]. As vasculitides are a significantly heterogenous group of diseases affecting potentially different organs, the pathogenesis of how they may cause weight loss and malnutrition varies [17]. For example, small- (e.g., ANCA-associated) and medium-vessel vasculitides (e.g., polyarteritis nodosa) may directly affect GI tract function, whereas other non-GI vasculitides may contribute to malnutrition through increased metabolic demand from disease activity.

14.1.2 GI Causes of Malnutrition and Weight Loss

Symptoms in any region of the GI tract can potentially cause malnutrition and weight loss due to potential effects on appetite. However, this relationship is complex and is often likely to be multi-factorial in origin. Some of the more common GI causes for under-nourishment in rheumatological conditions and vasculitis are shown in Table 14.1. As previously stated, GI symptoms have not been shown to be predictive of malnutrition in patients with SSc. However, in patients with SSc with significant weight loss it may be prudent to screen for GI disease which may be contributing to under-nourishment and may be treatable.

Disease of the small bowel is particularly likely to cause under-nourishment, weight loss and specific macro- and micronutrient deficiencies due to loss of function in this region. This can in turn affect gut function potentially leading to malabsorption through gut atrophy, impaired gastric acid secretion, reduced pancreatic

Table 14.1 GI abnormalities related to rheumatological/vasculitides conditions which can lead to malnutrition

Region of GI tract	Abnormality	Conditions which can present with this
Oesophagus	Oesophageal dysmotility	SSc
Stomach	Gastroparesis	Sjogren's syndrome [18]
Small bowel	Small intestinal bacterial overgrowth	Scleroderma
	Chronic intestinal pseudo-obstruction	Scleroderma, SLE, dermatomyositis [19]
	Coeliac disease	Association with RA, Sjogren's syndrome, SLE
	Crohn's disease	IBD associated arthropathy
Pancreas	Chronic pancreatitis	SLE [20], RA (likely medication-related effects) [21]
Large bowel	Colitis	IBD associated arthropathy

IBD inflammatory bowel disease, *SLE* systemic lupus erythematosus, *SSc* systemic sclerosis enzymes and small intestinal bacterial overgrowth [22]. Small intestinal bacterial overgrowth (SIBO) is defined by an excess of bacteria in the small bowel in quantities of >10^5 organisms/mL [23]. It commonly occurs in anatomically abnormal small bowel or in any condition which significantly affects small bowel motility. It can result in GI symptoms, such as pain and bloating, weight loss and specific deficiencies such as iron, calcium and magnesium as well as vitamin B12 and fat-soluble vitamins A, D, E and K. The prevalence of SIBO may be as high as 43% in unselected patients with SSc [24].

Amyloidosis can occur in any chronic inflammatory disorder. It results in amyloid deposition in several organs including the GI tract particularly the small bowel. This can result in symptoms such as diarrhoea and weight loss through dysmotility and protein losing enteropathy [25].

Coeliac disease can be associated with other autoimmune diseases such as RA and SLE and should be screened for in patients with rheumatological disease with weight loss. It is caused by an abnormal immune reaction to gluten ingestion leading to villous atrophy of the small bowel lining. This can lead to GI symptoms and deficiencies of iron, folate, vitamin B12, vitamin D, calcium, zinc, and copper [26].

14.1.3 Non-GI Causes of Malnutrition and Weight Loss

There are many non-GI factors which can lead to malnutrition or weight loss in rheumatological and vasculitis conditions. Several of these are listed in Table 14.2. Some of these are specific to certain rheumatological diseases. For example, xerostomia in Sjogren's syndrome may result in reduced oral intake, tooth decay and weight loss [28]. Microstomia, often seen in SSc has been reported to be associated with malnutrition [29].

Any active inflammatory condition can predispose to weight loss through increased energy consumption, and this has been found in several rheumatological conditions such as RA [30]. There is a growing body of evidence linking active

Table 14.2 Non-GI factors which can contribute to malnutrition in rheumatological and vasculitic conditions

Non-GI factors		Diseases
Oral	Reduced oral aperture	Systemic sclerosis
	Poor dentition	Sjogren's syndrome
	Temporomandibular joint dysfunction/disease	Rheumatoid arthritis, psoriatic arthritis
Loss of hand function		Any inflammatory arthropathy which affects the hands/upper limbs, systemic sclerosis with functional impairment from skin fibrosis and joint contractures [27]
Disease activity		All
Appetite disturbance		All
Mood disturbance		All

inflammation with anorexia (reduced appetite) and negative energy balance [31]. The term rheumatoid cachexia refers to loss of muscle mass with preserved fat mass [32]. This occurs in a pro-inflammatory state and can occur in other conditions such as IBD [33]. Furthermore, treatment of active inflammatory disease appears to reduce rates of weight loss and malnutrition in conditions such as RA and SLE. Neurocognitive impairment leading to weight loss can also occur in inflammatory conditions such as RA and SLE via several insults such as cerebral ischaemia and active disease [34].

14.1.4 Psychosocial Dimension

Health related quality of life (HRQOL) includes physical, social, and psychological domains and is frequently adversely affected by chronic disease including through pain which is experienced by many patients with rheumatological disease [35]. There is a significant psychosocial aspect of rheumatological conditions such as SSc [36]. This is multifactorial with contributors such as anxiety, depression, body image dissatisfaction and disease process. In all patients with intestinal failure (IF) the rates of anxiety and depression can be as high as 56% [37]. Intestinal failure occurs when the GI tract cannot absorb the necessary constituents to sustain life, requiring intravenous supplementation or replacement [38]. Patients with SSc are particularly at risk of IF [39]. The underlying rheumatological disease process may not be as important as factors such as lack of social support. In conditions such as RA pain can also be a risk factor for anxiety and depression [40].

14.2 Assessment

There is no single standardised approach to the assessment of malnutrition. Basic measurement of weight and height gives a snapshot assessment leading to calculation of body mass index (BMI). This is calculated as weight in kilograms divided by height in metres squared. The world health organisation classifies BMI from underweight to obesity as per Table 14.3. Weight or BMI trend within patients over time is more useful than a single reading.

The Malnutrition Universal Screening Tool ('MUST') (Fig. 14.1) is recommended for use by the British Association for Parenteral and Enteral Nutrition (BAPEN) to identify people who are malnourished, at risk of malnourishment or obese. It uses BMI, degree of weight loss and acute disease effect score to calculate an overall score determining a low, medium, or high risk of malnutrition [43]. It is the most widely used nutrition screening tool in the UK [44]. The 'MUST' has been validated in the hospital inpatient and outpatient settings and its validity is comparable to other nutritional screening tools [45, 46]. To calculate the BMI height

Table 14.3 Classification of nutrition status by BMI [41]

Body Mass Index (kg/m^2)	Nutritional status classification
Below 18.5	Underweight
18.5–24.9	Normal weight
25.0–29.9	Pre-obesity
30.0–34.9	Obesity class I
35.0–39.9	Obesity class II
Above 40	Obesity class III

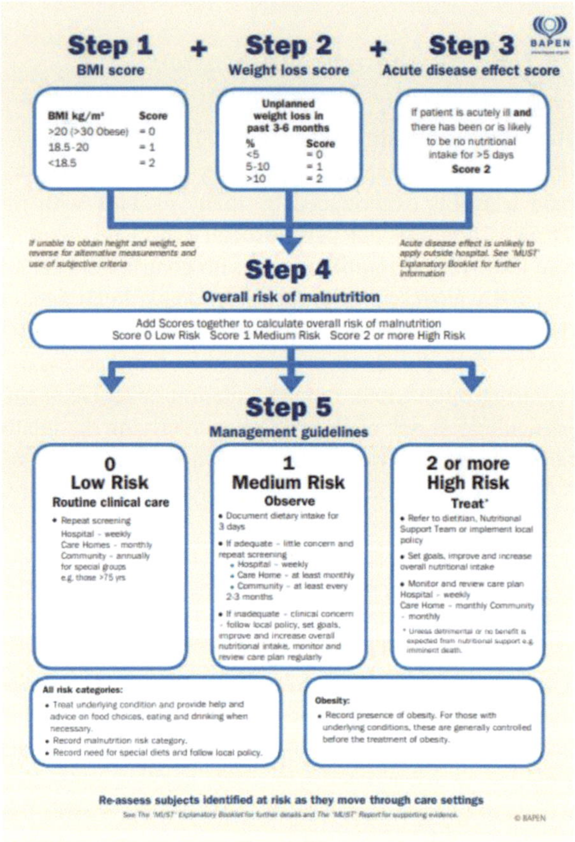

Fig. 14.1 The Malnutrition Universal Screening Tool ('MUST') is reproduced here with the kind permission of BAPEN (British Association for Parenteral and Enteral Nutrition). For further information on 'MUST' see www.bapen.org.uk [42]

should be measured using a free-standing stadiometer and weight measured using calibrated scales with shoes removed and minimal light clothing [47].

In the rheumatology setting the 'MUST' has been used to detect malnutrition in SSc patients [7, 48]. However, care should be taken when using the 'MUST' to assess for malnutrition in chronic disease as the weighting given to recent weight loss and, where appropriate, acute disease effect means that some patients may not score highly even when they are undernourished. The acute disease component is only used in patients who are admitted to hospital. Therefore, it is important to use other measurements.

The Subjective Global Assessment is a simple tool requiring no specific measurements which has been found to accurately assess nutrition in many patient groups [49]. It considers the medical history including factors such as weight loss, GI symptoms and functional deficit with physical examination findings.

14.2.1 Anthropometric Measurements

Ideally screening for nutrition should include more sensitive physical measures such as anthropometry. As well as BMI anthropometric measurements include body size and shape [50]. This gives an opportunity to monitor nutrition in disease states and importantly the effects of any interventions such as treatment of the disease itself or nutritional interventions [47]. In one study in patients with RA BMI alone was found to be a poor predictor of malnutrition [51]. Waist circumference may be used in the detection of obesity and can be used to predict cardiovascular risk and mortality [52]. Mid-upper arm circumference (MUAC) is a useful tool to detect undernourishment and can be used to calculate an estimate of BMI [53]. In hospitalised patients MUAC can predict outcomes such as length of stay and mortality [54]. Triceps skinfold thickness (Fig. 14.2) can be performed in the supine position and is reliable when the same callipers are used serially by the same observer to detect change over time. In tandem with MUAC, triceps skinfold thickness can be used to determine mid arm muscle circumference, which is a surrogate marker of fat-free mass [47]. These measurements have prognostic value in several disease states including critical illness [55]and HIV [56].

There is a strong evidence base for the use of handgrip dynamometry as part of nutritional assessment particularly in older adults [57]. As the name suggests this is a measurement of handgrip strength and is reproducible within patients when the same equipment and measurement protocol are followed. It relates to muscle mass and physical function [58] and can predict outcomes such as sarcopenia, hospital stay and mortality [57]. However, this measurement may be impractical in patients with rheumatological conditions affecting hand function or causing joint or digital pain. This should be considered when determining which anthropometric measurements to perform.

14.2.2 Bioelectrical Impedance Analysis

Bioelectrical impedance analysis (BIA) is a low-cost, safe, and effective way of measuring body composition. This is performed by passing a low voltage current through the patient's body and measuring the resistance present. This in turn gives estimates of total body water, fat free mass and dry lean mass. When measured serially within patient groups ideally the same measurement device should be used as there can be variation between devices [59]. BIA has been found to be comparable

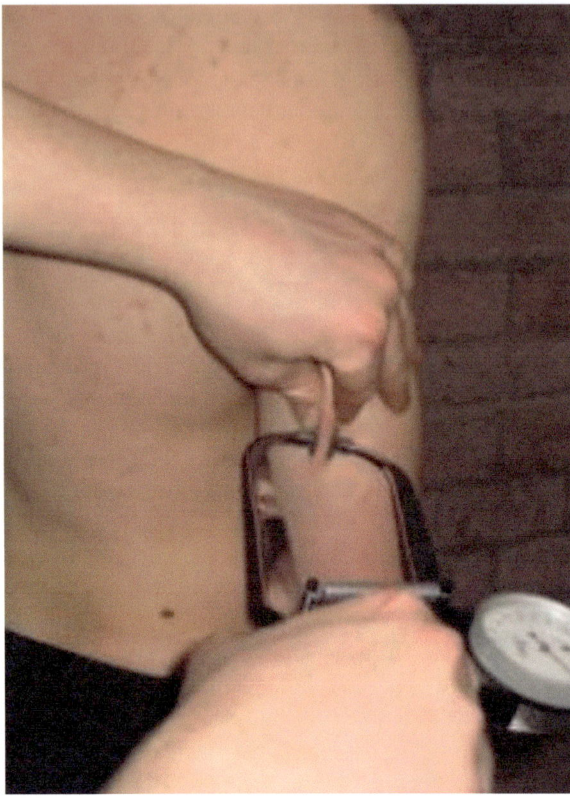

Fig. 14.2 Triceps skinfold thickness measurement with calliper

to computed tomography at the third lumbar vertebra level in several patient groups in the detection of sarcopenia or low muscle mass [60, 61]. In one study which followed up patients with SSc for 1 year, four site anthropometry was found to be similar to BIA in determining the risk of malnutrition [62].

14.2.3 Food Diaries

Food diaries are useful for dietetic assessment and allow for energy intake calculation and break down of diet to different components. They can be a useful adjunct particularly if nutritional intervention is warranted. Patients should be encouraged to complete these prospectively and technology such as mobile phone applications may aid this and be preferred over paper records by patients [63].

14.2.4 Combined Approach

Nutritional assessment should take into consideration several different measurements to gain an accurate picture of nutritional risk and more importantly to assess the value of nutritional interventions. There are no studies showing benefit of serial nutritional status measurement in patients with vasculitic and rheumatological diseases; however, one expert review recommended a blended approach of assessment at disease diagnosis and annual review [64]. In a study which included 36 patients with SSc, there was no correlation between intake and either predicted or measured (using a specialist monitor) energy expenditure [65].

It should be noted that there is no blood test which is a reliable marker of nutritional status in isolation although disturbance of electrolytes, iron, vitamins, and micronutrients may reflect a malabsorption state. Haemoglobin was found to be a poor marker of nutritional status in one study in SSc patients [66]. Although low serum albumin is often used as marker of nutritional status it is indicative of a pro-inflammatory state or protein-losing state and should not be misinterpreted as a reflection of nutrition [67]. In patients with severe anorexia nervosa or other states of starvation without inflammatory illness, serum albumin is frequently normal even in patients with a dangerously low BMI [68].

14.3 Approaches

14.3.1 General Measures

As in all clinical services, treatment of malnutrition in rheumatological and vasculitic diseases should involve a multi-disciplinary team (MDT) approach [69]. The suggested make up of this MDT is shown in Fig. 14.3 and the MDT may also be supported by pharmacists, dentists and surgeons depending on an individual patient's needs. The overall approach to assessment and treatment is suggested in a flowchart in Fig. 14.4. The suggested timing of nutritional assessment is at the time of underlying disease diagnosis, where there is significant clinical change in underlying disease or in the presence of GI symptoms or GI involvement. However, as stated, GI involvement is not predictive of malnutrition in patients with SSc and this may not be an indication for assessment in this patient group in the absence of weight loss.

Treatment of the underlying disease process has been shown to improve nutritional status in some conditions. In RA the proportion of patients with sarcopenia was 31.5% at diagnosis, compared with 8.7% 3 months after disease modifying treatment was commenced [8]. Issues with hand function such as digital ulceration in SSc and inflammatory arthropathies should benefit from treatment of the underlying disease, physiotherapy, and occupational therapy input. Therefore, a holistic

Fig. 14.3 Suggested multidisciplinary team (MDT) members

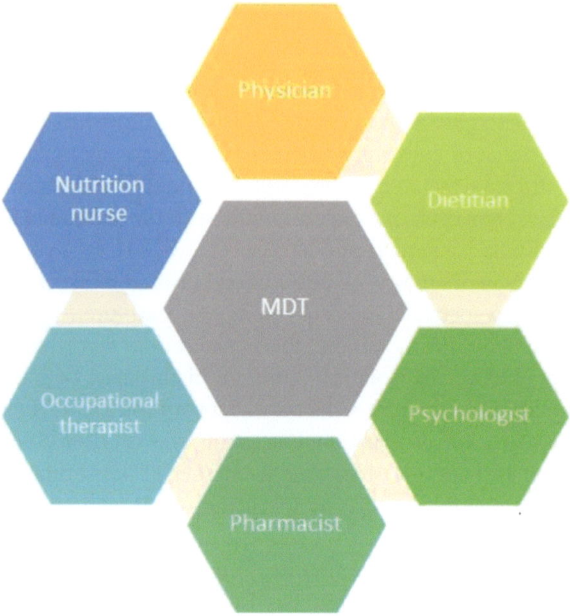

approach to these patient's care is essential. Oral conditions and problems with dentition may be improved with the involvement of a dentist or oral health physician.

If the patient has GI symptoms and/or evidence of malabsorption, then a gastroenterology opinion should be sought. This should assess for GI manifestations of the underlying rheumatological disease and co-existent unrelated GI disease. Specifically, SIBO should be suspected in patients with SSc or any rheumatological condition with small bowel involvement. This should be investigated with a glucose breath test and treated with antibiotics and response assessed [70]. If treatment trial is successful rotational antibiotics can be considered. If testing is negative but there is a strong clinical suspicion, it is still reasonable to give a trial of treatment.

Psychological comorbidity can affect appetite and energy intake and should be assessed in these patient groups. In SSc the prevalence of clinically significant depression has been found to be as high as 51–65% [71]. Psychology input has been found to be promising in other gastroenterology settings and should be considered in rheumatological patients who have psychological morbidity [72, 73].

14.3.2 *Dietary Counselling*

Any patient who is found to be undernourished should undergo dietetic assessment ideally utilising multiple assessment tools to give a true picture of the extent of malnourishment. The presence of malnutrition with or without GI symptoms may also prompt involvement of gastroenterologists for assessment of the presence of

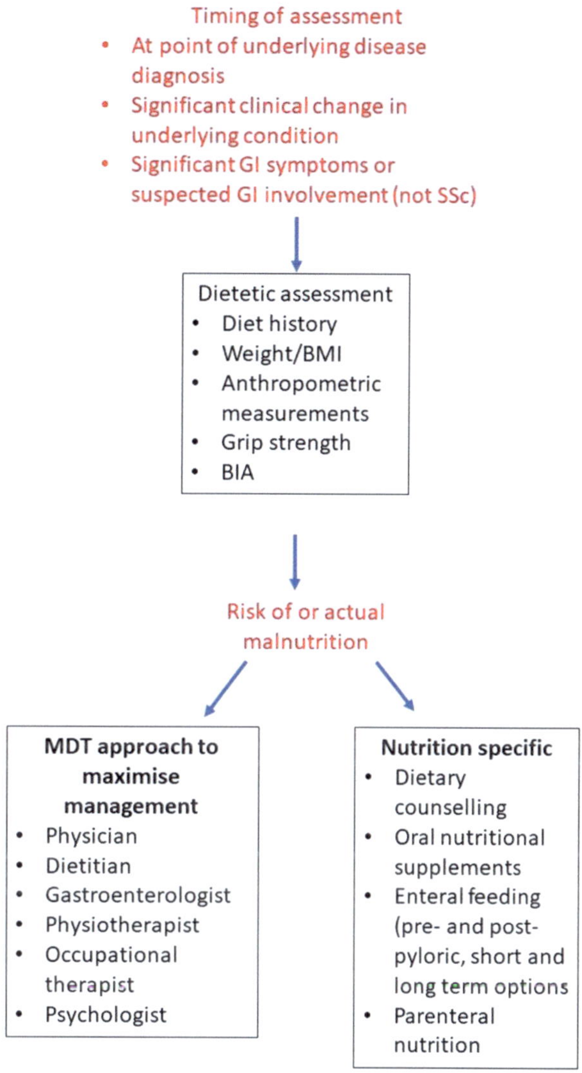

Fig. 14.4 Flowchart of overall suggested approach to risk of malnutrition in patients with rheumatic and vasculitic diseases. *SSc* systemic sclerosis, *'MUST'* malnutrition universal screening tool, *BMI* body mass index, *BIA* bioelectrical impedance analysis, *MDT* multi-disciplinary team

underlying GI disease. Dieticians may further assess patients using food diaries to understand whether there is an energy, protein and/or micronutrient deficiency. Initial dietary counselling may involve assisting the patient to increase their energy intake through food fortification, and extra meals or snacks. If this is not effective enough oral nutritional supplements (ONS) may be trialled.

ONS have been found to improve nutritional status and strength outcomes in patients with sarcopenia, dementia, and other conditions [74, 75]. Evidence for dietary counselling and use of ONS is scarce in rheumatological diseases and there remains much work to be done in this area.

14.3.3 Enteral Feeding

A step-wise approach to feeding should be taken with the ideal route being the oral route. There are several indications for feeding directly into the GI tract. These can include, but are not limited to oral disease, dysphagia, oesophageal dysmotility and gastroparesis. Potential enteral feeding routes are depicted in Fig. 14.5. Enteral feeding may also be used to provide supplementary macro and micronutrient provision where the patient is not able to tolerate the required dietary regimen orally or if ONS are found to be unpalatable. There are small case series in the use of artificial tube feeding in patients with SSc [77, 78].

14.3.4 Pre-pyloric Feeding

Naso-gastric (NG) feeding can be performed to provide additional macro and micronutrients, to overcome any GI tract issue proximal to the stomach or as a trial prior to permanent placement of a gastrostomy tube. NG tubes can be placed by a

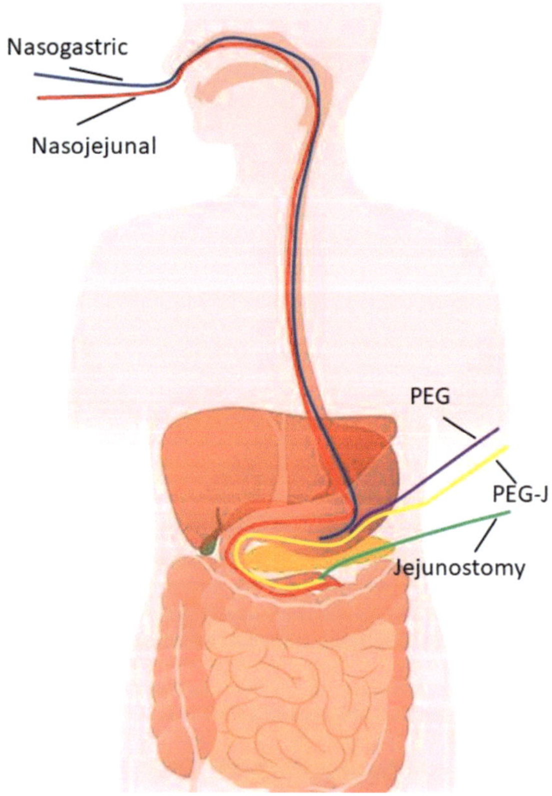

Fig. 14.5 Enteral feeding routes. PEG, percutaneous endoscopic gastrostomy; PEG-J, percutaneous endoscopic gastrostomy with jejunal extension. (Adapted with permission from [76])

competent health care professional at the bedside or radiologically. Position of the NG tube is then confirmed by aspirating gastric fluid to confirm that the pH is less than 5. If this is not possible a chest X-ray is performed to ensure that the NG tube tip is below the diaphragm. Generally, NG tubes are used for up to 4 weeks around which time a decision is made regarding a more permanent feeding solution.

Absolute contraindications to NG feeding include nasal trauma or surgery and relative contraindications to consider are coagulopathy, recently treated oesophageal varices and oesophageal strictures (which may necessitate radiologically guided placement).

When correctly placed NG tubes have a low complication rate. Very rarely they can cause oesophageal perforation and misplacement and subsequent use of an NG tube is generally considered a never event. However, they can easily dislodge and come out, necessitating replacement.

A gastrostomy is a feeding tube inserted directly through the wall of the stomach. This is most commonly performed at endoscopy when it is called a percutaneous endoscopic gastrostomy (PEG). Gastrostomy can also be performed radiologically (radiologically inserted gastrostomy or RIG) or rarely surgically. Indications for gastrostomy are similar to those of NG feeding but generally they are only placed if longer term feeding is indicated. Complications of placement are rare but significant such as bleeding and perforation of a viscous therefore patient selection is important and patients who are very malnourished may need a period of NG feeding to improve their nutrition status prior to gastrostomy placement. Longer term complications include infection or abscess at the PEG site and overgrowth of the stomach mucosa if the PEG is not cared for correctly, known as 'buried bumper'. This can be difficult to manage and often requires endoscopy assisted removal of the PEG. Patient and carer education and training can prevent the development of buried bumper syndrome.

Absolute contraindications to gastrostomy include abdominal varices and anatomical abnormalities where a large part of the stomach is in the chest (e.g., a type 3 or 4 hiatus hernia). Previous gastric surgery is a relative contraindication and patients such as these may require a RIG due to their altered anatomy. If endoscopy is contraindicated or impossible then a RIG may still be possible although passage of an NG tube is required to distend the stomach with air for the procedure. This is generally possible radiologically unless there is a pin hole stricture. Gastrostomy tubes can be displaced and should ideally be replaced with a spare device or a foley catheter as the stoma can close within 4 hours even in well-established tracts.

14.3.5 Post-pyloric Feeding

Naso-jejunal (NJ) tubes are used for post-pyloric feeding. They can be placed endoscopically or radiologically and can be displaced by vomiting. The main clinical reason for post-pyloric feeding would be a problem with the stomach such as gastroparesis or gastric outlet obstruction. The complications and contraindications are similar to that of NG tubes. In selected patients with SSc who have a risk of aspiration (such as those with oesophageal dysmotility) it may be appropriate to consider post-pyloric feeding if enteral feeding is required. However, ultimately patients with pan-enteric dysmotility may require long-term parenteral nutrition.

If, following a trial of NJ feeding, a more permanent post-pyloric feeding tube is required then a percutaneous endoscopic gastrostomy with jejunal extension (PEG-J) or surgical jejunostomy can be placed. This has been shown to be effective in delayed gastric emptying in small case series [79]. Jejunal extensions can be thread through an existing PEG radiologically or can be added at time of PEG insertion. As they have to pass through the PEG, they have a small diameter and therefore can block more easily. They can be displaced into the stomach. Surgical jejunostomy is placed laparoscopically directly into the wall of the jejunum. Complications include misplacement, infection and bleeding. Surgical jejunostomy has been demonstrated to contribute to improved nutritional status and overall health in patients with severe gastroparesis however the major complication rate can be as high as 54% [80].

14.3.6 Parenteral Nutrition

Parenteral nutrition (PN) may be necessary if the enteral route cannot be accessed or if the patient has a non-functioning GI tract, which can be for many reasons including malabsorption, dysmotility, or functional or anatomical short bowel syndrome (SBS). PN can provide all the energy, nitrogen, macro- and micro-nutrients that a patient requires. It can be delivered via a peripheral cannula on a very temporary bases or a peripherally inserted central catheter (PICC) but is ideally given via a dedicated central venous catheter. PN administration should be managed by a nutrition support team and may be used as a temporary measure for example pre-operatively or until an enteral route is established. However longer term PN delivery is managed by specialist intestinal failure units supported by home care companies to give home PN (HPN) in England. This is necessary due to the expert MDT approach required to manage these patients and the risk of potentially life-threatening complications which can occur with the use of PN (Table 14.4).

Various small case series exist in the use of PN for severe gastrointestinal involvement in patients with SSc. One larger study of 8 patients in whom PN was commenced for nutritional decline using the enteral route showed that HPN prolonged life and had a complication rate comparable to use in non-rheumatological diseases [39]. In a separate study of 25 patients with SSc requiring HPN had a very low complication rate and was found to be effective with a 5-year survival of 37% [82]. Patients with SLE and mixed connective tissue disease have also received HPN to overcome GI involvement and malnutrition [83]. In patients with rheumatological disease there may be complicating factors to take into account when considering HPN. Patients may not have the manual dexterity required to care for their own central venous catheter meaning that family members or home care company nurses may have to assist them [39]. Fluid balance may become challenging in patients

Table 14.4 Parenteral nutrition complications, adapted from BAPEN [81]

Insertion complications	Line complications	Metabolic (feed/intestinal failure) complications	
		Short-term	*Long-term*
Pneumothorax	Line sepsis	Refeeding syndrome	Liver disease
Bleeding	Thrombosis, phlebitis	Hyper/hypoglycaemia	Cholelithiasis
Misplacement	Occlusion	Electrolyte disturbances	Metabolic bone disease
	Dislodgement, fracture, leaking	Hypertriglyceridemia	Micronutrient imbalances
		Acute cholestasis	

with multisystem disease with cardiorespiratory involvement. In some patients it may be extremely difficult to administer sufficient energy and nitrogen without causing fluid overload and medications such as diuretics may only add to electrolyte imbalances.

14.3.7 Psychological Support and Therapies

Gastrointestinal involvement is common in SSc and can often lead to impaired quality of life and adversely affect the patient's social life [84]. There is strong evidence that psychosocial intervention can be beneficial in conditions such as chronic small bowel dysmotility which can be found in both SSc and SLE [22].

There are recommendations in conditions such as inflammatory bowel disease and GI dysmotility that the MDT should include input from psychologists and liaison psychiatrists who can provide different interventions [22, 85]. However, there is scant evidence even in these diseases for which type of psychological intervention is best.

14.4 Priorities for Future Research

Further work is needed to provide evidence for screening for and treating malnutrition in rheumatological and vasculitic diseases. In patients with GI involvement of their primary condition gastroenterology expertise should be sought and may well lead to dietetic assessment and treatment. However as described the reasons for malnutrition in these conditions is often multifactorial including underlying disease activity and psychological comorbidity therefore even patients without obvious GI involvement may require screening. Further evidence would be beneficial in driving service development to allow for more rigorous detection and treatment of malnutrition in these conditions. This could include the presence of dietitians in rheumatology outpatient clinics.

14.5 Conclusion

In conclusion, malnutrition in rheumatological and vasculitic disease is multifactorial and when screened for in certain conditions such as SSc it is very common. Rheumatological conditions which do not traditionally affect the GI tract can also result in malnutrition due to disease activity, psychological comorbidity, and other factors. Most of the available data are regarding SSc and future work should focus on other rheumatological and vasculitic conditions. There are several tools which can be used to detect the risk of, or actual malnutrition and its management should involve a multidisciplinary approach. Particular expertise is required in patients with intestinal failure due to the complications which can occur secondary to HPN and intestinal failure itself.

References

1. Malnutrition. https://www.who.int/news-room/questions-and-answers/item/malnutrition. Accessed 6 Jan 2022.
2. Saunders J, Smith T. Malnutrition: causes and consequences. Clin Med (Lond). 2010;10:624.
3. Cruz-Jentoft AJ, Sayer AA. Sarcopenia. Lancet. 2019;393:2636–46.
4. Baron M, Hudson M, Steele R, et al. Malnutrition is common in systemic sclerosis: results from the Canadian Scleroderma Research Group database. J Rheumatol. 2009;36:2737–43.
5. Hughes M, Heal C, Siegert E, Hachulla E, Airó P, Riccardi A, Distler O, Matucci-Cerinic M. Significant weight loss in systemic sclerosis: a study from the EULAR Scleroderma Trials and Research (EUSTAR) database. Ann Rheum Dis. 2020;79:1123–5.
6. Rosato E, Gigante A, Chiara Pellicano A, Villa A, Iannazzo F, Danilo FA, Muscaritoli M. Symptoms related to gastrointestinal tract involvement and low muscularity in systemic sclerosis. Clin Rheumatol. 2022;3:1–10.
7. Krause L, Becker MO, Brueckner CS, et al. Nutritional status as marker for disease activity and severity predicting mortality in patients with systemic sclerosis. Ann Rheum Dis. 2010;69:1951–7.
8. Ekici R, Erden A, Güven SC, Armağan B, Özdemir B, Karakaş Ö, Gök K, Omma A, Küçükşahin O, Erten Ş. Prevalence of sarcopenia and clinical implications in patients with newly diagnosed rheumatoid arthritis. Nutrition. 2021;90:111353.
9. Craig E, Cappelli LC. Gastrointestinal and hepatic disease in rheumatoid arthritis. Rheum Dis Clin N Am. 2018;44:89–111.
10. Arvikar SL, Fisher MC. Inflammatory bowel disease associated arthropathy. Curr Rev Musculoskelet Med. 2011;4:123.
11. Peluso R, Manguso F, Vitiello M, Iervolino S, Minno MND. Management of arthropathy in inflammatory bowel diseases. Ther Adv Chronic Dis. 2015;6:65.
12. Kopylov U, Starr M, Watts C, Dionne S, Girardin M, Seidman EG. Detection of Crohn disease in patients with spondyloarthropathy: the SpACE capsule study. J Rheumatol. 2018;45:498–505.
13. Stolwijk C, van Tubergen A, Castillo-Ortiz JD, Boonen A. Prevalence of extra-articular manifestations in patients with ankylosing spondylitis: a systematic review and meta-analysis. Ann Rheum Dis. 2015;74:65–73.
14. Rudwaleit M, Baeten D. Ankylosing spondylitis and bowel disease. Best Pract Res Clin Rheumatol. 2006;20:451–71.
15. Scaldaferri F, Pizzoferrato M, Lopetuso LR, et al. Nutrition and IBD: malnutrition and/or sarcopenia? A practical guide. Gastroenterol Res Pract. 2017;2017:8646495.

16. Gross WL, Trabandt A, Reinhold-Keller E. Diagnosis and evaluation of vasculitis. Rheumatology (Oxford). 2000;39:245–52.
17. Ahn E, Luk A, Chetty R, Butany J. Vasculitides of the gastrointestinal tract. Semin Diagn Pathol. 2009;26:77–88.
18. Hammar O, Ohlsson B, Wollmer P, Mandl T. Impaired gastric emptying in primary Sjögren's syndrome. J Rheumatol. 2010;37:2313–8.
19. Antonucci A, Fronzoni L, Cogliandro L, Cogliandro RF, Caputo C, de Giorgio R, Palloti F, Barbara G, Corinaldesi R, Stanghellini V. Chronic intestinal pseudo-obstruction. World J Gastroenterol. 2008;14:2953–61.
20. Jadhav P, Desai S, Jadhav J, Bichile L. Acute pancreatitis in rheumatology practice, with emphasis on systemic lupus erythematosus: a case series and newer concepts. Indian J Rheumatol. 2019;14:229.
21. Alkhayyat M, Abou Saleh M, Grewal MK, Abureesh M, Mansoor E, Simons-Linares CR, Abelson A, Chahal P. Pancreatic manifestations in rheumatoid arthritis: a national population-based study. Rheumatology (Oxford). 2021;60:2366–74.
22. Nightingale JMD, Paine P, McLaughlin J, Emmanuel A, Martin JE, Lal S. The management of adult patients with severe chronic small intestinal dysmotility. Gut. 2020;69:2074.
23. Khoshini R, Dai SC, Lezcano S, Pimentel M. A systematic review of diagnostic tests for small intestinal bacterial overgrowth. Dig Dis Sci. 2008;53:1443–54.
24. Marie I, Ducrotté P, Denis P, Menard JF, Levesque H. Small intestinal bacterial overgrowth in systemic sclerosis. Rheumatology (Oxford). 2009;48:1314–9.
25. Rowe K, Pankow J, Nehme F, Salyers W. Gastrointestinal amyloidosis: review of the literature. Cureus. 2017;9:e1228.
26. Al-Toma A, Volta U, Auricchio R, Castillejo G, Sanders DS, Cellier C, Mulder CJ, Lundin KEA. European Society for the Study of Coeliac Disease (ESsCD) guideline for coeliac disease and other gluten-related disorders. United European Gastroenterol J. 2019;7:583–613.
27. Sandler RD, Matucci-Cerinic M, Hughes M. Musculoskeletal hand involvement in systemic sclerosis. Semin Arthritis Rheum. 2019;50:329–34.
28. Wick JY. Xerostomia: causes and treatment. Consult Pharm. 2007;22:985–92.
29. Türk İ, Cüzdan N, Çiftçi V, Arslan D, Doğan MC, Unal İ. Malnutrition, associated clinical factors, and depression in systemic sclerosis: a cross-sectional study. Clin Rheumatol. 2020;39:57–67.
30. Fukuda W, Yamazaki T, Akaogi T, Hayashi H, Kusakabe T, Tsubouchi Y, Kawahito Y, Inoue M, Yoshikawa T. Malnutrition and disease progression in patients with rheumatoid arthritis. Mod Rheumatol. 2005;15:104–7.
31. Aviello G, Cristiano C, Luckman SM, D'Agostino G. Brain control of appetite during sickness. Br J Pharmacol. 2021;178:2096–110.
32. Roubenoff R, Roubenoff RA, Cannon JG, Kehayias JJ, Zhuang H, Dawson-Hughes B, Dinarello CA, Rosenberg IH. Rheumatoid cachexia: cytokine-driven hypermetabolism accompanying reduced body cell mass in chronic inflammation. J Clin Invest. 1994;93:2379–86.
33. Rajbhandary R, Khezri A, Panush RS. Rheumatoid cachexia: what is it and why is it important? J Rheumatol. 2011;38:406–8.
34. Meade T, Manolios N, Cumming SR, Conaghan PG, Katz P. Cognitive impairment in rheumatoid arthritis: a systematic review. Arthritis Care Res. 2018;70:39–52.
35. Megari K. Quality of life in chronic disease patients. Health Psychol Res. 2013;1:27.
36. Kwakkenbos L, Delisle VC, Fox RS, Gholizadeh S, Jewett LR, Levis B, Milette K, Mills SD, Malcarne VL, Thombs BD. Psychosocial aspects of scleroderma. Rheum Dis Clin N Am. 2015;41:519–28.
37. Ablett J, Vasant DH, Taylor M, Cawley C, Lal S. Poor social support and unemployment are associated with negative affect in home parenteral nutrition-dependent patients with chronic intestinal failure. JPEN J Parenter Enteral Nutr. 2018;43:534–9.
38. Lal S, Allan P. Intestinal failure: a review. F1000Res. 2018. https://doi.org/10.12688/F1000RESEARCH.12493.1/DOI

39. Brown M, Teubner A, Shaffer J, Herrick AL. Home parenteral nutrition—an effective and safe long-term therapy for systemic sclerosis-related intestinal failure. Rheumatology (Oxford). 2008;47:176–9.
40. Backman CL. Arthritis and pain. Psychosocial aspects in the management of arthritis pain. Arthritis Res Ther. 2006;8:221.
41. WHO/Europe | Nutrition—Body mass index—BMI. https://www.euro.who.int/en/health-topics/disease-prevention/nutrition/a-healthy-lifestyle/body-mass-index-bmi?source=post_page. Accessed 6 Jan 2022.
42. Todorovic V, Russell C, Elia M. THE "MUST" EXPLANATORY BOOKLET a guide to the "malnutrition universal screening tool" ('MUST') for adults. https://www.bapen.org.uk/pdfs/must/must_explan.pdf. Accessed 16 Feb 2022.
43. Malnutrition Universal Screening Tool. https://www.bapen.org.uk/pdfs/must/must_full.pdf. Accessed 11 Jan 2022.
44. Russell C, Elia M. Nutrition screening survey in the UK and Republic of Ireland in 2010. 2011. https://www.bapen.org.uk/pdfs/nsw/nsw-2011-report.pdf. Accessed 11 Jan 2022.
45. Parsons E. Nutritional care and the Malnutrition Universal Screening Tool (MUST). Br J Comm Nurs. 2011;16(5 suppl)
46. Stratton RJ, Hackston A, Longmore D, Dixon R, Price S, Stroud M, King C, Elia M. Malnutrition in hospital outpatients and inpatients: prevalence, concurrent validity and ease of use of the "malnutrition universal screening tool" ('MUST') for adults. Br J Nutr. 2004;92:799–808.
47. Madden AM, Smith S. Body composition and morphological assessment of nutritional status in adults: a review of anthropometric variables. J Hum Nutr Diet. 2016;29:7–25.
48. Preis E, Franz K, Siegert E, Makowka A, March C, Riemekasten G, Cereda E, Norman K. The impact of malnutrition on quality of life in patients with systemic sclerosis. Eur J Clin Nutr. 2018;72:504–10.
49. Baker JP, Detsky AS, Wesson DE, Wolman SL, Stewart S, Whitewell J, Langer B, Jeejeebhoy KN. Nutritional assessment. N Engl J Med. 2010;306:969–72.
50. Padilla CJ, Ferreyro FA, Arnold WD. Anthropometry as a readily accessible health assessment of older adults. Exp Gerontol. 2021;153:111464.
51. Elkan AC, Engvall IL, Tengstrand B, Cederholm T, Hafström I. Malnutrition in women with rheumatoid arthritis is not revealed by clinical anthropometrical measurements or nutritional evaluation tools. Eur J Clin Nutr. 2007;62:1239–47.
52. Taylor AE, Ebrahim S, Ben-Shlomo Y, Martin RM, Whincup PH, Yarnell JW, Wannamethee SG, Lawlor DA. Comparison of the associations of body mass index and measures of central adiposity and fat mass with coronary heart disease, diabetes, and all-cause mortality: a study using data from 4 UK cohorts. Am J Clin Nutr. 2010;91:547–56.
53. James WPT, Mascie-Taylor GCN, Norgan NG, Bistrian BR, Shetty PS, Ferro-Luzzi A. The value of arm circumference measurements in assessing chronic energy deficiency in Third World adults. Eur J Clin Nutr. 1994;48:883–94.
54. Powell-Tuck J, Hennessy EM. A comparison of mid upper arm circumference, body mass index and weight loss as indices of undernutrition in acutely hospitalized patients. Clin Nutr. 2003;22:307–12.
55. Sungurtekin H, Sungurtekin U, Oner O, Okke D. Nutrition assessment in critically ill patients. Nutr Clin Pract. 2008;23:635–41.
56. Villamor E, Saathoff E, Mugusi F, Bosch RJ, Urassa W, Fawzi WW. Wasting and body composition of adults with pulmonary tuberculosis in relation to HIV-1 coinfection, socioeconomic status, and severity of tuberculosis. Eur J Clin Nutr. 2006;60:163–71.
57. Bohannon RW. Muscle strength: clinical and prognostic value of hand-grip dynamometry. Curr Opin Clin Nutr Metab Care. 2015;18:465–70.
58. Itoh S, Shirabe K, Yoshizumi T, Takeishi K, Harimoto N, Ikegami T, Kawanaka H, Nishie A, Kamishima T, Maehara Y. Skeletal muscle mass assessed by computed tomography correlates to muscle strength and physical performance at a liver-related hospital experience. Hepatol Res. 2016;46:292–7.

59. Bellafronte NT, Batistuti MR, dos Santos NZ, Holland H, Romaõ EA, Chiarello PG. Estimation of body composition and water data depends on the bioelectrical impedance device. J Electr Bioimped. 2018;9:96–105.
60. Kopczynska M, Barrett MP, Cloutier A, Farrer K, Taylor M, Burden S, Lal S. Body composition in patients with type 2 intestinal failure. Nutr Clin Pract. 2021;37:137–45.
61. Jones DJ, Lal S, Strauss BJ, Todd C, Pilling M, Burden ST. Measurement of muscle mass and sarcopenia using anthropometry, bioelectrical impedance, and computed tomography in surgical patients with colorectal malignancy: comparison of agreement between methods. Nutr Cancer. 2019;72:1074–83.
62. Hvas CL, Harrison E, Eriksen MK, Herrick AL, McLaughlin JT, Lal S. Nutritional status and predictors of weight loss in patients with systemic sclerosis. Clin Nutr ESPEN. 2020;40:164–70.
63. Ji Y, Plourde H, Bouzo V, Kilgour RD, Cohen TR. Validity and usability of a smartphone image-based dietary assessment app compared to 3-day food diaries in assessing dietary intake among Canadian adults: randomized controlled trial. JMIR Mhealth Uhealth. 2020; https://doi.org/10.2196/16953.
64. Harrison E, Herrick AL, Mclaughlin JT, Lal S. Malnutrition in systemic sclerosis. Rheumatology (Oxford). 2012;51:1747–56.
65. Hughes M, Harrison AL, Herrick AL, McLaughlin JT, Lal S. The need to accurately measure energy intake and expenditure in patients with systemic sclerosis. J Scleroderma Relat Disord. 2022. [Accepted—in press].
66. Herrick AL, WHRFCDSDBJJMMI. Dietary intake of micronutrient antioxidants in relation to blood levels in patients with systemic sclerosis. J Rheumatol. 1996;23:650–3.
67. Bouillanne O, Hay P, Liabaud B, Duché C, Cynober L, Aussel C. Evidence that albumin is not a suitable marker of body composition-related nutritional status in elderly patients. Nutrition. 2011;27:165–9.
68. Mehler PS, Koutsavlis A. Anorexia nervosa, albumin, and inflammation. Am J Med. 2021;134:e401.
69. Recasens MA, Puig C, Ortiz-Santamaria V. Nutrition in systemic sclerosis. Rheumatol Clin. 2012;8:135–40.
70. Gyger G, Baron M. Gastrointestinal manifestations of scleroderma: recent progress in evaluation, pathogenesis, and management. Curr Rheumatol Rep. 2011;14:22–9.
71. Thombs BD, Taillefer SS, Hudson M, Baron M. Depression in patients with systemic sclerosis: a systematic review of the evidence. Arthritis Rheum. 2007;57:1089–97.
72. Ford AC, Quigley EMM, Lacy BE, Lembo AJ, Saito YA, Schiller LR, Soffer EE, Spiegel BMR, Moayyedi P. Effect of antidepressants and psychological therapies, including hypnotherapy, in irritable bowel syndrome: systematic review and meta-analysis. Am J Gastroenterol. 2014;109:1350–65.
73. Thakur ER, Shapiro J, Chan J, Lumley MA, Cully JA, Bradford A, El-Serag HB. A systematic review of the effectiveness of psychological treatments for IBS in gastroenterology settings: promising but in need of further study. Dig Dis Sci. 2018;63:2189–201.
74. Tangvik RJ, Bruvik FK, Drageset J, Kyte K, Hunskår I. Effects of oral nutrition supplements in persons with dementia: a systematic review. Geriatr Nurs. 2021;42:117–23.
75. Cramer JT, Cruz-Jentoft AJ, Landi F, Hickson M, Zamboni M, Pereira SL, Hustead DS, Mustad VA. Impacts of high-protein oral nutritional supplements among malnourished men and women with sarcopenia: a multicenter, randomized, double-blinded, controlled trial. J Am Med Dir Assoc. 2016;17:1044–55.
76. Human Digestive Organs Vector Illustration Stock Illustration—Download Image Now—iStock. https://www.istockphoto.com/vector/human-digestive-organs-vector-illustration-gm609440664-104438955?clarity=false. Accessed 12 May 2022.
77. Bharadwaj S, Tandon P, Gohel T, Corrigan ML, Coughlin KL, Shatnawei A, Chatterjee S, Kirby DF. Gastrointestinal manifestations, malnutrition, and role of enteral and parenteral nutrition in patients with scleroderma. J Clin Gastroenterol. 2015;49:559–64.

78. Fynne L, Kruse A, Borre M, Søndergaard K, Krogh K. Percutaneous endoscopic gastrostomy in patients with systemic sclerosis. Scand J Rheumatol. 2010;39:266–8.
79. Keld R, Kinsey L, Athwal V, Lal S. Pathogenesis, investigation and dietary and medical management of gastroparesis. J Hum Nutr Diet. 2011;24:421–30.
80. Tang DM, Friedenberg FK. Gastroparesis: approach, diagnostic evaluation, and management. Dis Mon. 2011;57:74–101.
81. Complication Management. https://www.bapen.org.uk/nutrition-support/parenteral-nutrition/complication-management. Accessed 26 Jan 2022.
82. Harrison E, Herrick AL, Dibb M, McLaughlin JT, Lal S. Long-term outcome of patients with systemic sclerosis requiring home parenteral nutrition. Clin Nutr. 2015;34:991–6.
83. Srinivasaiah N, Mottershead H, Magambo W, Jukes A, Harwood S, Hargest R, Hawthorne AB. Home parenteral nutrition (HPN): a Welsh experience. Proc Nutr Soc. 2010;69:156.
84. Gyger G, Baron M. Systemic sclerosis: gastrointestinal disease and its management. Rheum Dis Clin N Am. 2015;41:459–73.
85. Menichetti J, Fiorino G, Vegni E. Personalizing psychological treatment along the IBD journey: from diagnosis to surgery. Curr Drug Targets. 2018;19:722–8.

Chapter 15
GI Manifestations and Treatment Considerations of Rheumatological Disease in Older Adults

Sarah Theiner, Jason Perlmutter, Lavinia Salama, and Rebecca Stetzer

15.1 Introduction

Greater understanding of rheumatological diseases has paved the way for treatments that have dramatically improved the quality and longevity of patient's lives. The increasing size of the geriatric population necessitates incorporation of geriatric principles into routine medical practice [1]. Disease management for these older adults can be optimized by a big-picture approach guided by goals of care, which in turn requires exploration of details of functional and cognitive status. For older adults and those with multiple chronic conditions, manifestations of their rheumatologic disease will be just one aspect of the challenges they are facing. This holds true whether they recently presented with a rheumatic disease or have lived with their disease for decades. Furthermore, their rheumatologic-related symptoms may be a subset of multiple components of a geriatric syndrome, making evaluation and management of complaints complex, and frustrating to patients and clinicians alike.

S. Theiner
Santa Clara Valley Medical Center, Fruitdale, CA, USA

J. Perlmutter
Department of Internal Medicine, Albany Medical Center, Albany, NY, USA
e-mail: perlmuj@amc.edu

L. Salama
The Arnold & Marie Schwartz College of Pharmacy and Health Sciences, Long Island University, Brooklyn, NY, USA
e-mail: Lavinia.salama@liu.edu

R. Stetzer (✉)
Departments of Family Medicine, Neurology, Albany Medical Center, Albany, NY, USA
e-mail: stetzer@amc.edu

M. Tadros et al. (eds.), *GI Diseases Associated with Rheumatological and Vasculitic Conditions*, Clinical Gastroenterology,
https://doi.org/10.1007/978-3-032-07868-1_15

Approaching care of older adults using the "5Ms" of geriatrics can provide a framework to help optimize care of these complex patients.

15.2 Homeostenosis

Homeostasis is the maintenance of equilibrium within a system achieved by the physiologic balance of multiple interdependent factors, internal and external. Both the normal physiologic changes of aging and the stress imposed by multiple comorbid disease processes increase the energy needed to maintain homeostasis. This depletes the reserves available in times of stress. This state of homeo*stenosis* means that smaller insults can tip patients out of homeostasis into a state needing further support (such as hospitalization) or death [2]. Evaluating frailty status can help estimate the degree of homeostenosis present, allowing for better prediction of the impact a particular disease process or treatment may have on a complex patient.

15.3 Geriatric Syndromes

As opposed to a disease which may have multiple presenting symptoms caused by one underlying pathophysiologic process, a syndrome is a presenting problem that has multiple etiologies. There are multiple syndromes common to older adults that significantly impact daily functioning and quality of life. When evaluating a complaint, one cannot stop investigation after finding the first potential cause as it may be just one of the contributing factors. Common geriatric syndromes include falls, malnutrition and weight loss, incontinence, cognitive impairment and delirium. [3]. Including a geriatric review of systems (ROS) can help unearth these concerns and allow for a geriatrician's approach to rheumatologic disease processes [4, 5].

Geriatric Syndrome ROS

Mobility impairment

- Recent falls
- Fear of falling

Vision

Hearing

Incontinence

Constipation

Nutritional status

- weight loss
- dysphagia

Functional status

- Activities of Daily Living (ADLs)*
- Instrumental Activities of Daily Living (IADLs)**

Cognitive impairment

Depression/anxiety

Social support:

- formal/informal caregivers
- community support services (fall alert system, meal services, day program, etc)

*ADLs: bathing, dressing, toileting, transferring, continence, feeding [4].

**IADLs: Telephone/computer, shopping, food preparation, housekeeping, laundry, transportation, medication management, finance management [5].

15.4 Rheumatologic Contributions to Geriatric Syndromes

The clinical manifestations of rheumatological disease in older adults are an accumulation of damage from both active and chronic disease as well as long-term side effects of treatment. In older adults these processes are intermingled with age-related immune dysregulation and decline in organ function (homeostenosis) as well as comorbid medical conditions and treatment side effects. Common contributing GI manifestations of rheumatologic disease include xerostomia, oral ulcers, dental caries, dysphagia, aspiration, malabsorption, diarrhea, and fecal incontinence. These overlapping end organ manifestations can contribute to geriatric syndromes of weight loss, incontinence and falls and contribute to depression and social isolation.

Xerostomia, common in Sjogren's syndrome and scleroderma, can lead to dry, cracked lips as well as angular cheilitis, which may result in oral infections, especially candidiasis and oral mucositis [6]. Salivary dysfunction can also lead to difficulty speaking, recurrent dental caries, and challenges for denture-wearers as desiccated and friable tissue is more likely to develop lesions, making it hard for these patients to use their dentures [6]. Furthermore, in patients with scleroderma, fibrosis of facial, tongue and mucosal tissue can cause microstomia and impaired mastication and swallowing leading to poor nutritional intake [7, 8]. These effects are frequently compounded by drying side-effects of medications, particularly those with anticholinergic and antihistaminic properties. These changes contribute to the development of dental caries and dysphagia. The difficulties in swallowing and embarrassment of coughing while eating can restrict participation in social meals, contributing to malnutrition, weight loss and social isolation.

Dysphagia is common in scleroderma, Sjogren's disease, polymyositis and dermatomyositis and can also be seen in Behcet's disease [9]. This can interfere with normal food intake and medication adherence and increase susceptibility to aspiration pneumonia. Patients with atlantoaxial subluxation secondary to rheumatoid arthritis may develop dysphagia, and if the temporomandibular joint is involved, the patient's diet may be further impacted by pain and impaired mastication [9]. Candida esophagitis can be seen in scleroderma due to impaired peristalsis secondary to fibrosis of esophageal smooth muscle, immunosuppressive therapy, or chronic proton pump inhibitor (PPI) use [9].

When evaluating a complaint, one cannot stop investigation after finding the first potential cause as it may be just one of the contributing factors.

Rheumatologic disease-associated dysphagia is compounded by the increased risk of dysphagia with age. Studies in the US and Europe have found to the prevalence of dysphagia to be between 12% and 60% in older adults [10–13]. In addition to complications such as pill esophagitis, dysphagia can negatively impact medication compliance. In a survey of adults with difficulty swallowing pills, 14% have reported delays in taking their medications and 8% skipped doses completely. In long term care facilities, a study found that of patients experiencing difficulties swallowing capsules, 5% of patients regularly expectorated their medication, and 27% did not attempt to swallow their medications due to their dysphagia [14]. Some methods to improve compliance in patients with dysphagia include oral dissolving tablets, crushing medications, opening medications, or obtaining liquid alternatives [12]. Unfortunately, for many DMARDS and other anti-rheumatic medications, these strategies are not viable options for safe administration.

Systemic sclerosis can result in either diarrhea or constipation, and sphincter dysfunction can lead to incontinence. As the disease progresses, over 90% of patients will experience gut dysmotility and overall loss of absorption. Diarrhea is caused by malabsorption due to decreased surface area of atrophied intestinal epithelium, decreased permeability of the small intestines, as well as chronic interstitial edema. This may transition to constipation as smooth muscle is atrophied, causing dysmotility or even absent colonic peristalsis [15]. Collagen deposition may lead to malabsorption, pseudo-obstruction or cystoides intestinalis. The continued risk of bacterial colonization can result in small intestinal bacterial overgrowth [16, 17]. This can manifest as bloating, abdominal discomfort, diarrhea, weight loss, delirium, neuropathy, and worsening weakness and debility. These conditions can have devastating social consequences as people avoid the embarrassment of multiple trips to the bathroom or incontinent episodes.

Weight loss is a multifactorial issue in older adults with rheumatological disease due to a combination of xerostomia and dysphagia, malabsorption secondary to bacterial overgrowth, gastroparesis, medication side effects, and self-restriction from community meals due to dysphagia and diarrhea. The prevalence of malnutrition in patients with systemic scleroderma is approximately 15–58%, causing significant morbidity and mortality [18]. Monitoring for malnutrition includes weight and laboratory measurements, but questions about the various contributing factors allows for earlier detection and identifies opportunities for intervention.

15.5 Management of Geriatric Syndromes

Awareness of potential gastrointestinal manifestations of rheumatologic disease and their overlap with geriatric syndromes allows the clinician to monitor for these symptoms and take a proactive approach toward management. Nutrition screening tools such as the Malnutrition Universal Screening Tool (MUST) questionnaire and the Mini Nutritional Assessment (MNA) can assist in screening patients for malnutrition risk [19, 20]. Routine monitoring for geriatric syndromes of weight loss, dysphagia, constipation and incontinence, evaluation of medication side effects and deprescribing when possible, and encouraging regular visits with the dentist can help minimize eating and speech difficulties [6]. Speech therapists are particularly skilled at assessing and teaching patients appropriate swallowing techniques, and helping caregivers coach these modifications at home. Management of constipation is usually a dynamic process which needs to be modified according to changes in medical conditions, treatments, activity level, diet, and aging. Most importantly, taking a whole-person into account can help identify approaches that are person-specific rather than disease-specific. Interventions such as deprescribing, pull-up adult diapers, proper fitting of assistive devices, or identification of a "meal buddy" can have a profound impact on a frail adult's participation in group meals and improve nutrition status, strength, and ability to perform ADLs.

15.6 Atypical Gastrointestinal Presentations and Course of Rheumatological Disease in Older Adults

In older adults, rheumatological diseases can have atypical and more subtle presentations and a varied clinical course. For instance, Pautas et al. observed that older patients with dermatomyositis or polymyositis have a higher incidence of dysphagia (2.3-fold increase), of complicating bacteria pneumonia (4.2-fold increase), and of associated malignancy (2.5 to 5.2-fold increase) than younger patients [21]. Older patients were also found to have a more chronic disease course and poorer outcomes [1, 22]. Conversely, patients with elderly onset systemic lupus erythematous (EOSLE) were found to have a more indolent disease course and a better response to treatment with lower treatment doses and duration than younger onset SLE patients. Other studies have found that patient with EOSLE have different serological features and patterns of organ involvement. This includes prominent lung disease, musculoskeletal symptoms and serositis and lower incidence of renal disease, CNS involvement, lymphadenopathy, and cutaneous symptoms [1]. When older patients with SLE develop protein-losing enteropathy (PLE), there is concern for an exacerbation of protein wasting and worsening sarcopenia [21]. Older patients with systemic vasculitis like Eosinophilic Granulomatosis with Polyangiitis may develop an acute abdomen secondary to mesenteric artery involvement [23]. The possibility of severe complications compounded by underlying pre-existing morbidity can render these conditions rapidly fatal. Since physical exam findings may be muted in older adults, it is essential to maintain a high level of suspicion as early intervention for mesenteric ischemia will have better outcomes [24]. These more atypical disease presentations can mimic other conditions, and it may be challenging to identify their contribution to geriatric syndromes [1].

15.7 The 5M's of Geriatric Care

The 5M's of geriatric care was introduced by Mary Tinetti as a framework for approaching important aspects of care of older adults that go beyond disease management [25]. The 5M's stand for what matters most, medication, mentation, mobility and multi-complexity. Although many health systems have adopted a "4M" approach to geriatrics care, the 5th M of "multi-complexity" is a key consideration in clinical care, especially for those with conditions that have medical and social complexity. This approach helps guide clinicians to create evaluation and management plans within the context of specific medication considerations, functional status and social complexities so they can be focused on what brings meaning and joy to their patients' lives.

15.8 Matters Most

Managing multiple chronic conditions requires active balancing of disease manifestations and treatment burden. Understanding what brings meaning to our patients' lives allows us to discuss the harms and benefits of treatment within the context of their values and treatment goals. There is significant variation among patient goals of care, with some valuing longevity at almost all cost, while others prefer maintaining function or reducing symptoms so that they can engage in specific activities and relationships [26]. Asking questions such as, "what makes a good day good," "what goals do you have for your health," or "what symptoms interfere with your daily life?" can be a starting point for these conversations. Preferences and priorities may change over time, so it's important to revisit these conversations and adapt management plans as appropriate. Patient Priorities Care (patientprioritiescare.org) offers a comprehensive approach toward eliciting patients' health priorities and can help guide these conversations [27].

15.9 Multi-complexity

Multi-complexity refers to the medical complexity of the interactions among multiple chronic conditions and their treatments, various geriatric syndromes, frailty, and complex psychosocial situations. The ability to manage a complex medical regimen depends not just on a patient's cognition, functional status, and preferences, but also their financial resources, social supports, religious and cultural identity. Studies in older patients have found improved adherence to medications for patients living with a partner and for those with higher socio-economic status and education level [28]. Going back to the concept of homeostenosis, consider the manifestation of illness in the older adult. A frail patient on an immunosuppressive may develop delirium as a result of a fever. If living alone without routine support, they may not be able to seek the needed emergency care needed in this situation. Treatment plans must be developed with consideration of medical and social context, with extra support put in place for the most vulnerable.

15.10 Medication

The treatment of rheumatological diseases in geriatric patients is complicated by age-related changes in drug pharmacokinetics, drug pharmacodynamics, comorbid medical conditions, concurrent medications, increases in drug interactions and adverse effects. Drugs pharmacokinetic and pharmacodynamic parameters are altered with age due to declining renal function, fewer drug receptors, increase in potential for interactions between different receptors and changes to downstream signaling cascades that are activated following drug binding [29]. A key clinical pearl is that a decrease in serum albumin can lead to higher active drug levels at the same dose and mediation doses should be periodically reevaluated with any change in renal function. [29].

Polypharmacy is a common geriatric syndrome, with nearly 50% of patients on Medicare reporting taking five or more medications [26]. Older adults suffer more adverse drug reactions (ADR) than their younger counterparts, and polypharmacy increases this risk due to increased drug-drug and drug-disease interactions [30]. Percy et al. found that older adults taking six different medications were 14 times more likely to have an ADR than younger patients taking the same medications [31]. For example, older adults are at increased risk of complications due to non-steroidal anti-inflammatory drugs (NSAID) use including *Helicobacter pylori* infection, gastroesophageal reflux, pill-induced esophagitis, and peptic ulcer disease [29]. Polypharmacy can lead to burdensome treatments, monitoring regimens and worse outcomes including increase in falls and hospitalizations and a decrease in function and cognition. High anticholinergic load can contribute to geriatric syndromes by causing dry mouth, constipation, urinary retention, confusion, and falls. High cumulative anticholinergic use over a lifetime is associated with increased risk for dementia [32]. It is especially important to conduct thorough medication review to identify anticholinergic medications that can contribute to geriatric syndromes, which can help prompt deprescribing and improve outcomes. The ACB Calculator (acbcalc.com) is a useful online tool for assessing individual medication and total anticholinergic burden.

During treatment it is critical to review the patient's current medications, to consider if these medications are still beneficial, and to continue to assess if the current treatment plan is aligned with the patient's health goals. Given the ubiquity of polypharmacy in older patients it can be helpful to match medications and diagnoses and then assess if these medications are still of benefit. If appropriate, deprescribing should be attempted. Medications should be down-titrated slowly with close follow up to assess for recurrence of symptoms and tolerability. Additionally, new health complaints or geriatric syndrome worsening may be due to medication side effects. Routinely assessing for medication side effects can help prevent prescribing cascades, where new medications are started to treat existing medication side effects.

Anti-rheumatic drugs are often prescribed for the duration of a patient's life. Education about medications is frequently only done during treatment initiation. It is essential to re-educate patients and their caregivers verbally and in writing on medication indications, dosage, scheduling, side effects and warning signs of drug toxicity or failure. Table 15.1 details antirheumatic treatment considerations in geriatric patients. Many treatment guidelines are based on research in younger patients with few comorbidities so special consideration needs to be taken to assess whether medications will be of benefit to older adult patients given their decreased lifespan, comorbidities, and goals of care. Examination of the Beers Criteria for list of potentially inappropriate medications may help guide treatment choices [81]. Treatment decision can have a significant impact on mortality. For example, more deaths in older patients with SLE are caused by treatment complications such as infections and perforated peptic ulcers as compared to younger patients where death is related to the disease process [1]. Conversely, older adults may not be adequately treated due to concern about potential side effects. When a new medication needs to be started, a guiding principle in geriatric pharmacology is to "start low and go slow, but go!"

15.11 Mind

Attention to cognitive ability is essential prior to starting new treatment regimens, particularly if the regimen is complex or close monitoring is needed. Ask about each patient's system for taking medications (do they use a pill organizer or take pills directly from the bottles for each dose), how often they miss doses, and who manages refills. The mini-cog, which involves a 3-item recall and clock draw, is an efficient screening technique for cognitive impairment [82]. In addition, it is helpful to obtain collateral history about medication adherence from family, caregivers and the patient's pharmacy. Depression and anxiety screening should also be routine, as these conditions may interfere with adherence to treatment regimens.

Table 15.1 Considerations for using antirheumatic agents in geriatric populations[a]

Medication	Special consideration in older adults
Abatacept	Infections and malignancies (incidence is low) Patients with chronic obstructive pulmonary disease may be at higher risk of upper respiratory infections Adverse events including dizziness, headache, and hypertension can occur [33–35]
Antimuscarinic agents (e.g., pilocarpine and cevimeline hydrochloride)	Pilocarpine (systemic): older women have decreased hepatic clearance of this drug and increased incidence of urinary frequency, diarrhea, and dizziness [36, 37]
Azathioprine (AZA)	Myelosuppression, hepatotoxicity, hypersensitivity reactions and malignancy Nausea, and vomiting (dose-dependent) In geriatric populations, there is a risk for drug-drug interaction especially with allopurinol which can increase myelosuppression due to interference with AZA metabolism and angiotensin converting enzyme inhibitors which can increase risk of leukopenia and neutropenia due to competition for renal clearance [38–44]
Cyclophosphamide	Myelosuppression, hemorrhagic cystitis [45, 46]
Hydroxychloroquine	Increased risk for cardiomyopathy and QTc prolongation especially in combination with other QTc prolonging agents Retinal toxicity Headache and dizziness Nausea, vomiting, and diarrhea [47, 48]
IL-6 inhibitors (tocilizumab, sarilumab)	Infection Increased risk of GI perforation, particularly in patients with diverticulitis Herpes zoster reactivation has been reported [49–52]
JAK inhibitor (baricitinib, upadacitinib)	Herpes zoster reactivation has been reported. Tofacitinib and baricitinib can increase LDL levels, although the ratio of LDL:HDL remain stable Increased risk of serious heart-related events (e.g. heart attack), stroke, cancer, thrombosis, and death Possible increased risk for lymphomas and other malignancies Baricitinib is substantially renally excreted Tofacitinib is hepatically metabolized though CYP3A4 (major) and CYP2C19 (minor) Upadacitinib is hepatically metabolized though CYP3A4 [53–57]
Leflunomide	Limited evidence in geriatric population Long half-life: some experts recommend skipping the usual loading dose and considering alternate day dosing New onset or exacerbation of hypertension can impact common comorbid conditions such as heart failure and chronic kidney diseases Enterohepatic recycling can cause an erratic half-life of the drug especially in older adults who have altered hepatic function [58–61]
Methotrexate	Consider decreasing dosage due to physiologic age-related decrease in hepatic and renal function [62, 63]

(continued)

Table 15.1 (continued)

Medication	Special consideration in older adults
Mycophenolate mofetil and mycophenolate sodium	Up titration should be approached with caution due to the possible age-related physiologic decrease in hepatic, renal and cardiac function Older adults may be at an increased risk of myelosuppression, infections, gastrointestinal hemorrhage, and pulmonary edema [64, 65]
NSAIDs	Except for aspirin, NSAID are 99% albumin bound and hence in patients with poor nutritional status there may be increased unbound drug and adverse side effects [29] Mental status changes especially with indomethacin [66–68]
Rituximab	Risk of hypogammaglobulinemia, serious infections, malignancies, and cardiovascular events including hypertension and arrhythmias Infusion related reactions Rare but serious risk for progressive multifocal leukoencephalopathy (challenging to monitor due to non-specific symptoms that may already be present in geriatrics like altered mental status, weakness) [69, 70]
Steroids	Common (even with short-term use): increased appetite, insomnia (an already common co-morbidity in geriatrics), psychosis (geriatrics are at high risk of altered mental status/ mood disturbances), increase in glucose (caution in patients with diabetes), impaired wound healing, hypertension, GI disturbances (GI ulcers), increased risk of infection, fluid retention (caution in renal and heart failure) With long-term use: adrenal suppression, osteoporosis, glaucoma and Cushing's syndrome [29, 71]
Sulfasalazine	Prolonged plasma half-life of the drug and its metabolites expected in older adults with renal dysfunction Gastrointestinal toxicity (including nausea/ vomiting/ diarrhea, dyspepsia). Nephrotoxicity and hepatotoxicity (rare) [29, 72, 73]. Hemolytic anemia (in glucose-6-phosphate dehydrogenase deficiency) Contraindicated in sulfa-allergy Antifolate properties (not well defined), but since geriatrics often have folate deficiency consider monitoring
TNF inhibitors (infliximab, adalimumab, etanercept, golimumab)	Injection site reactions (most common adverse events (including rash, pain, and redness at the site Risk of infections (mostly URT infections) Risk of malignancies. Excluding non-melanoma skin cancers, the absolute risk of malignances with this class is low Chronic heart failure (CHF) exacerbations [74–80]

[a]Adapted, updated and expanded from Blumstein et al. [29]

15.12 Mobility

Older adults with rheumatologic disease are at risk for significant mobility compromise due to sequelae of the diseases themselves, potential medication side effects and normal processes of aging. The use of canes, walkers, and wheelchairs may allow patients to remain more independent for a longer time [29]. Many are reluctant to use mobility aids, so encouragement from clinicians can be helpful. Discussion of fall prevention, including supportive shoes with non-slip tread and environmental modifications, should be addressed periodically. Pain management, and hand arthritis in particular, should be addressed so modifications to pill delivery can be put in place if there is difficulty with opening bottles. Referrals to physical and occupational therapy can help support patients through these challenges.

15.13 Conclusion

Care of the older adult can be optimized by starting with an exploration of patients' health care priorities. This lens can then be used to approach details of disease-related complications within the context of geriatric syndromes, functional status and social supports. Taking a systematic "5M" approach brings a focus to goals of care, improves health-related quality of life, increases medication adherence and safety, and attempts to minimize burdens of rheumatic disease, both gastrointestinal and systemic, on older adults and their caregivers.

References

1. Diep JT, Gorevic PD. Geriatric autoimmune diseases: systemic lupus erythematosus, Sjogren's syndrome, and myositis. Geriatrics. 2005;60(5):32–8.
2. GN GL. Handbook of the biology of aging. San Diego: Academic; 2006.
3. Inouye SK, Studenski S, Tinetti ME, Kuchel GA. Geriatric syndromes: clinical, research, and policy implications of a core geriatric concept. J Am Geriatr Soc. 2007;55(5):780–91.
4. Katz S. Assessing self-maintenance: activities of daily living, mobility, and instrumental activities of daily living. J Am Geriatr Soc. 1983;31(12):721–7.
5. Lawton MP, Brody EM. Assessment of older people: self-maintaining and instrumental activities of daily living. Gerontologist. 1969;9(3):179–86.
6. Ship JA, Pillemer SR, Baum BJ. Xerostomia and the geriatric patient. J Am Geriatr Soc. 2002;50(3):535–43.
7. Albilia JB, Lam DK, Blanas N, Clokie CM, Sándor GK. Small mouths ... Big problems? A review of scleroderma and its oral health implications. J Can Dent Assoc. 2007;73(9):831–6.
8. Almadori A, Griffin M, Ryan CM, Hunt DF, Hansen E, Kumar R, et al. Stem cell enriched lipotransfer reverses the effects of fibrosis in systemic sclerosis. PLoS One. 2019;14(7):e0218068.
9. Kröner PT, Tolaymat OA, Bowman AW, Abril A, Lacy BE. Gastrointestinal manifestations of rheumatological diseases. Am J Gastroenterol. 2019;114(9):1441–54.

10. Lee JC, Gross BW, Rittenhouse KJ, Vogel AR, Vellucci A, Alzate J, et al. A bitter pill to swallow: dysphagia in cervical spine injury. J Surg Res. 2016;201(2):388–93.
11. Geller AI, Shehab N, Weidle NJ, Lovegrove MC, Wolpert BJ, Timbo BB, et al. Emergency department visits for adverse events related to dietary supplements. N Engl J Med. 2015;373(16):1531–40.
12. Morris H. Dysphagia in the elderly—a management challenge for nurses. Br J Nurs. 2006;15(10):558–62.
13. Lau ETL, Steadman KJ, Mak M, Cichero JAY, Nissen LM. Prevalence of Swallowing difficulties and medication modification in customers of community pharmacists. J Pharm Pract Res. 2015;45(1):18–23.
14. Wright D. Medication administration in nursing homes. Nurs Stand. 2002;16(42):33–8.
15. Marie I. Atteinte digestive au cours de la sclérodermie systémique. La Press Médicale. 2006;35(12):1952–65.
16. Sallam H, McNearney TA, Chen JDZ. Systematic review: pathophysiology and management of gastrointestinal dysmotility in systemic sclerosis (scleroderma). Aliment Pharm Therap. 2006;23(6):691–712.
17. Marie I, Ducrotté P, Denis P, Menard J-F, Levesque H. Small intestinal bacterial overgrowth in systemic sclerosis. Rheumatology. 2009;48(10):1314–9.
18. Bharadwaj S, Tandon P, Gohel T, Corrigan ML, Coughlin KL, Shatnawei A, et al. Gastrointestinal manifestations, malnutrition, and role of enteral and parenteral nutrition in patients with scleroderma. J Clin Gastroenterol. 2015;49(7):559–64.
19. Huhmann MB, Perez V, Alexander DD, Thomas DR. A self-completed nutrition screening tool for community-dwelling older adults with high reliability: a comparison study. J Nutr Health Aging. 2013;17(4):339–44.
20. Stratton RJ, Hackston A, Longmore D, Dixon R, Price S, Stroud M, et al. Malnutrition in hospital outpatients and inpatients: prevalence, concurrent validity and ease of use of the 'malnutrition universal screening tool' ('MUST') for adults. Br J Nutr. 2004;92(5):799–808.
21. Chen Z, Li M-T, Xu D, Yang H, Li J, Zhao J-L, et al. Protein-losing enteropathy in systemic lupus erythematosus: 12 years experience from a chinese academic center. PLoS One. 2014;9(12):e114684.
22. Pautas E, Cherin P, Piette JC, Pelletier S, Wechsler B, Cabane J, et al. Features of polymyositis and dermatomyositis in the elderly: a case-control study. Clin Exp Rheumatol. 2000;18(2):241–4.
23. Soowamber M, Weizman AV, Pagnoux C. Gastrointestinal aspects of vasculitides. Nat Rev Gastroenterol. 2017;14(3):185–94.
24. Ozden N, Gurses B. Mesenteric ischemia in the elderly. Clin Geriatr Med. 2007;23(4):871–87.
25. Tinetti M, Huang A, Molnar F. The geriatrics 5M's: a new way of communicating what we do. J Am Geriatr Soc. 2017;65(9):2115.
26. Ouellet GM, Ouellet JA, Tinetti ME. Principle of rational prescribing and deprescribing in older adults with multiple chronic conditions. Ther Adv Drug Saf. 2018;9(11):639–52.
27. Tinetti ME, Naik AD, Dindo L, Costello DM, Esterson J, Geda M, et al. Association of patient priorities-aligned decision-making with patient outcomes and ambulatory health care burden among older adults with multiple chronic conditions: a nonrandomized clinical trial. JAMA Intern Med. 2019;179(12):1688–97.
28. Uchmanowicz B, Chudiak A, Uchmanowicz I, Rosinczuk J, Froelicher ES. Factors influencing adherence to treatment in older adults with hypertension. Clin Interv Aging. 2018;13:2425–41.
29. Blumstein H, Gorevic PD. Rheumatologic illnesses: treatment strategies for older adults. Geriatrics. 2005;60(6):28–35.
30. Charlesworth CJ, Smit E, Lee DS, Alramadhan F, Odden MC. Polypharmacy among adults aged 65 years and older in the United States: 1988–2010. J Gerontol A Biol Sci Med Sci. 2015;70(8):989–95.
31. Percy LA, Fang MA. Geropharmacology for the rheumatologist. Rheum Dis Clin N Am. 2000;26(3):433–54, v–vi.

32. Gray SL, Anderson ML, Dublin S, Hanlon JT, Hubbard R, Walker R, et al. Cumulative use of strong anticholinergics and incident dementia: a prospective cohort study. JAMA Intern Med. 2015;175(3):401–7.
33. Abatacept: Drug Information, Lexicomp. In: UpToDate. Post: TW (Ed), UpToDate, Waltham, MA. Accessed 27 Apr 2022.
34. Orencia (abatacept), [package insert]. U.S. Food and Drug Administration website. https://www.accessdata.fda.gov/drugsatfda_docs/label/2013/125118s171lbl.pdf. Revised December 2013. Accessed 29 Apr 2022.
35. Alten R, Kaine J, Keystone E, Nash P, Delaet I, Genovese MC. Long-term safety of subcutaneous abatacept in rheumatoid arthritis: integrated analysis of clinical trial data representing more than four years of treatment. Arthritis Rheumatol. 2014;66(8):1987–97.
36. Salagen (pilocarpine hydrochloride). [package insert]. U.S. Food and Drug Administration website.https://www.accessdata.fda.gov/drugsatfda_docs/label/2003/020237s012lbl.pdf. Accessed 29 Apr 2022.
37. Pilocarpine: Drug Information, Lexicomp. In: UpToDate. Post: TW (Ed), UpToDate, Waltham, MA. Accessed 27 Apr 2022.
38. Prometheus Laboratories Inc. Imuran (azathioprine) [package insert]. U.S. Food and Drug Administration website. https://www.accessdata.fda.gov/drugsatfda_docs/label/2011/016324s034s035lbl.pdf. Revised May 2011. Accessed 26 Apr 2022.
39. Azathioprine: Drug Information, Lexicomp In: UpToDate Post: TW (Ed), UpToDate, Waltham. Accessed 27 Apr 2022.
40. Azathioprine: Drug Information, Lexicomp. In: UpToDate. Post: TW (Ed), UpToDate, Waltham. Accessed 27 Apr 2022.
41. Guidelines for monitoring drug therapy in rheumatoid arthritis. American College of Rheumatology Ad Hoc Committee on clinical guidelines. Arthritis Rheum. 1996;39(5):723–31.
42. Singh G, Fries JF, Spitz P, Williams CA. Toxic effects of azathioprine in rheumatoid arthritis. A national post-marketing perspective. Arthritis Rheum. 1989;32(7):837–43.
43. Gearry RB, Day AS, Barclay ML, Leong RW, Sparrow MP. Azathioprine and allopurinol: a two-edged interaction. J Gastroenterol Hepatol. 2010;25(4):653–5.
44. Madrazo L. Azathioprine-induced severe anemia potentiated by the concurrent use of allopurinol. Can Med Assoc J [Internet]. 2021. Available from: https://doi.org/10.1503/cmaj.201022.
45. Cyclophosphamide for injection, USP and Cyclophosphamide tablets, USP. [package insert]. U.S. Food and Drug Administration. https://www.accessdata.fda.gov/drugsatfda_docs/label/2012/012141s089lbl.pdf. Revised April 2012. Accessed 29 Apr 2022.
46. Cyclophosphamide: Drug Information, Lexicomp. In: UpToDate. Post: TW (Ed), UpToDate, Waltham. Accessed 27 Apr 2022.
47. Concordia Pharmaceuticals Inc. Plaquenil (hydroxychloroquine sulfate) [package insert]. U.S. Food and Drug Administration website. https://www.accessdata.fda.gov/drugsatfda_docs/label/2017/009768s037s045s047lbl.pdf. Revised January 2017. Accessed 26 Apr 2022.
48. Hydroxychloroquine. Drug Information, Lexicomp. In: UpToDate. Post: TW (Ed), UpToDate, Waltham. Accessed 27 Apr 2022.
49. Genetech Inc. Actemra (tocilizumab). [package insert]. U.S. Food and Drug Administration. https://www.accessdata.fda.gov/drugsatfda_docs/label/2013/125276s092lbl.pdf. Accessed 29 Apr 2022.
50. Tocilizumab: Drug Information, Lexicomp. In: UpToDate. Post: TW (Ed), UpToDate, Waltham. Accessed 27 Apr 2022.
51. Sarilumab: Drug Information, Lexicomp. In: UpToDate. Post: TW (Ed), UpToDate, Waltham. Accessed 27 Apr 2022.
52. Sanofi-Aventis U.S. LLC. Kevzara (sarilumab) injection. [package insert]. U.S. Food and Drug Administration. https://www.accessdata.fda.gov/drugsatfda_docs/label/2017/761037s000lbl.pdf. Accessed 30 Apr 2022.

53. Pfizer Labs. Xeljanz (tofacitinib) tablets and Xeljanz XR (tofacitinib) extended-release tablets. [package insert]. U.S. Food and Drug Administration. https://www.accessdata.fda.gov/drugsatfda_docs/label/2018/203214s018lbl.pdf. Revised may 2018. Accessed 29 Apr 2022.
54. Tofacitinib: Drug Information, Lexicomp. In: UpToDate. Post: TW (Ed), UpToDate, Waltham. Accessed 27 Apr 2022.
55. Eli Lilly and Company. Olumiant (baricitinib). [package insert]. U.S. Food and Drug Administration website. https://www.accessdata.fda.gov/drugsatfda_docs/label/2018/207924s000lbl.pdf. Accessed 30 Apr 2022.
56. AbbVie Ireland NL B.V. RINVQQ (upadacitinib). [package insert]. U.S. Food and Drug Administration website. https://www.accessdata.fda.gov/drugsatfda_docs/label/2019/211675s000lbl.pdf. Accessed 30 Apr 2022.
57. Administration USFaD. FDA requires warnings about increased risk of serious heart-related events, cancer, blood clots, and death for JAK inhibitors that treat certain chronic inflammatory conditions 2022 [updated January 2022. FDA Drug Safety Podcast for health care professionals from the Division of Drug Information]. Available from: https://www.fda.gov/drugs/fda-drug-safety-podcasts/fda-requires-warnings-about-increased-risk-serious-heart-related-events-cancer-blood-clots-and-death#:~:text=On%20September%201%2C%202021%2C%20based,medicines%20Xeljanz%20and%20Xeljanz%20XR.
58. Sanofi-Aventis U.S. LLC. Arava (leflunomide). [package insert]. U.S. Food and Drug Administration. https://www.accessdata.fda.gov/drugsatfda_docs/label/2011/020905s022lbl.pdf. Revised July 2011. Accessed 29 Apr 2022.
59. Leflunomide: Drug Information, Lexicomp. In: UpToDate. Post: TW (Ed), UpToDate, Waltham. Accessed 27 Apr 2022.
60. Chan J, Sanders DC, Du L, Pillans PI. Leflunomide-associated pancytopenia with or without methotrexate. Ann Pharmacother. 2004;38(7–8):1206–11.
61. Olivieri I, Palazzi C, Peruz G, Padula A. Management issues with elderly-onset rheumatoid arthritis: an update. Drugs Aging. 2005;22(10):809–22.
62. DAVA Pharmaceuticals, Inc. Methotrexate tablets [package insert]. U.S. Food and Drug Administration website. https://www.accessdata.fda.gov/drugsatfda_docs/label/2016/008085s066lbl.pdf. Accessed 26 Apr 2022.
63. Methotrexate. Drug Information, Lexicomp. In: UpToDate. Post: TW (Ed), UpToDate, Waltham. Accessed 27 Apr 2022.
64. Mycophenolate mofetil: Drug Information, Lexicomp. In: UpToDate. Post: TW (Ed), UpToDate, Waltham. Accessed 27 Apr 2022.
65. Mycophenolate sodium: Drug Information, Lexicomp. In: UpToDate. Post: TW (Ed), UpToDate, Waltham. Accessed 27 Apr 2022.
66. Hughes GR. The problems of using NSAIDs in the elderly. Scand J Rheumatol Suppl. 1991;91:19–25.
67. Phillips AC, Polisson RP, Simon LS. NSAIDs and the elderly. Toxicity and economic implications. Drugs Aging. 1997;10(2):119–30.
68. Solomon DH. Nonselective NSAIDs: overview of adverse effects. In: UpToDate. Post: TW (Ed), UpToDate, Waltham. Accessed 30 Apr 2022.
69. Genentech, Inc. Rituxan (rituximab). [package insert]. U.S. Food and Drug Administration. https://www.accessdata.fda.gov/drugsatfda_docs/label/2010/103705s5311lbl.pdf. Revised February 2010. Accessed 29 Apr 2022.
70. Rituximab: Drug Information, Lexicomp. In: UpToDate. Post: TW (Ed), UpToDate, Waltham. Accessed 27 Apr 2022.
71. Saag KM. Major side effects of systemic glucocorticoids. Drug Information, Lexicomp. In: UpToDate. Post: TW (Ed), UpToDate, Waltham. Accessed 27 Apr 2022.
72. Azulfidine (sulfasalazine tablets, USP). [package insert]. U.S. Food and Drug Administration. https://www.accessdata.fda.gov/drugsatfda_docs/label/2009/007073s124lbl.pdf. Revised 2009. Accessed April 29, 2022.

73. Sulfasalazine: Drug Information, Lexicomp. In: UpToDate. Post: TW (Ed), UpToDate, Waltham, MA. Accessed 27 Apr 2022.
74. Janssen Biotech, Inc. Remicade (infliximab). [package insert]. U.S. Food and Drug Administration website. https://www.accessdata.fda.gov/drugsatfda_docs/label/2013/103772s5359lbl.pdf. Revised November 2013. Accessed 29 Apr 2022.
75. Infliximab: Drug Information, Lexicomp. In: UpToDate. Post: TW (Ed), UpToDate, Waltham, MA. Accessed 27 Apr 2022.
76. Abbott Laboratories. Humira (adalimumab). [package insert]. U.S. Food and Drug Administration website. https://www.accessdata.fda.gov/drugsatfda_docs/label/2011/125057s0276lbl.pdf. Revised December 2011. Accessed 29 Apr 2022.
77. Adalimumab: Drug Information, Lexicomp. In: UpToDate. Post: TW (Ed), UpToDate, Waltham, MA. Accessed 27 Apr 2022.
78. Immunex Corporation. Enbrel (etanercept)[package insert]. U.S. Food and Drug Administration website. https://www.accessdata.fda.gov/drugsatfda_docs/label/2012/103795s5503lbl.pdf. Revised December 2012. Accessed 29 Apr 2022.
79. Etanercept: Drug Information, Lexicomp. In: UpToDate. Post: TW (Ed), UpToDate, Waltham, MA. Accessed 27 Apr 2022.
80. Micic D, Komaki Y, Alavanja A, Rubin DT, Sakuraba A. Risk of cancer recurrence among individuals exposed to antitumor necrosis factor therapy: a systematic review and meta-analysis of observational studies. J Clin Gastroenterol. 2019;53(1):e1–e11.
81. American Geriatrics Society 2019 Updated AGS Beers Criteria® for potentially inappropriate medication use in older adults. J Am Geriatr Soc. 2019;67(4):674–94.
82. Borson S, Scanlan J, Brush M, Vitaliano P, Dokmak A. The mini-cog: a cognitive 'vital signs' measure for dementia screening in multi-lingual elderly. Int J Geriatr Psychiatry. 2000;15(11):1021–7.

Part III
Treatment Considerations

Chapter 16
Probiotics and Dietary Recommendations for Rheumatologic Diseases

Madeleine E. Frech and Elizabeth R. Volkmann

16.1 Introduction

Nutrition is a cornerstone for health. While genetic factors play a role in autoimmune disease susceptibility, environmental factors (epigenetic modifiers), such as diet, contribute to the development of diverse disease states, from obesity and periodontal disease to rheumatic disease [1]. Several studies support the concept that diet directly stimulates or inhibits inflammatory processes and that diet has a central role in rheumatic disease management [2]. Modification of diet may be necessary as a result of gastrointestinal (GI) tract symptoms due to the underlying rheumatic disease. The role of specific nutrients and alteration of gut microbiota as an adjunct to standard therapeutic plans is gaining interest. Targeted investigations for etiologies of malnutrition are critical for wellness in treating patients with rheumatic disease.

16.2 Gastro-enteric Microbiota

Microbiota populate the lumen of the intestine and perform complex host-microorganism interactions that modulate immune response both within and outside of the gastrointestinal (GI) tract [3]. Most human immune cells reside in the gastrointestinal tract, and the microbiota plays a critical role in their differentiation and

M. E. Frech (✉)
University of Utah School of Medicine, Salt Lake City, UT, USA

E. R. Volkmann
David Geffen School of Medicine, Division of Rheumatology, Department of Medicine, University of California, Los Angeles, Los Angeles, CA, USA

M. Tadros et al. (eds.), *GI Diseases Associated with Rheumatological and Vasculitic Conditions*, Clinical Gastroenterology,
https://doi.org/10.1007/978-3-032-07868-1_16

maintenance of host homeostasis. Microbiota influences the host immune response through carbohydrate metabolism (degradation of polysaccharides and indigestible dietary fibers), which produces active metabolites through fermentation. These metabolites then modulate the innate and adaptive immune system through cellular differentiation and cytokine production. Gut microbial communities provide their human host nutritional support through the production of vitamins and amino acids. Gut microbiota dysbiosis occurs when there is an imbalance in the composition and function of intestinal microbes, and this imbalance has been linked to a number of chronic inflammatory diseases [4]. Furthermore, the microbiota can degrade the mucus on the intestinal epithelial barrier resulting in increased gut permeability. Failure of the intestinal microbiome to maintain gut homeostasis leads to negative changes in the host metabolism and is linked to rheumatic disease [3].

Metagenomics applies sequencing techniques to study genetic and genomic profiles to provide an outline of the microbial communities in the human gut, which reveal an association between low microbial diversity and several disease states, such as systemic lupus erythematosus [5]. Genetic associations with specific rheumatic diseases are associated with altered microbiota [6]. Stool and plasma studies of systemic autoimmune diseases, including systemic lupus erythematous, Sjogren's syndrome, and primary anti-phospholipid syndrome demonstrated pro-tolerogenic bacteria were reduced, while pathobiont genera were increased [7]. Asymptomatic subjects with an increased genetic risk score for RA likewise demonstrated an increased fecal abundance of *Prevotella* suggesting that prior to disease onset host genotype is associated with the microbiome [8]. Specific abnormalities in the gastrointestinal microbiota of patients with SSc from two geographically and ethnically distinct cohorts who demonstrated an increased abundance of *Clostridium were* associated with less severe gastrointestinal symptoms [9]. The microbiome plays a vital role in maintaining the immune system by consistently interacting with host immune cells, thus the long-term effect of immunosuppression on gut microbiome is unclear [10].

16.3 Probiotics

Probiotics are live or attenuated microorganisms that, when administered at a functional dose as a food or supplement, may confer a health benefit on the host to enhance intestinal barrier function [11]. In addition to vitamin synthesis and metabolism, probiotics act to competitively exclude pathogens, reinforce gut barrier function, and regulate intestinal transit.

The bacterial genera most often used in probiotic supplements include *Lactobacillus* and *Bifidobacterium* [12]. Unfortunately, because dietary supplements in the US do not undergo regulatory review by the Food and Drug Administration, the consumer has no way to know whether the supplement contains viable organisms at the time of purchase. Furthermore, it is unclear whether consumption of probiotic supplements leads to sustained colonization of these potentially beneficial microbes within the GI tract. For most disease states, results of randomized controlled trials of probiotic supplementation have yielded mixed results. Patients with rheumatic disease may take them without any medical advice, making it difficult to quantify their effect [13].

Probiotic studies may benefit from the analysis of the pretreatment microbiota to replete an organism that is of relatively low abundance and avoid additional levels of an already abundant organism; however, this is not commonly done in rheumatic disease studies. Thus, while studies evaluating probiotics in RA, SSc, or SpA demonstrate tolerability, there is minimal evidence of clinical benefit [6]. Furthermore, consistent results are not evidenced in randomized studies evaluating FMT in rheumatic disease by various routes (oral, duodenal, ileocolonoscopic, or enema) and highlight the importance of a control group in study design [6].

It is important to note that beneficial microbes naturally occur in certain food products, such as fermented dairy products and pickled vegetables. These food products contain a more diverse array of beneficial microbes, and their regular consumption may lead to more substantive changes in gut microbial composition than the use of a probiotic supplement with one or two species.

16.4 Nutrition as Medicine

Dietary intake is a key regulator of the structure and function of gut microbiota [14]. Fiber is the main source of microbiota-accessible carbohydrates in the diet of humans. Short-chain fatty acids (SCFA) (including acetate, butyrate, and propionate) represent the major metabolites of dietary fibers, which act both at a local level to improve intestinal mucosal immunity and at a systemic level as a source of energy for the liver and regulator of neuroendocrine processes [15]. The dietary effects of medium-chain fatty acids (MCFA) on the human microbiome have been studied in the context of inflammatory bowel disease (IBD) but require further investigation in rheumatic diseases. Moreover, dietary choline, which includes red meat, is metabolized by gut microbiota into derivatives that are associated with adverse cardiovascular events [16]. As such, alterations in diet could indirectly alter the downstream production and concentration of a variety of metabolites, which, in turn, could exert local and systemic immune-modulating effects.

While there are only a relatively small number of longitudinal randomized clinical control trials of dietary interventions on microbial and host metabolites (the metabolome) in humans, energy restriction and diets rich in fiber and vegetables are associated with health benefits. Modern Western diets, characterized by high consumption of salt, refined carbohydrates, added sugars, and red and processed meats, are associated with an increased risk of autoimmune disease [17]. While published literature does not provide high-level evidence of clinically meaningful effect sizes from individual dietary exposures on outcomes in rheumatic disease [18], nutritional counseling should be performed to educate patients on diet influences on obesity, cardiovascular risk, and malnutrition [19].

16.5 Specific Diet Recommendations in Rheumatic Disease

As shown in Table 16.1, dietary studies for risk of developing and management thereafter of rheumatic disease are most extensive in rheumatoid arthritis (RA) followed by systemic lupus erythematosus (SLE) [11, 20]. In the Nurses' Health Study (NHS) I (years 1984–2014), and II (years 1991–2015), adherence to higher dietary quality guidelines was associated with reduced RA risk in the subset of seropositive patients with earlier onset of RA (less than 55 years old) [21]. Moderate alcohol consumption and lower red meat intake were associated with decreased early-onset RA risk [21]. The empirical dietary inflammatory pattern (EDIP) diet includes nine anti-inflammatory food/beverage groups (beer, wine, tea, coffee, dark yellow vegetables, leafy green vegetables, snacks, fruit juice, and pizza) and excludes nine

Table 16.1 Dietary Intervention

Dietary intervention	Disease state	Location	Study design	Number of patients	Outcome	References
Mediterranean	RA SLE	US UK Greece Sweden Japan US Spain Germany	Cohort Parallel Groups Randomized Control Trial Randomized Parallel Groups Cohort Cohort Cross-sectional Cross-sectional	83,245 130 40 51 208 173,122 280 145	No association with RA risk Reduced RA disease activity Reduced RA disease activity Reduced RA disease activity MUFA reduces RA disease activity No association with SLE risk Reduced SLE disease activity and CV risk Reduced SLE activity when combined with physical activity and no tobacco	[26] [27] [31] [28] [29] [24] [30] [32]
EDIP	RA SLE	US US	Cohort Cohort	173,560 173,122	Lower RA risk in < 55 years of age No association with SLE risk	[23] [24]
DASH	SLE Gout RA	US US Iran	Cohort Cohort Cross-sectional	173,122 44,444 300	No association with SLE risk Lower risk of gout Reduced RA risk	[24] [37] [38]
Low FODMAP	SSc	France	Cohort	80	Low fructose diet improved GI symptoms	[42]

pro-inflammatory food/beverage groups (meat, red meat, organ meat, non-dark meat fish, other vegetables, refined grains, high-energy beverages, low-energy beverages, and tomatoes) based on their association with plasma levels of inflammatory biomarkers [22]. In RA, increasing EDIP scores were associated with increased risk of seropositive RA among women aged 55 years or below [23]. There was no association between EDIP scores or dietary quality of prudent or Western dietary pattern with incident cases of SLE [24]. However, a potential reduction in overall SLE risk with a high nut/legume diet was noted to warrant further studies [25].

While the Mediterranean Diet may not impact the risk of RA, it may control symptoms once a diagnosis is made [26]. The Mediterranean Diet is characterized by whole or minimally processed foods with a consistent intake of vegetables, fruits, nuts, legumes, whole grains, extra-virgin olive oil, and fish; moderate consumption of eggs, dairy products, lean meats, and alcohol; and small amounts of saturated fats, red meat, and refined carbohydrates. The Mediterranean Diet aims to provide antioxidants that modulate inflammation. In a pilot study, RA females following the Mediterranean Diet had improvement in pain and physical function at 3 months, and they had a reduction in global visual analog scale (VAS) and morning stiffness at 6 months [27]. In another study of stable, but active RA adjusting to a Mediterranean diet improved disease activity and physical function measured by composite disease activity index, a physical function index, quality of life measures, and reduced anti-inflammatory medication use [28]. In another study of Mediterranean diet in RA, the ratio of daily monounsaturated to saturated fatty acids intake significantly correlated to disease activity scores [29]. Greater adherence to the Mediterranean diet is associated with less disease activity and damage accrual in SLE [30]. The Mediterranean diet for RA and SLE is most effective for management of disease when combined with physical activity [31, 32] The Mediterranean diet has reduced skin severity in psoriasis, but musculoskeletal manifestations improvement on this diet were not reported in this study [33, 34]. While the mechanisms underlying the possible positive effects of the Mediterranean diet on the immune system are not yet fully elucidated, nutritional counseling on this diet is recommended in rheumatic disease [35].

The Dietary Approach to Stop Hypertension (DASH) diet includes high consumption of vegetables, nuts, legumes, fruits, low-fat dairy products, and whole grains, and low intake of sodium, sweetened beverages, and red and processed meats [36]. This diet has been studied in metabolic diseases, including gout, but did not demonstrate an association with risk of developing SLE [24, 37]. A small cross-sectional study identified a potential causal association between adherence to the DASH diet and lower risk of RA, which needs to be confirmed by prospective studies of high methodological quality [38]. Nonetheless, sodium reduction is recommended due to association with autoimmunity [35]. Outside of the DASH diet, one dietary study noted that low intakes of fiber and high intakes of ultra-transformed foods are associated with high SpA activity [39]. It is generally accepted that dietary interventions should be implemented in conjunction with standard medical therapies.

The low FODMAP diet restricts fermentable oligosaccharides, disaccharides, monosaccharides, and polyols, which are short-chain carbohydrates (sugars) that are poorly absorbed by the small intestine and thus cause bothersome GI symptoms. This diet restricts dairy-based, wheat-based, beans and lentils, and certain vegetables and fruits to minimize irritable bowel disease symptoms. Systemic sclerosis (SSc) studies report dietary modification, including low FODMAP, in the management of gastrointestinal symptoms [40]. One small study found that patients with SSc adhering to a low FODMAP diet had lower abundance of the pathobiont, *Enterococcus*, compared with patients not adhering to a low FODMAP diet [41].

Dietary recommendations for patients with rheumatic diseases require a personalized approach. The idea that there is one diet for all patients with rheumatic diseases is problematic for several reasons. Both patient-related factors and external factors may influence how the individual patient tolerates specific food products. For example, patients with SSc and Sjogren's disease often have poor dentition and xerostomia, and this may affect their tolerance to specific foods. In addition, treatment regimens that include acid suppression for gastroesophageal reflux may impact absorption of nutrients and contribute to small intestine bacterial overgrowth (SIBO). In patients with gastroparesis, fiber intake can worsen abdominal distention, bloating, and cramping [40]. For patients with SIBO or gastroparesis, a low residue diet restricts the ingestion of indigestible content of food material that remains in the gastrointestinal tract. Specifically, this diet includes eggs, refined grains, white rice, seafood, and poultry; limits dairy intakes; and entirely avoids high fiber-containing food and whole grains [42]. Thus, dietary recommendations must be individualized and may require both speech therapy and a nutritionist to properly guide the treating physician to avoid malnutrition.

16.6 Dietary Fasting, Caloric Reduction, and Supplements

The concept of dietary fasting in autoimmune disease is founded on the principle that the immune system is tightly regulated by nutrient availability and metabolism. A systematic review of 31 RA studies of medically supervised fasting followed by a vegetarian diet, including 4 controlled studies, found significant improvement in pain [43]. Independent of weight loss, a 12-week hypocaloric intervention provided suitable control of joint disease activity in patients with psoriatic arthritis (PsA) [44]. For patients with psoriatic arthritis, the Medical Board of the National Psoriasis Foundation weakly recommends vitamin D supplementation and dietary weight reduction with a hypocaloric diet in overweight and obese patients [45].

With restrictive diets, screening for vitamin D is required, followed by the appropriate action for replacement to support bone health. Further studies on vitamin D and targetable levels in rheumatic disease are needed [46]. For RA, the effects of fish oils (n = 17 studies) and omega-3 fatty acid supplements (n = 9 studies) are reported, but the interpretation of results is challenged by variable dosage of supplementation [47]. Similarly, while Omega-3 and curcumin supplementation is potentially promising for SpA, further study of dosing is required [48]. While the use of supplements as adjunct therapy in rheumatic disease requires better-designed and adequately powered studies for strong recommendations, it is clear that nutrition should be routinely addressed by the rheumatologist.

16.7 Conclusion

Understanding the role of the gut microbiome in rheumatic disease risk and modification of inflammatory outcomes is an area of active interest. Dietary intervention may improve symptoms of rheumatic diseases through modification of the gut microbiome, but further research is needed to understand the mechanism of action of these approaches. All patients with rheumatic diseases should undergo a comprehensive nutritional assessment followed by the implementation of personalized dietary recommendations.

References

1. Gioia C, Lucchino B, Tarsitano MG, Iannuccelli C, Di Franco M. Dietary habits and nutrition in rheumatoid arthritis: can diet influence disease development and clinical manifestations? Nutrients. 2020;12(5).
2. Paolino S, Pacini G, Patane M, Alessandri E, Cattelan F, Goegan F, Pizzorni C, Gotelli E, Cutolo M. Interactions between microbiota, diet/nutrients and immune/inflammatory response in rheumatic diseases: focus on rheumatoid arthritis. Reumatologia. 2019;57(3):151–7.
3. Abdollahi-Roodsaz S, Abramson SB, Scher JU. The metabolic role of the gut microbiota in health and rheumatic disease: mechanisms and interventions. Nat Rev Rheumatol. 2016;12(8):446–55.
4. Lynch SV, Pedersen O. The human intestinal microbiome in health and disease. N Engl J Med. 2016;375(24):2369–79.
5. Perez-Cobas AE, Gomez-Valero L, Buchrieser C. Metagenomic approaches in microbial ecology: an update on whole-genome and marker gene sequencing analyses. Microb Genom. 2020;6(8).
6. Stoll ML. Therapeutic alteration of the microbiota in rheumatic diseases: hype or potential? Best Pract Res Clin Rheumatol. 2022;36(4):101806.
7. Bellocchi C, Fernandez-Ochoa A, Montanelli G, Vigone B, Santaniello A, Quirantes-Pine R, Borras-Linares I, Gerosa M, Artusi C, Gualtierotti R, et al. Identification of a shared microbiomic and metabolomic profile in systemic autoimmune diseases. J Clin Med. 2019;8(9).
8. Wells PM, Adebayo AS, Bowyer RCE, Freidin MB, Finckh A, Strowig T, Lesker TR, Alpizar-Rodriguez D, Gilbert B, Kirkham B, et al. Associations between gut microbiota and genetic risk for rheumatoid arthritis in the absence of disease: a cross-sectional study. Lancet Rheumatol. 2020;2(7):e418–27.
9. Volkmann ER, Hoffmann-Vold AM, Chang YL, Jacobs JP, Tillisch K, Mayer EA, Clements PJ, Hov JR, Kummen M, Midtvedt O, et al. Systemic sclerosis is associated with specific alterations in gastrointestinal microbiota in two independent cohorts. BMJ Open Gastroenterol. 2017;4(1):e000134.
10. Palm NW, de Zoete MR, Flavell RA. Immune-microbiota interactions in health and disease. Clin Immunol. 2015;159(2):122–7.
11. Hill C, Guarner F, Reid G, Gibson GR, Merenstein DJ, Pot B, Morelli L, Canani RB, Flint HJ, Salminen S, et al. Expert consensus document. The International Scientific Association for

Probiotics and Prebiotics consensus statement on the scope and appropriate use of the term probiotic. Nat Rev Gastroenterol Hepatol. 2014;11(8):506–14.
12. Gupta V, Garg R. Probiotics. Indian J Med Microbiol. 2009;27(3):202–9.
13. Bungau SG, Behl T, Singh A, Sehgal A, Singh S, Chigurupati S, Vijayabalan S, Das S, Palanimuthu VR. Targeting probiotics in rheumatoid arthritis. Nutrients. 2021;13:10.
14. David LA, Maurice CF, Carmody RN, Gootenberg DB, Button JE, Wolfe BE, Ling AV, Devlin AS, Varma Y, Fischbach MA, et al. Diet rapidly and reproducibly alters the human gut microbiome. Nature. 2014;505(7484):559–63.
15. Han M, Wang C, Liu P, Li D, Li Y, Ma X. Dietary fiber gap and host gut microbiota. Protein Pept Lett. 2017;24(5):388–96.
16. Tang WH, Wang Z, Levison BS, Koeth RA, Britt EB, Fu X, Wu Y, Hazen SL. Intestinal microbial metabolism of phosphatidylcholine and cardiovascular risk. N Engl J Med. 2013;368(17):1575–84.
17. Zinocker MK, Lindseth IA. The Western diet-microbiome-host interaction and its role in metabolic disease. Nutrients. 2018;10(3).
18. Gwinnutt JM, Wieczorek M, Rodriguez-Carrio J, Balanescu A, Bischoff-Ferrari HA, Boonen A, Cavalli G, de Souza S, de Thurah A, Dorner TE, et al. Effects of diet on the outcomes of rheumatic and musculoskeletal diseases (RMDs): systematic review and meta-analyses informing the 2021 EULAR recommendations for lifestyle improvements in people with RMDs. RMD Open. 2022;8(2).
19. Cutolo M, Nikiphorou E. Nutrition and diet in rheumatoid arthritis. Nutrients. 2022;14(4).
20. Khanna S, Jaiswal KS, Gupta B. Managing rheumatoid arthritis with dietary interventions. Front Nutr. 2017;4:52.
21. Hu Y, Sparks JA, Malspeis S, Costenbader KH, Hu FB, Karlson EW, Lu B. Long-term dietary quality and risk of developing rheumatoid arthritis in women. Ann Rheum Dis. 2017;76(8):1357–64.
22. Tabung FK, Smith-Warner SA, Chavarro JE, Wu K, Fuchs CS, Hu FB, Chan AT, Willett WC, Giovannucci EL. Development and validation of an empirical dietary inflammatory index. J Nutr. 2016;146(8):1560–70.
23. Sparks JA, Barbhaiya M, Tedeschi SK, Leatherwood CL, Tabung FK, Speyer CB, Malspeis S, Costenbader KH, Karlson EW, Lu B. Inflammatory dietary pattern and risk of developing rheumatoid arthritis in women. Clin Rheumatol. 2019;38(1):243–50.
24. Barbhaiya M, Tedeschi S, Sparks JA, Leatherwood C, Karlson EW, Willett WC, Lu B, Costenbader KH. Association of dietary quality with risk of incident systemic lupus erythematosus in the nurses' health study and nurses' health study II. Arthritis Care Res. 2021;73(9):1250–8.
25. Tedeschi SK, Barbhaiya M, Sparks JA, Karlson EW, Kubzansky LD, Roberts AL, Willett WC, Lu B, Costenbader KH. Dietary patterns and risk of systemic lupus erythematosus in women. Lupus. 2020;29(1):67–73.
26. Hu Y, Costenbader KH, Gao X, Hu FB, Karlson EW, Lu B. Mediterranean diet and incidence of rheumatoid arthritis in women. Arthritis Care Res. 2015;67(5):597–606.
27. McKellar G, Morrison E, McEntegart A, Hampson R, Tierney A, Mackle G, Scoular J, Scott JA, Capell HA. A pilot study of a Mediterranean-type diet intervention in female patients with rheumatoid arthritis living in areas of social deprivation in Glasgow. Ann Rheum Dis. 2007;66(9):1239–43.
28. Skoldstam L, Hagfors L, Johansson G. An experimental study of a Mediterranean diet intervention for patients with rheumatoid arthritis. Ann Rheum Dis. 2003;62(3):208–14.
29. Matsumoto Y, Sugioka Y, Tada M, Okano T, Mamoto K, Inui K, Habu D, Koike T. Monounsaturated fatty acids might be key factors in the Mediterranean diet that suppress rheumatoid arthritis disease activity: the TOMORROW study. Clin Nutr. 2018;37(2):675–80.
30. Pocovi-Gerardino G, Correa-Rodriguez M, Callejas-Rubio JL, Rios-Fernandez R, Martin-Amada M, Cruz-Caparros MG, Rueda-Medina B, Ortego-Centeno N. Beneficial effect of

Mediterranean diet on disease activity and cardiovascular risk in systemic lupus erythematosus patients: a cross-sectional study. Rheumatology (Oxford). 2021;60(1):160–9.
31. Papandreou P, Gioxari A, Daskalou E, Grammatikopoulou MG, Skouroliakou M, Bogdanos DP. Mediterranean diet and physical activity nudges versus usual care in women with rheumatoid arthritis: results from the MADEIRA randomized controlled trial. Nutrients. 2023;15(3).
32. Vordenbaumen S, Kleefisch M, Sokolowski A, Dusing C, Richter JG, Brinks R, Schneider M, Chehab G. Beneficial effects associated to a healthy lifestyle in systemic lupus erythematosus: a cross-sectional study. Lupus. 2023;32(7):855–63.
33. Phan C, Touvier M, Kesse-Guyot E, Adjibade M, Hercberg S, Wolkenstein P, Chosidow O, Ezzedine K, Sbidian E. Association between Mediterranean anti-inflammatory dietary profile and severity of psoriasis: results from the NutriNet-Sante cohort. JAMA Dermatol. 2018;154(9):1017–24.
34. Barrea L, Balato N, Di Somma C, Macchia PE, Napolitano M, Savanelli MC, Esposito K, Colao A, Savastano S. Nutrition and psoriasis: is there any association between the severity of the disease and adherence to the Mediterranean diet? J Transl Med. 2015;13:18.
35. Alunno A, Carubbi F, Bartoloni E, Grassi D, Ferri C, Gerli R. Diet in rheumatoid arthritis versus systemic lupus erythematosus: any differences? Nutrients. 2021;13(3).
36. Akhlaghi M. Dietary Approaches to Stop Hypertension (DASH): potential mechanisms of action against risk factors of the metabolic syndrome. Nutr Res Rev. 2020;33(1):1–18.
37. Rai SK, Fung TT, Lu N, Keller SF, Curhan GC, Choi HK. The Dietary Approaches to Stop Hypertension (DASH) diet, Western diet, and risk of gout in men: prospective cohort study. BMJ. 2017;357:j1794.
38. Ghaseminasabparizi M, Nazarinia MA, Akhlaghi M. Adherence to the dietary approaches to stop hypertension dietary pattern and rheumatoid arthritis in Iranian adults. Public Health Nutr. 2021;24(18):6085–93.
39. Vergne-Salle P, Salle L, Fressinaud-Marie AC, Descamps-Deplas A, Montestruc F, Bonnet C, Bertin P. Diet and disease activity in patients with axial spondyloarthritis: SpondyloArthritis and NUTrition Study (SANUT). Nutrients. 2022;14(22).
40. Smith E, Pauling JD. The efficacy of dietary intervention on gastrointestinal involvement in systemic sclerosis: A systematic literature review. Semin Arthritis Rheum. 2019;49(1):112–8.
41. Vandeputte D, Joossens M. Effects of low and high FODMAP diets on human gastrointestinal microbiota composition in adults with intestinal diseases: a systematic review. Microorganisms. 2020;8(11).
42. Sorathia AZ, Sorathia SJ. Low residue diet. In: StatPearls. edn. Treasure Island. ineligible companies. Disclosure: Sufian Sorathia declares no relevant financial relationships with ineligible companies. 2023.
43. Muller H, de Toledo FW, Resch KL. Fasting followed by vegetarian diet in patients with rheumatoid arthritis: a systematic review. Scand J Rheumatol. 2001;30(1):1–10.
44. Leite BF, Morimoto MA, Gomes CMF, Klemz BNC, Genaro PS, Shivappa N, Hebert JR, Damasceno NRT, Pinheiro MM. Dietetic intervention in psoriatic arthritis: the DIETA trial. Adv Rheumatol. 2022;62(1):12.
45. Ford AR, Siegel M, Bagel J, Cordoro KM, Garg A, Gottlieb A, Green LJ, Gudjonsson JE, Koo J, Lebwohl M, et al. Dietary recommendations for adults with psoriasis or psoriatic arthritis from the Medical Board of the National Psoriasis Foundation: a systematic review. JAMA Dermatol. 2018;154(8):934–50.
46. Christodoulou S, Goula T, Ververidis A, Drosos G. Vitamin D and bone disease. Biomed Res Int. 2013;2013:396541.
47. Philippou E, Petersson SD, Rodomar C, Nikiphorou E. Rheumatoid arthritis and dietary interventions: systematic review of clinical trials. Nutr Rev. 2021;79(4):410–28.
48. Jadhav P, Jiang Y, Jarr K, Layton C, Ashouri JF, Sinha SR. Efficacy of dietary supplements in inflammatory bowel disease and related autoimmune diseases. Nutrients. 2020;12(7).

Chapter 17
Use of Proton Pump Inhibitor: Balancing Risks and Benefits

Sonia B. Samuel, Alla Turshudzhyan, Lavinia Salama, Jessica Farrell, Micheal Tadros, and Lee Shapiro

17.1 Introduction

Proton pump inhibitors (PPIs) were first introduced in the late 1980s and have become an integral part of clinical practice. PPIs have revolutionized the treatment of acid-related diseases, as they offered strong antisecretory properties that were shown to be superior to prior agents [1]. PPIs work by directly inhibiting active

S. B. Samuel
Department of Internal Medicine, Albany Medical Center, Albany, NY, USA
e-mail: samuels2@amc.edu

A. Turshudzhyan
Department of Internal Medicine and Gastroenterology, University of Connecticut, Farmington, CT, USA
e-mail: turshudzhyan@uchc.edu

L. Salama
School of Pharmacy, University of Wyoming, Laramie, WY, USA
e-mail: lsalama@uwyo.edu

J. Farrell
Department of Pharmacy Practice, Albany College of Pharmacy and Health Sciences, Albany, NY, USA

Division of Rheumatology, Albany Medical Center, Albany, NY, USA
e-mail: jessica.farrell@acphs.edu

M. Tadros (✉)
Division of Gastroenterology and Hepatology, Albany Medical College, Albany, NY, USA
e-mail: tadrosm1@amc.edu

L. Shapiro
Division of Rheumatology, Albany Medical College, Albany, NY, USA
e-mail: shapirl@amc.edu

M. Tadros et al. (eds.), *GI Diseases Associated with Rheumatological and Vasculitic Conditions*, Clinical Gastroenterology,
https://doi.org/10.1007/978-3-032-07868-1_17

parietal cells from secreting acid [2]. While PPIs are effective, they do have some limitations primarily related to short half-lives and meal-associated dosing, which may lead to poor compliance or breakthrough symptoms with incorrect usage [2]. For many years, PPIs were considered to have a limited side-effect profile, which contributed to a low threshold for initiating therapy. As a result, they became a first-line treatment for esophagitis, gastroesophageal reflux disease (GERD), peptic ulcer disease (PUD), Zollinger-Ellison syndrome (ZES), functional dyspepsia, Helicobacter pylori *(H. pylori)* infection, and many other conditions [3]. As clinicians became more comfortable with PPI therapy, their application extended to patients suffering from chronic dyspepsia related to various rheumatological conditions. Due to the chronic nature of rheumatologic conditions, many patients suffering from rheumatological dyspepsia were placed on long-term PPI therapy without clear expectation of the duration of therapy. Given the chronicity of dyspepsia in many of the rheumatological diseases and growing concerns of PPIs+, it is important to discuss the risks and benefits of long-term PPI use. It is especially important because inappropriate chronic PPI use has risen significantly in the last few decades [4] with some studies concluding that only half of patients on PPIs had an approved and appropriate indication [5].

17.2 General Overview of Proton Pump Inhibitors

PPIs are weak bases that suppress gastric acid secretion by irreversibly binding to the hydrogen/potassium adenosine triphosphatase (H+/K+ ATPase) of the gastric parietal cell, also known as the "proton pump" [6]. Common Food and Drug Administration (FDA) indications for PPIs include GERD, peptic ulcer disease, Zollinger-Ellison syndrome, erosive esophagitis, and *H. pylori*. In the United States (US), the available PPIs include esomeprazole, lansoprazole, omeprazole, dexlansoprazole, pantoprazole and rabeprazole [7]. Meta-analyses have studied the efficacy of esomeprazole, lansoprazole, omeprazole, pantoprazole and rabeprazole against each other, however results suggest there is no one PPI that has greater efficacy over the other [8]. These medications can therefore be prescribed interchangeably due to similar efficacy. Table 17.1 summarizes the pharmacokinetics of available PPIs [7, 9–11].

17.3 Benefits of PPI Therapy in Rheumatologic Diseases

PPIs are first line therapy for upper GI symptoms in patients suffering from rheumatological disorders such as GERD and esophagitis to increase patient quality of life by symptom management and reduce complication risk [12]. PPIs are also indicated in chronic NSAID use and concomitant steroid use to prevent upper GI bleeds and its associated complications. Guidelines from multiple societies including the

Table 17.1 Pharmacokinetics

PPI	Omeprazole	Esomeprazole	Lansoprazole	Dexlansoprazole	Pantoprazole	Rabeprazole
Available formulations	Capsule, tablet, packet for oral suspension	Capsule, tablet, packet for oral suspension, injection	Capsule, orally disintegrating tablet, suspension	Capsule	Tablet, packet for oral suspension, injection	Tablet, capsule sprinkle
Dose	20–80 mg daily	20–40 mg daily	15–30 mg daily	30–60 mg daily	20–40 mg daily	20–100 mg daily
Oral bioavailability (%)	30–40	64–90	80–85	NA	77	52
IV formulation	Yes	Yes	Yes	No	Yes	No
Time to plasma peak levels (Tmax) (h)	0.5–3.5	1.5	1.7	1–2	2–3	2–5
Elimination half-life (T1/2) (h)	0.5–1	1.3–1.6	1.6	1–2	1–1.9	1–2
Hepatic metabolism	Major: CYP2C19 Minor: CYP3A4	Major: CYP2C19 Minor: CYP3A4	Major: CYP2C19 Minor: CYP3A4	Major: CYP2C19 Minor: CYP3A4	Minor: CYP3A4 CYP2C19	Non-enzymatic reduction Minor: CYP2C19 and CYP3A4
Elimination	Renal	Renal	Renal/ fecal	Renal/ fecal	Renal	Renal
Renal dose adjustment	Not necessary	Not necessary	Not necessary	Not necessary	Not necessary	Not necessary
Affected by food	Yes, take before breakfast	Yes, take at least 60 min prior to breakfast	Yes, take before breakfast	No, take without regards to meals	No, take without regards to meals. Oral suspension: 30 min prior to meal	No, take without regards to meals Capsule sprinkle: 30 min prior to meal

American College of Gastroenterology (ACG) recommend when PPIs should be used for gastroprotection as seen in Fig. 17.1 [13–21]. The manifestation and treatment modalities of rheumatological diseases predispose patients to GI conditions; the most well studied rheumatologic disease requiring PPI therapy is systemic sclerosis but others are indicated for PPI use as well.

17.3.1 GERD/Esophagitis in Rheumatic Diseases

Many patients with connective tissue diseases (CTDs) are predisposed to GERD due to the underlying pathophysiology of the disease [22, 23]. Systemic sclerosis (SSc), also known as scleroderma, is a systemic connective tissue disease with a female predominance that commonly affects the esophagus. Smooth muscle atrophy and excess collagen deposition in the mucosal layers leads to lower esophageal sphincter (LES) hypotony and decreased pressure. This predisposes SSc patients to GERD affecting 50–90% of individuals [24–27]. Additionally, patients with mixed connective tissue disease (MCTD) and systemic lupus erythematous (SLE) were seen to have a hypotensive LES and decreased peristalsis on esophageal manometry

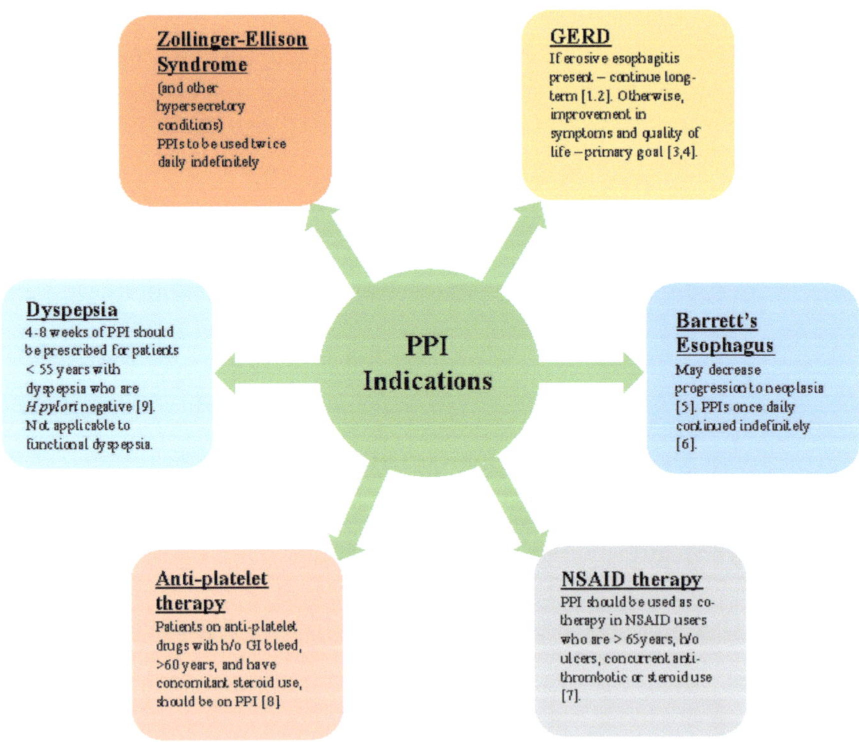

Fig. 17.1 Proton pump inhibitors indications

predisposing them to GERD as well [28, 29]. Due to the refluxed acidic gastric contents contributing to esophageal mucosal injury and its surrounding structures, uncontrolled long standing GERD can result in many complications including stricture formation, aspiration pneumonitis and Barrett's esophagus, a risk factor for esophageal adenocarcinoma, although low (0.1–0.6% a year) [12, 26, 30, 31]. Optimal management of GERD with PPIs is necessary to reduce gastric acid exposure, prevent pulmonary injury and decrease incidence of progression of metaplastic to high grade dysplasia [30]. Life-long PPI therapy is therefore recommended in patients with Barrett's esophagus and also in those with moderate to severe erosive esophagitis due to high rates of recurrence from PPI cessation [32].

Multiple studies demonstrate inadequately treated GERD are associated with an impaired quality of life in not only SSc patients, but also in patients with rheumatoid arthritis and Ehlers Danlos syndrome [23, 33, 34]. Hendel and colleagues showed scleroderma patients treated with omeprazole for up to 5 years had symptom relief and esophageal healing. Previous esophageal strictures regressed after 9 months without new stricture formation and led to improvement of dysphagia [25]. PPIs also treat low grade esophagitis as demonstrated in a retrospective study with 77% of patients showing complete healing on follow-up esophagogastroduodenoscopy (EGD) [35]. A prospective study evaluated the severity and frequency of GERD symptoms seen in SSc patients using a five dimensional scale for measurement: mobility, self-care, pain/discomfort, usual activity and anxiety/depression. Half the patients had complete response but those with refractory response had dysphagia associated with esophageal dysmotility [24]. PPIs assist with controlling GERD manifestations from increased acid exposure but have no role in esophageal motility impairment [26]. Iwata and colleagues demonstrated pre-dinner administration reduced the refractory symptoms in patients with connective tissue disease experiencing severe GERD. Patients are typically prescribed standard doses of PPIs and may increase to twice daily dosing or high doses dependent on response [22]. Overall, these patients may benefit from long term acid suppressive therapy to improve symptoms and reduce complications of acid reflux [29]. However, large scale randomized controlled trials (RCTs) for assessment of long-term PPI benefit in this patient population are lacking in literature [26].

Another complication of GERD is its role in recurrent micro-aspiration events. Studies suggest these events can lead to the development of interstitial lung disease (ILD), however there is no causal association [30, 31]. A prospective study demonstrated SSc patients with severe esophageal motility had increased risk of aspiration and higher frequency of ILD [36]. Aspiration pneumonitis resultant from GERD has potential contribution to SSc ILD [26, 37]. This is a notable concern because ILD is the leading cause of mortality in SSc patients. There are however limited studies that show efficacy of PPI use in SSc patients with ILD and further investigation is warranted [26].

17.3.2 Management of Adverse Effects of NSAIDs and Corticosteroid Therapy

Majority of patients with rheumatic conditions are prescribed NSAIDs and corticosteroids as the mainstay of treatment due to their anti-inflammatory and analgesic properties. However, they are at risk for upper GI complications as these treatment modalities can increase the risk of GI bleeding, gastroduodenal ulcers and perforation. Corticosteroids stimulate gastric acid secretion and suppresses prostaglandins in the gastric mucosa leading to increased susceptibility to mucosal injury [38]. Non-selective NSAIDs inhibit the enzyme cyclooxygenase (COX) activity, COX-1 of the gastric mucosa causing a disruption of the gastric mucosal barrier and decreasing its cytoprotective effects [39, 40]. One published study demonstrated almost 20% of patients with rheumatoid arthritis (RA) treated with NSAIDs had gastric mucosal injury. There is strong evidence that co-therapy with PPIs decreases the risk of ulcers and upper GI bleeding in arthritis patients [41]. Multiple RCTs demonstrate PPIs significantly reduced the risk of both gastric and endoscopic duodenal ulcers [42]. Patients who had poor adherence to PPIs and insufficient gastroprotective agents had a 1.8–4.0 fold increase of upper GI events. In a retrospective cross sectional observational study, for every 10% decrease in PPI adherence, the risk of upper GI bleeding and ulcers increased by 9% [41]. Therefore guidelines from the American Gastroenterology Association (AGA) and National Institutes of Health (NIH) recommend that PPIs are necessary to decrease GI complications in patients who are greater than age 65, take high dose or multiple NSAIDs and/or NSAID concomitant therapy with corticosteroids, anticoagulants or antiplatelets [40, 43]. PPIs should also be prescribed in patients with previous history of ulcers due to high risk of recurrence [40]. In patients with upper GI ulcers successfully treated with endoscopic hemostatic therapy, 3 days of high dose PPIs twice daily should follow. In accordance with the AGA guidelines, a conditional recommendation was made to continue twice daily PPI therapy for 2 weeks after index endoscopy [44]. Patients with idiopathic inflammatory myopathies and polymyalgia rheumatica (PMR) are susceptible to upper GI complications due to initial treatment with high dose corticosteroids [45, 46]. PMR patients may even remain on steroids greater than 2 years due to relapses [46]. Although there are no clear guidelines that suggest PPIs are indicated in patients taking steroids without NSAID use or additional risk factors, PPIs can still be considered in these patients for upper GI prophylaxis [46, 47]. Overall, PPIs are proven to be beneficial in rheumatic patients who take long term or high dose NSAIDs and with concomitant use of steroids for gastroprotective measures [40, 41, 43].

17.4 Risks Associated with PPI Therapy

Proton pump inhibitors have many benefits as discussed above but emerging studies address the safety concerns of PPI therapy, especially on long term use. Such concerns include nutritional and electrolyte abnormalities, calcinosis, enteric infections, gastric hyperplasia/neoplasia, kidney disease, bone fractures, cardiac events, dementia and many others. Majority of these associations are supported by observational studies which are susceptible to systematic errors of bias and confounding factors [48]. One cohort study associated PPI therapy with increased risk of mortality from a variety of diseases but had residual bias that likely overestimated worse health outcomes [49]. Although quality of evidence may be low, attention to the adverse side effects is worth noting in order to fully inform patients with rheumatic diseases of potential risks [48, 50].

17.4.1 Electrolyte/Mineral Deficiencies

PPI therapy is thought to cause vitamin and mineral deficiencies with proposed mechanisms seen in Table 17.2. Studies are controversial with the association of PPI use and vitamin B12 deficiency. Vitamin B12 requires a low pH environment for terminal ileum absorption but PPIs reduce the gastric acidic environment leading to impaired absorption [48, 51]. Large case control studies showed long term PPI use greater than 2–3 years was associated with a decline in vitamin B12 levels [47, 50]. However a cross sectional study showed no significant difference between chronic PPI therapy and decline in vitamin B12 levels [52].

Chronic PPI use can lead to hypomagnesemia. Although, the exact mechanism of how this occurs is not understood, it is hypothesized that PPIs lead to reduction in active magnesium (Mg^{2+}) absorption through transient receptor potential melastatin-6 and -7 (TRPM6/7) in the GI tract [53]. A 2014 meta-analysis included nine observational studies found a greater incidence of low magnesium levels in PPI users [54]. Magnesium levels returned to normal after PPIs were discontinued [50]. A retrospective single center cohort study showed a significant association with hypomagnesemia with concurrent use of tacrolimus (a commonly used medication in CTD patients) and PPI use. However the sample size was small which led to selection bias [55]. Nonetheless, hypomagnesemia can be life-threatening. Low magnesium can increase risk of cardiac arrythmia such as torsades de pointe [56]. Patients may also experience symptoms of muscle weakness, muscle cramps, seizures, tetany, delirium, weakness, and hypotension. Because magnesium (Mg^{2+}) is needed for potassium (K^+) absorption, patients may also present with hypokalemia and hypocalcemia [57]. In 2011, the Food and Drug Administration (FDA) recommended magnesium levels should be periodically checked in high risk cardiac patients and long term PPI users [58].

Table 17.2 Drug to Drug interactions with PPI use [100–110]

Medication/ supplements	Proposed mode of interaction with PPI	Effect	Clinical significance
Tacrolimus	Inhibition of tacrolimus metabolism by CYP2C19	Increases tacrolimus levels Rabeprazole or pantoprazole may be less likely to significantly interact	Not clinically significant Monitor therapy, tacrolimus dose may need to be decreased
Cyclosporine	Unknown	May increase cyclosporine concentration	Not clinically significant Monitor cyclosporine levels
Mycophenolate Mofetil (MMF)	The higher the gastric pH associated with PPI use, impairs the absorption of MMF	Decreased efficacy of MMF PPIs are less likely to affect the absorption of the enteric coated formulation of mycophenolate	Clinically significant Monitor MMF levels/ efficacy
Methotrexate (MTX)	Not fully understood, maybe due to the ability of PPI to inhibit renal hydrogen/potassium ATPase pump thus leading to inhibition of MTX clearance	Increases MTX bioavailability and toxicity	No clinically significant in the doses used for rheumatic conductions More significant toxicities in larger doses used in the management of oncological conditions
Calcium (Ca^{2+})	Calcium carbonate is an insoluble salt that requires the low gastric pH to help facilitate the release of ionized calcium and promote its absorption. Soluble forms of calcium such as calcium citrate are absorbed independent of gastric acid or pH	Lower absorption of insoluble calcium salt (i.e. calcium carbonate) Minimal effects on calcium citrate absorption	Clinical significance is dependent on nutritional status and form of Ca^{2+} Monitor Ca^{2+} levels and supplement with calcium citrate as needed
Iron	Dietary iron is present in food either in as heme (32%) or nonheme (64%). Absorption of nonheme iron is markedly improved by gastric acid and lower pH environments that allows the nonheme iron to dissociate and solubilize	Malabsorption of iron from diet which may lead to iron deficiency anemia	Clinical significance is dependent on nutritional status Monitor iron levels, hemoglobin (hgb), hematocrit (hct) and supplement as needed

(continued)

Table 17.2 (continued)

Medication/ supplements	Proposed mode of interaction with PPI	Effect	Clinical significance
Magnesium (Mg^{2+})	Exact mechanism of how this occurs is not understood, it is thought that PPIs lead to reduction in active magnesium (Mg^{2+}) absorption through transient receptor potential melastatin-6 and -7 (TRPM6/7) in the GI tract	Hypomagnesemia Possibly concurrent hypokalemia	Clinical significance is variable in the literature Monitor Mg^{2+}, K^+ levels and signs and symptoms of deficiency such as, confusion, muscle weakness, cramps, paresthesia, ataxia seizure
Vitamin B_{12} (Cobalamin)	Vitamin B_{12} is cleaved from dietary proteins by pepsin. Pepsin requires gastric acid to be activated from its pepsinogen precursor	Chronic gastric acid suppression by PPIs may lead to malabsorption of dietary vitamin B_{12} May lead to macrocytic anemia	Monitor B_{12} levels hemoglobin (hgb), hematocrit (hct) and supplement as needed
Vitamin C	PPIs lower the concentration of vitamin C in gastric juice and the proportion of the vitamin that is available in its active antioxidant form (ascorbic acid)	Decreased serum concentrations of vitamin C	Clinical significance is unknown Vitamin C supplementation is currently not recommended

Iron and calcium are elements thought to decline with PPI use due to gastric acid suppression decreasing intestinal absorption [48, 51]. A small retrospective cohort study associated chronic PPI therapy with iron deficiency due to a significant reduction in hemoglobin from baseline leading to anemia [59]. Yet, strong evidence based studies are lacking in this association as most evidence is in the form of case reports and small observational studies. Decreased calcium absorption was also seen in a randomized controlled trial studying elderly females using omeprazole [60]. These findings are significant as hypocalcemia can cause tetany, seizures, or laryngospasm.

17.4.2 Fractures

There are conflicting data over the use of PPI therapy and its association with fracture risk. Mechanisms also remain unclear. PPIs are thought to cause calcium malabsorption and/or increase bone resorption by increasing osteoclast activity or elicit gastrin induced parathyroid hyperplasia [56, 58]. Case controlled studies showed that dose and length of PPI use was associated with risk of bone fractures [51]. PPIs may decrease bone mineral density (BMD) leading to increased fracture risk particularly the hip [56]. In the United Kingdom, a study evaluating patients greater than age 50 showed hip fracture risk was dependent of PPI duration and dosage use with greater than 1 year of PPI use. The number needed to harm was 454, meaning 1 of 454 patients treated with a PPI for greater than 1 year would sustain a hip fracture [61]. A retrospective case control study showed older female patients with anti-neutrophil cytoplasmic antibodies (ANCA) associated vasculitis on glucocorticoid therapy had a higher risk of bone fractures with PPI use than those only on histamine 2 receptor antagonists (H2RAs) [62]. Furthermore, a meta-analysis that included 18 observational studies drew an association with PPI use and increased risk of fractures including the hip and spine [63].

Conversely, other case control studies found no relationship between dosage, PPI use and fracture incidence [64]. Prospective studies conducted in 2017 and 2019 found no significant association with BMD or fracture risk in short to medium term PPI use [56, 65, 66]. There was a previous warning on over the counter PPI use and bone fracture risk however in 2011, the FDA retracted the statement because evidence was lacking [48]. In the United States, a cohort study found no association between PPI use and increased fracture risk in rheumatoid arthritis patients. There is insufficient evidence to claim a cause and effect relationship between PPI therapy and fracture risk. The AGA recognizes chronic PPI therapy should not be used as an independent risk factor and indication for patients to have routine BMD assessments [67].

17.4.3 Calcinosis

Calcinosis is seen up to half of patients with scleroderma and also seen in dermatomyositis and other rheumatic conditions. Many mechanisms are hypothesized that suggests PPIs promote tissue calcification. A retrospective study of a cohort group found a significant association between PPI use and calcinosis with a dose response relationship in SSc patients. A prospective cohort study showed that higher and longer exposure to PPIs suggested increased likelihood of calcinosis [68].

17.4.4 Chronic Kidney Disease

PPIs are associated with acute and chronic kidney disease. Acute interstitial nephritis was the most observed acute kidney injury (AKI) seen in PPI users. In three large population studies conducted in Canada, New Zealand and the United States, those on PPI therapy had a greater than two-fold risk in developing AKI. Additionally, a large longitudinal retrospective cohort study including more than 190,000 patients saw a four-fold increase in AKI risk and 20% higher risk of incident chronic kidney disease (CKD) with PPI use [69]. The mechanism is unknown but theories suggest that PPIs or their metabolites deposit in the kidneys leading to an immune response and results in acute interstitial nephritis [50]. Further interstitial scarring and tubular atrophy leads to CKD [56]. Multiple retrospective studies support a positive association with CKD and PPI use with increased risk with higher PPI dose [47, 48]. The study by Xie et al. found in the veteran population that the risk of CKD and ESRD was higher in PPI users [70]. It was postulated that PPI induced AKI can serve as a warning for the progression of chronic renal outcomes. However a cohort study following veterans for 5 years found that PPI use can lead to increased risk of CKD and ESRD without an intervening AKI [71]. Fortunately, no reports currently exist suggesting PPI therapy increases the risk of scleroderma renal crisis.

17.4.5 Enteric Infections

PPIs are linked with increased risk for enteric infections including Clostridium difficile (CDI) and small intestinal bacterial overgrowth (SIBO). Chronic PPI therapy reduces stomach acidity altering the microbiota, decreasing bacterial flora diversity and increases survival of Clostridium difficile spores [48, 50]. The immunological barrier is also decreased due to chronic acid reduction [56]. Risk of developing recurrent CDI was seen in multiple retrospective studies but other studies showed no association [48]. One study showed hospitalized patients were 4.2 fold more likely to have recurrent disease with PPI use than those on H2RAs [72]. Three meta-analyses in 2012 found a significant association between PPI use and CDI infection with increased risk in patients on antibiotics [73–75]. However the high heterogeneity and publication bias weakened the results of the studies. CDI risk was also higher in elderly patients, those undergoing chemotherapy and in immunocompromised individuals [50].

Scleroderma patients are at increased risk for enteric infections due to decreased intestinal peristalsis leading to increased bacterial colonization [30]. Further acid suppression from PPI use allows for excess bacterial overgrowth and increased risk for SIBO [8]. Yet SIBO is not always observed and some studies suggest it is independent of intestinal dysmotility [26]. Spontaneous bacterial peritonitis (SBP) is another risk factor with PPI use. A retrospective case control study conducted in Montreal found an increased association of SBP and PPI use in cirrhotic patients than non-PPI users. Many had no clear or inappropriate indication of PPI use [76]. The American Association for the Study of Liver Diseases recommends unless PPIs are indicated, limitation of PPIs may help prevent SBP [77].

17.4.6 Pneumonia

Several controversial studies exist between the association of PPI therapy and developing community acquired pneumonia (CAP). Long term PPI therapy leads to bacterial overgrowth in the stomach which may increase risk of lung infection from micro-aspiration and bacterial translocation [50, 51]. A large meta-analysis with heterogeneity among the studies showed a significant association with those acquiring CAP while on PPI therapy. The risk increased with 1 month use, independent of patient age or PPI dose. PPIs were also found to increase likelihood of hospitalization [50, 78]. Another study suggested short term PPI use increases risk of CAP but its risk decreases with greater duration. Two day use of PPIs had an increased risk of developing CAP with an odds ratio of 6.53 which decreased to 3.21 over a 2 week duration [79]. However, a 2021 Korean nationwide cohort study showed that short term PPI use linked to pneumonia may be overestimated [56, 80]. Meta-analyses that studied long term PPI therapy did not find clinical significance between PPI use and CAP [51]. A large pharmacoepidemiologic cohort study included 35,000 patients which associated PPI use and increased risk of ventilator associated pneumonia. It was found mechanically ventilated patients developed pneumonia at higher rates when compared to those on H2RAs. Studies that suggest this association have low quality of evidence and likely high confounding factors [48, 81]. Additional studies are necessary to evaluate the association between pneumonia risk and PPI therapy.

17.4.7 Dementia

Some data suggests that there may be an association between chronic PPI use and increased risk of dementia but studies are controversial. The proposed hypothesis is the ability of PPIs to cross the blood brain barrier (BBB) where they increase the production and degradation of amyloid. PPIs decrease the acidity in lysosomes which inhibits the degradation of amyloid beta protein [48, 56]. Furthermore, the reduced levels of B12 and other nutrients as a result of chronic acid suppression poses as a potential hypothesis in the pathogenesis of PPI related dementia [82]. A longitudinal multicenter cohort study and large prospective cohort study found elderly patients had increased risk of dementia with PPI use [50, 83, 84]. In these large population based and epidemiological studies, significant limitations were present including inaccurate and missing diagnosis codes and absence of randomization which led to residual bias and confounding results [48]. They had small effect sizes with hazard ratio <2 so it was difficult to determine if the association between dementia and PPIs was valid or due to residual bias [43]. A meta-analysis consisting of six cohort studies in 2019 showed no statistical significance between PPI use and increased risk of dementia [85]. Another prospective population based cohort study over an average follow up of 7.5 years did not find an association [86]. Data is conflicting and strong evidence based studies are needed for further investigation.

17.4.8 Cardiovascular Adverse Events

PPI therapy is implicated in increased adverse cardiovascular events as a result of potential pharmacokinetic drug-drug interactions. PPIs, with recognition toward omeprazole, are competitive CYP450 inhibitors, targeting CYP2C19 and CYP3A4 [48, 50]. This is significant because clopidogrel, a commonly used antiplatelet drug after percutaneous intervention and prevention of cardiovascular (CV) events, undergoes metabolism by the cytochrome P450 system to its active form [50]. PPIs decrease the effectiveness of clopidogrel with studies showing a 40% increased risk of coronary artery stent occlusions with PPI use while on clopidogrel [51]. Systemic review and meta-analysis of observational studies showed that clopidogrel users on PPI therapy had increased mortality and adverse CV events compared with nonusers. However RCTs did not find any significant difference in ischemic events or mortality [47, 50]. In a study conducted in 2009, patients on clopidogrel had a 25% higher platelet reactivity while on PPI therapy than those without [87]. The US FDA issued a warning that same year to avoid concurrent administration of both omeprazole and clopidogrel due to concern of decreased clopidogrel beneficiary effect. The 2010 COGENT study, the only large scale prospective RCT, found no difference in cardiovascular endpoint between those who received omeprazole versus placebo. There was also a decreased risk of upper GI bleeds [48, 88]. Pantoprazole does not competitively inhibit the CYP450 system and may be a better alternative solution when prescribing a PPI with clopidogrel. A cohort study of around 20,000 patients evaluated patients on clopidogrel and PPI, with majority on pantoprazole, and saw no significance with increased risk of CV disease [89]. There is also no association with increased risk of coronary artery stent occlusions [51].

17.4.9 Mucosal Remodeling

Long-term PPI use has been associated with some histopathologic findings, such as parietal cell extension into the gland lumen, gastric fundic gland cystic dilation, and foveolar epithelial hyperplasia [90]. Endoscopically, these findings appear as white and flat elevated lesions, cobblestone-line mucosa, black pigmentation, fundic gland polyps, hyperplastic polyps [90, 91]. While it is important to educate clinicians on the appearance of these findings, the clinical significance of these new manifestations of mucosal remodeling remains unclear. These findings should be monitored closely in patients on chronic PPI therapy.

17.4.10 Further Gastric Mucosa Atrophy, Gastric Cancer Risk

Long term PPI therapy has a significant association with chronic atrophic gastritis. One of the studies found that incidence of atrophic gastritis rose from 1% to 25% in patients on long-term PPI therapy. Interestingly, majority of PPI related atrophic gastritis cases occurred in patients with preexisting gastritis, many of them with Helicobacter pylori infection [92]. Marked suppression of acid production within the stomach transforms the distribution of organisms, which subsequently leads to worsening of mucosal inflammation and atrophy further exacerbating acid suppression [93].

Besides increased risk of gastric mucosal atrophy, recent studies demonstrated that long-term PPI therapy increases risk of gastric cancer [94, 95]. It is theorized that decreased acid production and the hypergastrinemic state caused by long-term PPI use is what predisposes patients to gastric neoplasia [56, 94]. Hypergastrinemia causes enterochromaffin like cells to proliferate, subsequently leading to neoplastic chances and cancer progression [50, 56, 96]. One study found that 1–5 years of PPI therapy increases risk of fundic gland polyps by twofold and a 5-year PPI therapy increases risk by fourfold [50, 97]. While there is a growing concern of gastric neoplasia while on long-term PPI therapy, recent studies proposed that there are other malignancies PPI therapy may be associated with. Prolonged use of PPI causes increases in serum gastrin levels and bacterial overgrowth, which precipitates toxic bile salts [98]. These factors have been associated with increased risk of colorectal neoplasia. One of the studies concluded that prolonged use of PPIs may be associated with a modest risk of colorectal cancer [99].

17.4.11 Drug-Drug Interactions

Alterations in gastric pH, inhibition of hepatic cytochrome enzymes (particularly CYP2C19 and CYP3A4) and renal hydrogen/potassium ATPase pump are the predominant mechanisms by which PPIs interact with other medications. Mycophenolate mofetil (MMF) is a commonly used immunosuppressant in rheumatic disease and requires an acidic environment for adequate absorption. If alternative therapies cannot be used in rheumatic conditions, patients are encouraged to take their medications towards the end of the PPI dosing interval and be monitored closely. If possible, patients should take the first dose of MMF and wait at least 90 min before taking the PPI. Furthermore, malnutrition is a common complication of rheumatic conditions like in cases of systemic sclerosis. As discussed, PPIs can compromise the absorption of certain nutrients leading to additional vitamin and mineral deficiencies. Table 17.2 summarizes common interaction between PPIs and medications used in patients with rheumatic conditions [100–110].

There is a lack of RCTs to determine association of PPI therapy and adverse side effects. RCTs are warranted to clarify the controversial studies such as PPI therapy and its association with fractures, dementia, infections, etc. Observational studies support these findings but statistical significance does not take into account of certain biases and confounding factors. Although further investigation is merited, patients should be fully informed of the reported risks summarized in Table 17.3. Clinicians should also be aware of the potential drug to drug interactions with commonly used drugs to treat rheumatic conditions and monitor these patients closely. Administration of PPIs should be weighed carefully in each individual patient to tailor therapy to maximize benefits and reduce risks.

17.4.12 Strategies to Minimize Risks of PPI Use and Optimize Therapy

Prescribing proton pump inhibitors should be guided by evidence based data however many patients do not have clear indications for PPI use. In many scenarios, patients remain on PPI therapy inappropriately after being started on therapy during hospitalization for stress ulcer prophylaxis. Other patients may use PPI therapy for greater durations than indicated or stop PPI therapy prematurely due to lack of proper patient education. Patients may tailor PPI therapy to their own liking due to its safety profile but studies on adverse side effects are growing [43]. When prescribed PPIs, patients should have full understanding of its indication, how long and how much to use, other alternative medications and incorporate lifestyle modifications to optimize PPI therapy and minimize risks. Strategies of reducing risks are summarized in Table 17.3.

17.4.12.1 Strategy 1. Duration

According to the ACG, patients who have GERD, gastric ulcers, duodenal ulcer and *H. pylori* require only a short-term course with PPI therapy. On demand or intermittent therapy can be done for nonerosive reflux disease or mild erosive esophagitis [12]. It is recommended that standard dose PPI can be taken daily for at least 8 weeks, typically 30–60 min before the morning meal to maximize efficacy [12, 26]. Rheumatic disease patients who may benefit from long-term PPI treatment include those who develop refractory GERD, moderate to severe erosive esophagitis, Barrett's esophagus, history of NSAID induced bleeding ulcers and those actively receiving chronic anticoagulation therapy post GI bleed. Rheumatic disease patients who are receiving NSAID monotherapy or dual anti-platelet therapy (DAPT) may require long term PPI treatment if they have additional risk factors. Such risk factors include age greater than 65, receiving high dose NSAID therapy, concurrent corticosteroid use, peptic ulcer disease (PUD) and/or concurrent anticoagulation therapy [14, 43]. The European League against Rheumatism (EULAR) recommends PPI use for the prevention of SSc-related reflux disease, esophageal

Table 17.3 Proton pump inhibitors side effects and strategies

Reported PPI side effects	Proposed mechanisms/ theories	Supporting literature/ strength of literature	Strategies to reduce risk
Nutritional deficiencies: Vitamin B12 deficiency, iron deficiency, hypomagnesemia, hypocalcemia	Gastric acid suppression leads to decreased intestinal absorption of vitamins/minerals	Observational studies/Weak [47, 48, 50, 54, 55, 59, 60]	Monitor hemoglobin and iron Obtain vitamin B12 levels in elderly or malnourished and supplement as needed Obtain magnesium levels prior to PPI therapy and routinely checked in high risk cardiac patients and long term PPI users Incorporate calcium citrate into diet -Supplement minerals but not over recommended dietary allowance
Bone fracture	Calcium malabsorption -Increase bone resorption by increasing osteoclast activity and/or gastrin induced parathyroid hyperplasia	Observational studies/Weak [50, 51, 56, 61–64]	Incorporate calcium citrate, bisphosphonates and/or vitamin D if over age 65 with high risk factors Perform resistance and balance training exercises to prevent falls
Calcinosis	Promote tissue calcification	Observational studies/Weak [68]	Assess need for PPI use Consider H2RA therapy when appropriate
Acute intestinal nephritis and chronic kidney disease	PPIs or its metabolites deposit in kidneys leading to immune response	Observational studies/Weak [47, 48, 50, 69–71]	Monitor creatinine levels regularly and obtain routine urinalysis testing in high risk patients
Enteric infections: Clostridium difficile, Small intestinal bowel overgrowth, Spontaneous bacterial peritonitis	Decreases stomach acidity which alters gut microbiota, decrease bacterial flora diversity and decrease immunological barrier	Observational studies/Weak [26, 48, 50, 64, 74, 76]	Can add probiotic in patients with history of C. diff Restrict PPI use in cirrhotic patients unless medically indicated by evidence based data Consider H2RAs as an alternative for mild GERD

(continued)

Table 17.3 (continued)

Reported PPI side effects	Proposed mechanisms/ theories	Supporting literature/ strength of literature	Strategies to reduce risk
Community-acquired pneumonia	Increases bacterial overgrowth increases risk of pneumonia from micro-aspiration and bacterial translocation	Observational studies, RCTs/ Weak [50, 51, 56, 78–81]	Assess need for PPI use Counsel to reduce other risk factors as appropriate to individual patient
Dementia	-PPI cross blood brain barrier and increase amyloid production -Vitamin B12 malabsorption	Observational studies/Weak [44, 47, 48, 50, 83–86]	Incorporate vitamin B12 supplements if malnourished or for heavy alcohol consumers Counsel to reduce other risk factors as appropriate to individual patient
CV adverse events-coronary artery stent occlusions	Act as a competitive CYP450 inhibitor which decreases clopidogrel bioavailability	Observational studies, RCTs/ Weak [47, 48, 50, 87–89]	Use other PPIs such as pantoprazole due to minimal interaction with CYP450 system Temporal dosing with omeprazole and clopidogrel (12-15 hours apart) Substitute clopidogrel with ticagrelor or prasugrel Assess need for PPI use before changes are made
Atrophic gastritis/ Gastric cancer	Decreased acid production and hypergastrinemia cause mucosal inflammation and enterochromaffin cell proliferation	Observational studies, RCTs/ Weak [50, 92, 94–97]	Limit PPI use unless provided a clear indication
Colorectal cancer	Acid suppression and hypergastrinemia precipitates toxic bile salt linked to colorectal neoplasia	Observational studies/Weak [99]	Limit PPI use unless provided a clear indication

ulcers and strictures [111, 112]. The dose, frequency and duration of the PPI used is dependent on many factors including patient's presentation as well as esophageal endoscopic findings. Unfortunately not all patients will respond to PPI treatment successfully and is dependent on the GERD manifestation being treated [26]. Long-term use of PPIs may lead to rebound hyperacidity, also known as hypergastrinemia, when attempting to discontinue therapy. This rebound effect may occur with a short course of therapy of 8 weeks. Thus, rather than abrupt discontinuation, it is important to taper off PPI therapy. It can be accomplished over 2–4 weeks by reducing the PPI dose by 50% the first week until the lowest dose is reached and to continue the lowest dose for an additional week before discontinuation.

17.4.12.2 Strategy 2. Dosing

The circadian rhythm may influence gastric acid secretion and gastric motility. Gastric acid secretion peaks in a circadian fashion between 10 pm and 2 am [113, 114]. PPIs are typically administered in the morning before breakfast with a quick onset of action and are typically eliminated from the body within a few hours (see Table 17.1). This leaves the fragile GI tract susceptible to damage by nocturnal acid secretion, which may lead to several complications like erosive esophagitis. Using a combination of endoscopic findings and patient's clinical symptoms, the dose and frequency of PPIs may be increased to provide nocturnal gastric acid suppression [43, 113, 114]. Typically, once daily dosing of PPIs is used in the management of most gastric complications related to gastric acid. A higher dose acid suppression therapy may be warranted to avoid the risk of severe esophagitis and further complications. However, there is minimal evidence to support the use of twice daily PPI therapy [115].

In deciding whether the PPI dose should be increased, clinicians should evaluate the number of reflux episodes, the time of day in relation to PPI dose and symptom development and the severity of gastric symptoms. Additionally, clinicians can investigate the impact of chronic acid release on the GI mucosa using endoscopic findings to determine further therapeutic alterations.

In rheumatic disease patients who do not achieve relief of acid reflux symptoms with a once daily dosing regimen, the PPI dose may be increased, dose may be split in half and dosed twice daily, or the agent could be switched to another PPI with higher bioavailability and longer duration of action such as esomeprazole or rabeprazole [12, 26, 116]. Some studies suggest that twice daily PPI regimen produces significantly better gastric acid control compared to once daily regimen [116]. In SSc, patients often have lung involvement and with uncontrolled acid reflux, they may aspirate acid into their lungs especially at night. Thus, clinicians may choose to be aggressive and dose PPIs twice daily to target nocturnal acid release and protect the respiratory tract from further damage. Moreover, patients who suffer from breakthrough and/or nocturnal symptoms, once a day daily dosing of dexlansoprazole can be used. Its modified release formula increases the duration of acid suppression due to proximal small intestinal absorption and release to the distal small intestine hours later [26]. A prospective study was conducted in SSc patients using omeprazole 20 mg twice daily for the management of GERD. The results of the trial indicated that even with twice daily dosing, half the patients experienced PPI-partial GERD response which was defined as less than 50% improvement in the visual analogue scale (VAS) for symptom severity as well as acid reflux score by the frequency of symptoms using the frequency scale for symptoms of GERD (FSSG) [24]. Aggressive therapy using high dose PPIs may be warranted or using multiple therapies that have unique mechanism of actions to synergistically target acid suppression may be beneficial in the high-risk SSc patients. For SSc patients who continue to be symptomatic despite aggressive medical therapies, analysis of high-resolution manometry (HRM) and pH testing can provide better classification and quantification of esophageal pathologies, peristaltic dysfunction, and real-time acid exposure to the LES. Such complications may require surgical interventions or warrant therapies with different mechanisms [117, 118]. Esophageal 24-h pH/impedance monitoring is the gold standard for diagnosing GERD and can be particularly beneficial to detect nonacid reflux (with pH ≥ 4). This test may be performed after patients fail symptomatic control of their reflux after trialing PPI therapy for at least 8 weeks [119]. Once appropriate diagnosis of SSc complication is made, it may lead to discontinuation or dose reduction of PPI therapies. An algorithm shown in Fig. 17.2 can guide physicians on how to approach a patient with scleroderma with GERD symptoms.

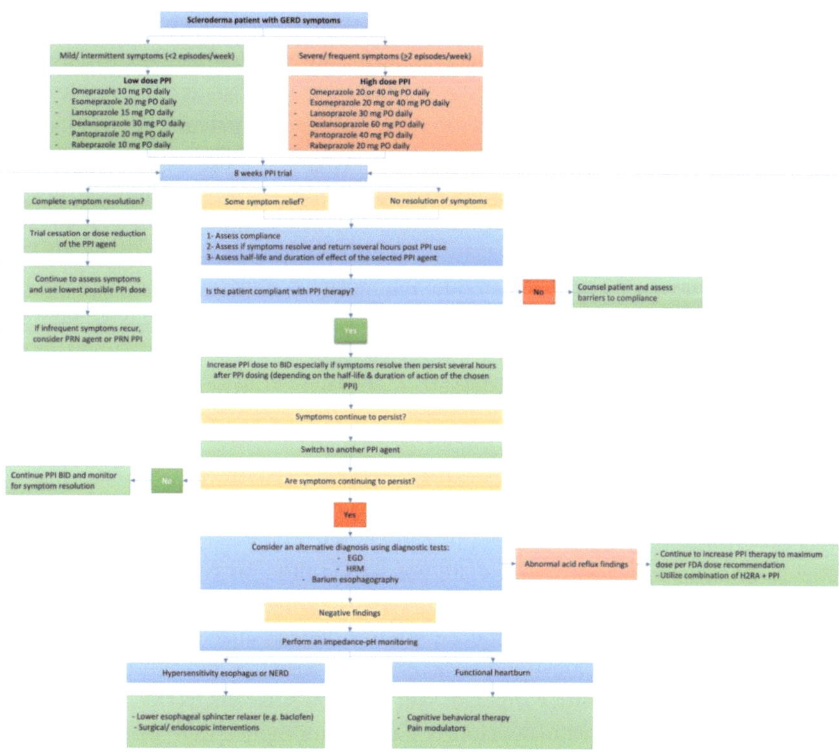

Fig. 17.2 Algorithm on how to approach a SSc patient with GERD symptoms

17.4.12.3 Strategy 3. Reducing Risks

Alternative Acid Suppressive and Synergistic Medications

Utilizing alternative or additional medications may help prevent escalating PPI dosing and potentially avoid chronic use in select patients. H2RAs are a suitable alternative acid suppressive medication for mild or occasional acid reflux symptoms however intermittent therapy is most effective as tolerance can develop [12]. Over the counter antacids such as calcium carbonate can also be trialed and used on-demand [43]. For patients on once daily PPI therapy who develop breakthrough reflux in the evening, H2RAs can be used at night as opposed to increasing the PPI to twice daily dosing. Some patients continue to have breakthrough nocturnal symptoms and therefore twice daily dosing of PPIs may be warranted in addition to H2RA use [8]. A prokinetic drug such as domperidone may be useful in refractory cases. One RCT found the addition of domperidone with twice daily PPIs improved patient quality of life [24]. However recent ACG guidelines recommend against prokinetic drugs if gastroparesis is not present. Baclofen, a GABA-B agonist, can also be used to improve GERD symptoms supported by RCTs [32]. Baclofen suppresses acid reflux and regurgitation by inhibiting transient LES relaxations and increasing its pressure [12, 30]. In accordance with ACG guidelines, baclofen is recommended if objective evidence of GERD is present but is not widely used. Another agent, buspirone has been studied in scleroderma patients due to its stimulatory properties on the esophagus and LES. A 4 week open label trial showed buspirone improved GERD symptoms but RCTs lack [120]. Sucralfate is another alternative but is recommended only in pregnancy showing benefit in a small RCT [32]. For those who respond successfully to PPI therapy but unable to take it long term, surgery may be the next best option. Laparoscopic fundoplication will provide symptom control but side effects such as bloating and dysphagia may occur [12]. Data for surgical treatment for scleroderma patients are limited providing mixed results. Laparoscopic roux-en-Y bypass (RYGB) is under investigation as a surgical alternative for SSc patients for its effectiveness on long term symptom control [121].

Reducing Bleeding Risk

Patients on chronic NSAID therapy are prescribed PPIs for NSAID bleeding prophylaxis. Bleeding risk can be minimized by appropriate NSAID selection and should be evaluated in high risk patients. Studies suggest selective COX2 inhibitors such as celecoxib may achieve the same effect as NSAIDs and PPI use to reduce upper GI complications [40]. Clinicians can consider selective COX-2 inhibitors as an alternative for those who developed bleeding complications from traditional NSAIDs. Patients should also be made aware of available combination pills such as naproxen-esomeprazole to increase patient adherence and medication compliance [122]. Misoprostol, a prostaglandin analogue, can be used as an alternative to PPIs for gastroprotection however use it limited due to frequent dosing and side effect tolerability [122, 123].

Reducing CV Events

PPIs may increase susceptibility of cardiovascular adverse events in patients on antiplatelet therapy by interfering with its metabolism via the CYP450 system. Omeprazole should be avoided in patients on clopidogrel therapy. Instead, pantoprazole is an acceptable alternative due to its minimal interaction with the CYP2C19 enzyme [50]. If there is still concern between concomitant use, competitive inhibition may be reduced by separating PPI and clopidogrel administration by 12–15 h [64]. Antiplatelet drugs such as ticagrelor or prasugrel are not dependent on the CYP2C19 enzyme and can be used in place of clopidogrel as well [50]. Before these changes are made, it should be evaluated whether there is an indication for PPI use while on antiplatelet therapy. In accordance with The American College of Cardiology Foundation and the American Heart Association, patients should only use PPI therapy while on DAPT if multiple risk factors are present for GI bleed [124].

Reducing Enteric Infections Risk

Gastric acid plays an important role in protecting the human body from pathogens colonizing the GI tract. Chronic acid suppression from PPI therapy can promote GI pathogen colonization and lead to infections like CDIs. It is important to take caution in patients who are immunocompromised who are receiving concomitant immunosuppressive therapy as they are at an increased risk of more severe infections or infection related complications [48, 125, 126]. An alternative for these patients with mild GERD could be to consider using H_2-receptor antagonists intermittently.

Reducing Fracture Risk

PPIs may have a role in increasing fracture risk. Bone protection with bisphosphonates and calcium and vitamin D supplementation can be considered in high risk populations. Rheumatic disease patients who require initial treatment with high dose steroids, for example PMR patients, fall into this high risk group. Patients who have additional risk factors including those age greater than 65, prior fragility fractures, osteopenia with increased fracture risk based on FRAX score, and T score of −2.5 and less in lumbar spine, femoral neck and total hip can be offered bisphosphonates as well [127, 128].

17.4.12.4 Strategy 4. Lifestyle Modifications and Dietary Supplementation

Patients can incorporate lifestyle changes to decrease need for PPI use. To reduce GERD symptoms, aggravating foods such as high fat, spicy and acidic foods, chocolate, and coffee carbonated beverages should be avoided [30, 32]. It is important to chew food well and avoid big bites [31]. Multiple small meals throughout the day is recommended while in the upright position during and after meals [29, 30]. Patients should be counseled to restrict alcohol intake and tobacco use to reduce symptoms. To reduce nocturnal acid reflux, it is necessary to avoid eating 2–3 h before bedtime. Elevating the head of the bed by at least 6 inches and sleeping on the left side will also aid in symptom relief [30, 32]. Overweight and obese patients are encouraged to lose weight to improve GERD symptoms [32]. Exercising can aid in weight loss and in addition to improving GERD symptoms, it can decrease falls and subsequently reduce fracture risk.

Chronic PPI use has been associated with increased risk of fractures due to increased likelihood of osteoporosis and malabsorption of calcium. Resistance and balance training exercises such as Tai Chi and back strengthening exercises should be encouraged to prevent falls and therefore fractures. Calcium and vitamin D can be incorporated into the diet as well to increase bone health [129]. Older rheumatic disease patients, especially those who are postmenopausal on chronic PPI therapy may have greater benefit from calcium supplementation [50]. Since water soluble calcium salts are not influenced by gastric acid for absorption, citrate formulation of calcium is encouraged over calcium carbonate in order to maximize calcium bioavailability [48, 57, 130]. PPIs can lead to decreased absorption of vitamin B12 and magnesium due to gastric acid suppression so dietary supplementation may be beneficial. It has been suggested that patients on chronic PPI therapy who consume a well-balanced diet may not experience B12 deficiency. Routine checks with vitamin B12 is likely unnecessary due to adequate vitamin B12 stores in the general population [48]. If vitamin and mineral supplementation are necessary, long term PPI users should not increase calcium, B12 or magnesium above the recommended dietary allowance according to the AGA [131].

17.5 Patient Education on PPI Use in the Short and Long Term Settings

Patient education plays an important role in PPI therapy. For the therapy to be successful, patients need to have a fundamental understanding of how the medication works and clear expectations of treatment. Prior to the therapy being initiated, indication for therapy as well as anticipated duration of treatment should be discussed with the patient. Whether the medication is started for an acute disease process or for a chronic medical issue, it is important to set realistic expectations for the patient.

Physicians prescribing PPIs should routinely re-evaluate the need for continuation of therapy and discuss goals of care with the patient. Whether PPIs are prescribed by the primary care physician, rheumatologist or gastroenterologist, they should follow the guidelines for PPI use to limit the side effects associated with these medications. There is a growing concern among patients regarding PPI side effects as PPIs have increasing media coverage. Specifically, many patients seem to be concerned with increased risk of fractures, pneumonia, diarrhea, and kidney disease but are unaware of the low quality of evidence behind these safety concerns. Working together with patients on modifiable risk factors and setting realistic goals for treatment plays a crucial role in treatment success and patient satisfaction.

17.6 Conclusion

Many patients with rheumatologic diseases suffer from chronic dyspepsia. Some of them have significant changes in the anatomy, predisposing them to these symptoms, while others depend on medications such as NSAIDs and corticosteroids to manage their chronic pain, which can worsen dyspepsia and/or increase their risk for GI ulcers. As a result, many patients with rheumatologic conditions are treated with PPI therapy long term. Since this class of medications was first introduced into clinical practice in the 1980s, we have gained substantial evidence on the side effect profile and can better navigate the risk and benefit discussion with patients. Providers should use evidence-based guidelines on PPI use when starting patients on therapy and routinely re-evaluate the need to continue therapy. Additionally, patient reassurance, education and setting of expectation will help decrease number of patients who lack appropriate indications and help more patients with rheumatologic diseases safely benefit from PPI therapy.

References

1. Satoh H. Discovery and development of proton pump inhibitors. Front Gastrointest Res. 2014;32:1–17.
2. Strand DS, Kim D, Peura DA. 25 years of proton pump inhibitors: a comprehensive review. Gut Liver. 2017;11(1):27–37.
3. Lassen AT. Acid-related disorders and use of antisecretory medication. Dan Med Bull. 2007;54(1):18–30.
4. Walker MJ, Crews NR, El-Halabi M, Fayad NF. Educational intervention improves proton pump inhibitor stewardship in outpatient gastroenterology clinics. Gastroenterol Res. 2019;12(6):305–11.
5. Batuwitage BT, Kingham JG, Morgan NE, Bartlett RL. Inappropriate prescribing of proton pump inhibitors in primary care. Postgrad Med J. 2007;83(975):66–8.
6. Schnoll-Sussman F, Niec R, Katz PO. Proton pump inhibitors: the good, bad, and ugly. Gastrointest Endosc Clin N Am. 2020;30(2):239–51.

7. Sachs G, Shin JM, Howden CW. Review article: the clinical pharmacology of proton pump inhibitors. Aliment Pharmacol Ther. 2006;23(Suppl 2):2–8.
8. Kaniecki T, Abdi T, McMahan ZH. A practical approach to the evaluation and management of gastrointestinal symptoms in patients with systemic sclerosis. Best Pract Res Clin Rheumatol. 2021;35(3):101666.
9. Graham DY, Tansel A. Interchangeable use of proton pump inhibitors based on relative potency. Clin Gastroenterol Hepatol. 2018;16(6):800–8 e7.
10. Ishizaki T, Horai Y. Review article: cytochrome P450 and the metabolism of proton pump inhibitors—emphasis on rabeprazole. Aliment Pharmacol Ther. 1999;13(Suppl 3):27–36.
11. Chubineh S, Birk J. Proton pump inhibitors: the good, the bad, and the unwanted. South Med J. 2012;105(11):613–8.
12. Sollano JD, Romano R, IbaÒez-Guzman L, Antoinette M, Ocampo SD, Policarpio AA, et al., editors. Clinical practice guidelines on the diagnosis and treatment of gastroesophageal reflux disease (GERD);2015.
13. Kahrilas PJ, Shaheen NJ, Vaezi MF, American Gastroenterological Association I, Clinical P, Quality Management C. American Gastroenterological Association Institute technical review on the management of gastroesophageal reflux disease. Gastroenterology. 2008;135(4):1392–413, 413 e1–5.
14. Katz PO, Gerson LB, Vela MF. Guidelines for the diagnosis and management of gastroesophageal reflux disease. Am J Gastroenterol. 2013;108(3):308–28; quiz 29.
15. Hungin AP, Rubin GP, O'Flanagan H. Long-term prescribing of proton pump inhibitors in general practice. Br J Gen Pract. 1999;49(443):451–3.
16. Van Soest EM, Siersema PD, Dieleman JP, Sturkenboom MC, Kuipers EJ. Persistence and adherence to proton pump inhibitors in daily clinical practice. Aliment Pharmacol Ther. 2006;24(2):377–85.
17. Singh S, Garg SK, Singh PP, Iyer PG, El-Serag HB. Acid-suppressive medications and risk of oesophageal adenocarcinoma in patients with Barrett's oesophagus: a systematic review and meta-analysis. Gut. 2014;63(8):1229–37.
18. Shaheen NJ, Falk GW, Iyer PG, Gerson LB, American College of G. ACG clinical guideline: diagnosis and management of Barrett's esophagus. Am J Gastroenterol. 2016;111(1):30–50. quiz 1
19. Lanza FL, Chan FK, Quigley EM, Practice Parameters Committee of the American College of G. Guidelines for prevention of NSAID-related ulcer complications. Am J Gastroenterol. 2009;104(3):728–38.
20. Bhatt DL, Scheiman J, Abraham NS, Antman EM, Chan FK, Furberg CD, et al. ACCF/ACG/AHA 2008 expert consensus document on reducing the gastrointestinal risks of antiplatelet therapy and NSAID use: a report of the American College of Cardiology Foundation Task Force on Clinical Expert Consensus Documents. Circulation. 2008;118(18):1894–909.
21. Talley NJ, American Gastroenterological A. American Gastroenterological Association medical position statement: evaluation of dyspepsia. Gastroenterology. 2005;129(5):1753–5.
22. Iwata A, Ikeda K, Hirose K, Takatori H, Takahashi K, Sanayama Y, et al. Pre-dinner administration increases the efficacy of proton pump inhibitors on refractory GERD symptoms in connective tissue disease patients. Mod Rheumatol. 2013;23(2):357–64.
23. Nampei A, Shi K, Ebina K, Tomita T, Sugamoto K, Yoshikawa H, et al. Prevalence of gastroesophageal reflux disease symptoms and related factors in patients with rheumatoid arthritis. J Clin Biochem Nutr. 2013;52(2):179–84.
24. Foocharoen C, Chunlertrith K, Mairiang P, Mahakkanukrauh A, Suwannaroj S, Namvijit S, et al. Prevalence and predictors of proton pump inhibitor partial response in gastroesophageal reflux disease in systemic sclerosis: a prospective study. Sci Rep. 2020;10(1):769.
25. Hendel L, Hage E, Hendel J, Stentoft P. Omeprazole in the long-term treatment of severe gastro-oesophageal reflux disease in patients with systemic sclerosis. Aliment Pharmacol Ther. 1992;6(5):565–77.

26. Carlson DA, Hinchcliff M, Pandolfino JE. Advances in the evaluation and management of esophageal disease of systemic sclerosis. Curr Rheumatol Rep. 2015;17(1):475.
27. Ebert EC. Esophageal disease in scleroderma. J Clin Gastroenterol. 2006;40(9):769–75.
28. Daruwala C, Mercogliano G, Harder TP. Gastrointestinal manifestations of systemic lupus erythematosus and scleroderma. Clin Med Gastroenterol. 2009;2:CGast.S2264.
29. Fitzgerald RC, Triadafilopoulos G. Esophageal manifestations of rheumatic disorders. Semin Arthritis Rheum. 1997;26(4):641–66.
30. Nagaraja V, McMahan ZH, Getzug T, Khanna D. Management of gastrointestinal involvement in scleroderma. Curr Treatm Opt Rheumatol. 2015;1(1):82–105.
31. Denaxas K, Ladas SD, Karamanolis GP. Evaluation and management of esophageal manifestations in systemic sclerosis. Ann Gastroenterol. 2018;31(2):165–70.
32. Katz PO, Dunbar KB, Schnoll-Sussman FH, Greer KB, Yadlapati R, Spechler SJ. ACG clinical guideline for the diagnosis and management of gastroesophageal reflux disease. Am J Gastroenterol. 2021.
33. Bodukam V, Hays RD, Maranian P, Furst DE, Seibold JR, Impens A, et al. Association of gastrointestinal involvement and depressive symptoms in patients with systemic sclerosis. Rheumatology (Oxford). 2011;50(2):330–4.
34. Zeitoun JD, Lefevre JH, de Parades V, Sejourne C, Sobhani I, Coffin B, et al. Functional digestive symptoms and quality of life in patients with Ehlers-Danlos syndromes: results of a national cohort study on 134 patients. PLoS One. 2013;8(11):e80321.
35. Lundell LR, Dent J, Bennett JR, Blum AL, Armstrong D, Galmiche JP, et al. Endoscopic assessment of oesophagitis: clinical and functional correlates and further validation of the Los Angeles classification. Gut. 1999;45(2):172–80.
36. Marie I, Dominique S, Levesque H, Ducrotte P, Denis P, Hellot MF, et al. Esophageal involvement and pulmonary manifestations in systemic sclerosis. Arthritis Rheum. 2001;45(4):346–54.
37. Patti MG, Gasper WJ, Fisichella PM, Nipomnick I, Palazzo F. Gastroesophageal reflux disease and connective tissue disorders: pathophysiology and implications for treatment. J Gastrointest Surg. 2008;12(11):1900–6.
38. Tsujimoto S, Mokuda S, Matoba K, Yamada A, Jouyama K, Murata Y, et al. The prevalence of endoscopic gastric mucosal damage in patients with rheumatoid arthritis. PLoS One. 2018;13(7):e0200023.
39. Drini M. Peptic ulcer disease and non-steroidal anti-inflammatory drugs. Aust Prescr. 2017;40(3):91–3.
40. Gwee KA, Goh V, Lima G, Setia S. Coprescribing proton-pump inhibitors with nonsteroidal anti-inflammatory drugs: risks versus benefits. J Pain Res. 2018;11:361–74.
41. Henriksson K, From J, Stratelis G. Patient-reported adherence to coprescribed proton pump inhibitor gastroprotection in osteoarthritis, rheumatoid arthritis, and ankylosing spondylitis patients using nonsteroidal anti-inflammatory drugs. Patient Prefer Adherence. 2014;8:1611–7.
42. Scheiman JM. The use of proton pump inhibitors in treating and preventing NSAID-induced mucosal damage. Arthritis Res Ther. 2013;15(Suppl 3):S5.
43. Laine L, Nagar A. Long-term PPI use: balancing potential harms and documented benefits. Am J Gastroenterol. 2016;111(7):913–5.
44. Laine L, Barkun AN, Saltzman JR, Martel M, Leontiadis GI. ACG clinical guideline: upper gastrointestinal and ulcer bleeding. Am J Gastroenterol. 2021;116(5):899–917.
45. Malik A, Hayat G, Kalia JS, Guzman MA. Idiopathic inflammatory myopathies: clinical approach and management. Front Neurol. 2016;7:64.
46. Leung JL, Owen CE, Buchanan RRC, Liew DFL. Management of polymyalgia rheumatica in older people. J Pharm Pract Res. 2019;49(5):493–500.
47. Dharmarajan TS. The use and misuse of proton pump inhibitors: an opportunity for deprescribing. J Am Med Dir Assoc. 2021;22(1):15–22.

48. Jaynes M, Kumar AB. The risks of long-term use of proton pump inhibitors: a critical review. Ther Adv Drug Saf. 2019;10:2042098618809927.
49. Brown JP, Tazare JR, Williamson E, Mansfield KE, Evans SJ, Tomlinson LA, et al. Proton pump inhibitors and risk of all-cause and cause-specific mortality: a cohort study. Br J Clin Pharmacol. 2021;87(8):3150–61.
50. Eusebi LH, Rabitti S, Artesiani ML, Gelli D, Montagnani M, Zagari RM, et al. Proton pump inhibitors: risks of long-term use. J Gastroenterol Hepatol. 2017;32(7):1295–302.
51. Thomson AB, Sauve MD, Kassam N, Kamitakahara H. Safety of the long-term use of proton pump inhibitors. World J Gastroenterol. 2010;16(19):2323–30.
52. den Elzen WP, Groeneveld Y, de Ruijter W, Souverijn JH, le Cessie S, Assendelft WJ, et al. Long-term use of proton pump inhibitors and vitamin B12 status in elderly individuals. Aliment Pharmacol Ther. 2008;27(6):491–7.
53. Perazella MA. Proton pump inhibitors and hypomagnesemia: a rare but serious complication. Kidney Int. 2013;83(4):553–6.
54. Cheungpasitporn W, Thongprayoon C, Kittanamongkolchai W, Srivali N, Edmonds PJ, Ungprasert P, et al. Proton pump inhibitors linked to hypomagnesemia: a systematic review and meta-analysis of observational studies. Ren Fail. 2015;37(7):1237–41.
55. Hanaoka H, Kikuchi J, Kaneko Y, Seki N, Tsujimoto H, Chiba K, et al. Proton pump inhibitor and tacrolimus uses are associated with hypomagnesemia in connective tissue disease: a potential link with renal dysfunction and recurrent infection. Front Pharmacol. 2021;12:616719.
56. Yibirin M, De Oliveira D, Valera R, Plitt AE, Lutgen S. Adverse effects associated with proton pump inhibitor use. Cureus. 2021;13(1):e12759.
57. Ahmed A, Clarke JO. Proton Pump Inhibitors (PPI). StatPearls. Treasure Island (FL);2021.
58. Benmassaoud A, McDonald EG, Lee TC. Potential harms of proton pump inhibitor therapy: rare adverse effects of commonly used drugs. CMAJ. 2016;188(9):657–62.
59. Sarzynski E, Puttarajappa C, Xie Y, Grover M, Laird-Fick H. Association between proton pump inhibitor use and anemia: a retrospective cohort study. Dig Dis Sci. 2011;56(8):2349–53.
60. O'Connell MB, Madden DM, Murray AM, Heaney RP, Kerzner LJ. Effects of proton pump inhibitors on calcium carbonate absorption in women: a randomized crossover trial. Am J Med. 2005;118(7):778–81.
61. Yang YX, Lewis JD, Epstein S, Metz DC. Long-term proton pump inhibitor therapy and risk of hip fracture. JAMA. 2006;296(24):2947–53.
62. Miyano S, Michihata N, Sada KE, Uda K, Matsui H, Fushimi K, et al. Comparison of fracture risk between proton pump inhibitors and histamine-2 receptor antagonists in ANCA-associated vasculitis patients: a nested case-control study. Rheumatology (Oxford). 2021;60(4):1717–23.
63. Zhou B, Huang Y, Li H, Sun W, Liu J. Proton-pump inhibitors and risk of fractures: an update meta-analysis. Osteoporos Int. 2016;27(1):339–47.
64. Laria A, Zoli A, Gremese E, Ferraccioli GF. Proton pump inhibitors in rheumatic diseases: clinical practice, drug interactions, bone fractures and risk of infections. Reumatismo. 2011;63(1):5–10.
65. Moayyedi P, Eikelboom JW, Bosch J, Connolly SJ, Dyal L, Shestakovska O, et al. Safety of proton pump inhibitors based on a large, multi-year, randomized trial of patients receiving rivaroxaban or aspirin. Gastroenterology. 2019;157(3):682–91 e2.
66. Targownik LE, Goertzen AL, Luo Y, Leslie WD. Long-term proton pump inhibitor use is not associated with changes in bone strength and structure. Am J Gastroenterol. 2017;112(1):95–101.
67. Lai SW, Kuo YH, Liao KF. Association between proton pump inhibitors therapy and fracture risk in patients with rheumatoid arthritis. Ann Rheum Dis. 2020;79(12):e156.
68. Host LV, Campochiaro C, Afonso A, Nihtyanova SI, Denton CP, Ong VH. High proton pump inhibitor exposure increases risk of calcinosis in systemic sclerosis. Rheumatology (Oxford). 2021;60(2):849–54.

69. Hart E, Dunn TE, Feuerstein S, Jacobs DM. Proton pump inhibitors and risk of acute and chronic kidney disease: a retrospective cohort study. Pharmacotherapy. 2019;39(4):443–53.
70. Xie Y, Bowe B, Li T, Xian H, Balasubramanian S, Al-Aly Z. Proton pump inhibitors and risk of incident CKD and progression to ESRD. J Am Soc Nephrol. 2016;27(10):3153–63.
71. Xie Y, Bowe B, Li T, Xian H, Yan Y, Al-Aly Z. Long-term kidney outcomes among users of proton pump inhibitors without intervening acute kidney injury. Kidney Int. 2017;91(6):1482–94.
72. Cadle RM, Mansouri MD, Logan N, Kudva DR, Musher DM. Association of proton-pump inhibitors with outcomes in Clostridium difficile colitis. Am J Health Syst Pharm. 2007;64(22):2359–63.
73. Kwok CS, Arthur AK, Anibueze CI, Singh S, Cavallazzi R, Loke YK. Risk of Clostridium difficile infection with acid suppressing drugs and antibiotics: meta-analysis. Am J Gastroenterol. 2012;107(7):1011–9.
74. Janarthanan S, Ditah I, Adler DG, Ehrinpreis MN. Clostridium difficile-associated diarrhea and proton pump inhibitor therapy: a meta-analysis. Am J Gastroenterol. 2012;107(7):1001–10.
75. Tleyjeh IM, Bin Abdulhak AA, Riaz M, Alasmari FA, Garbati MA, AlGhamdi M, et al. Association between proton pump inhibitor therapy and clostridium difficile infection: a contemporary systematic review and meta-analysis. PLoS One. 2012;7(12):e50836.
76. Ratelle M, Perreault S, Villeneuve JP, Tremblay L. Association between proton pump inhibitor use and spontaneous bacterial peritonitis in cirrhotic patients with ascites. Can J Gastroenterol Hepatol. 2014;28(6):330–4.
77. Runyon BA. Introduction to the revised American Association for the Study of Liver Diseases Practice Guideline management of adult patients with ascites due to cirrhosis 2012. Hepatology. 2013;57(4):1651–3.
78. Lambert AA, Lam JO, Paik JJ, Ugarte-Gil C, Drummond MB, Crowell TA. Risk of community-acquired pneumonia with outpatient proton-pump inhibitor therapy: a systematic review and meta-analysis. PLoS One. 2015;10(6):e0128004.
79. Sarkar M, Hennessy S, Yang YX. Proton-pump inhibitor use and the risk for community-acquired pneumonia. Ann Intern Med. 2008;149(6):391–8.
80. Lee SW, Ha EK, Yeniova AO, Moon SY, Kim SY, Koh HY, et al. Severe clinical outcomes of COVID-19 associated with proton pump inhibitors: a nationwide cohort study with propensity score matching. Gut. 2021;70(1):76–84.
81. MacLaren R, Reynolds PM, Allen RR. Histamine-2 receptor antagonists vs proton pump inhibitors on gastrointestinal tract hemorrhage and infectious complications in the intensive care unit. JAMA Intern Med. 2014;174(4):564–74.
82. Kuller LH. Do proton pump inhibitors increase the risk of dementia? JAMA Neurol. 2016;73(4):379–81.
83. Gomm W, von Holt K, Thome F, Broich K, Maier W, Fink A, et al. Association of proton pump inhibitors with risk of dementia: a pharmacoepidemiological claims data analysis. JAMA Neurol. 2016;73(4):410–6.
84. Haenisch B, von Holt K, Wiese B, Prokein J, Lange C, Ernst A, et al. Risk of dementia in elderly patients with the use of proton pump inhibitors. Eur Arch Psychiatry Clin Neurosci. 2015;265(5):419–28.
85. Li M, Luo Z, Yu S, Tang Z. Proton pump inhibitor use and risk of dementia: systematic review and meta-analysis. Medicine (Baltimore). 2019;98(7):e14422.
86. Gray SL, Walker RL, Dublin S, Yu O, Aiello Bowles EJ, Anderson ML, et al. Proton pump inhibitor use and dementia risk: prospective population-based study. J Am Geriatr Soc. 2018;66(2):247–53.
87. Gilard M, Arnaud B, Cornily JC, Le Gal G, Lacut K, Le Calvez G, et al. Influence of omeprazole on the antiplatelet action of clopidogrel associated with aspirin: the randomized, double-blind OCLA (Omeprazole CLopidogrel Aspirin) study. J Am Coll Cardiol. 2008;51(3):256–60.

88. Bhatt DL, Cryer BL, Contant CF, Cohen M, Lanas A, Schnitzer TJ, et al. Clopidogrel with or without omeprazole in coronary artery disease. N Engl J Med. 2010;363(20):1909–17.
89. Ray WA, Murray KT, Griffin MR, Chung CP, Smalley WE, Hall K, et al. Outcomes with concurrent use of clopidogrel and proton-pump inhibitors: a cohort study. Ann Intern Med. 2010;152(6):337–45.
90. Kim GH. Proton pump inhibitor-related gastric mucosal changes. Gut Liver. 2021;15(5):646–52.
91. Takahari K, Haruma K, Ohtani H, Kiyoto S, Watanabe A, Kamada T, et al. Proton pump inhibitor induction of gastric cobblestone-like lesions in the stomach. Intern Med. 2017;56(20):2699–703.
92. Klinkenberg-Knol EC, Festen HP, Jansen JB, Lamers CB, Nelis F, Snel P, et al. Long-term treatment with omeprazole for refractory reflux esophagitis: efficacy and safety. Ann Intern Med. 1994;121(3):161–7.
93. Eissele R, Brunner G, Simon B, Solcia E, Arnold R. Gastric mucosa during treatment with lansoprazole: Helicobacter pylori is a risk factor for argyrophil cell hyperplasia. Gastroenterology. 1997;112(3):707–17.
94. Waldum HL, Sordal O, Fossmark R. Proton pump inhibitors (PPIs) may cause gastric cancer—clinical consequences. Scand J Gastroenterol. 2018;53(6):639–42.
95. Poulsen AH, Christensen S, McLaughlin JK, Thomsen RW, Sorensen HT, Olsen JH, et al. Proton pump inhibitors and risk of gastric cancer: a population-based cohort study. Br J Cancer. 2009;100(9):1503–7.
96. Joo MK, Park JJ, Chun HJ. Proton pump inhibitor: the dual role in gastric cancer. World J Gastroenterol. 2019;25(17):2058–70.
97. Jalving M, Koornstra JJ, Wesseling J, Boezen HM, Kleibeuker JH. Increased risk of fundic gland polyps during long-term proton pump inhibitor therapy. Aliment Pharmacol Ther. 2006;24(9):1341–8.
98. van Soest EM, van Rossum LG, Dieleman JP, van Oijen MG, Siersema PD, Sturkenboom MC, et al. Proton pump inhibitors and the risk of colorectal cancer. Am J Gastroenterol. 2008;103(4):966–73.
99. Abrahami D, McDonald EG, Schnitzer ME, Barkun AN, Suissa S, Azoulay L. Proton pump inhibitors and risk of colorectal cancer. Gut. 2022;71(1):111–8.
100. Wedemeyer RS, Blume H. Pharmacokinetic drug interaction profiles of proton pump inhibitors: an update. Drug Saf. 2014;37(4):201–11.
101. Lorf T, Ramadori G, Ringe B, Schworer H. The effect of pantoprazole on tacrolimus and cyclosporin A blood concentration in transplant recipients. Eur J Clin Pharmacol. 2000;56(5):439–40.
102. Iwamoto T, Monma F, Fujieda A, Nakatani K, Katayama N, Okuda M. Hepatic drug interaction between tacrolimus and lansoprazole in a bone marrow transplant patient receiving voriconazole and harboring CYP2C19 and CYP3A5 heterozygous mutations. Clin Ther. 2011;33(8):1077–80.
103. Hosohata K, Masuda S, Ogura Y, Oike F, Takada Y, Katsura T, et al. Interaction between tacrolimus and lansoprazole, but not rabeprazole in living-donor liver transplant patients with defects of CYP2C19 and CYP3A5. Drug Metab Pharmacokinet. 2008;23(2):134–8.
104. Takahashi K, Yano I, Fukuhara Y, Katsura T, Takahashi T, Ito N, et al. Distinct effects of omeprazole and rabeprazole on the tacrolimus blood concentration in a kidney transplant recipient. Drug Metab Pharmacokinet. 2007;22(6):441–4.
105. Castellote E, Bonet J, Lauzurica R, Pastor C, Cofan F, Caralps A. Does interaction between omeprazole and cyclosporin exist? Nephron. 1993;65(3):478.
106. Doesch AO, Mueller S, Konstandin M, Celik S, Erbel C, Kristen A, et al. Proton pump inhibitor co-medication reduces active drug exposure in heart transplant recipients receiving mycophenolate mofetil. Transplant Proc. 2010;42(10):4243–6.

107. Knorr JP, Sjeime M, Braitman LE, Jawa P, Zaki R, Ortiz J. Concomitant proton pump inhibitors with mycophenolate mofetil and the risk of rejection in kidney transplant recipients. Transplantation. 2014;97(5):518–24.
108. Vakily M, Amer F, Kukulka MJ, Andhivarothai N. Coadministration of lansoprazole and naproxen does not affect the pharmacokinetic profile of methotrexate in adult patients with rheumatoid arthritis. J Clin Pharmacol. 2005;45(10):1179–86.
109. Suzuki K, Doki K, Homma M, Tamaki H, Hori S, Ohtani H, et al. Co-administration of proton pump inhibitors delays elimination of plasma methotrexate in high-dose methotrexate therapy. Br J Clin Pharmacol. 2009;67(1):44–9.
110. Heidelbaugh JJ. Proton pump inhibitors and risk of vitamin and mineral deficiency: evidence and clinical implications. Ther Adv Drug Saf. 2013;4(3):125–33.
111. Kowal-Bielecka O, Landewe R, Avouac J, Chwiesko S, Miniati I, Czirjak L, et al. EULAR recommendations for the treatment of systemic sclerosis: a report from the EULAR Scleroderma Trials and Research group (EUSTAR). Ann Rheum Dis. 2009;68(5):620–8.
112. Hansi N, Thoua N, Carulli M, Chakravarty K, Lal S, Smyth A, et al. Consensus best practice pathway of the UK scleroderma study group: gastrointestinal manifestations of systemic sclerosis. Clin Exp Rheumatol. 2014;32(6 Suppl 86):S-214-21.
113. Levin E, Kirsner JB, Palmer WL. Twelve-hour nocturnal gastric secretion in uncomplicated duodenal ulcer patients; before and after healing. Proc Soc Exp Biol Med. 1948;69(1):153–6.
114. Feldman M, Richardson CT. Total 24-hour gastric acid secretion in patients with duodenal ulcer. Comparison with normal subjects and effects of cimetidine and parietal cell vagotomy. Gastroenterology. 1986;90(3):540–4.
115. Janiak P, Thumshirn M, Menne D, Fox M, Halim S, Fried M, et al. Clinical trial: the effects of adding ranitidine at night to twice daily omeprazole therapy on nocturnal acid breakthrough and acid reflux in patients with systemic sclerosis--a randomized controlled, cross-over trial. Aliment Pharmacol Ther. 2007;26(9):1259–65.
116. Khalaf M, Abdul-Hussein M, Castell D. Are twice daily proton pump inhibitors better than once daily in suspected GERD?: 429. Am J Gastroenterol. 2016;111:S192.
117. Carlo-Stella N, Belloli L, Barbera R, Gambaro C, Rando G, Malesci A, et al. Gastroesophageal reflux and lung disease in systemic sclerosis. Am J Respir Crit Care Med. 2009;179(12):1167. author reply -8
118. Savarino E, Bazzica M, Zentilin P, Pohl D, Parodi A, Cittadini G, et al. Gastroesophageal reflux and pulmonary fibrosis in scleroderma: a study using pH-impedance monitoring. Am J Respir Crit Care Med. 2009;179(5):408–13.
119. Villa N, Vela MF. Impedance-pH testing. Gastroenterol Clin N Am. 2013;42(1):17–26.
120. Karamanolis GP, Panopoulos S, Denaxas K, Karlaftis A, Zorbala A, Kamberoglou D, et al. The 5-HT1A receptor agonist buspirone improves esophageal motor function and symptoms in systemic sclerosis: a 4-week, open-label trial. Arthritis Res Ther. 2016;18:195.
121. Yan J, Strong AT, Sharma G, Gabbard S, Thota P, Rodriguez J, et al. Surgical management of gastroesophageal reflux disease in patients with systemic sclerosis. Surg Endosc. 2018;32(9):3855–60.
122. Chaplin S, Hawkins T, Emery P. NSAIDs for RA, osteoarthritis and ankylosing spondylitis. Prescriber. 2011;22.
123. Hawkey CJ, Karrasch JA, Szczepanski L, Walker DG, Barkun A, Swannell AJ, et al. Omeprazole compared with misoprostol for ulcers associated with nonsteroidal antiinflammatory drugs. Omeprazole versus Misoprostol for NSAID-induced Ulcer Management (OMNIUM) Study Group. N Engl J Med. 1998;338(11):727–34.
124. Ali Khan M, Howden CW. The role of proton pump inhibitors in the management of upper gastrointestinal disorders. Gastroenterol Hepatol (N Y). 2018;14(3):169–75.
125. Wilhelm SM, Rjater RG, Kale-Pradhan PB. Perils and pitfalls of long-term effects of proton pump inhibitors. Expert Rev Clin Pharmacol. 2013;6(4):443–51.

126. Johnson DA, Oldfield EC. Reported side effects and complications of long-term proton pump inhibitor use: dissecting the evidence. Clin Gastroenterol Hepatol. 2013;11(5):458–64; quiz e37–8.
127. Paskins Z, Whittle R, Sultan AA, Muller S, Blagojevic-Bucknall M, Helliwell T, et al. Risk of fracture among patients with polymyalgia rheumatica and giant cell arteritis: a population-based study. BMC Med. 2018;16(1):4.
128. Tu KN, Lie JD, Wan CKV, Cameron M, Austel AG, Nguyen JK, et al. Osteoporosis: a review of treatment options. P T. 2018;43(2):92–104.
129. Senderovich H, Tang H, Belmont S. The role of exercises in osteoporotic fracture prevention and current care gaps. Where are we now? Recent updates. Rambam Maimonides Med J. 2017;8(3).
130. Sheen E, Triadafilopoulos G. Adverse effects of long-term proton pump inhibitor therapy. Dig Dis Sci. 2011;56(4):931–50.
131. Freedberg DE, Kim LS, Yang YX. The risks and benefits of long-term use of proton pump inhibitors: expert review and best practice advice from the American Gastroenterological Association. Gastroenterology. 2017;152(4):706–15.

Chapter 18
Gastrointestinal Drugs in Scleroderma and GI Dysmotility

Dia Shah, Dharma Ayer, Dareen S. Chuy, Shahad Almahmoud, Kainat Akhtar, Jessica Farrell, and Micheal Tadros

18.1 Introduction

Scleroderma is an autoimmune and noninflammatory vasculopathy with collagen deposition and fibrosis [1]. There are two types of sclerodermas: diffuse and limited [1]. Diffuse scleroderma covers larger areas of the skin, progresses quicker, has more severe symptoms, and involves internal organs earlier in the disease process [1]. Limited scleroderma covers smaller areas of the skin, progresses slower, involves internal organs later in the disease process, and has been formerly known as CREST Syndrome [1]. CREST Syndrome stands for Calcinosis, Raynaud's syndrome, Esophageal dysmotility, Sclerodactyly, and Telangiectasia [2]. Scleroderma and gastrointestinal manifestations have been shown to be correlated [3–5].

GI dysmotility is a diffuse process that involves the entire GI tract and includes but is not limited to esophageal dysmotility, gastroparesis, small bowel dysfunction, and anorectal dysfunction [6]. GI dysfunction is frequent in scleroderma, with over 90% of patients with scleroderma having multiple variations of gastrointestinal

D. Shah · D. Ayer · D. S. Chuy · K. Akhtar
Albany Medical College, Albany, NY, USA

S. Almahmoud
Department of Pharmacy Practice, Albany College of Pharmacy and Health Sciences, Albany, NY, USA

J. Farrell (✉)
Department of Pharmacy Practice, Albany College of Pharmacy and Health Sciences, Albany, NY, USA

Division of Rheumatology, Albany Medical Center, Albany, NY, USA
e-mail: Jessica.Farrell@acphs.edu

M. Tadros
Division of Gastroenterology and Hepatology, Albany Medical College, Niskayuna, NY, USA

M. Tadros et al. (eds.), *GI Diseases Associated with Rheumatological and Vasculitic Conditions*, Clinical Gastroenterology,
https://doi.org/10.1007/978-3-032-07868-1_18

dysfunction, and it is the third highest cause of death in scleroderma patients [4]. Scleroderma patients with GI involvement have impaired quality of life due to poor prognosis [4]. Additionally, esophageal reflux, heartburn, and dysphagia can be worsened by Barrett's esophagus, esophageal stenosis, and esophageal cancer, which lead to a worse prognosis in patients with scleroderma [4].

Drugs commonly used for GI dysmotility can be broken down into three categories based off which part of the GI tract they mainly affect: the foregut (Gastric dysmotility), antidiarrheals/antibiotics (Small intestinal dysmotility), and the colonic dysmotility. Commonly used GI dysmotility drugs in scleroderma include H2 receptor antagonists, Proton Pump inhibitors, pro-kinetic agents, antibiotics, laxatives, cholinergic agonists, opioid reversal agents, antidiarrheals, and secretagogues. Yet, there are limitations with these drugs which may be attributed to various drug interactions as well as side effects that may affect other aspects of scleroderma. Side effects include dizziness, headaches, increased risk of *C. difficile* infection, effects on absorption of vitamins/minerals and other medications, constipation, hyperprolactinemia, drowsiness, restlessness, depression, and GI distress [3]. Lastly, in advanced disease, therapeutic effects become dramatic, potentially causing hospitalization and parental feeding [3]. Even though various drugs are utilized for individuals with scleroderma and GI dysmotility, there is no universally successful treatment.

18.2 Gastric Dysmotility

18.2.1 Bethanechol

18.2.1.1 Background/Mechanism of Action

Cholinergic agonists are used for parasympathetic suppression, and they are muscarinic stimulants, such as bethanechol [5]. Bethanechol is a muscarinic agonist of M2 and M3 receptors, and it does not cause nicotinic or cardiac effects, lending proof to its efficacy in treatment of gastrointestinal dysmotility [7]. Muscarinic receptors are located throughout the upper gastrointestinal tract. This class of drugs can be broken down into direct-acting and indirect-acting cholinergic drugs, with bethanechol being an example of a direct-acting cholinergic agents [8].

Bethanechol acts as a direct stimulant of muscarinic receptors, enhances lower esophageal sphincter (LES) pressure, and augments the amplitude of contractions in the distal esophagus [5]. It has been shown that step doses (increased doses) of bethanechol cause an analogous stepwise stimulation of antral and duodenal motor activity [9]. As a direct-acting muscarinic receptor agonist, it acts by amplifying the effect of acetylcholine directly at the postganglionic cholinergic receptors, thereby improving esophageal peristaltic pressures [10]. Bethanechol has been used in the past in the treatment of Gastroesophageal Reflux Disease (GERD), yet its implications in treating GI dysmotility in scleroderma may vary since the causes of GERD are multifactorial [10].

18.2.1.2 Side Effects

Although bethanechol does not cause cardiac and nicotinic side effects, its side effects are explained by stimulation of muscarinic receptors by acetylcholine [7]. Examples of side effects due to high cholinergic activity include abdominal cramps and diarrhea, which have specifically been shown as frequent and common complications of bethanechol administration [7]. Other noncardiac cholinergic side effects include lacrimation, sweating, dizziness, salivation, facial flushing, chills, diaphoresis, and fecal and urinary urgency [7]. Due to its plethora of cholinergic side effects, the administration of bethanechol is contraindicated in various conditions including hyperthyroidism, peptic ulcer disease, asthma, coronary artery disease, epilepsy, parkinsonism, bradycardia, and hypotension [5]. However, in scleroderma patients with overlap Sjogren's syndrome, the side effect profile may improve symptoms associated with Sjogren's.

18.2.1.3 Utility and Implications in Scleroderma

In scleroderma, gastrointestinal motility issues are linked to the presence of autoantibodies targeting the muscarinic-3 receptor (M3-R). Supporting its effectiveness stepwise, bethanechol induced a rise in colon smooth muscle strip contractions, which was directly proportional to its concentration, and this effect was lessened by the presence of scleroderma intravenous immunoglobulins [11]. In a study on the utility of prokinetic agents in managing of scleroderma-related GI dysmotility, patients treated with bethanechol demonstrated increased LES pressure and distal esophageal contraction amplitude [5].

18.2.1.4 Conclusion

While cholinergic agonists such as bethanechol do show promise in the treatment of scleroderma induced GI dysmotility, it is important to assure that it is not contraindicated due to a patient's other conditions [5]. Since muscarinic receptors are widely located within and outside of the GI tract, the variety of side effects caused by cholinergic toxicity must be outweighed prior to initiating bethanechol [7]. The use of bethanechol in scleroderma associated GI dysmotility has not yet been widely studied, but with more knowledge regarding safety implications, it may a promising therapeutic approach [5, 7].

18.2.2 Promotility Agents

18.2.2.1 Background/Mechanism of Action

Prokinetic agents facilitate esophageal motility by increasing LES pressure, supporting the rationale that they may improve reflux control and GERD refractory to proton pump inhibitor treatment [12]. Prokinetic agents, a class of promotility agents, have been proposed to treat conditions with severe constipation-predominant symptoms. Two examples of prokinetic agents for the treatment of GI dysmotility include metoclopramide and cisapride. Of note, cisapride was withdrawn from the U.S. market July 14, 2000 due to significant safety concerns and is only available through a limited-access protocol with the manufacturer.

Metoclopramide, a D2-receptor antagonist and 5-HT_4 agonist higher is usually the first-line treatment for gastroparesis [13]. Metoclopramide is often to treat GERD and gastroparesis by increasing gastric motility [14]. Metoclopramide is also approved to combat nausea and vomiting in chemotherapy patients, as well as serve as prophylaxis in postoperative patients [14]. The next recommendation is typically domperidone, a D2 receptor antagonist, which may be used when there are symptoms of gastroparesis or reflux despite previous acid suppression. Domperidone may be preferred in long-term management as there are limited, but still present, cardiac side effects in comparison to other prokinetic agents [15]. However, domperidone is still not an approved medication by the US Food and Drug Administration (FDA) but may be acquired by the completion of Investigational New Drug Application (IND) [16]. Another prokinetic agent, prucalopride is a selective 5-HT_4 receptor agonist which can also stimulate GI motility, and generally has lower risk of cardiac arrhythmias compared to cisapride [5]. Finally, prucalopride is another prokinetic agent discussed in the laxative section.

Cisapride is a serotonin (5-HT4) agonist which acts as a parasympathomimetic. When the receptor signaling pathway is activated, cisapride initiates the release of acetylcholine neurotransmitters in the enteric nervous system. Cisapride enhances motility of the upper GI tract without influencing gastric, biliary, and pancreatic secretions. Additionally, cisapride increases the amplitude and tone of gastric antral contractions as well as peristalsis in the duodenum and jejunum. Along with that, cisapride relaxes the pyloric sphincter and duodenal bulb, allowing cisapride to increase gastric emptying and intestinal transit time. It is important to note that while cisapride increases LES tone, it has negligible effects on colon and gallbladder motility as well as no acetylcholinesterase, muscarinic receptor, and nicotinic receptor stimulation.

18.2.2.2 Side Effects

Cisapride carries a boxed warning for serious cardiac arrhythmias including ventricular tachycardia, ventricular fibrillation, torsade de pointes, and QT prolongation which greatly limits use as a common treatment for GI dysmotility in scleroderma [17]. Due to this warning, cisapride is only available through a limited-access protocol requiring physicians to be registered to prescribe therapy and patients must meet specific criteria.

Dopamine receptor blockers, such as metoclopramide, increase the risk of extrapyramidal side effects including dystonia, dyskinesia, Parkinsonism, and most importantly tardive dyskinesia [5]. Tardive dyskinesia (TD) is generally associated with the use of antipsychotics, which also serve as dopamine receptor antagonists [18]. TD has a poorly understood pathophysiology, but it mainly involves the lower face and jaw muscles and has a negative effect on walking and breathing [18]. TD decreases quality of life and since it is usually irreversible, the use of metoclopramide should be monitored and administered with caution [18]. Lastly, metoclopramide can also cause QT interval prolongation, predisposing to torsades de pointes [5].

18.2.2.3 Utility and Implications in Scleroderma

Acutely, esophageal dysmotility can lead to GERD and erosive esophagitis, as well as strictures and Barrett's esophagus if left untreated [3]. Although clinical trials still show limited efficacy, prokinetic agents have been indicated to alleviate GERD symptoms and gastroparesis in scleroderma by enhancing gastric emptying [3]. Combining prokinetic agents with acid-blocking medications, such as proton pump inhibitors, may be beneficial in early-stage disease, reducing symptoms and minimizing the risk of tissue damage [3]. However, their impact diminishes in later stages characterized by prominent smooth muscle atrophy [3]. Metoclopramide (prokinetic agent) and erythromycin (promotility antibiotic) contribute to controlling GERD by increasing LES tone and facilitating gastric emptying [3]. Although other agents such as cisapride and domperidone have been reported to improve symptoms, their use is tightly regulated due to associated toxicities [3].

Gastroparesis is characterized by prolonged gastric emptying and abnormal gastric motility not caused by a mechanical obstruction and is present in about 50% of scleroderma patients [3]. Prokinetic agents are the primary intervention of gastroparesis, along with antiemetics [3]. Prokinetic agents such as subcutaneous octreotide, metoclopramide, domperidone, cisapride, and erythromycin also serve as a secondary intervention in the treatment of intestinal pseudo-obstruction in scleroderma, in combination with broad-spectrum antibiotics [3, 19]. The utility of prokinetic agents such as metoclopramide, erythromycin, and cisapride may increase LES tone, gastric emptying, and dysphagia in scleroderma patients, yet there is insufficient data supporting the effectiveness due to wide ranges of toxicities [12]. Despite the presence of toxicity, patients treated with appropriately dosed metoclopramide had a significant reduction of reflex episodes as well as a normalization of LES pressure (refer to Table 18.1 for dosage) [12].

18.2.2.4 Conclusion

Overall, prokinetic agents show promising outcomes in enhancing gastric motility, gastric emptying, and LES tone and pressure in patients with scleroderma [3, 14, 18, 19]. It is imperative that agents such as metoclopramide and cisapride be used with caution in scleroderma patients, and with minimization of cofactors and comorbidities [3, 14, 18, 19].

18.2.3 Buspirone

18.2.3.1 Background/Mechanism of Action

Buspirone is a 5-hydroxytryptamine 1A (5-HT1A) receptor and 5-hydroxytryptamine 2 (5-HT2) receptor antagonist and has moderate affinity for dopamine D_2 receptors [20]. It is approved for generalized anxiety disorder, but because it has been shown to increase LES pressure, it had shown promise in the treatment of gastrointestinal dysfunction [5]. Buspirone has an active role in treating esophageal dysmotility, GERD, and early satiety by increasing esophageal peristalsis, gastric accommodation, and LES pressure [5].

18.2.3.2 Side Effects

Side effects of buspirone include excessive excitement, dizziness, headaches, and nervousness [5]. Buspirone has also been associated with rare cases of drug-induced movement disorders, including dyskinesia and akathisia. Serotonin syndrome has been associated with buspirone when co-administered with another or multiple serotonergic agents. Serotonin syndrome is characterized by autonomic dysfunction, altered mental status, and neuromuscular excitation due to excessive stimulation of the serotonin receptors [21].

Table 18.1 Summary of gastrointestinal drugs for GI dysmotility in Scleroderma

Medication name	Class	Dosing	Side effects	Clinical pearls for use in scleroderma
Section 1—Gastric dysmotility				
Bethanechol	Muscarinic (Cholinergic) agonist of M2 and M3 receptors	10–50 mg 3–4 times daily. Dose adjustment is not required	Diaphoresis, abdominal cramps, diarrhea, lacrimation, salivation, facial flushing, chills, fecal and urinary urgency, and asthma exacerbation	Can increase lower esophageal sphincter (LES) pressure and distal esophageal contraction amplitude
Metoclopramide	Dopamine receptor (D2 receptor) antagonist	5–10 mg 3–4 times daily administered prior to meals and at bedtime. Dose adjustment is required	Dystonia, dyskinesia, parkinsonism, tardive dyskinesia, QT interval prolongation	Indicated in esophageal dysmotility, refractory GERD, gastroparesis May increase LES tone, gastric emptying, and dysphagia in scleroderma patients Insufficient data support the effectiveness in Scleroderma

(continued)

Table 18.1 (continued)

Medication name	Class	Dosing	Side effects	Clinical pearls for use in scleroderma
Buspirone	5-hydroxytryptamine 1A (5-HT1A) receptor and 5-hydroxytryptamine 2 (5-HT2) receptor antagonist	10 mg before meals three times daily	Serotonin syndrome, excessive excitement, dizziness, headaches, and nervousness	Indicated for refractory GERD, oesophageal dysmotility, early satiety Caution with serotonin syndrome Can increase in the resting LES pressure in 80% of scleroderma patients Effective combination therapy with PPIs in scleroderma with refractory GERD
Sections 2—Small intestinal dysmotility				
Loperamide	Antidiarrheal	4 mg, followed by 2 mg after each loose stool; maximum: 16 mg/day	Dizziness, constipation, abdominal cramps, nausea	Can assist in inhibiting peristalsis and secretions in patients with scleroderma
Diphenoxylate with atropine	Antimotility agent	Initial: Diphenoxylate 5 mg/atropine sulfate 0.05 mg (2 tablets or 10 mL) 4 times daily until control achieved	Abdominal distress, anorexia, gingival swelling, nausea, non-Hirschsprung megacolon, paralytic ileus, toxic megacolon, vomiting, pruritus, urticaria	
Erythromycin	Promotility antibiotic	Oral: 250–500 mg (base) 3 times daily before meals	Nausea, diarrhea, abdominal pain, bloating, and loss of appetite	Enhance gastric motility, gastric emptying, and LES tone

(continued)

Table 18.1 (continued)

Medication name	Class	Dosing	Side effects	Clinical pearls for use in scleroderma
Metronidazole	Promotility antibiotic	Oral: 500 mg every 12 h	Nausea, vaginitis, Headache	Enhance gastric motility, gastric emptying, and LES tone
Rifaximin	Promotility antibiotic	Oral: 550 mg 3 times daily	Peripheral edema, nausea, ascites, dizziness, fatigue	Enhance gastric motility, gastric emptying, and LES tone
Section 3—Colonic dysmotility				
Senna	Stimulant laxative	Oral: 17.2 mg once daily; maximum: 34.4 mg twice daily	Abdominal cramps, diarrhea, nausea, vomiting	Many patients with scleroderma have SIBO. Some of these patients may have a hard time with fiber intake due to underlying SIBO, Thus, laxatives may be useful in patients who have slow transit of stool
Bisacodyl	Stimulant laxative	Oral: 5–15 mg once daily	Abdominal cramps, diarrhea, headache	
Polyethylene glycol	Osmotic laxative	Oral: 17 g dissolved in 240 mL (8 oz) of liquid once daily	Abdominal cramps, abdominal distention, abdominal pain, bloating, diarrhea, nausea, stomach discomfort, hypersensitivity, rectal bleeding (rare)	
Docusate sodium	Stool softener	Oral: 50–360 mg once daily or in divided doses	Diarrhea, abdominal cramping, rectal bleeding (rare)	

(continued)

Table 18.1 (continued)

Medication name	Class	Dosing	Side effects	Clinical pearls for use in scleroderma
Prucalopride	5-HT4 receptor agonist	Oral: 2 mg once daily	Nausea, abdominal pain, diarrhea, headache, dizziness	Data showed positive effects on gastrointestinal motility. The drug may be particularly helpful in cases of dysmotility that have been refractory to other agents
Linaclotide	Guanylate Cyclase-C (GC-C) Agonist	Oral: 72–145 mcg once daily	Diarrhea, abdominal pain, GERD, nausea, bowel urgency	Treatment option for refractory lower gastrointestinal symptoms in scleroderma
Lubiprostone	Chloride channel activator	Oral: 24 mcg twice daily	Diarrhea, nausea, headache	May be considered in scleroderma patients who have not adequately responded to other prokinetic agents that have been more well-studied in this population
Pyridostigmine	Reversible acetylcholinesterase inhibitor	Oral: 90–180 mg every 12 h or as needed	Diarrhea, increased peristalsis, vomiting, asthenia	Can be considered to treat refractory gastrointestinal disease in scleroderma, especially in those with prominent constipation symptoms

(continued)

Table 18.1 (continued)

Medication name	Class	Dosing	Side effects	Clinical pearls for use in scleroderma
Section 4—Other considerations				
Methylnaltrexone	Peripherally—acting opioid antagonist	450 mg once daily	Abdominal pain, flatulence, nausea	Low-dose naltrexone was safe and effective in treating pruritis associated with scleroderma The combination of oxycodone/naloxone can be useful to provide pain relief in patients with digital ulcers
Naloxegol		12.5–25 mg once daily		

18.2.3.3 Utility and Implications in Scleroderma

Buspirone showed a significant increase in the resting LES pressure in 80% of scleroderma patients suffering from esophageal symptoms refractory to PPI therapy [20]. Additionally, when administered for 4 weeks, an increase in LES pressure was also noted, supporting the role of buspirone in long-term treatment [20]. Another study showed that buspirone improved esophageal hypomotility and hypotensive LES in scleroderma patients and that buspirone treatment increased LES pressure to a greater extent than domperidone [22]. Interestingly, buspirone was shown to have a more effective outcome in patients with less severe esophageal dysfunction as opposed to more severely affected [23]. Within the same study as well as multiple others, buspirone increased LES resting pressure, and decreased heartburn and regurgitation in scleroderma patients [5, 23]. Due to the efficacy of buspirone in treating heartburn and regurgitation in addition to LES hypomotility, buspirone is an effective combination therapy with PPIs in scleroderma with refractory GERD [5].

18.2.3.4 Conclusion

Overall, buspirone administration shows consistent responses in increasing LES resting pressure and upper gastrointestinal symptoms in scleroderma patients [24]. It is important to be aware of the risk of CNS related side effects such as dizziness and headaches when administering buspirone to treat gastrointestinal dysfunction dysmotility as these side effects may exacerbate underlying comorbidities, for example increasing the risk of falls in SSc patient with osteopenia/osteoporosis [5].

18.3 Small Intestinal Dysmotility

18.3.1 Antidiarrheals

18.3.1.1 Background/Mechanism of Action

Antidiarrheal drugs are those that help minimize symptoms of diarrhea by working to improve the consistency, frequency, and weight of stool. Loperamide is a common anti-diarrheal agent that acts by binding mu-opioid receptors [25]. Diphenoxylate is a active ingredient in many combination antimotility agents and is a common therapy in conditions like IBS (diarrhea prominent) [26]. Opioid receptors, including the most predominant mu-opioid receptors (MOR), delta opioid receptors (DOR), and kappa opioid receptors (KOR), are localized to enteric neurons, interstitial cells of Cajal, and immune cells in the GI tract. In humans, these receptors are linked to the inhibition of acetylcholine (ACh) release from certain inhibitory motor neurons as well as purine/norepinephrine release from these motor neurons, which can contribute to dysmotility patterns, including those present in scleroderma patients. Thus, opioid receptor agonists can serve as effective antidirrheals [27]. Diphenoxylate is also an opioid agonist that acts on the enteric nervous system (ENS) by blocking the release of ACh, thereby inhibiting motility action of the ENS. It enhances active absorption by acting on delta receptors [28]. In practice, for the use of antidiarrheals in patients with SSc, it may be important to consider testing for small intestinal bacterial overgrowth (SIBO) prior to antidiarrheal use to prevent exacerbation of any GI symptoms [29].

18.3.1.2 Side Effects

Common adverse effects associated with loperamide include cramps, nausea, dry mouth, and flatulence [25]. High-dose loperamide has shown reports of toxicity due euphoric effects from its opioid properties [30]. Additionally, high dose loperamide has been associated with cardiac toxicity due to inhibition of cardiac potassium and sodium channels [31]. Diphenoxylate is an opioid agonist with misuse potential. Thus it is used in combination with a dose of atropine which competitively inhibits ACh receptors [28]. Reported adverse effects include abdominal distress, sedation, confusion, headache, depression, malaise and urticaria. Caution should be used in patients with dehydration/electrolyte imbalances, as inhibiting peristalsis may lead to fluid retention in the intestine aggravating dehydration and electrolyte imbalance.

18.3.1.3 Utility and Implications in Scleroderma

Diarrhea is frequently reported in patients with scleroderma and may be due to many factors including SIBO and constipation overflow, and may contribute to fecal incontinence in these patients [32]. The use of antidiarrheals such as loperamide and diphenoxylate can assist in inhibiting peristalsis and secretions in patients with scleroderma [33]. From existing reviews, it evident that loperamide may serve as a beneficial anti-diarrheal, however it must be used cautiously to prevent against the risk of pseudo-obstruction [3, 26]. Diphenoxylate in preparation with atropine may also be used as an alternative anti-diarrheal. However, due to diphenoxylate/atropine potential adverse effects, loperamide is more widely used [28].

18.3.1.4 Conclusion

Anti-diarrheals, such as the commonly administered loperamide, can be used for scleroderma patients with diarrhea. Though these are commonly recommended or prescribed, there are limited clinical trials directly investigating the efficacy of these drugs on treating GI dysmotility specifically in scleroderma patients.

18.3.2 Antibiotics

18.3.2.1 Background/Mechanism of Action

Antibiotics, in the context of GI, may help in alleviating bacterial overgrowth in conditions such as SIBO and ameliorating nutritional deficiencies [34]. Antibiotics are a useful treatment options for scleroderma patients. Small intestinal bacterial overgrowth (SIBO) occurs with a 39% prevalence in patients with scleroderma and can have a range of associated symptoms. Thus, antibiotics may be useful treatment options in patients with scleroderma who also suffer from GI dysmotility [35, 36]. For example, erythromycin, is an antibiotic widely used in treat chest infections and skin conditions, which has also been tested to see gastric emptying in scleroderma patients with GI motility issues.

18.3.2.2 Side Effects

Most antibiotics can cause gastrointestinal side effects including nausea, diarrhea, abdominal pain, bloating, and loss of appetite. This is due to negative effects on gut flora, even cases such as treating GI bacteria overgrowth [37].

18.3.2.3 Utility and Implications in Scleroderma

Rifaximin, a drug commonly used to treat traveler's diarrhea and IBS symptoms has been effective in the management of diarrhea and other symptoms in patients scleroderma patients with SIBO. However, SIBO often recurs, and may require multiple courses of antibiotics. Thus, further measures for bacterial stabilization may be needed to promote normal gut motility and prevent recurrence of SIBO in scleroderma patients [38]. Additionally, rifaximin may be limited in its use to it being difficult to acquire and expensive [39]. Thus, other antibiotics are often used first. Another study investigated the effectiveness of the antibiotic metronidazole and probiotic *Saccharomyces boulardii* in treating patients with SSc and SIBO. The patients were either given metronidazole (M group), *Saccharomyces boulardii* (SB group), or both (M+SB group). The results revealed that SIBO was eradicated in 55% of the M+SB group, 33% of the SB group, and 25% of the M group. Thus, it was concluded that the antibiotic Metronidazole as part of a combination therapy can help improve gastrointestinal symptoms in patients with SSc [40].

Scleroderma patients often have emptying abnormalities related to the esophagus and stomach and may have small intestine dysfunction [41]. One particular study tested the effects of the antibiotic erythromycin on 12 scleroderma patients. The treatment was administered for weeks, at a 250 mg oral dose three times daily. Additionally, the effects of a single IV dose prior to the oral treatment was also evaluated. The effects were measured by sonography after a meal. Single IV administration reduced gastric emptying while accelerating gallbladder emptying, while the oral 4 week treatment also has similar effects. Overall, erythromycin was found to help stimulate GI motility in patients with scleroderma by accelerating and reducing both gastric and gallbladder emptying time along with GI symptoms [42].

18.3.2.4 Conclusion

Evidence shows that the use of antibiotics such as rifaximin, metronidazole, and erythromycin can help in patients facing SIBO or GI dysmotility due to scleroderma. Supplementation of these antibiotics with probiotics may also be beneficial in helping alleviate GI manifestations in scleroderma/SSc patients [43]. Increasing relevant trials and optimization of antibiotic treatments for the may help mor effectively ameliorate GI dysmotility in scleroderma patients.

18.4 Colonic Dysmotility

18.4.1 Laxatives

18.4.1.1 Background/Mechanism of Action

Laxatives are a type of medication frequently used as a treatment for constipation, secondary to lifestyle modification. There are various types of laxatives classified by their mechanism of action, including stimulant, osmotic and surface active agents, that may be used in patients with scleroderma [44]. Osmotic laxatives have poor gut absorption and pull water into the content of stool. This allows softening of the stool, making it easier to pass [45]. Examples of osmotic laxatives include lactulose, sorbitol, and polyethylene glycol (PEG) [44]. Stimulant laxatives act on the mucosa of the intestines, helping stimulate contractions and increase secretion of both water and electrolytes [46]. Common examples include bisacodyl and senna [44]. Surface active agents, such as docusate, reduce the surface tension of oil and water within stool, allowing for movement of these into the stool to help in managing constipation [47].

18.4.1.2 Side Effects

Osmotic laxatives may cause partial ion absorption which can lead to metabolic disturbances [48]. Additional common side effects include bloating, abdominal cramps, and intestinal gas [49]. Stimulant laxatives are known to cause abdominal pain, may cause muscular injury, electrolyte disturbances, risk of dehydration, and possible carcinogenic risk [44, 50]. The use of docusate can cause irritation if taken in syrup or liquid formulations. Additionally abdominal pain, nausea and vomiting, and potential hypersensitivity may result from docusate use [47].

18.4.1.3 Utility and Implications in Scleroderma

Many patients with scleroderma have SIBO as mentioned previously. Some of these patients may have a hard time with fiber intake due to underlying SIBO, Thus, osmotic laxatives (e.g. PEG) may be useful in patients who have slow transit of stool [3, 51]. Stimulant laxatives, such as senna and bisacodyl, are usually preferred over osmotic laxatives due to the potential to worsen existing electrolyte imbalances and need for dose escalation [52]. Additionally, stimulant laxatives are often effective in combination with stool softeners [3]. However, patients need to be educated on the risk of diarrhea with stimulant laxatives and subsequent dehydration and electrolyte disturbances. Additionally, caution should be used in patients with overlap Sjogren's syndrome due to exacerbation of dryness.

18.4.1.4 Conclusion

Though it is well-established that many patients with scleroderma have GI manifestations, including constipation, clinical trials on optimized laxative treatment in patients with scleroderma are limited [53]. Further research and evaluation of laxatives discussed in this section may provide a better understanding of laxative drugs that work best for scleroderma patients with constipation.

18.4.2 Prucalopride

18.4.2.1 Background/Mechanism of Action

Prucalopride is a 5-HT4 receptor agonist that has demonstrated efficacy as a colonic prokinetic agent [54]. Receptor binding on presynaptic cholinergic neurons leads to acetylcholine release that promotes longitudinal smooth muscle contraction. Studies have conversely shown that 5-HT_4 agonism promotes relaxation of colonic circular smooth muscle. In all, induction of longitudinal propulsive contraction with decreased circular contraction facilitates forward motility [54].

18.4.2.2 Side Effects

Reported side effects with prucalopride treatment include headache, nausea, abdominal pain, and diarrhea [55]. Prucalopride also has a greater selectivity for the 5-HT_4 receptor compared to other similar drugs, such as cisapride, causing it to have a more favorable cardiovascular profile [5, 55]. Specifically in scleroderma patients, reported side effects comparably include headache, abdominal pain, dizziness, and sensation of feeling sick [56].

18.4.2.3 Utility and Implications in Scleroderma

A case report presented by Boeckxstaens, et al. demonstrated the beneficial use of prucalopride in two patients with scleroderma and secondary disordered motility that were refractory to laxatives, octreotide, and other prokinetic agents [57].

The first patient was a 60-year-old female with chronic scleroderma involving severe constipation and incontinence with paradoxical diarrhea. Other symptoms included dysphagia, early satiety, and abdominal distention. Treatment with prucalopride 2 mg once a day led to increased appetite, decreased abdominal distention, daily defecation, and decreased fecal incontinence. Manometry studies showed increased postprandial motility in the antrum and the duodenum; total colonic transit time also decreased [57]. The second patient was a 30-year-old female with scleroderma and Sjögren's syndrome with symptoms of dysphagia, loss of appetite, abdominal pain, and abdominal distention. Initiation of prucalopride 2 mg once a day led to increased appetite, decreased abdominal distention, and normalization of defecation. Postprandial motility increased in the antrum and small intestine, and colonic transit time decreased with treatment [57]. In both patients, treatment had little to no effect on dysphagia [57].

An open-label crossover study of prucalopride also has demonstrated its efficaciousness in scleroderma, finding treatment to be significantly associated with increased intestinal evacuation and improvement in University of California Los Angeles gastrointestinal tract (UCLA GIT) 2.0 questionnaire scores for constipation, reflux, and bloating. Orocecal transit times were significantly decreased with treatment [56].

18.4.2.4 Conclusion

Prucalopride is an effective agent with observed effects on improving overall GI motility but also demonstrable utility in scleroderma patients. The drug may be particularly helpful in cases of dysmotility that have been refractory to other agents. Care should be taken to counsel patients on prominent side effects—headaches, abdominal pain, and diarrhea (a predicted effect of the therapeutic prokinetic actions of the drug).

18.4.3 Linaclotide

18.4.3.1 Background/Mechanism of Action

Linaclotide is a granulate cyclase (GC-C) selective agonist that has prosecretory and prokinetic actions and has been used to treat refractory constipation in other GI disorders, such as inflammatory bowel syndrome (IBS). In activating GC-C, there is an increase in cyclic guanosine monophosphate (cGMP) that promotes intestinal fluid secretion. Specifically as a second messenger, cGMP activates the Cystic Fibrosis Transmembrane Conductance Regulator (CFTR) channel, causing secretion of chloride and bicarbonate ions into the lumen of the intestine; fluid is secreted in turn, and motility is enhanced [58]. Linaclotide's effects on motility have been well-studied in IBS, particularly the constipation predominant subtype (IBS-C), showing significant symptom relief in accordance with FDA response end points [59, 60].

18.4.3.2 Side Effects

In studies of IBS patients, diarrhea was the most common side effect to cause discontinuation of linaclotide use [59] and was a statistically significant side effect that differed from placebo groups [60]. Other reported side effects of significance include abdominal pain and flatulence [59]. In scleroderma patients, common reported side effects similarly include diarrhea, cramping, and bloating, with a potential dose-dependent effect [61].

18.4.3.3 Utility and Implications in Scleroderma

Studies investigating the utility of linaclotide directly in patients with scleroderma are limited. One retrospective case series analysis was conducted of clinical data from patients at the Johns Hopkins Scleroderma Center who were treated with linaclotide for refractory lower GI disease [61]. Treatment response to the medication was characterized by improvement in number of bowel movements, stool consistency, ease of evacuation, and/or associated symptoms (e.g., abdominal pain, bloating, distention). Patients were treated with linaclotide for a mean of 22.6 months, and 90.3% of patients had a treatment repsonse [61].

18.4.3.4 Conclusion

Linaclotide is an agent with indications for stimulation of motility in cases of chronic constipation. Its side effect profile has been reported as safe, and it has shown promise in treating refractory lower GI symptoms in scleroderma. However, further studies and clinical trials are certainly needed to further elucidate its applications in this patient population.

18.4.4 Lubiprostone

18.4.4.1 Background/Mechanism of Action

Traditionally, lubiprostone has been characterized as an activator of type 2-chloride channels (ClC-2) in enteric epithelial cells. In the GI tract, activation of ClC-2 leads to an efflux of chloride ions into the lumen, causing sodium ions to follow suit via a paracellular route. Secretion of water follows similarly through a paracellular path to maintain isotonicity [62]. However, more recent data suggests that lubiprostone may actually act through the Prostaglandin E2 receptor 4 (EP4 receptor) to increase

CFTR-dependent chloride secretion, while internalization of ClC-2 channels causes decreased chloride ion reabsorption. Nevertheless, the net effect of the drug is chloride and fluid secretion into the intestinal lumen, causing peristalsis, colonic relaxation, and decreased transit times [63]. The drug's positive effects on motility in healthy patients have been demonstrated in a study by Camilleri, et al., particularly finding decreased intestinal and colonic transit times [64].

18.4.4.2 Side Effects

The most common reported side effect of lubiprostone is dose-dependent nausea, which may be secondary to distention due to increased intestinal fluid secretion [63]. Studies evaluating the safety profile of lubiprostone have supported that it is well-tolerated, with low to no incidence of serious adverse effects. A study in healthy participants reported that the most frequent side effects were nausea, vomiting, and abdominal cramps [63]. In IBS-C patients, lubiprostone has been found to cause nausea, diarrhea, urinary tract infection, sinusitis, and abdominal distention [65]. In chronic constipation patients, lubiprostone has been found to cause headache, nausea, diarrhea, abdominal distention, and abdominal pain [66].

18.4.4.3 Utility and Implications in Scleroderma

To date, there is scarce literature on the application of lubiprostone in patients with scleroderma, especially in testing its effects in this population via clinical trial. However, lubiprostone has been well-studied in treating chronic constipation, which may be a GI manifestation of scleroderma. It is currently FDA-approved for the treatment of chronic idiopathic constipation (CIC) at 24 g twice a day. In the treatment of constipation, lubiprostone has positive effects on spontaneous bowel movements, stool consistency, straining, and constipation severity [67, 68].

18.4.4.4 Conclusion

A trial of lubiprostone perhaps may be considered in scleroderma patients who have not adequately responded to other prokinetic agents that have been more well-studied in this population. Given its efficaciousness and FDA approval in treating CIC, its use in scleroderma may reasonably be comparable. However, more substantial research and clinical trials are needed to form stronger, evidence-based treatment recommendations.

18.4.5 *Pyridostigmine*

18.4.5.1 Background/Mechanism of Action

Pyridostigmine is a reversible acetylcholinesterase inhibitor; it increases acetylcholine concentrations at synapses, enhancing transmission at neuromuscular junctions [69]. While it is primarily indicated for the treatment of myasthenia gravis, it has shown some promise in treating GI dysmotility, as acetylcholine is a primary excitatory neurotransmitter in intestinal smooth muscle [70]. A study of pyridostigmine treatment in patients with severe constipation or recurrent pseudo-obstruction found that all patients with pseudo-obstruction had significant improvement in reported symptoms [71]. Another study investigating treatment of pyridostigmine versus bisacodyl (standard treatment) in chronic constipation found that pyridostigmine improved symptoms similarly to bisacodyl with regard to weekly defecation frequency, pain score, time of defection, and Bristol Stool Form Scale [69].

18.4.5.2 Side Effects

In a study of pyridostigmine treatment in scleroderma patients, the most commonly reported side effect of therapy was diarrhea; less commonly reported side effects included abdominal pain, nausea, bloating, and dizziness [70]. Other studies in different patient populations support pyridostigmine being overall well-tolerated; some side effects that were attributed to therapy included headache, bloating, dry mouth, nausea, and mild muscle twitching [71, 72]. While not a common side effect, cholinergic toxicity is a possibility with this agent, and patients should be cautioned regarding signs [5].

18.4.5.3 Utility and Implications in Scleroderma

Research delineating the efficacy of pyridostigmine treatment in scleroderma is limited. Ahuja, et al. did evaluate its use in this population through a retrospective case series analysis of scleroderma patients with GI symptoms refractory to first-line therapy who were treated with pyridostigmine for at least four weeks [70]. Responders were defined as having a documented clinical benefit by the treating physician or as a response from the patient. 51.6% of patients had self-reported symptomatic improvement; the most common improved symptom was constipation [70].

18.4.5.4 Conclusion

Pyridostigmine has the potential to successfully treat refractory GI disease in scleroderma, especially in those with prominent constipation symptoms. Studies have supported that it is well-tolerated, with a low-risk safety profile. Trialing pyridostigmine for its prokinetic effects after established first-line therapies may be beneficial; nevertheless, more research is needed in those with scleroderma to better understand its potential.

18.5 Other Considerations

18.5.1 Opioids and Opioid Reversal Agents

18.5.1.1 Background/Mechanism of Action

A high concentration of opioid receptors is found within the enteric nervous system, in addition to immune and muscular cells [73]. Along with their role in the transmission of pain signals, opioid receptors in intestines and stomach also have a role in transmission of signals important for motor gastrointestinal function [73]. The release of opioid peptides causes activation of opioid receptors in the gastrointestinal tract leading to an increase in sphincter tone, blocked peristalsis, and inhibited gastric emptying [74].

Opioid reversal agents serve as a peripheral and selective opioid antagonist in the treatment of constipation in chronic illness refractory to laxatives [75]. An example of a peripherally acting mu-opioid receptor antagonist is methylnaltrexone which displaces opioids from mu-receptors in the GI tract, improving constipation symptoms induced and enhanced by opioid receptor binding [75]. Naloxegol is another example which also serves as a peripherally acting selective mu-opioid receptor antagonist to prevent opioid induced constipation [75]. Both methylnaltrexone and naloxegol can be used in the treatment of chronic constipation in chronic illness for patients who do not have an effective or prolonged response to laxatives [75].

18.5.1.2 Side Effects

General side effects of most opioids include respiratory depression, decrease GI motility, nausea, vomiting, constipation, sedation, and bloating [76]. With respect to the usage of opioids such as tramadol and oxycodone on pain treatment in scleroderma specifically, oxycodone showed efficacy with limited side effects. Side effects were characterized as itching, nausea, dizziness, and constipation.

The most common adverse effect of naloxone, an opioid reversal agent, is acute opioid withdrawal [77]. Due to opioids' highly addictive potential, the administration of an opioid reversal agent acutely may precipitate acute opioid withdrawal symptoms such as agitation, nausea, vomiting, diarrhea, irritability, and anxiety [77].

18.5.1.3 Utility and Implications in Scleroderma

Opioid reversal agents have not been studied deeply in treating gastrointestinal symptoms associated with scleroderma. Yet, digital ulcers are a common complication in patients with scleroderma, often causing severe pain and decreased quality of life [78]. A case report was done to report the efficacy and safety of oxycodone/naloxone in treating digital ulcers in patients with scleroderma [78]. The findings showed that the combination therapy caused adequate pain relief and increased adherence to therapy [78]. Additionally, a systematic review was done to explore the utility of naltrexone in various dermatologic conditions, including scleroderma [79]. It was shown that low-dose naltrexone was safe and effective in pruritis associated with scleroderma, and there more information needed to elucidate appropriate dosing and long-term treatment recommendations [79].

18.5.1.4 Conclusion

Evidently, the utility of opioid antagonists and reversal agents has not been widely implicated in treating GI dysmotility in scleroderma. Despite their benefits in treating other complications of scleroderma, there is insufficient data to form a conclusion regarding opioid reversal agents' ability to treat scleroderma induced gastric dysmotility.

18.5.1.5 Overall Conclusions

Scleroderma is a connective tissue disorder involving thickening and hardening of the skin. In localized cases it affects the skin, muscles, and bones. In diffuse scleroderma, involvement of internal organs is often present and as reviewed in this chapter, gastrointestinal manifestations occur in up to 90% of patients with systemic sclerosis (SSc). These GI manifestations include but are not limited to GERD, gastroparesis, SIBO, dysphagia, and fecal incontinence [80].

Many medications that are used for GI dysmotility have not been thoroughly reviewed in their effectiveness in SSc patients. However, many medications commonly prescribed for different GI dysmotility disorders are still prescribed for SSc patients. In this chapter, we categorized the many drugs into three major sections based on their primary targets: gastric dysmotility, small intestinal dysmotility, and colonic dysmotility. For gastric dysmotility, bethanechol, metoclopramide, and buspirone may be more frequently prescribed in patients with SSc. Commonly prescribed drugs for GERD are various promotility agents, though certain drugs need to be used with much caution due to side effects such as cisapride. With small intestinal dysmotility, antidiarrheals such as loperamide are frequently prescribed through further studies may need to be conducted to gauge the true effectiveness of this medication in the context of SSc. Antibiotics may also be used, helping with gastric motility, emptying, and LES tone. Finally, drugs for colonic dysmotility that include prucalopride and pyridostigmine which have been better evaluated in their used for this specific patient population. Overall, despite the existence of numerous medical therapies for GI dysmotility, many still need to be optimized specifically in the context of treating patients with SSc.

References

1. Rongioletti F, Ferreli C, Atzori L, Bottoni U, Soda G. Scleroderma with an update about clinico-pathological correlation. G Ital Dermatol Venereol. 2018;153:208–15. https://doi.org/10.23736/s0392-0488.18.05922-9.
2. Lauritano D, Bussolati A, Baldoni M, Leonida A. Scleroderma and CREST syndrome: a case report in dentistry. Minerva Stomatol. 2011;60:443–65.
3. Nagaraja V, McMahan ZH, Getzug T, Khanna D. Management of gastrointestinal involvement in scleroderma. Curr Treatm Opt Rheumatol. 2015;1:82–105. https://doi.org/10.1007/s40674-014-0005-0.
4. Li B, et al. Esophageal dysfunction in systemic sclerosis: an update. Rheumatol Ther. 2021;8:1535–49. https://doi.org/10.1007/s40744-021-00382-0.
5. Cheah JX, Khanna D, McMahan ZH. Management of scleroderma gastrointestinal disease: lights and shadows. J Scleroderma Relat Disord. 2022;7:85–97. https://doi.org/10.1177/23971983221086343.
6. Deane AM, Chapman MJ, Reintam Blaser A, McClave SA, Emmanuel A. Pathophysiology and treatment of gastrointestinal motility disorders in the acutely ill. Nutr Clin Pract. 2019;34:23–36. https://doi.org/10.1002/ncp.10199.
7. Law NM, Bharucha AE, Undale AS, Zinsmeister AR. Cholinergic stimulation enhances colonic motor activity, transit, and sensation in humans. Am J Physiol Gastrointest Liver Physiol. 2001;281:G1228–37. https://doi.org/10.1152/ajpgi.2001.281.5.G1228.
8. Pakala RS, Brown KN, Preuss CV. StatPearls. StatPearls Publishing Copyright © 2023, StatPearls Publishing LLC; 2023.
9. Katschinski M, et al. Gastrointestinal motor and secretory responses to cholinergic stimulation in humans. Differential modulation by muscarinic and cholecystokinin receptor blockade. Eur J Clin Investig. 1995;25:113–22. https://doi.org/10.1111/j.1365-2362.1995.tb01535.x.
10. Agrawal A, Hila A, Tutuian R, Mainie I, Castell DO. Bethanechol improves smooth muscle function in patients with severe ineffective esophageal motility. J Clin Gastroenterol. 2007;41:366–70. https://doi.org/10.1097/01.mcg.0000225542.03880.68.
11. Kumar S, et al. Role of muscarinic-3 receptor antibody in systemic sclerosis: correlation with disease duration and effects of IVIG. Am J Physiol Gastrointest Liver Physiol. 2016;310:G1052–60. https://doi.org/10.1152/ajpgi.00034.2016.
12. Voulgaris TA, Karamanolis GP. Esophageal manifestation in patients with scleroderma. World J Clin Cases. 2021;9:5408–19. https://doi.org/10.12998/wjcc.v9.i20.5408.

13. Miller JB, Gandhi N, Clarke J, McMahan Z. Gastrointestinal involvement in systemic sclerosis: an update. J Clin Rheumatol. 2018;24:328–37. https://doi.org/10.1097/rhu.0000000000000626.
14. Isola S, Hussain A, Dua A, Singh K, Adams N. StatPearls. StatPearls Publishing Copyright © 2023, StatPearls Publishing LLC; 2023.
15. Shah AA, Wigley FM. My approach to the treatment of scleroderma. Mayo Clin Proc. 2013;88:377–93. https://doi.org/10.1016/j.mayocp.2013.01.018.
16. Ortiz A, et al. Cardiovascular safety profile and clinical experience with high-dose domperidone therapy for nausea and vomiting. Am J Med Sci. 2015;349:421–4. https://doi.org/10.1097/maj.0000000000000439.
17. Barbey JT, Lazzara R, Zipes DP. Spontaneous adverse event reports of serious ventricular arrhythmias, QT prolongation, syncope, and sudden death in patients treated with cisapride. J Cardiovasc Pharmacol Ther. 2002;7:65–76. https://doi.org/10.1177/107424840200700202.
18. Takeuchi H, Mori Y, Tsutsumi Y. Pathophysiology, prognosis and treatment of tardive dyskinesia. Ther Adv Psychopharmacol. 2022;12:20451253221117313. https://doi.org/10.1177/20451253221117313.
19. Sjogren RW. Gastrointestinal features of scleroderma. Curr Opin Rheumatol. 1996;8:569–75. https://doi.org/10.1097/00002281-199611000-00012.
20. Denaxas K, Ladas SD, Karamanolis GP. Evaluation and management of esophageal manifestations in systemic sclerosis. Ann Gastroenterol. 2018;31:165–70. https://doi.org/10.20524/aog.2018.0228.
21. Wang RZ, Vashistha V, Kaur S, Houchens NW. Serotonin syndrome: preventing, recognizing, and treating it. Cleve Clin J Med. 2016;83:810–7. https://doi.org/10.3949/ccjm.83a.15129.
22. Karamanolis GP, et al. Beneficial effect of the 5-HT1A receptor agonist buspirone on esophageal dysfunction associated with systemic sclerosis: a pilot study. United European Gastroenterol J. 2015;3:266–71. https://doi.org/10.1177/2050640614560453.
23. Karamanolis GP, et al. The 5-HT1A receptor agonist buspirone improves esophageal motor function and symptoms in systemic sclerosis: a 4-week, open-label trial. Arthritis Res Ther. 2016;18:195. https://doi.org/10.1186/s13075-016-1094-y.
24. Schutyser W, Cruyt L, Vulsteke JB, Lenaerts JL, De Langhe E. The role of high-resolution manometry in the assessment of upper gastrointestinal involvement in systemic sclerosis: a systematic review. Clin Rheumatol. 2020;39:149–57. https://doi.org/10.1007/s10067-019-04794-w.
25. Sahi N, Nguyen R, Santos C. StatPearls. StatPearls Publishing Copyright © 2023, StatPearls Publishing LLC; 2023.
26. Nassar M, et al. Gastrointestinal involvement in systemic sclerosis: an updated review. Medicine (Baltimore). 2022;101:e31780. https://doi.org/10.1097/md.0000000000031780.
27. Galligan JJ, Sternini C. Insights into the role of opioid receptors in the GI tract: experimental evidence and therapeutic relevance. Handb Exp Pharmacol. 2017;239:363–78. https://doi.org/10.1007/164_2016_116.
28. Jain M, Wylie WP. StatPearls. StatPearls Publishing Copyright © 2023, StatPearls Publishing LLC; 2023.
29. Tansel A, Levinthal DJ. Understanding our tests: hydrogen-methane breath testing to diagnose small intestinal bacterial overgrowth. Clin Transl Gastroenterol. 2023;14:e00567. https://doi.org/10.14309/ctg.0000000000000567.
30. Wu PE, Juurlink DN. Clinical review: loperamide toxicity. Ann Emerg Med. 2017;70:245–52. https://doi.org/10.1016/j.annemergmed.2017.04.008.
31. Eggleston W, et al. Loperamide toxicity: recommendations for patient monitoring and management. Clin Toxicol (Philadelphia, Pa). 2020;58:355–9. https://doi.org/10.1080/15563650.2019.1681443.
32. Thoua NM, Schizas A, Forbes A, Denton CP, Emmanuel AV. Internal anal sphincter atrophy in patients with systemic sclerosis. Rheumatology (Oxford). 2011;50:1596–602. https://doi.org/10.1093/rheumatology/ker153.

33. Butt S, Emmanuel A. Systemic sclerosis and the gut. Expert Rev Gastroenterol Hepatol. 2013;7:331–9. https://doi.org/10.1586/egh.13.22.
34. Sorathia SJ, Chippa V, Rivas JM. StatPearls. StatPearls Publishing Copyright © 2023, StatPearls Publishing LLC; 2023.
35. Morrisroe K, Baron M, Frech T, Nikpour M. Small intestinal bacterial overgrowth in systemic sclerosis. J Scleroderma Relat Disord. 2020;5:33–9. https://doi.org/10.1177/2397198319863953.
36. Polkowska-Pruszyńska B, Gerkowicz A, Szczepanik-Kułak P, Krasowska D. Small intestinal bacterial overgrowth in systemic sclerosis: a review of the literature. Arch Dermatol Res. 2019;311:1–8. https://doi.org/10.1007/s00403-018-1874-0.
37. Mohsen S, Dickinson JA, Somayaji R. Update on the adverse effects of antimicrobial therapies in community practice. Can Fam Physician. 2020;66:651–9.
38. Cheah JX, Khanna D, McMahan ZH. Management of scleroderma gastrointestinal disease: lights and shadows. J Scleroderma Related Disord. 2022;7:85–97. https://doi.org/10.1177/23971983221086343.
39. Shah ED, et al. Comparing costs and outcomes of treatments for irritable bowel syndrome with diarrhea: cost-benefit analysis. Clin Gastroenterol Hepatol. 2022;20:136–144.e131. https://doi.org/10.1016/j.cgh.2020.09.043.
40. García-Collinot G, et al. Effectiveness of Saccharomyces boulardii and metronidazole for small intestinal bacterial overgrowth in systemic sclerosis. Dig Dis Sci. 2020;65:1134–43. https://doi.org/10.1007/s10620-019-05830-0.
41. Di Ciaula A, et al. Gastrointestinal symptoms and motility disorders in patients with systemic scleroderma. BMC Gastroenterol. 2008;8:7. https://doi.org/10.1186/1471-230X-8-7.
42. Fiorucci S, Distrutti E, Gerli R, Morelli A. Effect of erythromycin on gastric and gallbladder emptying and gastrointestinal symptoms in scleroderma patients is maintained medium term. Am J Gastroenterol. 1994;89:550–5.
43. Luquez-Mindiola A, Atuesta AJ, Gómez-Aldana AJ. Gastrointestinal manifestations of systemic sclerosis: an updated review. World J Clin Cases. 2021;9:6201–17. https://doi.org/10.12998/wjcc.v9.i22.6201.
44. Bashir A, Sizar O. StatPearls. StatPearls Publishing Copyright © 2023, StatPearls Publishing LLC; 2023.
45. Gordon M, MacDonald JK, Parker CE, Akobeng AK, Thomas AG. Osmotic and stimulant laxatives for the management of childhood constipation. Cochrane Database Syst Rev. 2016;2016:Cd009118. https://doi.org/10.1002/14651858.CD009118.pub3.
46. Sayuk GS, Waldman SA, Brenner DM. Mechanisms of action of current pharmacologic options for the treatment of chronic idiopathic constipation and irritable bowel syndrome with constipation. Off J Am Coll Gastroenterol | ACG. 2022;117:S6–S13. https://doi.org/10.14309/ajg.0000000000001687.
47. Hannoodee S, Patel P, Annamaraju P. StatPearls. StatPearls Publishing Copyright © 2023, StatPearls Publishing LLC; 2023.
48. Xing JH, Soffer EE. Adverse effects of laxatives. Dis Colon Rectum. 2001;44:1201–9. https://doi.org/10.1007/BF02234645.
49. Sumida K, Yamagata K, Kovesdy CP. Constipation in CKD. Kidney Int Rep. 2020;5:121–34. https://doi.org/10.1016/j.ekir.2019.11.002.
50. Noergaard M, Traerup Andersen J, Jimenez-Solem E, Bring Christensen M. Long term treatment with stimulant laxatives—clinical evidence for effectiveness and safety? Scand J Gastroenterol. 2019;54:27–34. https://doi.org/10.1080/00365521.2018.1563806.
51. Pittman N, et al. Treatment of small intestinal bacterial overgrowth in systemic sclerosis: a systematic review. Rheumatology. 2018;57:1802–11. https://doi.org/10.1093/rheumatology/key175.
52. McFarlane IM, et al. Gastrointestinal manifestations of systemic sclerosis. Rheumatology (Sunnyvale). 2018;8 https://doi.org/10.4172/2161-1149.1000235.

53. Shreiner AB, Murray C, Denton C, Khanna D. Gastrointestinal manifestations of systemic sclerosis. J Scleroderma Relat Disord. 2016;1:247–56. https://doi.org/10.5301/jsrd.5000214.
54. Wong BS, Manabe N, Camilleri M. Role of prucalopride, a serotonin (5-HT(4)) receptor agonist, for the treatment of chronic constipation. Clin Exp Gastroenterol. 2010;3:49–56. https://doi.org/10.2147/ceg.s8091.
55. Camilleri M, Kerstens R, Rykx A, Vandeplassche L. A placebo-controlled trial of prucalopride for severe chronic constipation. N Engl J Med. 2008;358:2344–54. https://doi.org/10.1056/NEJMoa0800670.
56. Vigone B, et al. Preliminary safety and efficacy profile of prucalopride in the treatment of systemic sclerosis (SSc)-related intestinal involvement: results from the open label cross-over PROGASS study. Arthritis Res Ther. 2017;19:145. https://doi.org/10.1186/s13075-017-1340-y.
57. Heim RA, et al. Alternative splicing of rat tropoelastin mRNA is tissue-specific and developmentally regulated. Matrix. 1991;11:359–66. https://doi.org/10.1016/s0934-8832(11)80207-6.
58. Thomas RH, Allmond K. Linaclotide (Linzess) for irritable bowel syndrome with constipation and for chronic idiopathic constipation. P T. 2013;38:154–60.
59. Rao S, et al. A 12-week, randomized, controlled trial with a 4-week randomized withdrawal period to evaluate the efficacy and safety of linaclotide in irritable bowel syndrome with constipation. Am J Gastroenterol. 2012;107:1714–24. https://doi.org/10.1038/ajg.2012.255; quiz p 1725
60. Chey WD, et al. Linaclotide for irritable bowel syndrome with constipation: a 26-week, randomized, double-blind, placebo-controlled trial to evaluate efficacy and safety. Am J Gastroenterol. 2012;107:1702–12. https://doi.org/10.1038/ajg.2012.254.
61. Dein EJ, Wigley FM, McMahan ZH. Linaclotide for the treatment of refractory lower bowel manifestations of systemic sclerosis. BMC Gastroenterol. 2021;21:174. https://doi.org/10.1186/s12876-021-01738-0.
62. Lacy BE, Levy LC. Lubiprostone: a novel treatment for chronic constipation. Clin Interv Aging. 2008;3:357–64. https://doi.org/10.2147/cia.s2938.
63. Wilson N, Schey R. Lubiprostone in constipation: clinical evidence and place in therapy. Ther Adv Chronic Dis. 2015;6:40–50. https://doi.org/10.1177/2040622314567678.
64. Camilleri M, et al. Effect of a selective chloride channel activator, lubiprostone, on gastrointestinal transit, gastric sensory, and motor functions in healthy volunteers. Am J Physiol Gastrointest Liver Physiol. 2006;290:G942–7. https://doi.org/10.1152/ajpgi.00264.2005.
65. Chey WD, et al. Safety and patient outcomes with lubiprostone for up to 52 weeks in patients with irritable bowel syndrome with constipation. Aliment Pharmacol Ther. 2012;35:587–99. https://doi.org/10.1111/j.1365-2036.2011.04983.x.
66. Lembo AJ, et al. Long-term safety and effectiveness of lubiprostone, a chloride channel (ClC-2) activator, in patients with chronic idiopathic constipation. Dig Dis Sci. 2011;56:2639–45. https://doi.org/10.1007/s10620-011-1801-0.
67. Barish CF, Drossman D, Johanson JF, Ueno R. Efficacy and safety of lubiprostone in patients with chronic constipation. Dig Dis Sci. 2010;55:1090–7. https://doi.org/10.1007/s10620-009-1068-x.
68. Johanson JF, Morton D, Geenen J, Ueno R. Multicenter, 4-week, double-blind, randomized, placebo-controlled trial of lubiprostone, a locally-acting type-2 chloride channel activator, in patients with chronic constipation. Am J Gastroenterol. 2008;103:170–7. https://doi.org/10.1111/j.1572-0241.2007.01524.x.
69. Soufi-Afshar I, Moghadamnia A, Bijani A, Kazemi S, Shokri-Shirvani J. Comparison of pyridostigmine and bisacodyl in the treatment of refractory chronic constipation. Caspian J Intern Med. 2016;7:19–24.
70. Ahuja NK, Mische L, Clarke JO, Wigley FM, McMahan ZH. Pyridostigmine for the treatment of gastrointestinal symptoms in systemic sclerosis. Semin Arthritis Rheum. 2018;48:111–6. https://doi.org/10.1016/j.semarthrit.2017.12.007.

71. O'Dea CJ, Brookes JH, Wattchow DA. The efficacy of treatment of patients with severe constipation or recurrent pseudo-obstruction with pyridostigmine. Color Dis. 2010;12:540–8. https://doi.org/10.1111/j.1463-1318.2009.01838.x.
72. Bharucha AE, et al. Pilot study of pyridostigmine in constipated patients with autonomic neuropathy. Clin Auton Res. 2008;18:194–202. https://doi.org/10.1007/s10286-008-0476-x.
73. Mosińska P, Zielińska M, Fichna J. Expression and physiology of opioid receptors in the gastrointestinal tract. Curr Opin Endocrinol Diabetes Obes. 2016;23:3–10. https://doi.org/10.1097/med.0000000000000219.
74. Holzer P. Opioid receptors in the gastrointestinal tract. Regul Pept. 2009;155:11–7. https://doi.org/10.1016/j.regpep.2009.03.012.
75. Manabat ML. Intestinal motility disorders medication; 2020.
76. LiverTox: clinical and research information on drug-induced liver injury. National Institute of Diabetes and Digestive and Kidney Diseases; 2012.
77. Roy K, Bhattacharyya P, Deb I. Naloxone precipitated morphine withdrawal and clock genes expression in striatum: a comparative study in three different protocols for the development of morphine dependence. Neurosci Lett. 2018;685:24–9. https://doi.org/10.1016/j.neulet.2018.07.023.
78. Ughi N, Crotti C, Ingegnoli F. Effectiveness and safety of oxycodone/naloxone in the management of chronic pain in patients with systemic sclerosis with recurrent digital ulcers: two case reports. Clin Interv Aging. 2016;11:307–11. https://doi.org/10.2147/cia.S102577.
79. Ekelem C, Juhasz M, Khera P, Mesinkovska NA. Utility of naltrexone treatment for chronic inflammatory dermatologic conditions: a systematic review. JAMA Dermatol. 2019;155:229–36. https://doi.org/10.1001/jamadermatol.2018.4093.
80. Odonwodo A, Badri T, Hariz A. StatPearls. StatPearls Publishing Copyright © 2024, StatPearls Publishing LLC; 2024.

Chapter 19
Adverse Effects of Commonly Used Drugs to Treat Rheumatologic Conditions

Patrick J. Tempera, Joo Hye Park, and Nour A. Parsa

19.1 Nonsteroidal Antiinflammatory Drugs

Nonsteroidal antiinflammatory drugs (NSAIDs) have numerous medical indications including pain relief from discomfort associated with chronic conditions such as rheumatoid arthritis, osteoarthritis, juvenile arthritis, psoriatic arthritis, systemic lupus erythematosus, rheumatic fever, gout and gouty arthritis, and ankylosing spondylitis, among many other conditions. They are also readily available and easy to access [1].

Unfortunately, NSAIDs come with relatively high rates of gastrointestinal (GI) side effects. The medication alters mucus and bicarbonate secretions, reduces mucosal blood flow, affects neutrophilic function and leukocyte adherence to endothelium, and alters endothelial function. NSAID-induced prostaglandin reduction is central to most upper GI injuries, and the NSAID lesions correlate well with the medication's capacity to inhibit cyclooxygenase (COX) activity, thereby reducing mucosal prostaglandins. The majority of NSAIDs are nonspecific COX inhibitors that inhibit both the constitutively expressed COX1 and the inducible COX2

P. J. Tempera
Department of Medicine, Albany Medical Center, Albany, NY, USA
e-mail: temperp@amc.edu

J. H. Park
Department of Medicine, Division of Gastroenterology, Albany Medical Center, Albany, NY, USA
e-mail: parkj5@amc.edu

N. A. Parsa (✉)
Department Medicine, Division of Gastroenterology, Loma Linda University Medical Center, Loma Linda, CA, USA
e-mail: nparsa@llu.edu

M. Tadros et al. (eds.), *GI Diseases Associated with Rheumatological and Vasculitic Conditions*, Clinical Gastroenterology,
https://doi.org/10.1007/978-3-032-07868-1_19

isoenzymes of COX as seen in Fig. 19.1. While selective COX2 inhibitors do reduce the potential for NSAID induced side effects, this risk is not fully eliminated [1, 2].

The small bowel is unusual in that it is also affected by NSAIDs via a different mechanism. In NSAID-induced enteropathy, unlike upper GI injuries, the etiology is not primarily COX inhibition, as mentioned above. It is the enterohepatic circulation and the role of gut bacteria that are mostly responsible for small intestinal and some colonic lesions. The role of enteric flora is complex given that probiotics seem to be protective, while treatment with broad spectrum antibiotics may reduce the severity of NSAID-induced enteropathy. The lesions may be due to increased permeability of the mucosa, direct damage of intestinal cells, and uncoupling of oxidative phosphorylation [4]. Ultimately, NSAIDs can affect the entire GI tract and cause a wide range of adverse events that have clinical implications, as discussed further below.

NSAID use can induce ulcers and erosions in the esophagus, stomach, small bowel and colon. These lesions can lead to dyspepsia, bleeding, and anemia if they are extensive or unaddressed for a significant amount of time. Pill esophagitis, esophagitis dissecans and perforation are additional potential sequelae of NSAID use in the esophagus. Rarely, they can lead to esophageal perforation if the damage affects the majority of the tissue layers [1].

In the small bowel, NSAIDs can cause ulcers and erosions in the duodenum and distal ileum as well as diaphragm disease, which is multiple thin, concentric stenosing strictures that can lead to intermittent or complete bowel obstruction. The pathogenesis of diaphragm disease is not well understood, but it is thought that injury to enterocytes and villous microcirculation, and the subsequent inflammatory reaction leads to ulceration, which then develops circumferential fibrosis. The fibrosis results in the formation of strictures that resemble a "diaphragm" [5].

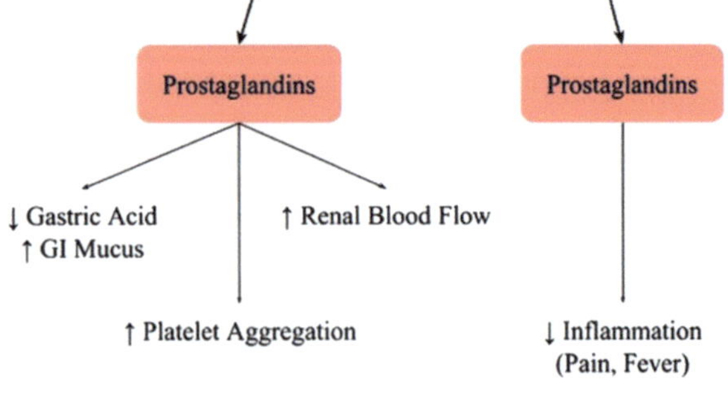

Fig. 19.1 Prostaglandin pathway with COX-1 and COX-2 inhibition. [3]

In the colon, NSAIDs can cause erosion, ulcers, and focal colitis. NSAIDs are also associated with collagenous and lymphocytic colitis (which are subsets of microscopic colitis). The pathogenesis leading to microscopic colitis likely begins with injury to both the mucosal layer and enterocytes in the intestinal barrier, leading to physiological dysfunction and increased intestinal permeability, which could lead to enhanced exposure to luminal triggers and acute inflammation. Like in the small bowel, NSAIDs can also cause diaphragm disease, particularly in the right colon. Last but not least, ischemic colitis can develop due spasms of the microvasculature as a consequence of inflammatory processes that include the release of vasoconstricting leukotrienes, free radicals, platelet thrombi, tumor necrosis factor-a, among other molecules [1, 6, 7].

Hepatic toxicity is another known side effect of NSAIDs. Injuries usually manifest as one of two patterns: acute hepatitis (with jaundice, nausea, fever, and elevated transaminase levels) and chronic active hepatitis (with abnormal labs and histopathology of the liver). The two predominant mechanisms of action for liver injury are hypersensitivity and metabolic aberration. Patients who have experienced hepatotoxicity from one NSAID often suffer the same reaction if the drug is reinitiated or with a similar drug with identical structure. Metabolic aberrations could be due to genetic polymorphisms and varied susceptibility to a spectrum of drugs related to mitochondrial impairment and oxidative stress [8].

19.2 Steroids

Glucocorticoids play an important role in the management of many rheumatologic diseases, with their therapeutic effects ranging from pain relief in arthritides, to disease-modifying effects in rheumatoid arthritis, and to strong immunosuppressive actions in vasculitides and systemic lupus erythematosus [9].

The effects of glucocorticoids are achieved by various different mechanisms. In low-dose therapy, genomic mechanisms lead to changes in gene expression via transactivation (where two activated glucocorticoid-cytosolic glucocorticoid receptor complexes bind to the promoter of glucocorticoid-regulated genes activate the synthesis of certain regulatory proteins) and transrepression (where the glucocorticoid-cytosolic glucocorticoid receptor monomer complexes interfere with the activity of proinflammatory transcription factors in order to downregulate synthesis of proinflammatory proteins). Genomic processes require at least thirty minutes before changes can be observed in regulatory protein synthesis, but usually it will take hours to days for changes to occur at the cell, tissue or organ level. In very high-dose therapy, nongenomic mechanisms also occur, effects of which are evident within minutes. These nongenomic mechanisms occur via the glucocorticoid receptors in the cytosol, cell membrane as well as nonspecific interactions with membranes of cells and organelles. The size of genomic effects of glucocorticoid preparations defines their dose equivalence. Dexamethasone and betamethasone are the most potent preparations, followed by methylprednisolone, predniso(lo)ne, cortisol and cortisone [9, 10].

Glucocorticoids, however, come with adverse effects like any medication, which are more frequent with chronic use and with higher doses. Gastrointestinal side effects that can be associated with glucocorticoid use include GI irritation (nausea, vomiting, mild abdominal pain or discomfort), peptic ulcer disease (PUD), GI bleed, and pancreatitis, which are discussed further below. It is important to note that intravenous (IV) and oral versions of glucocorticoids (particularly methylprednisolone) seem to be equally tolerated regardless of administration route [11, 12].

Current literature regarding the risk of PUD and GI bleeding is conflicting in patients who are on glucocorticoid monotherapy. Some studies show no increased risk of PUD for patients on glucocorticoid monotherapy regardless of dose while others find PUD to be a rare complication. Patients who are taking glucocorticoids may experience more symptoms of gastric irritation than those who are not, but several studies showed that these symptoms did not translate into an increased risk for PUD. Similarly, the data regarding the risk of GI bleed with glucocorticoid use is inconsistent between studies. However, glucocorticoid therapy with concomitant NSAID use has been shown to increase the risk of peptic ulcer disease and gastrointestinal bleeding and should be avoided in the majority of cases. Adding proton pump inhibitor therapy is generally recommended if it is necessary to take glucocorticoids with NSAID, as well as patients who have other reasons to be at high risk of developing PUD or GI bleed [9, 10].

Cases of glucocorticoid-induced bowel perforation and pancreatitis are conflicting as well, with some studies supporting the association while others unable to find a significant correlation. Other factors such as the inflammatory disease itself might also play a role [9].

19.3 Colchicine

As a drug that induces mitotic arrest, colchicine is commonly used in the treatment of gouty arthritis, Behcet's disease, and familial Mediterranean fever. The effects of this medication are seen in the proliferative compartments of the gastrointestinal glands, sparing the mature superficial epithelium and favoring the small bowel and antrum [1].

Common side effects include abdominal cramping, bloating, pain, vomiting, and diarrhea due to hyperperistalsis. These symptoms are usually mild and reversible with dose tapering or discontinuation of the drug. Other possible side effects include melena and peptic ulcers. Studies have reported effects on the liver in the form of increased liver enzymes, hepatitis, hepatotoxicity, and other hepatic abnormalities but without statistical significance.

Colchicine toxicity, usually in patients with renal insufficiency, can lead to a cholera-like syndrome associated with dehydration and shock. High or supratherapeutic doses may cause malabsorption of fat, D-xylose, and vitamins as well as erosions in stomach and duodenum [13, 14].

19.4 Febuxostat

Febuxostat is used for the treatment of gout, uric acid nephropathy, and hyperuricemia that is caused by malignancy and anti-cancer therapies. Mechanistically, it works by lowering serum uric acid levels which is beneficial in preventing gouty attacks. One of the main gastrointestinal complications associated with febuxostat is minor liver function test abnormalities. Liver test abnormalities have been reported in 2–13% of patients using febuxostat, however, these levels are mild-to-moderate and self-limiting after drug discontinuation. In performed clinical trials, these liver test abnormalities were the major reason for discontinuation. It is important to note that within these same clinical trials, there were no reports of jaundice or acute hepatitis. It is proposed that the reasoning behind this elevation in liver function testing is due to febuxostat's hepatic metabolism, the major pathway being glucuronidation with minor metabolism via the CYP 450 system [15]. These minor elevations in liver tests are self-limited and resolve with cessation of the drug but have also been shown to resolve with drug continuation. There have been no instances of acute liver failure or chronic liver injury ever reported. The exact mechanism by which the metabolism of Febuxostat causes minor liver test elevations is not completely known. Additionally, a second well documented gastrointestinal side effect of febuxostat is diarrhea which was illustrated in the CONFIRMS trial. This trial compared individuals with moderate renal impairment who were receiving allopurinol versus febuxostat as urate-lowering agents. It was shown that those individuals receiving febuxostat experienced higher rates of diarrhea when compared to its counterpart receiving allopurinol [16]. The exact mechanism by which Febuxostat causes diarrhea is now known. Further investigation as to why this may occur has not been adequately studied and its cause of diarrhea has only been observed as an association during clinical trials.

19.5 Pegloticase

Pegloticase is a commonly used rheumatologic medication for patients with chronic refractory and symptomatic gout. It functions as a recombinant DNA-produced enzyme that allows for urate clearance by the kidney, decreasing serum uric acid concentrations and alleviating the symptoms and complications of gout. Common gastrointestinal side effects of pegloticase include nausea, vomiting, and constipation. Due to its polypeptide structure, it is metabolized by serum and tissue proteases and is unlikely to be directly hepatotoxic. Thus far, there have been no published case reports of hepatotoxicity due to pegloticase. The medication label does not currently list liver injury as a potential side effect. Based on this data, pegloticase has a likelihood score of E translating to being an unlikely cause of clinically apparent liver injury [17, 18].

19.6 Analgesics

Along with the importance of medications specifically designed to curb the pathophysiology involved with rheumatologic disease, downstream and outward symptoms are also important therapeutic targets, such as pain. Adequate pain management is an important aspect in the treatment of patients with rheumatologic disease such as rheumatoid arthritis that can cause debilitating pain. In patients who have poor pain control, opioids are often used. Interestingly, no randomized controlled clinical trials exist that have examined the efficacy and benefit/risk ratio of opioids used in rheumatoid arthritis [19]. Although further randomized controlled trial studies are needed to determine the best use of opioids in rheumatoid arthritis, targeted use of existing opioid treatments are often still used to reduce pain [20]. However, many randomized clinical studies examining opioid use in musculoskeletal pain, like osteoarthritis, have extended the use of opioids.

Opioids are widely used for pain associated with rheumatologic disease and gastrointestinal side effects often coincide and limit their use. Due to where opioid receptors are located in the human body, specifically for our purposes within the GI tract and central nervous system, common side effects include nausea, vomiting, gastroesophageal reflux, and constipation. Once digested, opioid metabolites bind to opioid receptors on the enteric nervous circuitry controlling motility and secretion [21]. Once activated, these receptors inhibit gastric emptying, reduce mucosal secretion, and increase fluid reabsorption creating an environment conducive to constipation [22]. One strategy to combat such side effects is to use peripherally active opioid-receptor antagonists. These will serve to block the unwanted peripheral side effects without affecting the centrally based analgesic response [23]. An example of such a medication is Methylnaltrexone which is a peripherally targeting antagonist of the mu-opioid receptors in the tissues of the GI tract.

Nausea and vomiting are caused by activity of opioid receptors in the central nervous system and GI tract together and are thought to affect 25% of individuals treated with opioids [19]. There is reduction in gastric motility and activation of the chemoreceptor trigger zone as well as vestibular sensitivity that results in nausea with vomiting as the end motor consequence of nausea [19].

Although opioids have been shown to effectively control pain, it of course must be noted that opioid-associated GI side effects are an important health problem with both patient and economic consequences that must be considered by health professionals before opting for their use [24].

19.7 Muscle Relaxants

In addition to NSAIDs and analgesics, muscle relaxants have also been used to treat pain associated with rheumatologic disease. These include but are not limited to antispasmodic benzodiazepines and antispasmodic non-benzodiazepines such as cyclobenzaprine, methocarbamol, and tizanidine as well as anti-spasticity drugs like baclofen and dantrolene [25].

In terms of gastrointestinal side effects, asymptomatic elevations in serum aminotransferase levels have been observed. Muscle relaxant agents that have been linked to show direct liver toxicity leading to acute liver injury include chlorzoxazone and dantrolene. Although there have not been any formal prospective studies to date demonstrating AST and ALT elevations, rare instances do implicate chlorzoxazone as the culprit of liver disease. In these cases, there is consistency in presentation showing that there is a latency period of 1–4 weeks with a hepatocellular disease pattern, elevations in ALT, and jaundice. Recovery is rapid once the drug is discontinued. The cause of hepatocellular injury is thought to be due to a hypersensitivity reaction. Clinically, when dantrolene therapy is used, liver injury is estimated to occur in one to two per thousand treated persons. Mild, asymptomatic elevations in serum aminotransferases are most commonly seen. However, more serious rare cases show sudden onset jaundice, nausea and fatigue, with rapid progression to fever, rash, and eosinophilia [26]. Recovery will fully occur in 1–3 months. Although benzodiazepines may have very little to no adverse hepatic side effects, it has been shown that benzodiazepines can promote gastroesophageal reflux by reducing lower esophageal sphincter pressure. In the 1980, it was shown that patients receiving benzodiazepines had a 18.9% reduction in lower esophageal pressure [27]. However, a more recent study performed, Corley et al, studied the relationship between medications known to lower esophageal pressure and Barrett's esophagus but did not find any correlation associated with benzodiazepines specifically [27].

19.8 Allopurinol

Allopurinol is a urate-lowering medication that can be used for prevention of tumor lysis syndrome, prevention of recurrent calcium nephrolithiasis in hyperuricosuria and when managing patients with gout. It undergoes metabolism in the liver and modifies into its active form, oxypurinol. By doing so, allopurinol and oxypurinol inhibit enzymes that make uric acid thus helping in patients with gout. In a particular study performed by Ryu et al., they found that 5% of al allopurinol users experience adverse events and a further 2% of this population will experience gastrointestinal side effects that include nausea, vomiting, diarrhea, intermittent abdominal pain, epigastric pain, dyspepsia, GI bleeding, pancreatitis, stomatitis, and salivary gland swelling [28]. Unfortunately, the exact mechanism between allopurinol and the listed GI side effects has not been adequately researched and requires further investigation. The known GI side effects experienced with allopurinol are associations observed in the patient population.

19.9 Bisphosphonates

Bisphosphonates are commonly used to treat osteoporosis in patients with rheumatological diseases to address bone loss. The medications are formulated as large pills that have an increased propensity to cause mucosal damage, which is likely mediated by the generation of oxygen radicals. The most common side effect is upper GI discomfort, which is the main reason for suspending therapy among patients taking this medication, particularly postmenopausal women. Endoscopic findings in the stomach are usually limited to erosions [1].

Less commonly, these medications can cause esophagitis ("pill esophagitis") more proximally in the GI tract. The incidence of esophagitis is low (1.5%) and usually occurs as a result of taking the medication incorrectly in addition to direct topical injury. Lack of sufficient water intake with pills and reclined position while taking the pill are associated with higher risk of esophageal injury. The lesion develops in the mid and distal esophagus usually within 1 month of therapy, but it can also at 2–12 months. Although most patients who experience drug-induced pill esophagitis cases have no underlying abnormality in the anatomy of the esophagus, the condition is more common in areas of esophageal narrowing due to intrinsic structural issues (e.g. vascular ring, esophageal web) or extrinsic compression (e.g. site of aortic arch, left mainstem bronchus, gastroesophageal junction, or left atrial enlargement). Bisphosphonates can also rarely cause esophageal dissecans superficialis [29, 30].

Another potential side effect is the development of Barrett's esophagus (BE), especially in patients with underlying gastroesophageal reflux disease or active use of proton pump inhibitors. The pathophysiology is thought to be similar to the inflammatory process that gives rise to esophagitis and esophageal erosions from bisphosphonate use. Given that BE is a known premalignant precursor lesion to esophageal adenocarcinoma, this association could suggest an increased risk of esophageal cancer in patients who use oral bisphosphonates [31].

19.10 Sulfasalazine

In the setting of rheumatologic disease, sulfasalazine is used in the treatment of rheumatoid arthritis and ankylosing spondylitis. It is not known whether sulfasalazine or its metabolites, sulfapyridine and mesalazine, are directly involved. Pharmacodynamically it is known, however, that sulfasalazine, sulfapyridine, and mesalazine inhibit cytokine release and IgM and IgG production. Twenty to thirty percent of patients with rheumatoid arthritis treated with sulfasalazine will discontinue treatment courses due to adverse side effects and about two-thirds involve the gastrointestinal tract or central nervous system. After ingestion, sulfasalazine is absorbed in the small intestine intact until it reaches the large intestine and bacterial enzymes cleave the parent drug into its metabolites. Sulfasalazine is overall well tolerated but gastrointestinal side effects including nausea, vomiting, dyspepsia, and anorexia have been reported. Due to this, enteric coated sulfasalazine tablets have replaced the standard formulation markedly reducing the incidence of adverse gastrointestinal effects [32]. The etiology of sulfasalazine and its known gastrointestinal side effects are not clear and requires further investigation. The gastrointestinal side effects associated with sulfasalazine use are known due to observation within the patient population.

19.11 Leflunomide

Leflunomide has been shown in many clinical trials that it can control the signs and symptoms of rheumatoid arthritis as well as the slowing of joint damage progression. Once it is ingested, it is converted to its active metabolite teriflunomide which inhibits lymphocyte enzymes decreasing T-cell proliferation [33]. When using leflunomide, up to 15% of individuals will develop asymptomatic elevations in serum aminotransferases. However, leflunomide has been shown to be associated with clinically apparent liver injury associated with diarrhea in rare cases. This usually arises after 1–6 months of continued treatment and will subside within 1 week after discontinuation. Additionally, it is imperative that patients using leflunomide be screened for hepatitis B status. Leflunomide has been associated with reactivation of hepatitis B in patients with rheumatoid arthritis who are also HBsAg positive. Reactivation is thought to be due to immunosuppression which allows for HBV replication and subsequent immune reaction leading to increase in viral antigens. It is highly recommended to monitor liver serum enzymes monthly for the first 6 months and then every other month. Patients with HBsAg, anti-HBc without HBsAg, or have rises in HBV DNA levels should be provided antivirals. Without prophylaxis, the frequency of re-activation is 50% in HBsAg patients [34].

19.12 Potassium Supplements

Potassium, among other physiologic electrolytes, participate in the homeostasis and electrophysiology of nerve impulses. Therapeutically, potassium has shown to reduce pain and inflammation in rheumatoid arthritis. Adhering to a potassium supplementation regimen, it has been shown in controlled trials that potassium can decrease pain and arthritis. These controlled studies suggest that there is a link between potassium supplementation and cortisol status that then helps decrease inflammation and pain experienced in rheumatoid arthritis [35]. However, there are gastrointestinal side effects associated with potassium supplementation including esophageal, gastric, small bowel ulcerations, as well as stenotic lesions [36]. An exact mechanism of action is not known, however, it is thought that these symptoms are due to the irritating and potentially erosive nature of potassium ions to the gastrointestinal mucosal lining [36].

19.13 Iron

Iron supplementation is commonly used in rheumatological diseases in the setting of iron deficiency anemia. Common side effects of oral iron therapy (most commonly ferrous sulfate) include constipation as well as mucosal injuries such as erosions in esophagus and stomach (and rarely duodenum), mucosal erythema and discoloration of mucosa, and reactive gastropathy with associated iron deposition, all of which can manifest as nausea, vomiting, and epigastric discomfort [1].

The majority of patients with iron deposition in their upper GI tract demonstrate corrosive mucosal injury as erosions and ulcerations. The corrosive effect may be due to ferrous and ferric iron catalyzing the formation of reactive oxygen metabolites. Other forms of mucosal injury include epithelial distortion and ischemia, which can result from iron-containing thrombi in the microvasculature. However, it is not entirely clear if iron deposition is the primary or secondary event in relation to the mucosal injuries. It has been shown that there are cases of oral iron-related injuries where ulceration precedes the initiation of iron supplementation. Iron-associated GI mucosal injury is likely the result of a combination of pre-existing mucosal damage and trapped therapeutic iron that has prolonged contact with the GI tract mucosa [37–39].

19.14 Herbal Supplements (Table 19.1)

Photograph of evening primrose [41]
Photograph of feverfew [42]
Photograph of perennial vine [43]
Photograph of ginger [44]

19.15 Antimuscarinic Agents and Hydroxychloroquine

For individuals suffering from oral dryness experienced in Sjogren Syndrome, pilocarpine and cevimeline are two agents that stimulate muscarinic receptors within the salivary glands leading to increased secretory function. When compared to

Table 19.1 Herbal supplements and their associated GI adverse effects [40]

Herbal supplement	Where supplement is found	Mechanism and rheumatologic disease treated	GI side effect(s)
Gammalinolenic acid	Oils of evening primrose, borage seed, black currant seed (Fig. 19.2)	Effective in decreasing joint inflammation in RA and sicca symptoms in SS	Soft stools, constipation, flatulence, belching, elevated serum transaminases
Harpagophytum Extract	Harpagophytum perennial plant	Used for arthritis due to anti-inflammatory effects	Mild gastrointestinal disturbance in patients with gastric or duodenal ulcers and gallstones
Salix app.	Constituent of willow tree bark that yields salicylic acid	When extracted contains analgesic properties to help with rheumatic pain	Gastric irritation
Tanacetum parthenium	Aromatic herb feverfew (Fig. 19.3)	Leaves chewed has anti-inflammatory properties for RA inhibiting TXB2, leukotriene B4, TNF-alpha, IL-1	Oral ulcers, nausea, vomiting, diarrhea, flatulence
Tripterygium wilfordii Hook F	Perennial vine with active substance derived from the root (Fig. 19.4)	Inhibits the production of cytokines by blocking proinflammatory genes; used in RA, SLE, ankylosing spondylitis, psoriasis, leprosy, and nephropathy	Diarrhea, nausea, vomiting, xerostomia, oral ulcers, gastritis, abdominal pain, weight gain, weight loss
Zingiber officinale	"Gingers" (Fig. 19.5)	Inhibitor of prostaglandin and leukotriene synthesis and production of TNF-alpha	Dyspepsia, nausea

pilocarpine in random controlled trials, cevimeline has been shown to have a higher frequency of nausea and sweating [45].

Hydroxychloroquine is a well known anti-malarial drug but it has been used to treat rheumatologic diseases such as SLE, rheumatoid arthritis, and Sjogren Syndrome. There are not many gastrointestinal side effects associated with hydroxychloroquine. However, if genetic polymorphisms are present within the hepatic cytochrome responsible for metabolism, a variability of adverse side effects may manifest of which could be hepatically related [46, 47]. Additionally, there have been reports of dyspepsia, abdominal cramps and dysgeusia depending on the brand of hydroxychloroquine used. A study performed in 2017, Srinivasa et al., determined that gastrointestinal side effects due to hydroxychloroquine may be brand-related. However, a controlled prospective study would be required to further explore and test formally [48].

19.16 Tetracyclines

In the field of rheumatology, tetracyclines are used as off-label medications for anti-inflammatory treatment of rheumatoid arthritis. Tetracyclines, particularly doxycycline, are associated with pill esophagitis, which can present as dysphagia, odynophagia, and retrosternal pain that resolve after cessation of the drug. As mentioned previously, pill esophagitis can arise due to patient related factors with incorrect techniques when taking the medications as well as direct effects on the mucosa and esophageal anatomical factors. Women appear affected twice as often as men.

Tetracyclines can also cause erosions, ulcers, sloughed mucosa and hemorrhage, which can be seen on endoscopy. In general, effects on the stomach are less common, but doxycycline has been suggested to cause a reactive gastropathy variant where white adherent gastric exudate extends beyond the antrum (although histology is more similar to GAVE) [39, 49].

In the colon, tetracyclines can infrequently cause pseudomembranous colitis by disrupting the balance of intestinal flora, allowing the toxin-producing bacterium *clostridioides difficile* to proliferate [49, 50].

19.17 Misoprostol

Misoprostol is used in the prevention and treatment of NSAID-induced gastric ulcers in patients taking NSAIDs and at high risk for ulceration, such as older patients with rheumatoid arthritis. Misoprostol is a prostaglandin analogue, while NSAIDs suppress mucosal prostaglandin synthesis, thereby contributing to the creation of ulcers. However, aside from misoprostol's gastric mucosal protective effects, there are also several gastrointestinal side effects associated with its use. The most frequently encountered side effects are self-limiting diarrhea and abdominal pain thought to be due to exposure to the misoprostolic acid released during its metabolism. Misoprostol is also associated with nausea/vomiting, heartburn, regurgitation, difficulty swallowing, constipation and less commonly bloating [51–53].

19.18 Summary Table

Medication name	Indication(s)	Side effect(s)	Side effect management
NSAIDs	RA, OA, juvenile arthritis, SLE, rheumatic fever, gout, gouty arthritis, ankylosing spondylitis for pain relief	Esophagus: ulcers, erosions, pill esophagitis, esophagitis dissecans, perforation; small bowel: ulcers, erosions, diaphragm disease; colon: ulcers, erosions, focal colitis; liver: acute hepatitis, chronic active hepatitis	Cessation of NSAID use, procedural intervention if needed
Steroids	Pain relief in arthritides, disease-modifying effects, immunosuppressive actions	GI irritation, peptic ulcer disease, bleeding, pancreatitis	Concomitant PPI use, drug cessation, procedural intervention if needed
Colchicine	Gouty arthritis, Behcet's disease, familial Mediterranean fever	Abdominal cramping, bloating, vomiting, diarrhea, cholera-like syndrome, malabsorption, erosions, melena, peptic ulcers, elevated transaminases	Drug cessation
Febuxostat	Gout, uric acid nephropathy, hyperuricemia	Liver function test abnormalities, diarrhea	Drug cessation
Pegloticase	Chronic refractory and symptomatic gout	Nausea, vomiting, constipation	Drug cessation and symptom management
Analgesics	Pain management in in patients with poor pain control	Nausea, vomiting, GERD, constipation	Peripherally active opioid-receptor antagonists, concomitant anti-constipation medications, symptom management, drug cessation
Muscle Relaxants	Pain control	Asymptomatic elevations in aminotransferase levels, hepatotoxicity due to hypersensitivity reaction in dantrolene use, GERD in benzodiazepine use	Drug cessation

Medication name	Indication(s)	Side effect(s)	Side effect management
Allopurinol	Gout	Nausea, vomiting, diarrhea, intermittent abdominal pain, epigastric pain, dyspepsia, GI bleeding, pancreatitis, stomatitis, salivary gland swelling	Symptom management and drug cessation
Bisphosphonates	Osteoporosis	Upper GI discomfort, erosions, esophagitis, Barrett's esophagus, esophageal dissecans superficialis, esophageal cancer	Drug cessation
Sulfasalazine	Rheumatoid arthritis and ankylosing spondylitis	Nausea, vomiting, dyspepsia, anorexia	Symptom management, drug cessation
Leflunomide	Rheumatoid arthritis, slowing of joint damage progression	Asymptomatic elevations in aminotransferase levels, diarrhea, reactivation of hepatitis B in rheumatoid arthritis who are also HBsAg positive	Drug cessation, antivirals
Potassium Supplements	Reduction of pain and inflammation in RA	Ulcers in the esophagus, stomach, and small bowel; stenotic lesions	Drug cessation
Iron	Iron deficiency anemia in setting of rheumatologic disease	Constipation, erosions, mucosal erythema, discoloration of mucosa, reactive gastropathy, naura, vomiting, and epigastric discomfort	Symptom management, drug cessation
Herbal Supplements	Anti-inflammatory properties, pain control	Constipation, diarrhea, gastric irritation, ulcers, liver enzyme elevations	Symptom management, drug cessation
Pilocarpine and Cevimeline	Oral dryness in Sjogren Syndrome	Nausea	Drug cessation, symptom management
Hydroxychloroquine	SLE, RA, SS	Dyspepsia, abdominal cramps and dysgeusia	Drug cessation
Tetracyclines	Anti-inflammatory	Pill esophagitis, dysphagia, odynophagia, retrosternal pain, erosions, ulcers, sloughed mucosa, hemorrhage, pseudomembranous colitis	Drug cessation
Misoprostol	NSAID-induced gastric ulcers	Diarrhea, abdominal pain, nausea, vomiting, heartburn, regurgitation, difficulty swallowing, bloating	Symptom management, drug cessation

References

1. De Petris G, Gatius Caldero S, Chen L, Xiao S, Dhungel BM, Wendel Spizcka AJ, Lam-Himlin D. Histopathological changes in the gastrointestinal tract due to drugs: an update for the surgical pathologist (Part I of II). Int J Surg Pathol. 2014:120–8.
2. Harirforoosh S, Asghar W, Jamali F. Adverse effects of nonsteroidal antiinflammatory drugs: an update of gastrointestinal, cardiovascular and renal complications. J Pharm Pharm Sci. 2013:821–47.
3. Haley RM, von Recum HA. Localized and targeted delivery of NSAIDs for treatment of inflammation: a review. Exp Biol Med (Maywood). 2019:433–44.
4. Tacheci I, Bradna P, Douda T, Bastecka D, Kopacova M, Rejchrt S, Bures J. NSAID-induced enteropathy in rheumatoid arthritis patients with chronic occult gastrointestinal bleeding: a prospective capsule endoscopy study. Gastroenterol Res Pract. 2013:1–10.
5. So H, Bloomfield I. Small bowel obstruction due to non-steroidal anti-inflammatory drug-induced diaphragm disease: a case report. Cureus. 2018:2350.
6. Lucendo AJ. Drug exposure and the risk of microscopic colitis: a critical update. Drugs R D. 2017:79–89.
7. Stolte M, Karimi D, Vieth M, Volkholz H, Dirschmid K, Rappel S, Bethke B. Strictures, diaphragms, erosions or ulcerations of ischemic type in the colon should always prompt consideration of nonsteroidal anti-inflammatory drug-induced lesions. World J Gastroenterol. 2005:5828–33.
8. Bindu S, Mazumder S, Bandyopadhyay U. Non-steroidal anti-inflammatory drugs (NSAIDs) and organ damage: a current perspective. Biochem Pharmacol. 2020:1–20.
9. Van der Goes MC, Jacobs JW, Bijlsma JW. The value of glucocorticoid co-therapy in different rheumatic diseases—positive and adverse effects. Arthritis Res Ther. 2014:1–13.
10. Strehl C, Ehlers L, Gaber T, Buttgereit F. Glucocorticoids-all-rounders tackling the versatile players of the immune system. Front Immunol. 2019:1–20.
11. Caplan A, Fett N, Rosenbach M, Werth VP, Micheletti RG. Prevention and management of glucocorticoid-induced side effects: a comprehensive review: Gastrointestinal and endocrinologic side effects. J Am Acad Dermatol. 2017:11–6.
12. Liu S, Liu X, Chen S, Xiao Y, Zhuang W. Oral versus intravenous methylprednisolone for the treatment of multiple sclerosis relapses: a meta-analysis of randomized controlled trials. PLoS One. 2017:1–13.
13. Iacobuzio-Donahue CA, Lee EL, Abraham SC, Yardley JH, Wu T. Colchicine toxicity: distinct morphologic findings in gastrointestinal biopsies. Am J Surg Pathol. 2001:1067–73.
14. Stewart S, Yang KC, Atkins K, Dalbeth N, Robinson P. Adverse events during oral colchicine use: a systematic review and meta-analysis of randomised controlled trials. Arthritis Res Ther. 2020:1–15.
15. LiverTox: Clinical and Research Information on Drug-Induced Liver Injury [Internet]. Bethesda (MD): National Institute of Diabetes and Digestive and Kidney Disease; 2018. Febuxostat. [cited 2021 Nov 15. Available from: ncbi.nlm.nih.gov/books/NBK548645/.
16. Becker MA, Schumacher HR, Espinoza LR, Wells AF, MacDonald P, Lloyd E, Lademacher C. The urate-lowering efficacy and safety of febuxostat in the treatment of the hyperuricemia of gout: the CONFIRMS trial. Arthritis Res Ther. 2010;
17. LiverTox: Clinical and Research Information on Drug-Induced Liver Injury [Internet]. Bethesda (MD): National Institute of Diabetes and Digestive and Kidney Diseases; 2018. Pegloticase. [cited 2021 Nov 15]. Available from: ncbi.nlm.nih.gov/books/NBK548768/.
18. Zimmerman HJ. Drugs used to treat gout. Drugs used to treat rheumatic and musculospastic disease. In: Zimmerman HJ, editor. Hepatotoxicity: the adverse effects of drugs and other chemicals on the liver. 2nd ed. Philadelphia: Lippincott; 1999. p. 543–4.
19. Griessinger N, Sittl R, Jost R, Schaefer M, Likar R. The role of opioid analgesics in rheumatoid disease in the elderly population. Drugs Aging. 2003:571–83.

20. Walsh DA, McWilliams DF. Mechanisms, impact and management of pain in rheumatoid arthritis. Nat Rev Rheumatol. 2014:581–92.
21. Holzer P. Opioid receptors in the gastrointestinal tract. Regul Pept. 2009:11–7.
22. Rausch T, Jansen T. Gastrointestinal side effects of opioid analgesics. US Pharmacol. 2012:36–9.
23. Cook SF, Lanza L, Zhou X, Sweeney CT, Goss D, Hollis K, Mangel AW, Fehnel SE. Gastrointestinal side effects in chronic opioid users: results from a population-based survey. Aliment Pharmacol Ther. 2008:1224–32.
24. Boswell K, Kwong WJ, Kavanagh S. Burden of opioid-associated gastrointestinal side effects from clinical and economic perspectives: a systematic literature review. J Opioid Manage. 2010:269–89.
25. Richards BL, Whittle SL, Buchbinder R. Muscle relaxants for pain management in rheumatoid arthritis. Cochrane Database Syst Rev. 2012; https://doi.org/10.1002/14651858.CD008922.pub2.
26. LiverTox: Clinical and Research Information on Drug-Induced Liver Injury [Internet]. Bethesda (MD): National Institute of Diabetes and Digestive and Kidney Diseases; 2018. Muscle Relaxants. [cited 2021 Nov 15]. Available from: ncbi.nlm.nih.gov/books/NBK548375/.
27. Tutuian R. Adverse effects of drugs on the esophagus. Best Pract Res Clin Gastroenterol. 2010:91–7.
28. Ryu H, Song R, Kim HW, Kim JH, Lee EY, Lee YJ, Song YW, Lee EB. Clinical risk factors for adverse events in allopurinol users. J Clin Pharmacol. 2013:211–6.
29. Guttman OR, Zachos M. Drug-induced esophageal injury with an occult vascular ring. Paediatr Child Health. 2011:554–6.
30. Saleem F, Sharma A. Drug induced esophagitis. StatPearls Publishing; 2021.
31. Lin D, Kramer JR, Ramsey D, Alsarraj A, Verstovsek G, Rugge M, Parente P, Graham DY, El-Serag HB. Oral bisphosphonates and the risk of Barrett's esophagus: case-control analysis of US veterans. Am J Gastroenterol. 2013:1576–83.
32. Plosker GL, Croom KF. Sulfasalazine: a review of its use in the management of rheumatoid arthritis. Drugs. 2005:1825–49.
33. Alfaro-Lara R, Espinosa-Ortega H, Arce-Salinas C. Systemic review and meta-analysis of the efficacy and safety of leflunomide and methotrexate in the treatment of rheumatoid arthritis. Reumatologia. Clinica. 2017:133–9.
34. LiverTox: Clinical and Research Information on Drug-Induced Liver Injury [Internet]. Bethesda: National Institute of Diabetes and Digestive and Kidney Diseases; 2018. Leflunomide. [cited 2021 Nov 15]. Available from: ncbi.nlm.nih.gov/books/NBK548725.
35. Kianifard T, Chopra A. A therapeutic role for potassium (K) to reduce pain and complications related to the cardiovascular system and bone in rheumatoid arthritis (RA): a clinical research perspective. Rheumatol Res. 2018;3(1):1–12. https://doi.org/10.22631/rr.2017.69997.1035.
36. Mihalchik AL, Rogers EN. Classes of compounds with GI tract toxicity. In: Toxicology of the gastrointestinal tract 2018 Oct 26. CRC Press. p. 383–420.
37. Ji H, Yardley JH. Iron medication-associated gastric mucosal injury. Arch Pathol Lab Med. 2004:821–2.
38. Sahebzamani FM, Berarducci A, Murr MM. Malabsorption anemia and iron supplement induced constipation in post-Roux-en-Y gastric bypass (RYGB) patients. J Am Assoc Nurse Pract. 2013:634–40.
39. Cancelo-Hidalgo MJ, Castelo-Branco C, Palacios S, Haya-Palazuelos J, Ciria-Recasens M, Manasanch J, Perez-Edo L. Tolerability of different oral iron supplements: a systematic review. 2013:291–303. -Iron-.
40. Setty AR, Sigal LH. Herbal medications commonly used in the practice of rheumatology: mechanisms of action, efficacy, and side effects. Semin Arthritis Rheum. 2005:773–84.
41. Evening Primrose Oil [Internet]. National Center for Complementary and Integrative Health: National Institute of Health; 2020. Available from: https://www.nccih.nih.gov/health/evening-primrose-oil.

42. Feverfew [Internet]. National Center for Complementary and Integrative Health: National Institute of Health; 2020. Available from: https://www.nccih.nih.gov/health/feverfew.
43. Thunder God Vine [Internet]. National Center for Complementary and Integrative Health: National Institute of Health; 2021. Available from: https://www.nccih.nih.gov/health/thunder-god-vine.
44. Ginger [Internet]. National Center for Complementary and Integrative Health: National Institute of Health; 2020. Available from: https://www.nccih.nih.gov/health/ginger.
45. Brito-Zerón P, Retamozo S, Kostov B, Baldini C, Bootsma H, De Vita S, Dörner T, Gottenberg JE, Kruize AA, Mandl T, Ng WF, Seror R, Tzioufas AG, Vitali C, Bowman S, Mariette X, Ramos-Casals M. Efficacy and safety of topical and systemic medications: a systematic literature review informing the EULAR recommendations for the management of Sjögren's syndrome. Rheum Musculoskelet Dis Open. 2019;
46. Olsen NJ, Schleich MA, Karp D. Multifaceted effects of hydroxychloroquine in human disease. Semin Arthritis Rheum. 2013:264–72.
47. Eljaaly K, Alireza KH, Alshehri S, Al-Tawfiq JA. Hydroxychloroquine safety: a meta-analysis of randomized controlled trials. Travel Med Infect Dis. 2020;
48. Srinivasa A, Tosounidou S, Gordon C. Increased incidence of gastrointestinal side effects in patients taking hydroxychloroquine: a brand-related issue? J Rheumatol. 2017:398.
49. De Petris G, Gatius Caldero S, Chen L, Xiao S, Dhungel BM, Wendel Spizcka AJ, Lam-Himlin D. Histopathological changes in the gastrointestinal tract due to drugs: an update for the surgical pathologist (Part II of II). Int J Surg Pathol. 2014:202–11.
50. Slimings C, Riley TV. Antibiotics and healthcare family-associated *Clostridioides difficile* infection: systematic review and meta-analysis 2020 update. J Antimicrob Chemother. 2021:1676–88.
51. Kim JW. NSAID-induced gastroenteropathy. Korean. J Gastroenterol. 2008:134–41.
52. Silverstein FE, Graham DY, Senior JR, Davies HW, Struthers BJ, Bittman RM, Geis GS. Misoprostol reduces serious gastrointestinal complications in patients with rheumatoid arthritis receiving nonsteroidal anti-inflammatory drugs. a randomized, double-bline, placebo-controlled trial. Ann Intern Med. 1995:241–9.
53. Taha AS, McCloskey C, McSkimming P, McConnachie A. Misoprostol for small bowel ulcers in patients with obscure bleeding taking aspirin and non-steroidal anti-inflammatory drugs (MASTERS): a randomized, double-blind, placebo-controlled, phase 3 trial. Lancet. 2018:469–76.

Chapter 20
Immune Modulating and Immunosuppressive Drugs

Barrett O. Attarha, Radhika Sharma, Vinit H. Majmudar, Lee Shapiro, Andrew Flint, and Peter Ghali

20.1 Introduction

A plethora of medications within multiple classes exist for the treatment of immune-mediated rheumatologic and non-rheumatologic diseases. Many, but not all these medications are parenterally administered, and so are not necessarily dependent on an intact gastrointestinal (GI) tract for their absorption. Clinically, the route of administration is a key determinant in drug selection, especially in patients with active gastrointestinal disease. For instance, in Crohn's disease with small bowel involvement, intravenous biologics may be favored due to impaired mucosal absorption. Understanding pharmacokinetic profiles in altered GI anatomy or function is

B. O. Attarha · P. Ghali
Department of Medicine, Division of Gastroenterology, University of Florida Jacksonville, Jacksonville, FL, USA
e-mail: barrett.attarha@jax.ufl.edu; peter.ghali@jax.ufl.edu

R. Sharma
Department of Medicine, University of Florida Jacksonville, Jacksonville, FL, USA
e-mail: Radhika.Sharma@jax.ufl.edu

V. H. Majmudar (✉)
Department of Medicine, Division of Gastroenterology, Albany Medical Center, Albany, NY, USA
e-mail: majmudv@amc.edu

L. Shapiro
Department of Medicine, Division of Rheumatology, Albany Medical Center, Albany, NY, USA
e-mail: shapirl@amc.edu

A. Flint
Department of Medicine, University of Florida Jacksonville, Jacksonville, FL, USA
e-mail: Andrew.Flint@jax.ufl.edu

M. Tadros et al. (eds.), *GI Diseases Associated with Rheumatological and Vasculitic Conditions*, Clinical Gastroenterology,
https://doi.org/10.1007/978-3-032-07868-1_20

critical for optimizing therapeutic outcomes. Nevertheless, in some cases, alteration of the GI tract or a functional change, as can be seen in bowel inflammation, can affect the absorption and pharmacokinetics of these medications. Furthermore, GI tract side effects are fairly ubiquitous in immune modulating drugs. In this chapter, we briefly review the mechanism of action, side effects, and issues related to absorption of the major classes of medications used in the treatment of immune mediated diseases.

20.2 Anti-TNF Medications

Tumor necrosis factor (TNF) is a multifaceted cytokine and adipokine that plays a key role in the host immune system. **TNF is expressed in two forms: membrane-bound and soluble.** It is rapidly expressed within minutes of stress or injury and serves as a signal to regulate immune cells. The subsequent response to this is via IL-1 and IL-6 production [1]. TNF is a main regulator of the inflammatory process itself, leading to a diverse and complex response [2]. Both forms are biologically active. TNF acts on two receptors, TNF Receptor 1 (TNFR1) and TNF Receptor 2 (TNFR2) [3]. TNFR1 is widely present while TNFR2 is found on lymphocytes and endothelial cells. The two forms of TNF do not act exclusively on either receptor, but membrane-bound TNF acts more on TNFR2 and soluble TNF on TNFR1. While the TNFR1 mediated response is pro-inflammatory and apoptotic, TNFR2 signaling is anti-inflammatory and can promote wound healing. Once TNFR1 is activated, the classic activation of nuclear factor kappa-B (NFK-B) follows, with its ensuing inflammatory cascade (Fig. 20.1). As a result, the benefit of anti-TNF medications is mainly via the TNFR1 pathway. The main anti-TNF therapies in use today are infliximab, adalimumab, golimumab, certolizumab pegol, and etanercept.

20.2.1 Side Effects

TNF-inhibitors are generally well tolerated with minimal side effects. Non-gastrointestinal adverse reactions include local skin irritation from injection sites, infusion reactions, headaches, anemia, upper respiratory tract infections, sinusitis, cough, pharyngitis, and, rarely, serious infections, malignancies (especially lymphomas), worsening of established congestive heart failure, drug-induced lupus (<1%), demyelinating disorders, and skin reactions [4]. Gastrointestinal side effects include transaminitis, diarrhea, nausea, and abdominal pain. The transaminitis can be mild and non-specific, or can reflect underlying liver disease. Diarrhea can be difficult to distinguish from worsening inflammatory bowel disease in those patients

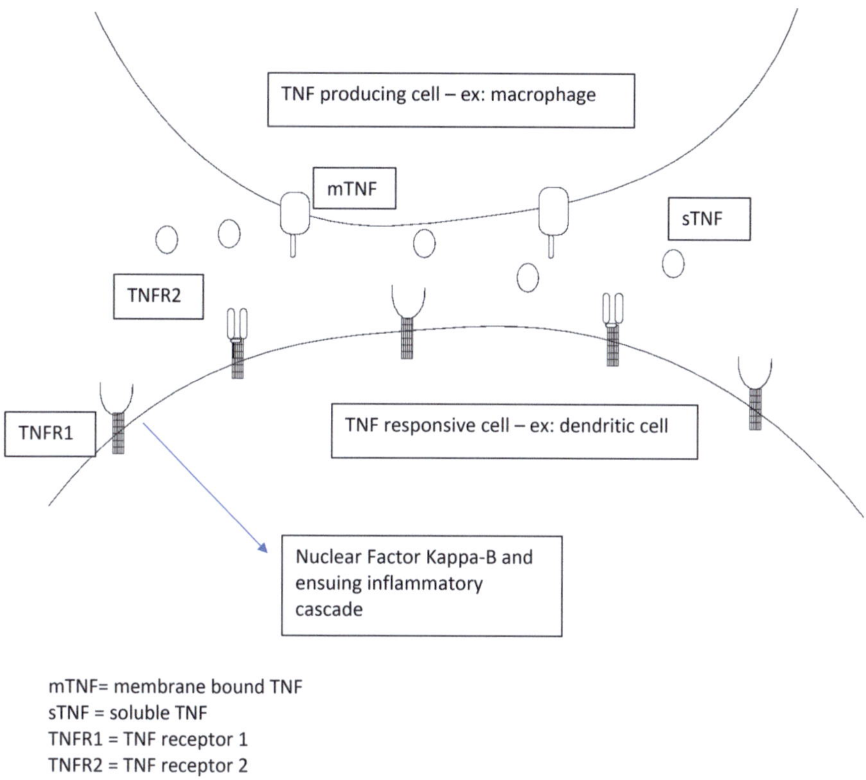

Fig. 20.1 Simplified schematic of the action of TNF
mTNF membrane bound TNF, *sTNF* soluble TNF, *TNFR1* TNF receptor 1, *TNFR2* TNF receptor 2

taking anti-TNFs for that indication, and can even reflect a paradoxical worsening of IBD due to the medication [5]. There have also been reports of colitis induced specifically by etanercept used for diseases other than IBD, and this has not been found with other anti-TNF medications [6]. Clinicians should assess fecal calprotectin and perform stool studies when diarrhea emerges during anti-TNF therapy to differentiate disease flare from paradoxical drug-induced colitis. Paradoxical colitis is most commonly reported with etanercept and rarely with monoclonal antibodies like infliximab. The risk of infections is higher and more common in those who are on multiple immunosuppressive agents. Screening for hepatitis B and C, as well as tuberculosis is recommended as these infections can reactivate while on therapy. It is also recommended to screen for endemic fungal infections in areas with high incidences of these types of infections prior to initiation of therapy. Of note, there are no controlled trials in assessing the safety of anti-TNF therapy in pregnancy or lactation by the FDA.

20.2.2 GI Absorption

Current anti-TNF therapy is administered intravenously or intramuscularly, and thus does not rely on the gastrointestinal system for initial absorption, which can be helpful in the setting of active inflammatory bowel disease where absorption may be greatly impaired. However, significant levels of anti-TNF medications can be detected in the stool of actively inflamed patients, often reflecting subtherapeutic levels of the medication in the blood [7]. Thus, the importance of therapeutic drug monitoring has emerged as an important tool in evaluating the cause of lack of response. In patients with severe mucosal inflammation, loss of drug in stool correlates with subtherapeutic serum trough levels.

20.2.3 Conclusion

The mechanisms of action and the exact signaling pathways of the anti-TNF therapies continue to be elucidated. Anti-TNF therapy works via several different processes which can explain their wide utility in a variety of diseases. The success and failure of this class of drugs can reflect the extent to which the underlying targeted mechanisms are at play in individual patients and may represent future opportunities to personalize therapy. Even within class, different medications may be preferentially more effective on certain mechanisms, or have higher affinity for specific TNF receptors, leading to different outcomes. The class is generally safe and has a long track-record of use. Nevertheless, minor side effects are common, and these include GI side effects. Some of these GI side effects can be unexpected in non-GI disease patients, and in GI patients can be difficult to distinguish from the underlying disease. It is important to have a high index of suspicion when a paradoxical worsening of GI symptoms follows the administration of this class of medication.

20.3 Anti-IL-12/23

Classically, Th cells are divided into Th1, Th2, and Th17. Different diseases result from each of these profiles. For example, Crohn's disease usually exhibits a Th1 profile, while ulcerative colitis exhibits a Th2 profile. Collagen-induced arthritis is a Th1-mediated disease [8] while rheumatoid arthritis may be affected by all three pathways, with Th1 and Th17 predominating [9–11]. Interleukin (IL)-12 and interleukin-23 induce inflammation in the adaptive pathway of immune response. IL-12 shifts the response towards a Th1 profile, while IL-23 stimulates the differentiation of naïve Th cells to Th17 cells, with a subsequent inflammatory cascade (Fig. 20.2). IL-23 also supports the maintenance of Th17 memory cells, linked to disease chronicity and relapse in psoriasis and inflammatory bowel disease (IBD). Thus,

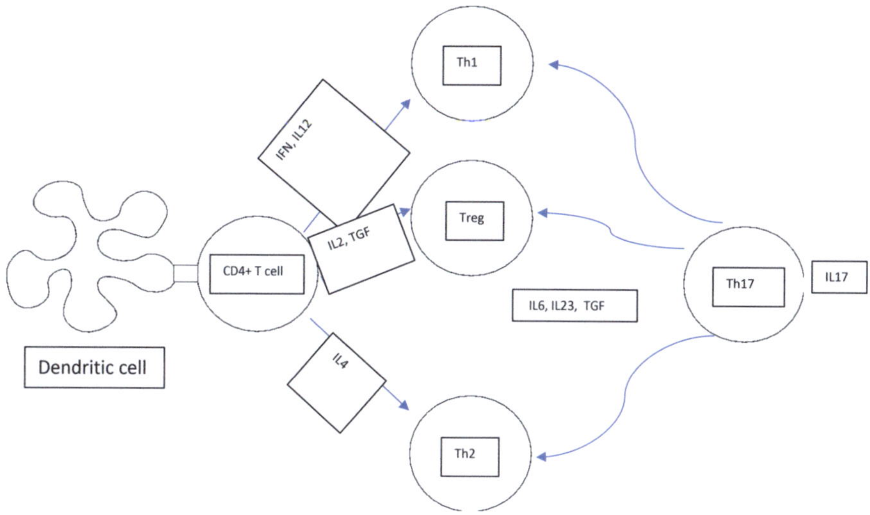

Fig. 20.2 Simplified schematic of differentiation of T-helper cells

IL-23–specific antibodies may offer better disease control compared to dual IL-12/23 inhibition in some patients. This pattern is implicated in the pathogenesis of Crohn's disease, seronegative spondyloarthritis, psoriasis, and multiple sclerosis [12]. Both IL-12 and IL-23 belong to the same family and share the subunit p40 and a common pathway. Therapies targeting IL-12 and IL-23 block the p40 subunit, halting the inflammatory cascade [13]. Ustekinumab is the primary treatment in this class and acts as an anti-p40 antibody. IL-12 and IL-23 have both pro- and anti-inflammatory roles, but IL-23 is more strongly linked to inflammation in diseases such as Crohn's, psoriasis, and multiple sclerosis. Thus, IL-23–specific antibodies, like briakinumab, have been developed and are currently under investigation. Nonetheless, the precise roles and interactions of these interleukins remain unclear.

Interleukins are mainly produced by antigen-presenting cells (APCs) such as dendritic cells and macrophages. IL-23 is notably abundant in the small intestine, especially in the terminal ileum [14].

20.3.1 Side Effects

Like other biologic therapies, adverse events from IL-12 and IL-23 inhibitors include serious infections, malignancies, and major cardiovascular events (associated with briakinumab in psoriasis patients) [15]. Ustekinumab crosses the placenta, but no increased incidence of infant infections has been reported. Gastrointestinal side effects (abdominal pain, nausea, vomiting, diarrhea) are rare and usually mild. Similar to anti-TNF medications, paradoxical worsening of inflammatory bowel disease has been reported with ustekinumab [16], challenging differentiation from underlying disease flare when indicated for IBD. Serious gastrointestinal events are exceedingly rare, though acute cholecystitis has been documented [17].

20.3.2 GI Absorption

As with anti-TNF therapy, IL-12/IL-23 p40 inhibitors are administered intravenously or subcutaneously, avoiding gastrointestinal absorption issues. This is ideal in inflammatory bowel disease, where GI tract absorption can be significantly impaired. Therapeutic drug monitoring for this drug class is emerging, although anti-drug antibody (ADA) formation does not seem problematic. Nonetheless, preliminary data suggest a potential role for therapeutic drug monitoring to optimize efficacy [18].

20.3.3 Conclusion

Anti-IL-12/IL-23 therapy has demonstrated safety and efficacy. Blocking the p40 subunit provides significant anti-inflammatory benefits, especially in diseases driven by Th1 and Th17 pathways. Selective targeting of IL-23 alone might offer therapeutic advantages over combined IL-12/23 blockade, although further studies are needed. Side effects are rare and typically mild, making this class attractive for Crohn's disease and psoriatic arthritis.

20.4 IL-17 Inhibitors

As discussed above different diseases are associated with different Th profiles. Stimulation by transforming growth factor-B (TGF-B) and IL-6 makes native CD4+ T-cells differentiate into Th17, which induces IL-17A which is proinflammatory, and associated with psoriasis. IL-17 is also implicated in the pathogenesis of rheumatoid arthritis, ankylosing spondylitis, Crohn's disease, Ulcerative Colitis, and multiple sclerosis [19].

20.4.1 Mechanism of Action

IL-17 inhibiting agents include secukinumab, brodalumab, ixekizumab. Secukinumab is an IL-17A inhibitor approved for use in psoriasis. It has been found that there are elevated levels of IL-17A in the lamina propria in patients with Crohn's Disease and Ulcerative Colitis. This suggests that this interleukin plays a role in the inflammatory process of the disease. IL-17A mRNA is enriched in the gastrointestinal mucosa of patients with active inflammatory bowel disease. This makes this a potentially useful target for therapeutic intervention.

However, data is contradictory as IL-17 has also been shown to be helpful in the repair of the intestinal wall, production of mucus by intestinal goblet cells, and maintaining homeostasis of the intestinal tract [20, 21]. So, blocking this interleukin could lead to questionable bowel wall integrity and aggravate inflammation.

20.4.2 GI Side Effects

Since IL-17 is responsible for the recruitment of neutrophils, blocking it may leave patients at increased risk of contracting infections, whether from bacteria, fungi, or yeast. Most data is from patients taking it for psoriasis, and there have been reports of these patients developing digestive adverse effects like bowel inflammation, diarrhea, and other digestive symptoms [20]. There have even been case reports documenting newly diagnosed IBD or IBD exacerbations while on this therapy [20, 21] It is unclear whether IL-17 inhibitors can actually cause Ulcerative Colitis in a patient who did not have it, or simply trigger an undiagnosed IBD exacerbation. Nevertheless, it is advisable to take a thorough history to exclude IBD, and to exclude any family history of IBD before deciding to initiate this therapy for any indication (i.e. not just those with Inflammatory Bowel Disease). Furthermore, it is advisable to measure fecal calprotectin levels prior to starting, and for those with elevated levels, referral to Gastroenterology for colonoscopy may be advised [22]. In clinical practice, patients with positive fecal calprotectin or a family history of IBD should undergo colonoscopy before starting IL-17 inhibitors. This preemptive strategy can help identify subclinical disease and avoid exacerbation.

20.4.3 GI Absorption

IL-17 inhibitors are administered intravenously or intramuscularly, and do not rely on a healthy or intact GI tract for absorption.

20.4.4 Conclusion

IL-17 is broadly implicated in a wide range of inflammatory and immune diseases, ranging from the central nervous system, to skin, to the GI tract. While it is involved in a pro-inflammatory cascade and presents an attractive therapeutic target, its effect on gut health is unclear. It is found in inflamed gut mucosa, but also seems to play a protective role. When used, particular attention to close surveillance of the health of the GI tract needs to be paid. This should include a baseline clinical and biochemical assessment and monitoring on therapy. If GI symptoms develop with its use, referral to Gastroenterology should be made, with consideration for testing fecal calprotectin and endoscopy.

20.5 IL-1

IL-1 was described in 1979, initially thought to be a single molecule but subsequently differentiated into several cytokines. The observation that IL-1 could affect cells from various parts of the body introduced new insights into cytokine involvement in disease pathogenesis [23]. IL-1 inhibitors include anakinra, canakinumab, and rilonacept, used variably for rheumatoid arthritis, Still's disease, juvenile arthritis, and other inflammatory diseases.

20.5.1 Mechanism of Action

IL-1 is a potent proinflammatory cytokine that reduces tissue damage and lowers pain thresholds, playing a central role in inflammation and immune processes. Two primary cytokines comprise IL-1: IL-1α and IL-1β. Both bind to IL-1 receptor type 1 (IL-1 R1). Myeloid cells such as macrophages, mast cells, and neutrophils produce IL-1β, while IL-1α is derived from gene duplication of IL-1β [24]. IL-1β is predominantly involved in systemic inflammation, whereas IL-1α mediates local inflammatory responses. Activation of IL-1 via IL-1 R1 triggers a febrile response and downstream production of other inflammatory cytokines like IL-6 [25].

IL-1 inhibitors vary in their mechanism: anakinra and rilonacept block both IL-1α and β, whereas canakinumab selectively blocks IL-1β [26]. Anakinra is a receptor antagonist, while rilonacept is a soluble decoy receptor. Development of neutralizing antibodies with IL-1 antagonists occurs notably with anakinra in approximately 10% of cases, potentially limiting long-term efficacy and warranting clinical awareness [26].

20.5.2 Side Effects

Common adverse effects of IL-1 inhibitors include injection site reactions and increased infection risk, similar to other biologics. Rarely, reports exist of hepatitis progression to symptomatic liver disease with histologic foci of hepatocellular necrosis, particularly associated with anakinra [27]. Gastrointestinal side effects are not frequently reported as significant concerns with IL-1 inhibitors.

20.5.3 GI Absorption

IL-1 inhibitors are administered intravenously or subcutaneously, independent of GI absorption.

20.5.4 Conclusion

IL-1 is integral to inflammatory cascades and immune regulation. IL-1 inhibition effectively mitigates inflammation in various disease states, with anakinra most extensively studied. Overall, this class demonstrates a favorable safety profile. Clinicians should remain vigilant about the potential development of neutralizing antibodies, especially with anakinra.

20.6 JAK Inhibitors

Janus kinase (JAK) proteins are tyrosine kinases binding cytokine receptors, mediating intracellular immune responses. JAK inhibitors are widely utilized in rheumatologic diseases, inflammatory bowel disorders, and hematologic conditions. Clinical JAK inhibitors include tofacitinib, baricitinib, peficitinib, upadacitinib, and filgotinib.

20.6.1 Mechanism of Action

JAK inhibitors target four JAK receptor-associated tyrosine kinases: JAK1, JAK2, JAK3, and TYK2. JAK kinases normally facilitate transphosphorylation of proteins, influencing immune activity [28]. The JAK signaling pathway begins externally with cytokine-ligand binding to a heterodimeric receptor, triggering intracellular transphosphorylation. Phosphorylated JAK receptors recruit and activate STAT proteins, forming complexes that dimerize, enter the nucleus, and regulate gene transcription [29]. Recognition of mutated JAK signaling pathways in immunodeficiencies, like severe combined immunodeficiency, has guided therapeutic development [30].

JAK inhibitors bind reversibly or irreversibly to intracellular JAK proteins, inhibiting phosphorylation and subsequent STAT activation by occupying ATP-binding pockets. Each inhibitor exhibits differing JAK selectivity, influenced by binding affinity and concentration [31]. Upadacitinib and filgotinib exhibit higher affinity for JAK1; however, upadacitinib also targets TYK2. Recently developed selective TYK2 inhibitors, such as deucravacitinib, have emerged, representing advancements since the original drafting of this chapter [31].

20.6.2 GI Side Effects

Generally mild, GI side effects primarily include nausea. Tofacitinib specifically associates with diarrhea [32]. Serious risks include GI perforation, especially concomitant with NSAID or steroid use, contraindicating use in patients with diverticulitis or prior perforation [33, 34]. Transaminase elevation can occur, typically resolving upon dosage reduction or discontinuation.

20.6.3 GI Absorption

JAK inhibitors are absorbed across the GI tract. Studies demonstrate colonic tissue and plasma concentration equilibrium, suggesting minimal impact from altered bowel anatomy [35]. Because CYP3A4 metabolizes JAK inhibitors, co-administration with CYP3A inhibitors or inducers significantly alters drug levels, necessitating vigilant monitoring for drug interactions [36].

Immunosuppressive drugs

20.7 Calcineurin Inhibitors

Calcineurin inhibitors (CNIs), introduced clinically in the early 1980s, are pivotal immunosuppressive agents, particularly in transplantation and autoimmune disease management. Major CNIs include cyclosporine, tacrolimus, pimecrolimus, and voclosporin [37].

20.7.1 Mechanism of Action

CNIs inhibit calcineurin, a phosphatase vital for T-cell activation and cytokine production (IL-2, TNF-alpha, IL-3, IL-4, CD40L, interferon-gamma) [38]. CNIs form complexes with immunophilins, binding and inhibiting calcineurin, impairing T-cell activation, as shown in Fig. 20.3. Cyclosporine binds cyclophilin-1; tacrolimus and pimecrolimus bind FK-binding proteins. CNIs may induce renal fibrosis via transforming growth factor-β upregulation [39].

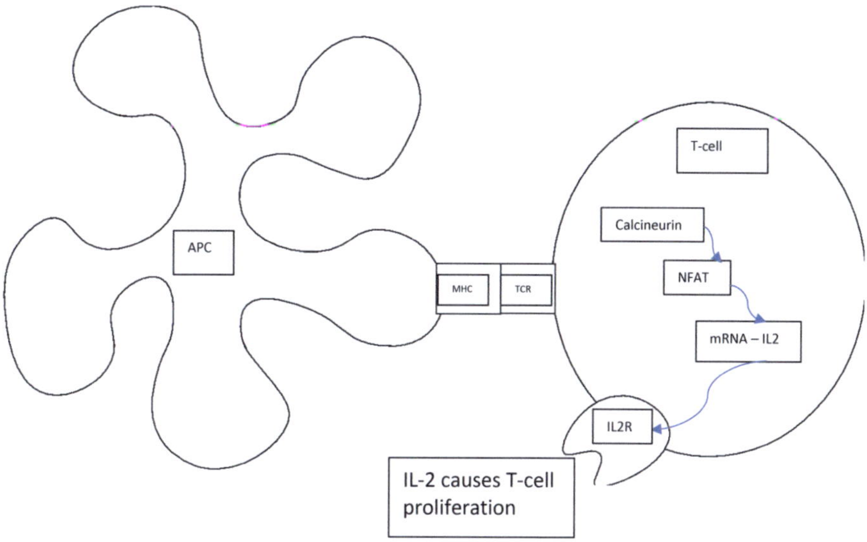

APC = Antigen presenting cell
MHC = Major histocompatibility complex
TCR = T-cell receptor
NFAT = Nuclear Factor of activated T-Cells
IL2R = IL2 Receptor

Fig. 20.3 Simplified schematic of mechanism of action of calcineurin inhibitors*APC* antigen presenting cell, *MHC* major histocompatibility complex, *TCR* T-cell receptor, *NFAT* nuclear factor of activated T-cells, *IL2R* IL2 Receptor

20.7.2 Side Effects

Major CNI side effects include nephrotoxicity (acute kidney injury, chronic kidney disease), hypertension, neurotoxicity, hepatotoxicity, metabolic disturbances, malignancies, and infections due to immunocompromise. Tacrolimus uniquely associates with increased gastrointestinal side effects; cyclosporine-specific adverse effects include hirsutism and gingival hyperplasia [40]. Side effect profiles can be seen in Table 20.1.

20.7.3 GI Absorption

CNIs exhibit erratic absorption, affected by CYP3A enzyme variability and P-glycoprotein efflux variability, requiring regular therapeutic monitoring, especially with altered bowel anatomy [41–45]. A table depicting possible drug-drug interactions that may affect CNI's is shown in Table 20.2.

Table 20.1 Side effects of Calcineurin inhibitors

Tacrolimus predominant	Cyclosporine predominant	Common with both
New onset diabetes	Hypertension	Chronic Kidney Disease
Nausea and Vomiting	Gingival hyperplasia	Headache
Diarrhea	Hirsutism	Tremors/seizures
Anorexia	Dyslipidemia	Increased infection risk
Abdominal pain	Hyperuricemia and gout	Malignancy risk
Alopecia		Hypomagnesemia
Hyperkalemia		Metabolic acidosis
		Peripheral neuropathy
		Pancreatitis
		Hemolytic uremic syndrome
		Posterior reversible encephalopathy syndrome

Table 20.2 Common medications metabolized via Cyp 3A4 pathway and at risk for Drug-Drug interactions with CNIs and Sirolimus

Drug	Effect on CNI levels
Azole antifungals (Ketoconazole, Fluconazole, Itraconazole, Voriconazole)	Increase[a]
Macrolide antibiotics[b]	Increase
Calcium Channel Blockers	Increase
Metronidazole	Increase
Ritonavir	Severe increase[a]
HMG co-A reductase inhibitors	Increase
Grapefruit juice	Increase
Rifampin	Decrease
Rifabutin	Decrease
Phenytoin	Decrease
Carbamazepine	Decrease
Phenobarbital	Decrease
Omeprazole	Decrease
Caspofungin	Decrease
St John's Wort	Decrease

[a]These medications always require dose adjustment prior to initiation
[b]Clarithromycin and Erythromycin; Azithromycin does NOT cause interactions

20.8 mTOR Inhibitors

In the early 1960s, rapamycin (sirolimus) was discovered as a fermentation product of *Streptomyces hygroscopicus* bacteria isolated from Rapa-Nui (Easter Island) [46]. Initially employed as an antifungal, rapamycin was later recognized for its potent immunosuppressive properties. The molecular target of rapamycin, mTOR (mechanistic target of rapamycin), is a serine-threonine protein kinase regulating cellular growth, proliferation, and metabolism. Two widely known complexes involving mTOR are mTOR complex 1 (mTORC1) and mTOR complex 2 (mTORC2). These complexes regulate cellular processes responding to environmental and hormonal cues, such as nutrients, growth factors, and stressors [47].

mTOR inhibitors include sirolimus, everolimus, and temsirolimus, primarily developed as immunosuppressive agents, but now also utilized in cancer therapies and autoimmune diseases.

20.8.1 Mechanism of Action

Sirolimus binds FK binding protein (FKBP), similar to tacrolimus, but rather than inhibiting calcineurin, the sirolimus-FKBP complex inhibits mTOR, preventing cytokine-induced T- and B-cell activation and proliferation. This blockade arrests cell cycles at the G1 phase, affecting cellular proliferation. Additionally, mTOR inhibition reduces proliferation of arterial smooth muscle cells and endothelial cells, beneficial in preventing graft atherosclerosis and intimal hyperplasia post-coronary stenting.

Second-generation mTOR inhibitors—temsirolimus and everolimus—are sirolimus analogs developed to improve bioavailability. Both share similar mechanisms, approved for renal cell carcinoma treatment, while everolimus also serves in kidney and liver transplantation [46].

20.8.2 Side Effects

Sirolimus and related mTOR inhibitors have extensive side-effect profiles. Hematologic effects include anemia, thrombocytopenia, and leukopenia. Anemia is generally mild and reversible; thrombotic microangiopathy and hepatic artery thrombosis in liver transplant recipients prompted a "black box warning" against early postoperative use [48, 49].

Metabolic effects include hyperlipidemia, hypercholesterolemia, and diabetes mellitus. Regular monitoring of lipids and glucose is recommended. Notably, interstitial pneumonitis may develop, necessitating drug discontinuation.

Impaired wound healing is well-described; thus, caution is required during surgical procedures. It is common practice to discontinue these agents perioperatively. Gastrointestinal side effects include diarrhea, constipation, dyspepsia, nausea, vomiting, mouth ulcers, and delayed ulcer healing.

mTOR inhibitors also have nephrotoxic potential, presenting as acute kidney injury or proteinuria, particularly when combined with calcineurin inhibitors [50]. Additional adverse effects include teratogenicity, impaired spermatogenesis, angioedema, vasculitis, acneiform eruptions, folliculitis, and hidradenitis suppurativa.

20.8.3 GI Absorption

mTOR inhibitors are orally administered and their absorption is significantly affected by high-fat meals. They undergo extensive hepatic metabolism via cytochrome P450 and P-glycoprotein. Consequently, drug levels can be highly variable, requiring consistent therapeutic monitoring [46].

20.8.4 Conclusion

mTOR inhibitors play essential roles in immunosuppression and cancer therapy. Their extensive side-effect profile necessitates careful patient monitoring. Despite these challenges, they remain invaluable in clinical management when utilized judiciously.

20.9 Steroids

Glucocorticoids, produced naturally by the adrenal cortex, were clinically introduced in the 1940s. They exert profound anti-inflammatory effects but also have numerous adverse effects. Common formulations include methylprednisolone, hydrocortisone, cortisone acetate, prednisone, and dexamethasone.

20.9.1 Mechanism of Action

Glucocorticoids bind cytoplasmic receptors, forming complexes translocating to the nucleus to alter protein synthesis, directly or indirectly reducing pro-inflammatory cytokine production [51].

Glucocorticoid receptors are also present in intestinal mucosal cells, where steroids can increase digestive capacity but also predispose to gastric lesions by inhibiting prostaglandin synthesis. While physiologic glucocorticoid levels maintain mucosal integrity, prolonged or elevated doses are catabolic and ulcerogenic [52, 53]. Thus, glucocorticoids contribute to stress ulcers frequently seen in intensive care patients. Interestingly, glucocorticoids released during NSAID treatment can mitigate NSAID-related gastric injury via cooperative interactions [54].

20.9.2 GI Side Effects

Steroids commonly cause gastrointestinal disturbances, including increased gastric contractions, altered transit time, and reduced villous height, potentially impairing nutrient and drug absorption. Histologically, reductions in mast cell populations may suppress innate intestinal immunity.

20.9.3 GI Absorption in Altered GI Tracts

Exogenous glucocorticoids are absorbed primarily in the stomach, small intestine, and colon. Crohn's patients exhibit variable prednisolone plasma concentrations due to reduced gut surface from inflammation or resection [55]. Ileal resection or active inflammation reduces oral steroid bioavailability, hence budesonide, with high first-pass metabolism, may be preferred in localized ileocecal disease.

20.9.4 Conclusion

Steroids remain highly effective immune modulators but require careful attention due to gastrointestinal and systemic toxicities. Their absorption variability underscores the need for tailored approaches in patients with altered GI anatomy.

20.10 Chapter Conclusion

In this chapter, a broad overview of mechanisms of action, side effects, and GI absorption issues associated with key immunomodulatory and immunosuppressive drug classes was provided. Understanding these diverse drug mechanisms and profiles enables optimal therapeutic decision-making. As oral formulations increasingly emerge, clinicians must carefully consider GI anatomy and function. Personalized medicine, integrating genetic polymorphisms and microbiome profiling, will further optimize therapy selection, underscoring interdisciplinary collaboration between pharmacy and specialty teams. Future immunotherapy advancements likely will emphasize targeted selectivity, improved tissue specificity, and reduced systemic adverse effects, supporting the continued evolution of precision pharmacology.

References

1. Monaco C, Nanchahal J, Taylor P, Feldmann M. Anti-TNF therapy: past, present and future. Int Immunol. 2015;27(1):55–62. https://doi.org/10.1093/intimm/dxu102.
2. Bradley J. TNF-mediated inflammatory disease. J Pathol. 2008;214(2):149–60. https://doi.org/10.1002/path.2287.
3. Billmeier U, Dieterich W, Neurath MF, Atreya R. Molecular mechanism of action of anti-tumor necrosis factor antibodies in inflammatory bowel diseases. World J Gastroenterol. 2016;22(42):9300. https://doi.org/10.3748/wjg.v22.i42.9300.
4. Bendtzen K. Immunogenicity of anti-TNF-α biotherapies: I. Individualized medicine based on immunopharmacological evidence. Front Immunol. 2015:6. https://doi.org/10.3389/fimmu.2015.00152.
5. Cleynen I, Vermeire S. Paradoxical inflammation induced by anti-TNF agents in patients with IBD. Nat Rev Gastroenterol Hepatol. 2012;9(9):496–503. https://doi.org/10.1038/nrgastro.2012.125.
6. Korzenik J, Larsen MD, Nielsen J, Kjeldsen J, Nørgård BM. Increased risk of developing Crohn's disease or ulcerative colitis in 17 018 patients while under treatment with anti-TNFα agents, particularly etanercept, for autoimmune diseases other than inflammatory bowel disease. Aliment Pharmacol Ther. 2019;50(3):289–94. https://doi.org/10.1111/apt.15370.
7. Brandse JF, van den Brink GR, Wildenberg ME, et al. Loss of infliximab into feces is associated with lack of response to therapy in patients with severe ulcerative colitis. Gastroenterology. 2015;149(2):350–5.e2. https://doi.org/10.1053/j.gastro.2015.04.016.
8. Hughes C, Wolos JA, Giannini EH, Hirsch R. Induction of T helper cell hyporesponsiveness in an experimental model of autoimmunity by using nonmitogenic anti-CD3 monoclonal antibody. J Immunol. 1994;153(7):3319–25. http://www.ncbi.nlm.nih.gov/pubmed/8089501.
9. Kiely PDW. The Th1-Th2 model—what relevance to inflammatory arthritis? Ann Rheum Dis. 1998;57(6):328–30. https://doi.org/10.1136/ard.57.6.328.
10. van Roon JAG. Th2 mediated regulation in RA and the spondyloarthropathies. Ann Rheum Dis. 2002;61(11):951–4. https://doi.org/10.1136/ard.61.11.951.
11. Chen J, Li J, Gao H, et al. Comprehensive evaluation of different T-helper cell subsets differentiation and function in rheumatoid arthritis. J Biomed Biotechnol. 2012;2012:1–6. https://doi.org/10.1155/2012/535361.
12. Schurich A, Raine C, Morris V, Ciurtin C. The role of IL-12/23 in T cell–related chronic inflammation: implications of immunodeficiency and therapeutic blockade. Rheumatology. 2018;57(2):246–54. https://doi.org/10.1093/rheumatology/kex186.
13. Xavier RJ, Podolsky DK. Unravelling the pathogenesis of inflammatory bowel disease. Nature. 2007;448(7152):427–34. https://doi.org/10.1038/nature06005.
14. Jefremow A, Neurath MF. All are equal, some are more equal: targeting IL 12 and 23 in IBD—a clinical perspective. ImmunoTargets Ther. 2020;9:289–97. https://doi.org/10.2147/ITT.S282466.
15. Kashani A, Schwartz DA. The expanding role of anti-IL-12 and/or anti-IL-23 antibodies in the treatment of inflammatory bowel disease. Gastroenterol Hepatol (N Y). 2019;15(5):255–65. http://www.ncbi.nlm.nih.gov/pubmed/31360139.
16. Puig L. Paradoxical reactions: anti-tumor necrosis factor alpha agents, ustekinumab, secukinumab, ixekizumab, and others. 2018:49–63. https://doi.org/10.1159/000479475.
17. Sandborn WJ, Feagan BG, Danese S, et al. Safety of ustekinumab in inflammatory bowel disease: pooled safety analysis of results from phase 2/3 studies. Inflamm Bowel Dis. 2021;27(7):994–1007. https://doi.org/10.1093/ibd/izaa236.
18. Restellini S, Khanna R, Afif W. Therapeutic drug monitoring with ustekinumab and vedolizumab in inflammatory bowel disease. Inflamm Bowel Dis. 2018;24(10):2165–72. https://doi.org/10.1093/ibd/izy134.
19. Yang J, Sundrud MS, Skepner J, Yamagata T. Targeting Th17 cells in autoimmune diseases. Trends Pharmacol Sci. 2014;35(10):493–500. https://doi.org/10.1016/j.tips.2014.07.006.

20. Fauny M, Moulin D, D'Amico F, et al. Paradoxical gastrointestinal effects of interleukin-17 blockers. Ann Rheum Dis. 2020;79(9):1132–8. https://doi.org/10.1136/annrheumdis-2020-217927.
21. Ju J, Dai Y, Yang J, et al. Crohn's disease exacerbated by IL-17 inhibitors in patients with psoriasis: a case report. BMC Gastroenterol. 2020;20(1):340. https://doi.org/10.1186/s12876-020-01474-x.
22. D'Amico F, Bonovas S, Danese S, Peyrin-Biroulet L. Review article: faecal calprotectin and histologic remission in ulcerative colitis. Aliment Pharmacol Ther. 2020;51(7):689–98. https://doi.org/10.1111/apt.15662.
23. Aarden L, Brunner T, Cerottini J, et al. Revised nomenclature for antigen-nonspecific T cell proliferation and helper factors. J Immunol. 1979;123(6):2928–9. http://www.ncbi.nlm.nih.gov/pubmed/91646.
24. Mantovani A, Dinarello CA, Molgora M, Garlanda C. Interleukin-1 and related cytokines in the regulation of inflammation and immunity. Immunity. 2019;50(4):778–95. https://doi.org/10.1016/j.immuni.2019.03.012.
25. Dayer JM, de Rochemonteix B, Burrus B, Demczuk S, Dinarello CA. Human recombinant interleukin 1 stimulates collagenase and prostaglandin E2 production by human synovial cells. J Clin Invest. 1986;77(2):645–8. https://doi.org/10.1172/JCI112350.
26. Dinarello CA, Simon A, van der Meer JWM. Treating inflammation by blocking interleukin-1 in a broad spectrum of diseases. Nat Rev Drug Discov. 2012;11(8):633–52. https://doi.org/10.1038/nrd3800.
27. Canna S, Frankovich J, Higgins G, et al. Acute hepatitis in three patients with systemic juvenile idiopathic arthritis taking interleukin-1 receptor antagonist. Pediatr Rheumatol. 2009;7(1):21. https://doi.org/10.1186/1546-0096-7-21.
28. Lin CM, Cooles FA, Isaacs JD. Basic mechanisms of JAK inhibition. Mediterr J Rheumatol. 2020;31(Suppl 1):100. https://doi.org/10.31138/mjr.31.1.100.
29. Darnell JE, Kerr Ian M, Stark GR. Jak-STAT pathways and transcriptional activation in response to IFNs and other extracellular signaling proteins. Science (80-). 1994;264(5164):1415–21. https://doi.org/10.1126/science.8197455.
30. Macchi P, Villa A, Giliani S, et al. Mutations of Jak-3 gene in patients with autosomal severe combined immune deficiency (SCID). Nature. 1995;377(6544):65–8. https://doi.org/10.1038/377065a0.
31. Berg J, Tymoczko J, Stryer L. Biochemsitry: The Michaelis-Menten Model accounts for the kinetic properties of many enzymes, 5th edn; 2002.
32. Wollenhaupt J, Lee E-B, Curtis JR, et al. Safety and efficacy of tofacitinib for up to 9.5 years in the treatment of rheumatoid arthritis: final results of a global, open-label, long-term extension study. Arthritis Res Ther. 2019;21(1):89. https://doi.org/10.1186/s13075-019-1866-2.
33. Xie F, Yun H, Bernatsky S, Curtis JR. Brief report: risk of gastrointestinal perforation among rheumatoid arthritis patients receiving tofacitinib, tocilizumab, or other biologic treatments. Arthritis Rheumatol. 2016;68(11):2612–7. https://doi.org/10.1002/art.39761.
34. Fleischmann R, Mysler E, Hall S, et al. Efficacy and safety of tofacitinib monotherapy, tofacitinib with methotrexate, and adalimumab with methotrexate in patients with rheumatoid arthritis (ORAL Strategy): a phase 3b/4, double-blind, head-to-head, randomised controlled trial. Lancet. 2017;390(10093):457–68. https://doi.org/10.1016/S0140-6736(17)31618-5.
35. Rogler G. Efficacy of JAK inhibitors in Crohn's disease. J Crohn's Colitis. 2020;14(Supplement_2):S746–54. https://doi.org/10.1093/ecco-jcc/jjz186.
36. Lefevre PLC, Vande Casteele N. Clinical pharmacology of Janus kinase inhibitors in inflammatory bowel disease. J Crohn's Colitis. 2020;14(Supplement_2):S725–36. https://doi.org/10.1093/ecco-jcc/jjaa014.
37. Safarini OA, Keshavamurthy C, Patel P. Calcineurin Inhibitors; 2022. http://www.ncbi.nlm.nih.gov/pubmed/32644421.
38. Azzi JR, Sayegh MH, Mallat SG. Calcineurin Inhibitors: 40 years later, can't live without …. J Immunol. 2013;191(12):5785–91. https://doi.org/10.4049/jimmunol.1390055.

39. Shin G-T, Khanna A, Ding R, et al. In vivo expression of transforming growth factor-1 in humans. Transplantation. 1998;65(3):313–8. https://doi.org/10.1097/00007890-199802150-00003.
40. Multicenter FK506 Liver Study Group U. A comparison of tacrolimus (FK 506) and cyclosporine for immunosuppression in liver transplantation. N Engl J Med. 1994;331(17):1110–5. https://doi.org/10.1056/NEJM199410273311702.
41. Plosker GL, Foster RH. Tacrolimus. Drugs. 2000;59(2):323–89. https://doi.org/10.2165/00003495-200059020-00021.
42. Riordan M, Oreschak K, Peters LL, Aquilante CL, Ambardekar AV. Bariatric surgery is associated with decreased calcineurin inhibitor time in therapeutic range after heart transplantation. Transplant Proc. 2021;53(2):681–5. https://doi.org/10.1016/j.transproceed.2021.01.020.
43. Huang L, Wang J, Yang J, et al. Impact of CYP3A4/5 and ABCB1 polymorphisms on tacrolimus exposure and response in pediatric primary nephrotic syndrome. Pharmacogenomics. 2019;20(15):1071–83. https://doi.org/10.2217/pgs-2019-0090.
44. Christians U, Strom T, Zhang YL, et al. Active drug transport of immunosuppressants. Ther Drug Monit. 2006;28(1):39–44. https://doi.org/10.1097/01.ftd.0000183385.27394.e7.
45. Möller A, Iwasaki K, Kawamura A, et al. The disposition of 14C-labeled tacrolimus after intravenous and oral administration in healthy human subjects. Drug Metab Dispos. 1999;27(6):633–6. http://www.ncbi.nlm.nih.gov/pubmed/10348790.
46. Santulli G, Totary-Jain H. Tailoring mTOR-based therapy: molecular evidence and clinical challenges. Pharmacogenomics. 2013;14(12):1517–26. https://doi.org/10.2217/pgs.13.143.
47. Kennedy BK, Lamming DW. The mechanistic target of rapamycin: the grand ConducTOR of metabolism and aging. Cell Metab. 2016;23(6):990–1003. https://doi.org/10.1016/j.cmet.2016.05.009.
48. Soefje SA, Karnad A, Brenner AJ. Common toxicities of mammalian target of rapamycin inhibitors. Target Oncol. 2011;6(2):125–9. https://doi.org/10.1007/s11523-011-0174-9.
49. Nguyen LS, Vautier M, Allenbach Y, et al. Sirolimus and mTOR inhibitors: a review of side effects and specific management in solid organ transplantation. Drug Saf. Published online March 13, 2019. https://doi.org/10.1007/s40264-019-00810-9.
50. Klümpen H-J, Beijnen JH, Gurney H, Schellens JHM. Inhibitors of mTOR. Oncologist. 2010;15(12):1262–9. https://doi.org/10.1634/theoncologist.2010-0196.
51. Becker DE. Basic and clinical pharmacology of glucocorticosteroids. Anesth Prog. 2013;60(1):25–32. https://doi.org/10.2344/0003-3006-60.1.25.
52. Black HE. The effects of steroids upon the gastrointestinal tract. Toxicol Pathol. 1988;16(2):213–22. https://doi.org/10.1177/019262338801600214.
53. Filaretova L, Podvigina T, Bagaeva T, Morozova O. Dual action of glucocorticoid hormones on the gastric mucosa: how the gastroprotective action can be transformed to the ulcerogenic one. Inflammopharmacology. 2009;17(1):15–22. https://doi.org/10.1007/s10787-008-8046-3.
54. Filaretova LP, Podvigina TT, Bagaeva TR, Tanaka A, Takeuchi K. Gastroprotective action of glucocorticoid hormones during NSAID treatment. Inflammopharmacology. 2005;13(1–3):27–43. https://doi.org/10.1163/156856005774423746.
55. Shaffer JA, Williams SE, Turnberg LA, Houston JB, Rowland M. Absorption of prednisolone in patients with Crohn's disease. Gut. 1983;24(3):182–6. https://doi.org/10.1136/gut.24.3.182.

Chapter 21
Investigational Therapies for Scleroderma Gastrointestinal Disease

Dharma Ayer, Dia Shah, Steven Sica, Kate Kennelly, Micheal Tadros, and Jessica Farrell

21.1 Introduction

Systemic sclerosis (SSc), or scleroderma, is a heterogenous autoimmune disorder that can vary dramatically in clinical presentation and severity. Among its systemic effects, gastrointestinal (GI) involvement is one of the most common complications, affecting up to 90% of patients [1]. GI involvement can be anywhere from the oral cavity to the anus and contributes to both the mortality and morbidity of the disorder [2]. Common GI symptoms in SSc include esophageal dysmotility, meteorism, dysphagia, gastroesophageal reflux disease (GERD), vomiting, diarrhea, constipation and small intestinal bacterial overgrowth (SIBO) [3]. About 8% of patients with SSc present with severe involvement that directly contributes to the disease morbidity and mortality [4]. Additionally, in a survey assessing the impact of GI on SSc patients, approximately 72% of respondents reported that GI involvement significantly affected their quality of life [5]. This underscores the profound burden of GI

D. Ayer · D. Shah
Albany Medical College, Albany, NY, USA

S. Sica · J. Farrell (✉)
Department of Pharmacy Practice, Albany College of Pharmacy and Health Sciences, Albany, NY, USA

Division of Rheumatology, Albany Medical Center, Albany, NY, USA
e-mail: Jessica.Farrell@acphs.edu

K. Kennelly
Department of Pharmacy Practice, Albany College of Pharmacy and Health Sciences, Albany, NY, USA

M. Tadros
Division of Gastroenterology and Hepatology, Albany Medical College, Niskayuna, NY, USA
e-mail: tadrosm1@amc.edu

M. Tadros et al. (eds.), *GI Diseases Associated with Rheumatological and Vasculitic Conditions*, Clinical Gastroenterology,
https://doi.org/10.1007/978-3-032-07868-1_21

complications in SSc and highlights the importance of effective symptom management to improve overall well-being.

The management of GI manifestations in SSc is complex and frequently involves multidisciplinary approaches. Due to the broad clinical spectrum of SSc, effective management often requires collaboration among rheumatologists, gastroenterologists, and other specialists. A team-based approach can ensure that referrals are fast-tracked and that all aspects of the disease, including GI symptoms, are managed more effectively [6]. First-line treatment strategies for GI symptoms tend to focus on symptom control and supportive measures, including proton pump inhibitors (PPIs) for GERD, antibiotics for SIBO, prokinetics for gastroparesis, and laxatives for constipation [2]. Commonly used medications for treating various symptoms include omeprazole/pantoprazole domperidone, cisapride, prucalopride, buspirone, and octreotide [7, 8]. Despite existing first-line therapies, many patients remain resistant, highlighting a critical need for more novel treatment options.

Newer treatment options being investigated for SSc and its GI symptoms include IVIG, potassium-competitive acid blockers, and immune-based therapies [7, 9]. Nevertheless, many of these therapies still need to be optimized or further investigated in SSc patients. Numerous studies emphasize a significant gap in the availability of randomized controlled trials assessing pharmacologic treatments specifically for systemic sclerosis (SSc) populations [5]. This lack of robust, targeted research limits evidence-based advancements in managing SSc-related complications. Increased research, along with education and active patient involvement in care are needed to optimize outcomes from these therapies and better understand the role they can play in managing the many symptoms of SSc.

21.2 Approved Therapies Under Investigation in SSc

21.2.1 Intravenous Immunoglobulin (IVIG)

Raja et al. report 15 patients with systemic sclerosis (SSc) who were treated with IVIG for an average duration of 2.3 years and showed a significant reduction in gastroesophageal reflux frequency and intensity ($P = 0.006$, $P = 0.013$) and a marked improvement in overall GI function, as evidenced by the Gastrointestinal Tract (GIT) 2.0 score ($P = 0.002$). One patient with chronic intestinal pseudo-obstruction experienced complete resolution of symptoms, including abdominal distension, diarrhea, malabsorption, electrolyte imbalances, and dependence on enteral feeding following IVIG administration. The pathophysiology of GI dysmotility in SSc is driven by both myogenic and neurogenic dysfunction, where autoantibodies interfere with muscarinic neurotransmission in smooth muscle cells. By neutralizing these autoantibodies, IVIG plays a key role in addressing the underlying cause of GI dysfunction. Beyond GI benefits, IVIG has proven efficacy in treating SSc-related inflammatory myopathy and skin fibrosis by modulating profibrotic cytokines, including IL-4 and TGF-β, reducing fibrosis in affected tissues, thus further reinforcing its role in modifying disease pathology. Patients receiving IVIG demonstrated sustained improvement in muscle strength, as reflected in enhanced Medical Research Council (MRC) sum scores with each treatment cycle. Given the overwhelming clinical evidence supporting IVIG's ability to improve GI symptoms in SSc, timely approval of IVIG therapy is crucial to manage this patient's refractory GI symptoms, reduce the risk of complications, and enhance her quality of life [10].

Matsuda et al. published a case series that reports the response of GI symptoms in three cases of SSc-myositis overlap who received IVIG treatment. In the first case, a 54-year-old female with diffuse cutaneous systemic sclerosis (dcSSc) suffered from severe GI dysfunction, including constipation, abdominal distention, and significant weight loss, and was unresponsive to standard therapy with corticosteroids and cyclophosphamide. Upon initiation of IVIG, her intestinal peristalsis improved almost immediately, reducing gas retention and allowing her to resume oral intake within a month. After 12 courses of IVIG, her body weight increased significantly, and her GI symptoms improved to the extent that she voluntarily requested less frequent dosing. Beyond GI benefits, IVIG also contributed to the management of her myositis and overall systemic disease. This case highlights IVIG as a highly effective therapy for severe refractory scleroderma-associated GI dysmotility, justifying its necessity in similar cases [11].

In the second case, a 71-year-old female with diffuse cutaneous systemic sclerosis (dcSSc) experienced severe GI dysfunction, including dysphagia, constipation, and significant weight loss. The patient remained resistant to corticosteroids, immunosuppressants, and multiple GI medications. Despite requiring total parenteral nutrition (TPN) for malnutrition, the addition of IVIG led to a remarkable improvement in her dysphagia and intestinal function, as evidenced by reduced intestinal gas on imaging. After eight courses of IVIG, she was able to discontinue TPN without recurrence of GI symptoms. Beyond GI benefits, IVIG also contributed to the management of her ILD and myositis. This case strongly supports IVIG as an essential therapy for refractory scleroderma-associated GI dysmotility, enabling patients to regain normal oral intake and avoid long-term TPN dependence [11].

In the third case, a 62-year-old female with diffuse cutaneous systemic sclerosis (dcSSc) suffered from severe abdominal distention due to scleroderma-associated intestinal pseudo-obstruction (SSc-IPO), which was unresponsive to standard GI therapies. Upon initiation of IVIG, her bowel motility improved rapidly, resolving abdominal distention and allowing her to gradually resume oral intake. Though she initially required TPN for intestinal rest, continued IVIG therapy led to sustained improvements in bowel function and a notable weight gain over 6 months. Additionally, IVIG was used to manage concurrent myocarditis. This case underscores IVIG's critical role in restoring GI motility in refractory SSc-IPO, preventing prolonged TPN dependency, and improving overall patient outcomes [11].

A systematic review of 12 studies involving 266 adults with SSc examined the use of IVIG therapy in treating the condition. The findings demonstrated that IVIG effectively alleviated GI symptoms, while also improving skin thickening, muscle, and joint pain. Notably, IVIG offered a corticosteroid-sparing benefit, with all studies showing a significant reduction in corticosteroid dosage. Additionally, patient-reported outcomes, including improvements in the health assessment questionnaire, further supported the clinical efficacy of IVIG. The therapy has a low risk of adverse effects when administered following recommended guidelines, making it a valuable treatment option for refractory SSc with GI involvement. This evidence strongly supports the use of IVIG for managing scleroderma-associated GI dysmotility, particularly as an adjunct therapy for uncontrolled disease [12].

21.2.2 Potassium-Competitive Acid Blockers (P-CABs)

Severe gastroesophageal reflux disease (GERD) is unfortunately one of the early manifestations seen with scleroderma. GERD is often present with esophageal dysmotility, which can manifest into more serious complications. For example, peptic esophagitis, erosive esophagitis, esophageal ulcerations, fistulae formation and such situations may contribute to the potential development of Barrett's esophagus or esophageal adenocarcinoma [13]. Omeprazole administered twice daily or alternative proton pump inhibitors (PPIs) are commonly used to treat esophageal dysmotility in patients with systemic scleroderma. However, PPIs have many limitations, including a slow onset of action, influence with CYP450 polymorphisms, unsatisfactory effects at night and instability to acidic conditions. Therefore, potassium competitive acid blockers (P-CABs) were developed to provide rapid and long-lasting effects [14]. P-CABs competitively inhibit the binding of potassium ions to the H+/K+ATPase enzyme system on gastric parietal cells. Unlike PPIs, P-CABs are not prodrugs and do not require modifications to become active compounds. They do not degrade in acidic environments and can accumulate in the secretory canaliculi of gastric parietal cells. These properties allow P-CABs to provide sustained and potent acid-inhibitory effects, surpassing conventional PPIs [15]. Side effects seen with long term acid suppression include hypergastrinemia, pneumonia, small bowel bacterial overgrowth and Clostridium difficile infections [16]. More specifically, the novel P-CAB named vonoprazan showed side effects of nausea, vomiting, constipation, abdominal pain, skin rashes and heartburn [9]. However, side effects seen with vonoprazan are similar to that of conventional PPIs and many clinical trials that studied the use of vonoprazan for the treatment of gastric and duodenal ulcers, reflux esophagitis, NSAID associated ulcers and Helicobacter pylori eradication displayed satisfactory effects and safety profiles [17].

At first, imidazopyridine derivatives were developed, but the presence of an imidazole ring correlated with hepatotoxicity in human clinical studies and therefore did not show statistical significance over conventional PPIs [18]. Subsequently, pyrimidine derivatives, such as vonoprazan and revaprazan were synthesized without the imidazole ring and are currently the only P-CABs on the market at this time. Vonoprazan is an orally formulated P-CAB that does not require enteric coating, due to being acid-stable and administration is not influenced by meals because of its fast absorption. Additional benefits of vonoprazan include its high affinity, long term stability at the site of action and slow clearance, which leads to accumulation of the drug in gastric parietal cells. Vonoprazan can accumulate in parietal cells in both acidic and neutral conditions because there is no acidic environment requirement needed for activation. Vonoprazan has also been shown to have an acid dissociation constant (pKa) of 9.3, which is higher than the dissociation constant of conventional PPIs and other P-CABs. Vonoprazan reaches a maximum plasma concentration in less than 2 h after oral administration and has a half-life of 9 h. Compared to the 2 h half-life seen with conventional PPIs, vonoprazan has the ability to block acid secretion for a longer period of time [19].

A statistical analysis was performed to demonstrate the comparison between vonoprazan and conventional PPIs. Vonoprazan was concluded to be superior to PPIs, in the aspects that P-CABs provided maximal acid suppression after 1 day of dosing, there was no influence of CYP2C19 polymorphisms, there was no influence on the rate of absorption in the presence or absence of a meal and they maintained a greater stability in acidic conditions. Vonoprazan also showed a greater percent at reducing acid at night, eradicating H. pylori infections, healing severe reflux esophagitis and treating PPI-refractory GERD [20].

The Nagasaki University Hospital Ethics Committee approved a study to assess the efficacy of vonoprazan for the management of systemic scleroderma related gastroesophageal reflux disease. The study included 15 patients with scleroderma related to GERD. A total of 7 participants were treated with a 20 mg/day dose of vonoprazan and 8 participants were treated with a 10 mg/day dose of vonoprazan. During the study, 4/8 participants in the 10 mg/day group had a dose increase to 20 mg/day after 4–17 weeks, due to insufficient effects seen with 10 mg/day. The Frequency Scale for the Symptoms of GERD (FSSG) score was established to correctly identify GERD and determine disease severity and treatment efficacy in the patients. The FSSG questionnaire was completed at baseline and after at least 4 weeks of treatment. An FSSG score greater than 8 was indicative of GERD. Further monitoring was performed with a 2-h pH monitoring catheter and esophageal motility was assessed using an esophageal high-resolution manometry (HRM) catheter. The data was then analyzed with JMP software. The mean baseline total FSSG, acid reflux and dysmotility scores were 25.2, 14.1 and 11.1, respectively. The mean total FSSG, acid reflux and dysmotility scores 4–28 weeks after vonoprazan treatment were reduced to 9.6, 4.6 and 4.8, respectively. A significant improvement in the mean total and acid reflux FSSG scores were observed, with an unexpected improvement in the mean dysmotility score. A pH > 4 holding time ratio (HTR) reached 63.3% of the participants treated with the 10 mg/day dose and a pH > 4 HTR reached 83.4% of the participants treated with the 20 mg/day dose. Therefore, a starting dose of 20 mg/day was shown to be more appropriate than starting at the 10 mg/day dose. The results from the study concluded that scleroderma patients with GERD, including those refractory to conventional PPI therapy experienced significant relief from symptoms when treated with 20 mg/day of vonoprazan [9].

A study was published in Sage Journals that investigated the efficacy of vonoprazan in patients with systemic scleroderma and proton pump inhibitor refractory reflux esophagitis. A total of 10 participants were selected from the systemic sclerosis database. Reflux esophagitis was evaluated by an endoscopy and GERD related symptoms were assessed by a frequency scale questionnaire that was answered before and after switching the participants' therapy from a PPI to vonoprazan. After switching the participants' therapies, endoscopic findings of reflux esophagitis were significantly improved, with a *P*-value of 0.033. In addition, six patients achieved mucosal healing. The total frequency scale for the GERD related symptoms were significantly reduced, with a *P*-value of 0.043. Vonoprazan was well tolerated and was continued for an average of 15.5 months. Therefore, the study concluded that vonoprazan is a potential treatment option for treating proton pump inhibitor refractory reflux esophagitis in patients with systemic scleroderma [21].

As stated previously, vonoprazan and revaprazan are the only P-CABs available on the market. Vonoprazan was approved in the U.S. for erosive GERD in November 2023 and non-erosive GERD in July 2024. Revaprazan is only available in South Korea and India. Furthermore, additional P-CAB formulations are in the process of coming to market. For example, tegoprazan is in phase III trials in South Korea and in phase I trials in Japan [14].

21.2.3 Eculizumab

Eculizumab is a monoclonal antibody directed against the complement component C5. Eculizumab is currently primarily in case studies and small-scale research for its use in SSc associated renal crisis. A systematic review demonstrated that from 17 patients treated with Eculizumab, 82.3% had significantly improved hematologic parameters with a less consistent and significant effect on renal recovery [22]. A case report also revealed the utility of complement activation and eculizumab on SSc renal crisis. Immunofluorescence studies showed C1q and C4d endothelial deposits of renal arterioles on kidney biopsy demonstrating classical pathway activations. Eculizumab blocked C5b-9 deposition and autopsy showed normal coronary arteries and myocardial vasculature despite the presence of diffuse patchy interstitial fibrosis also known as scleroderma-related cardiomyopathy [23]. Eculizumab is now also being studied for its role in treating complement associated disorders in conjunction with SSc, such as thrombotic microangiopathy. There are no clinical trials or large scale studies currently on this treatment, and while it is not yet a primary treatment of SSc renal crisis, it is used as a rescue therapy [24, 25].

21.3 Pipeline Therapies

21.3.1 Lenabasum

Lenabasum has undergone phase II and phase III trials as a possible treatment option for systemic sclerosis. Lenabasum (formally known as anabasum) is a synthetic small molecule drug that is administered orally. It works by binding selectively to the cannabinoid type 2 receptors that are expressed on activated immune cells and fibroblasts. By causing agonism of the cannabinoid type 2 receptors, an endogenous cascade is triggered which leads to a reduction of inflammatory mediators. The reduction of inflammatory mediators helps to resolve inflammation and fibrosis and may help with the chronic inflammation of the GI tract. In addition, animal and human studies have suggested that the drug may decrease gene expression and proteins that are responsible for inflammation and fibrosis [26]. Many chronic disease states of the Gl system such as inflammatory bowel disease have proven that several genes are expressed within the GI tract, suggesting that lenabasum may be a beneficial option for GI complications with SSc [27, 28].

Lenabasum is the first therapy studied that does not suppress the immune system but still increases bacterial clearance; offering a unique place in practice. During clinical trials 84% of patients were receiving background immunosuppressive drugs because most current therapies are immunosuppressive options [26]. It is favorable to have a possible treatment option that does not have additional immunosuppression effects.

A phase II, randomized, placebo-controlled trial was performed in 9 different US SSc clinics that studied the safety and efficacy of lenabasum in adults with systemic sclerosis. The trial included patients between 18 and 69 years old and met the 2013 ACR/European League Against Rheumatism classification criteria for SSc. Patients in this trial had diffuse cutaneous systemic sclerosis for ≤6 years in duration and were being treated with the standard of care. Patients taking cyclophosphamide within 3 months of starting, rituximab within 6 months of starting, or glucocorticoid dosages of greater than 10 mg prednisone or equivalent a day within 28 days before day 1 were excluded from the trial. However, doses of non-immunosuppressive medications for SSc that were needed to stabilize the patient ≥28 days before day 1 were deemed okay. Patients were not allowed to use other cannabinoid drugs during the trial. When considering lenabasum as a possible treatment for GI complications of SSc, it is important to note, that patients with GI dysmotility that required total parenteral nutrition or hospitalization in the 6 months before the first day of the study were excluded from this trial [29]. Lenabasum was taken by mouth twice a day with 8–16 h between doses. The patients had visits to assess safety and efficacy on days 1, 15, and end of weeks 4, 8, 12, and 16. Appropriate lab tests were performed along with physical examinations. The adverse event profile when compared to placebo was 63% vs. 60% respectively. There were no serious or severe adverse events observed. The serum concentrations of lenabasum were found to increase proportionately with the dose, however this had no effect on adverse event response. Dizziness, fatigue, headache, arthralgia, upper respiratory tract infection, nausea, and decreased FVC were adverse events that occurred in ≥10% of patients in the total 16-week study [29].

The efficacy of lenabasum was evaluated using the CRISS score and the change from baseline in patient global assessment and physician global assessment scores. At week 8 of the trial, improvement in CRISS scores was observed in the treatment group and increased overtime. Both patient global assessment and physician global assessment scores also improved with lenabasum treatment. Skin biopsy specimens were collected at baseline and at week 12 to assess gene expression [29]. The genes associated with inflammation and fibrosis were found to have reduced expression after lenabasum treatment. In addition, fundamental inflammatory and fibrotic pathways were impacted in the pathogenesis of SSc [30].

Genetic heterogeneities that may contribute to gut inflammation include NOD2/CARD15, TNFSF15, ATG16L1, IL23R, and IRGM [27, 28]. In the recent phase III study of lenabasum The University of California at Los Angeles Scleroderma Clinical Trial (UCLA SCTC) Consortium Gastrointestinal Tract symptoms questionnaire (GIT 2) was used as a tertiary efficacy outcome. The questionnaire was used to assess patients with irritable bowel syndrome, inflammatory bowel disease, and other common GI disorders. The questionnaire is measured by a scale that consists of eight domains regarding gastroesophageal reflux, disrupted swallowing, diarrhea, bowel incontinence/soilage, nausea and vomiting, constipation, belly pain, and gas/bloat/flatulence. The study outcomes assessed change from baseline to week 26 and week 52. Unfortunately, the study was terminated early due to inability to meet its primary endpoint and therefore results have not been posted [31]. However, due to the data showing lenabasum causes reduction of inflammatory and fibrotic gene expression and the introduction of the UCLA SCTC questionnaire, further investigations must be performed to look at the effects of lenabasum on GI complications in patients with SSc as it may pose as a successful treatment option.

21.3.2 EHP-101

EHP-101 is an investigational aminoquinone derivative of CBD which has activity for the cannabinoid receptor type 2 (CB2), proliferatory-activated receptor gamma (PPARγ), and the hypoxia-inducible factor -1 (HIF-1). Given EHP-101's targets, it is thought to work in a few different ways to benefit patients with SSc. By working on the CB2 receptor, which is a in the endocannabinoid system which functions to maintain homeostasis in the body, it is thought that CB2 modulation would produce the potential for regulation of neuroprotection, inflammation, immunomodulation, and vascular responses without inducing any psychotropic effects. The PPARγ receptor is a nuclear receptor which is responsible for assisting in regulation of cell growth, lipid metabolism and blood glucose. The receptor is broadly expressed throughout the body and has been known to prevent inflammation, dermal fibrosis and loss of adipose tissue. EHP-101 can partially activate PPARγ, which should help to mitigate negative effects associated with full activation. The proposed mechanism for benefit of HIF in patients with SSc is unknown at this time, as it appears to be more beneficial for multiple sclerosis patients [32].

A phase II clinical trial (NCT04166552) was designed to evaluate the safety, tolerability, and preliminary efficacy of EHP-101 in patients with diffuse cutaneous systemic sclerosis. Participants were randomized to receive either EHP-101 or a placebo over an 84-day treatment period, with a 28-day follow-up. However, the trial was suspended as of September 16, 2023, due to the sponsor ceasing operations [33].

21.3.3 GS-248

GS-248 is an investigational drug which is currently undergoing phase II clinical trials for its use in Raynaud's phenomenon in systemic sclerosis patients. GS-248 is a prostaglandin-E synthase inhibitor which exhibits its action in systemic sclerosis by blocking prostaglandin E synthase-1 (mPGES-1). mPGES-1 is pro-inflammatory and drives inflammation by activating release of prostaglandin E2. GS-248 also has vasodilatory action, leading to widening of the blood vessels and proposed improved blood flow to the GI tissues. However, recent findings suggest that GS-248 may not provide significant symptomatic relief compared to placebo in patients SSc-related Raynaud's. These results highlight the need for further research to fully understand GS-248's therapeutic potential [34].

21.3.4 AVID 200

AVID200 is a TGF-beta inhibitor which functions like an antibody and is currently in a Phase 1 trial under investigation for SSc [35, 36]. Penn Medicine is currently in the process of an open-label study to assess the safety, tolerability, and preliminary efficacy of AVID 200 in SSc patients to identify doses to continue to Phase 2 [37]. AVID200 is unique because it is a TGF-beta receptor ectodomain-IgG Fc fusion protein that inhibits immunosuppression by neutralizing TFG-beta 1 and TGF-beta 3 [38].

21.3.5 FCR001 Allogenic Cell Therapy

Allogenic FCR001 is a stem cell therapy composed of hematopoietic stem cells (HSCs), facilitating cells (CD8+/TCR- cells), and $\alpha\beta TCR^{+}$ T cells. It was designed to help support HSC transplantation while minimizing the risk of graft-versus-host-disease (GvHD) [39]. The therapy has been trialed in living-donor kidney transplant, successfully achieving tolerance and chimerism. Notably, it has also reduced relapse rates of underlying autoimmune disease in patients who received therapy, compared to those who received a graft without FCR001 [40]. Previous studies of SSc patients treated with autologous hematopoietic stem cell (HSC) transplants have demonstrated long-term benefits and reduced treatment-related mortality [41]. A phase I/II trial was developed to asses FCR001 cell therapy in adults with diffuse cutaneous SSc (dcSSc) at risk for organ failure [42]. Nevertheless, the full therapeutic potential of allogeneic FCR001 remains unclear for SSc, as clinical trials evaluating efficacy have not yet been completed.

21.3.6 CM-101

CM-101 is a humanized monoclonal antibody that prevents inflammation and fibrosis caused by CCL24 [43].

Elevated serum CCL24 levels have been associated with increased disease SSc, making it a potentially critical protein biomarker for novel therapeutic strategies [44]. The role of CM-101 in various inflammatory diseases, including SSc are currently under investigation. Mouse models from preclinical studies of non-alcoholic steatohepatitis (NASH), primary sclerosing cholangitis (PSC), and SSc have demonstrated the potential anti-inflammatory and anti-fibrotic activity of CM-10 [45–47]. Particularly, in a bleomycin (BLM) induced mouse model of dermal fibrosis and pulmonary fibrosis CM-101 had significant effects in attenuating fibrosis [45]. Additionally, in humans, Phase 1b studies in patients with metabolic dysfunction-associated steatotic liver disease (MASLD) without metabolic dysfunction-associated steatohepatitis (MASH) showed decreased liver inflammatory markers after 15 weeks (five doses) of CM-101 therapy [43]. Nevertheless, despite preclinical evidence of CM-101 potential in mouse models, clinical trials evaluating the efficacy of CM-101 in SSc have not yet been conducted.

21.4 Conclusion

The various therapies being developed and investigated for their utility in treating SSc highlight promising options to help treatment-resistant patients. The immunomodulatory effects of IVIg have shown potential in improving skin scores and symptoms associated with SSc. P-CABs, such as vonoprazan, offer an alternative to conventional PPIs for treating GERD in SSc patients by providing acid suppression, even in refractory cases. Lenabasum, which is a cannabinoid receptor agonist that works by reducing inflammation and fibrosis without suppressing the immune system making it a valuable option for treating GI complications in SSc. Many other investigational therapies including GS-248, AVID-200, FCR001, and CM-101 are also being researched for their potential use in SSc patients. There are also novel immunomodulatory therapies like Eculizumab that are additionally being studied. Despite advancements in understanding and treating systemic sclerosis (SSc), there remains a critical need for more targeted clinical trials to explore and validate therapies, particularly for treatment-resistant cases, to improve outcomes and address unmet patient needs.

References

1. Volkmann ER, Andréasson K, Smith V. Systemic sclerosis. Lancet. 2023;401:304–18. https://doi.org/10.1016/s0140-6736(22)01692-0.
2. Shreiner AB, Murray C, Denton C, Khanna D. Gastrointestinal manifestations of systemic sclerosis. J Scleroderma Relat Disord. 2016;1:247–56. https://doi.org/10.5301/jsrd.5000214.
3. Nassar M, et al. Gastrointestinal involvement in systemic sclerosis: an updated review. Medicine (Baltimore). 2022;101:e31780. https://doi.org/10.1097/md.0000000000031780.
4. McFarlane IM, et al. Gastrointestinal manifestations of systemic sclerosis. Rheumatology (Sunnyvale). 2018;8. https://doi.org/10.4172/2161-1149.1000235.
5. Bandini G, et al. Significant gastrointestinal unmet needs in patients with Systemic Sclerosis: insights from a large international patient survey. Rheumatology. 2023;63:e92–3. https://doi.org/10.1093/rheumatology/kead486.
6. Farina N, et al. The role of the multidisciplinary health care team in the management of patients with systemic sclerosis. J Multidiscip Healthc. 2022;15:815–24. https://doi.org/10.2147/jmdh.S295478.
7. Cheah JX, Khanna D, McMahan ZH. Management of scleroderma gastrointestinal disease: Lights and shadows. J Scleroderma Relat Disord. 2022;7:85–97. https://doi.org/10.1177/23971983221086343.
8. Nagaraja V, McMahan ZH, Getzug T, Khanna D. Management of gastrointestinal involvement in scleroderma. Curr Treatm Opt Rheumatol. 2015;1:82–105. https://doi.org/10.1007/s40674-014-0005-0.
9. Tabuchi M, et al. Use of vonoprazan for management of systemic sclerosis-related gastroesophageal reflux disease. Biomed Rep. 2021;14:25. https://doi.org/10.3892/br.2020.1401.
10. Raja J, Nihtyanova SI, Murray CD, Denton CP, Ong VH. Sustained benefit from intravenous immunoglobulin therapy for gastrointestinal involvement in systemic sclerosis. Rheumatology (Oxford). 2016;55:115–9. https://doi.org/10.1093/rheumatology/kev318.
11. Matsuda KM, et al. Rapid improvement of systemic sclerosis-associated intestinal pseudo-obstruction with intravenous immunoglobulin administration. Rheumatology (Oxford). 2023;62:3139–45. https://doi.org/10.1093/rheumatology/kead093.
12. Koczanowski S, et al. Role of intravenous immunoglobulins in systemic sclerosis (SSc): a systematic literature review. Semin Arthritis Rheum. 2024;68:152471. https://doi.org/10.1016/j.semarthrit.2024.152471.
13. Postlethwaite AE, Harris LJ, Raza SH, Kodura S, Akhigbe T. Pharmacotherapy of systemic sclerosis. Expert Opin Pharmacother. 2010;11:789–806. https://doi.org/10.1517/14656561003592177.
14. Oshima T, Miwa H. Potent potassium-competitive acid blockers: a new era for the treatment of acid-related diseases. J Neurogastroenterol Motil. 2018;24:334–44. https://doi.org/10.5056/jnm18029.
15. Wang YK, et al. Current pharmacological management of gastroesophageal reflux disease. Gastroenterol Res Pract. 2013;2013:983653. https://doi.org/10.1155/2013/983653.
16. Kinoshita Y, Ishimura N, Ishihara S. Advantages and disadvantages of long-term proton pump inhibitor use. J Neurogastroenterol Motil. 2018;24:182–96. https://doi.org/10.5056/jnm18001.

17. Mizokami Y, et al. Vonoprazan prevents ulcer recurrence during long-term NSAID therapy: randomised, lansoprazole-controlled non-inferiority and single-blind extension study. Gut. 2018;67:1042–51. https://doi.org/10.1136/gutjnl-2017-314010.
18. Rawla P, Sunkara T, Ofosu A, Gaduputi V. Potassium-competitive acid blockers—are they the next generation of proton pump inhibitors? World J Gastrointest Pharmacol Ther. 2018;9:63–8. https://doi.org/10.4292/wjgpt.v9.i7.63.
19. Inatomi N, Matsukawa J, Sakurai Y, Otake K. Potassium-competitive acid blockers: advanced therapeutic option for acid-related diseases. Pharmacol Ther. 2016;168:12–22. https://doi.org/10.1016/j.pharmthera.2016.08.001.
20. Ashida K, et al. Randomised clinical trial: a dose-ranging study of vonoprazan, a novel potassium-competitive acid blocker, vs. lansoprazole for the treatment of erosive oesophagitis. Aliment Pharmacol Ther. 2015;42:685–95. https://doi.org/10.1111/apt.13331.
21. Shirai Y, Kawami N, Iwakiri K, Kuwana M. Use of vonoprazan, a novel potassium-competitive acid blocker, for the treatment of proton pump inhibitor-refractory reflux esophagitis in patients with systemic sclerosis. J Scleroderma Relat Disord. 2022;7:57–61. https://doi.org/10.1177/23971983211021747.
22. Farrukh L, Steen VD, Shapiro L, Mehta S. Studying the role of C5-inhibition therapy in scleroderma renal crisis-induced thrombotic microangiopathy—a review of literature. Semin Arthritis Rheum. 2023;63:152256. https://doi.org/10.1016/j.semarthrit.2023.152256.
23. Devresse A, et al. Complement activation and effect of eculizumab in scleroderma renal crisis. Medicine (Baltimore). 2016;95:e4459. https://doi.org/10.1097/md.0000000000004459.
24. Del Galdo F, et al. EULAR recommendations for the treatment of systemic sclerosis: 2023 update. Ann Rheum Dis. 2024. https://doi.org/10.1136/ard-2024-226430.
25. Toker Dincer Z, et al. Targeting complement dysregulation: eculizumab in scleroderma renal crisis management-a case-based review. Rheumatol Int. 2024;44:3135–40. https://doi.org/10.1007/s00296-024-05689-z.
26. Corbus Pharmaceuticals announces topline results from resolve-1 phase 3 study of lenabasum for treatment of systemic sclerosis. Corbus Pharmaceuticals Holdings, Inc. 2020. Retrieved December 19, 2021, from https://www.corbuspharma.com/press-releases/detail/341/corbus-pharmaceuticals-announces-topline-results-from.
27. Park SC, Jeen YT, Genetic studies of inflammatory bowel disease-focusing on Asian patients. Cells. 2019;8. https://doi.org/10.3390/cells8050404.
28. Blumberg RS. Inflammation in the intestinal tract: pathogenesis and treatment. Dig Dis. 2009;27:455–64. https://doi.org/10.1159/000235851.
29. Spiera R, et al. Safety and efficacy of lenabasum in a phase II, randomized, placebo-controlled trial in adults with systemic sclerosis. Arthritis Rheumatol. 2020;72:1350–60. https://doi.org/10.1002/art.41294.
30. McMahan ZH, Volkmann ER. An update on the pharmacotherapeutic options and treatment strategies for systemic sclerosis. Expert Opin Pharmacother. 2020;21:2041–56. https://doi.org/10.1080/14656566.2020.1793960.
31. Spiera R, et al. A randomised, double-blind, placebo-controlled phase 3 study of lenabasum in diffuse cutaneous systemic sclerosis: RESOLVE-1 design and rationale. Clin Exp Rheumatol. 2021;39(Suppl 131):124–33. https://doi.org/10.55563/clinexprheumatol/i80zh7.
32. García-Martín A, et al. Cannabinoid derivatives acting as dual PPARγ/CB2 agonists as therapeutic agents for systemic sclerosis. Biochem Pharmacol. 2019;163:321–34. https://doi.org/10.1016/j.bcp.2019.02.029.
33. Emerald Health Pharmaceuticals, I. Evaluation of Safety, Tolerability and Preliminary Efficacy of EHP-101 in Diffuse Cutaneous Systemic Sclerosis. 2023. https://clinicaltrials.gov/study/NCT04166552.
34. Tornling G, et al. A phase 2 trial investigating the efficacy and safety of the mPGES-1 inhibitor vipoglanstat in systemic sclerosis-related Raynaud's. Rheumatology. 2024;64:704–13. https://doi.org/10.1093/rheumatology/keae049.

35. Lafyatis R, et al. THU0329 safety, target engagement, and initial efficacy of AVID200, a first-in-class potent and isoform-selective inhibitor of TGF-beta 1 and 3, in patients with diffuse cutaneous systemic sclerosis (DCSSC): a phase 1 dose escalation study. Ann Rheum Dis. 2020;79:394–5. https://doi.org/10.1136/annrheumdis-2020-eular.1753.
36. Phase 1 open-label study to determine the safety and tolerability of Avid200, a transforming growth factor B inhibitor, in diffuse cutaneous systemic sclerosis. Phase 1 Open-Label Study to Determine the Safety | Clinical Research Studies Listing. Available at: https://clinicalresearch.pennmedicine.org/us/en/listing/6258/phase-1-open-label-study/.
37. Clinical trial finder. Safety and Tolerability Study of AVID200 in Pts With Diffuse Cutaneous Systemic Sclerosis—Arthritis Foundation. Available at: https://trials.arthritis.org/trials/NCT03831438.
38. Deng Z, et al. TGF-β signaling in health, disease and therapeutics. Sign Transduct Target Ther. 2024;9:61. https://doi.org/10.1038/s41392-024-01764-w.
39. Khanna D, Krieger N, Sullivan KM. Improving outcomes in scleroderma: recent progress of cell-based therapies. Rheumatology (Oxford). 2023;62:2060–9. https://doi.org/10.1093/rheumatology/keac628.
40. Krieger N, et al. Immune tolerance via FCR001 cell therapy compared with maintenance immunosuppression for kidney transplantation: real-world evidence analysis of safety and efficacy. Clin Transpl. 2023;37:e15074. https://doi.org/10.1111/ctr.15074.
41. Del Papa N, Pignataro F, Zaccara E, Maglione W, Minniti A. Autologous hematopoietic stem cell transplantation for treatment of systemic sclerosis. Front Immunol. 2018;9:2390. https://doi.org/10.3389/fimmu.2018.02390.
42. A Safety and Efficacy Study of FCR001 in Adults With Rapidly Progressive Diffuse Cutaneous Systemic Sclerosis (FREEDOM-3)—ClinicalTrials.gov. 2021. https://clinicaltrials.gov/study/NCT05098145.
43. Mor A, et al. Targeting CCL24 in inflammatory and fibrotic diseases: rationale and results from three CM-101 phase 1 studies. Drug Saf. 2024;47:869–81. https://doi.org/10.1007/s40264-024-01436-2.
44. De Lorenzis E, et al. Serum CCL24 as a biomarker of fibrotic and vascular disease severity in systemic sclerosis. Arthritis Care Res. 2024;76:1269–77. https://doi.org/10.1002/acr.25344.
45. Mor A, et al. Blockade of CCL24 with a monoclonal antibody ameliorates experimental dermal and pulmonary fibrosis. Ann Rheum Dis. 2019;78:1260–8. https://doi.org/10.1136/annrheumdis-2019-215119.
46. Segal-Salto M, et al. A blocking monoclonal antibody to CCL24 alleviates liver fibrosis and inflammation in experimental models of liver damage. JHEP Rep. 2020;2:100064. https://doi.org/10.1016/j.jhepr.2019.100064.
47. Greenman R, et al. The role of CCL24 in primary sclerosing cholangitis: bridging patient serum proteomics to preclinical data. Cells. 2024;13. https://doi.org/10.3390/cells13030209.

Index

M. Tadros et al. (eds.), *GI Diseases Associated with Rheumatological and Vasculitic Conditions*, Clinical Gastroenterology,
https://doi.org/10.1007/978-3-032-07868-1

R

MIX
Papier aus verantwortungsvollen Quellen
Paper from responsible sources
FSC® C105338

If you have any concerns about our products,
you can contact us on
ProductSafety@springernature.com

In case Publisher is established outside the EU,
the EU authorized representative is:
Springer Nature Customer Service Center GmbH
Europaplatz 3, 69115 Heidelberg, Germany

Printed by Libri Plureos GmbH
in Hamburg, Germany